D1611785

# Encyclopedia of Folk Medicine

# Encyclopedia of
# Folk Medicine

## Old World and New World Traditions

Gabrielle Hatfield

A B C ● C L I O

Santa Barbara, California    Denver, Colorado    Oxford, England

Library of Congress Cataloging-in-Publication Data

Hatfield, Gabrielle.
    Encyclopedia of folk medicine : old world and new world traditions /
Gabrielle Hatfield.
      p. ; cm.
    Includes bibliographical references and index.
    ISBN 1-57607-874-4 (hardcover : alk. paper) ISBN 1-57607-825-6 (eBook)
    1. Alternative medicine—Encyclopedias. 2. Traditional
    medicine—Encyclopedias.
    [DNLM: 1. Medicine, Traditional—Encyclopedias—English. WB 13 H362e
    2004] I. Title.

    R733.H376 2004
    615.8'8'03—dc22

2003022101

08   07   06   05   04   10  9  8  7  6  5  4  3  2  1

ABC-CLIO, Inc.
130 Cremona Drive, P.O. Box 1911
Santa Barbara, California 93116-1911

This book is printed on acid-free paper. ∞
Manufactured in the United States of America

To my husband, John, with love.

# Contents

# Guide to Related Topics

**People**
Bartram, John
Black, William George
Hand, Wayland D.
Josselyn, John
Thomson, Samuel
Blacksmith
Colonists
Healer
Medicine man
Midwife
Seventh son
Specialist
Witch

**Ailments**
Abortion
Abscesses
Acne
Anemia
Arthritis
Asthma
Backache
Bad breath
Baldness
Bed-wetting
Bites and stings
Bleeding
Blisters
Boils
Breast problems
Bruises
Burns
Cancer

Chapped skin
Chilblains
Childbirth
Colds
Colic
Constipation
Consumption
Contraception
Corns
Coughs
Cramp
Croup
Cuts
Deafness
Depression
Diabetes
Diarrhea
Dizziness
Dropsy
Drunkenness
Dysentery
Earache
Eczema
Epilepsy
Erysipelas
Eye problems
Felons
Fevers
Fractures
Freckles
Frostbite
Gout
Gravel and stone
Hair problems

Hay fever
Headache
Heart trouble
Heartburn
Hiccups
Hives
Hunger
Indigestion
Insect bites and stings
Jaundice
King's Evil
Lumbago
Mad dog, bite of
Menopause
Menstrual problems
Migraine
Nausea
Nosebleed
Palsy
Piles
Plague
Poison ivy, Poison oak
Pregnancy
Quinsy
Rheumatism
Rickets
Ringworm
St. Anthony's fire (Erysipelas)
Scrofula
Scurvy
Shingles
Sleeplessness
Smallpox
Snake bite
Sore feet
Sore throat
Spots
Sprains
Sunburn
Teething
Tetters
Toothache
Tuberculosis
Warts
Whooping cough
Worms

Wounds
Wrinkles

**Healing Agents**
Acorn
Alder
Aloe vera
Amber
Apple
Ash
Balm of Gilead
Beans
Bee
Birch
Black cohosh
Blackberry
Blackthorn
Blood
Bloodroot
Bogbean
Boneset
Bread
Bryony
Burdock
Buttercups
Button snakeroot
Cabbage
Catnip
Caul
Cayenne
Chamomile
Cherry
Chickweed
Columbo
Comfrey
Corn
Cowslip
Cricket
Dandelion
Dead man's hand
Dew
Dock
Dog
Earth
Echinacea
Eggs
Elder

Elm
Eryngo
Excreta
Fat
Figwort
Fish
Flax
Forge water
Foxglove
Garlic
Ginger
Ginseng
Gold
Golden seal
Hawthorn
Hemlock
Hemlock spruce
Holly
Honey
Hops
Horehound
Houseleek
Ivy
Jimson weed
Lobelia
Mallow
Mandrake
Milk
Mistletoe
Molds
Moss
Mouse
Mugwort
Mullein
Nettle
Onion
Otter
Peach
Pine
Plantain
Poke
Poppy
Potato
Poultice
Prickly ash
Puffball

Rose
Rowan
St. John's wort
Sarsaparilla
Sassafras
Silverweed
Skull
Snail
Snake
Snow
Soda
Sphagnum moss
Spider
Spit
Stinging nettle
Thornapple
Thyme
Toads and frogs
Tobacco
Tonic
Tormentil
Urine
Valerian
Vinegar
Water
Willow
Yarrow
Yew

**Ideas**
Amulet
Color
Concepts of disease
Doctrine of signatures
Evil eye
Moon
Sympathetic magic
Transference

**Cultural Traditions**
African tradition
Celtic tradition
Mexican tradition
Native American tradition
Shakers

# Acknowledgments

I would like to thank all those who have helped in the preparation of this work. I am grateful to Jennifer Westwood for initiating the idea; to my editor Bob Neville for his help, patience, and encouragement; and to Simon Mason for seeing the project through to completion. I also wish to acknowledge gratefully financial support from the Author's Foundation.

Not least, I wish to thank my husband, John, and my family for their encouragement and support.

## NOTES ON SOURCES

Each entry is provided with a full bibliography. Manuscript sources are given reference numbers where these exist. In the case of manuscripts in private hands, the name of the owner is given.

The amazing resource of the Folklore Archives at the University of California at Los Angeles includes a vast database of North American folk remedies. These are referred to as UCLA Folklore Archives.

# Introduction

Examples in this book are drawn from the folk medicine of Britain and Ireland and from that of North America. Any attempt to define folk medicine is fraught with difficulty. William George Black was the first person to use the term in print, and he defined it as "meant to comprehend the subjects of charms, incantations, and those habits relating to the preservation of health, or the cure of disease, which were and are practiced by the more superstitious and old-fashioned" (Black 1878). To modern ears this sounds patronizing, and such social condescension would not be acceptable to most people today. Although folklore studies have moved on, it is surprising to find how neglected this particular area of folklore has been, particularly in Britain. Historians of medicine have on the whole neglected it as a subject hardly worthy of mention; they have concentrated instead on the history of official medicine, assuming that, in the words of the highly respected historian Singer, folk medicine is "usually medieval or renaissance medicine misunderstood" (Singer 1961: xlvii). However, there is much more to folk medicine than this. Far from representing an ignorant version of orthodox medicine, it should be regarded as the origin of all types of medical practice. It predates any form of official medicine and includes self-treatment as well as treatment by community healers.

Its being based largely on oral traditions

accounts in part for the relatively slight attention it has received from students of the written word. Since the practice of folk medicine is, at least in many parts of Britain, fast becoming obsolete, it is almost too late now to attempt to record the whole corpus of information for posterity. The fact that folk medicine embraces a wide variety of disciplines, from anthropology and religion to botany, zoology, and pharmaceutical science, may be another reason why it has been understudied as a subject.

Yet much of orthodox medicine has had its roots in folk medicine, and folk medicine far predates any kind of official medicine. The subject that we now call ethnobotany was born when the first human hunter-gatherers discovered that certain plants were toxic and could be used to man's advantage. This was long before written records existed. It seems safe to assume that empirical knowledge of plant and animal foods and medicines was passed on from one generation to the next as oral tradition within any one community. Thus began what Stuart has called the "longest clinical trial in human history" (Stuart 1979: 10).

Systems of official medicine began once recognized healers emerged within a community, but at any given time in history and any given place, official and folk medicine have coexisted, sometimes peacefully and sometimes at war with each other. In Britain rivalry between official and folk medicine was so extreme that it led during the eighteenth century to the abandonment of many native plant remedies by the medical profession. Increasing levels of education led to devaluation of the "old wives tales" of earlier generations, and this process has culminated in our modern society, where we are no longer self-reliant in treating even minor illness and depend instead on pills for all ills. Reaction against technological medicine and an increasing awareness of side effects of modern drugs has produced a resurgence of interest among the middle classes in so-called natural remedies. Unfortunately, this interest is often ill informed. When such remedies were used by our forebears they were hedged around with practical limitations. But knowledge of exact methodology, never written down, has often been lost. In this secondary "return to nature" we lack our forebears' detailed knowledge, and what was for them a safe remedy can be lethal in ignorant hands. There is probably no such thing as a perfectly safe remedy, natural or otherwise. Medicine in all its forms is a risky business and doubtless has always been. All these are reasons for preserving such knowledge as we still have of all forms of folk medicine.

Any collection of folk medicine is kaleidoscopic in nature, the fragments of information within it making different patterns depending on the viewpoint. The picture in British folk medicine is complex. In North America, it is even more so.

It is still sometimes possible to trace a particular remedy to one tradition of healing, such as the Native American tradition or the Celtic tradition. Over the centuries, communities have obviously borrowed information from each other, so that distinctions between disparate traditions have become increasingly blurred. Confusing the picture further, official medicine has borrowed from folk medicine, and vice versa. For every folk remedy that we have today on record, there are many that have been

forgotten, as the chain of oral tradition has been snapped. For all these reasons, generalizations in folk medicine are largely meaningless. The best we can do is to attempt to record for posterity what is left.

Folk medicine has had no scribes to record it in the past, and attempts retrospectively to interpret it are destined to failure. As Thompson has pointed out, too much of written history is "a description of social relations as they may be seen from above" (Thompson 1991: 21). We have no clear idea of past folk concepts of disease but are forced to infer these from the remedies used and their manner of use. In every field it is only the educated and the literate who have recorded their theories. In folk medicine this has sometimes led to misleading attribution to folk medicine of ideas that were actually formulated by the learned rather than the folk. An example is the doctrine of signatures.

Within our incomplete reservoir of information on folk medicine it is possible to detect some recurrent themes. One of these is the idea of transference of disease to an inanimate object (such as a stone or water [see entry]), or to an animal (such as a dog [see entry]), or to a plant (such as an apple [see entry] tree). In an extension of this idea, a disease may be "left behind" by a "passing-through ceremony," such as the cure for hernia, which involves passing under a blackberry arch. Wart remedies in particular are rich in examples of transference. They also illustrate several other themes common in folk medicine, such as the idea of sympathetic magic and of like curing like, sometimes described as "homeopathic magic." (Thus, the warty toad [see entry] can be a cause of warts.) Many folk remedies involve some kind of measurement or counting; Wayland D. Hand gives numerous examples from North Carolina (Hand 1961: xxix–xxx). A British example is to cut as many notches in an elder stick as you have warts and dispose of the stick. Many, too, have a built-in time element: rub the wart with meat and bury the meat; as it decays, the warts will disappear. For a child suffering from asthma, plug some of its hair into a hole bored in a tree above their head; when the child grows beyond it, the asthma will disappear.

It is in the nature of human study to categorize information, but there is much in folk medicine that does not lend itself to this treatment. Partly because our recorded information is so incomplete, and partly because the roots of folk medicine are so dispersed in time and place, many folk remedies can only be described as "miscellaneous."

In British plant medicine it is nevertheless possible to distinguish between the truly traditional, orally preserved folk medicine, practiced on the whole by those too poor to afford, or too remote from, official medical help; and the "book" medicine of official practitioners. The numerous printed books on do-it-yourself medicine occupy a position intermediate between folk and official medicine.

The origin of folk medicine in Britain is complex; in North America it is even more so. The Native American tradition is a vast subject in its own right, and one in which it is difficult, and perhaps meaningless, to attempt to separate treatment by healers from domestic folk medicine. Every subsequent wave of colonists to North America took with it its own folk medical traditions, some of which have become incorporated into what we might call "general" folk medicine. As in Britain, the role of printed information in American folk medicine is a difficult one to define. In fact, it is even more difficult in North America than in Britain, since many colonists came from backgrounds where they would have depended on official medical aid. They brought with them orthodox medical books of their day and depended on these in conditions where little else was available by way

of medical help. These books include some British orthodox medical texts, such as Thomas Phaire's *The Boke of Children* (first published in London in 1553 and subsequently reprinted) and texts of domestic medicine, such as John Wesley's *Primitive Physic* (London, 1781) and Culpeper's *English Physician* (London, 1652). In Britain these would not be regarded today as folk medicine in the strict sense, whereas in North America they have all gone into the giant melting pot of introduced traditions and information that has become today's North American folk medicine. Almanacs and books of domestic medicine abounded during the nineteenth century. These were a mix of official and folk medicine. Some, such as J. C. Gunn's *New Family Physician* (New York, 1869) were written by doctors but became immensely popular and ran into numerous editions. Indeed, in North America the dividing lines between "trained" doctors, herbalists, and folk practitioners are almost impossible to draw precisely. Some of the Shaker practitioners went on to become orthodox practitioners. Samuel Thomson, whose experience began in folk medicine, became a famous herbalist, profoundly influencing not only North American but also British herbalism (Griggs 1997: 166–187).

As with all aspects of folklore, there is a danger that the subject is misrepresented by an emphasis on the bizarre and, indeed, by a misunderstanding on the part of the recorders who are rarely themselves the users of folk medicine. The contrasting strands of practicality and credulity that characterize folk medicine are fascinating. In this book, emphasis has been placed on actual recorded folk remedies, which allow the "folk" to speak for themselves.

Nolan in Ireland and Hufford in Pennsylvania have both emphasized the community aspect of folk medicine. Nolan describes "healing and helping taking place every day" in rural communities (Nolan

1988: 55), while Hufford describes folk medicine as "community resources for dealing with illness" (Hufford 1992: 15). This caring aspect of folk medicine is another cogent reason for preserving our knowledge of it.

British folk medicine can be compared to a fabric composed of several interwoven strands. In North America, folk medicine is more like a patchwork. Just as with a quilt it is sometimes possible to recognize from a scrap the source of the original material, so in folk medicine the origin of a particular remedy may be traceable to one tradition. A whole quilt, composed of scraps, is an art form in its own right. Similarly, the corpus of folk medicine, with its contributions from many cultures and eras, is something more than the sum of its parts. It is a rich mosaic worth preserving for posterity. It is hoped that this book will arouse further interest and curiosity in this once undervalued aspect of human culture.

## References

Black, William George. *Journal of the British Archaeological Association* 34 (1878): 327–332.

Griggs, Barbara. *New Green Pharmacy: The Story of Western Herbal Medicine.* London: Vermilion, 1997.

Hand, Wayland D. Introduction to *The Frank C. Brown Collection of North Carolina Folklore.* Durham, NC: Duke University Press, 1961.

Hufford, David J. *Folk Medicine in Contemporary America: In Herbal and Magical Medicine.* Edited by James Kirkland, Holly F. Matthews, C. W. Sullivan III, and Karen Baldwin. Durham, NC, and London: Duke University Press, 1992.

Nolan, Peter W. "Folk Medicine in Rural Ireland." *Folk Life* 27 (1988–1999): 44–56.

Singer, Charles. Introduction to *Leechdoms, Wortcunning and Starcraft of Early England.* Collected and edited by Rev. Thomas Oswald Cockayne. London: Holland Press, 1961.

Stuart, Malcolm, ed. *The Encyclopedia of Herbs and Herbalism.* London: Orbis, 1979.

Thompson, E. P. *Customs in Common.* Suffolk: Merlin Press, 1991.

*See also* **Apple; Asthma; Black, William George; Blackberry; Celtic tradition; Colonists; Concepts of disease; Doctrine of signatures; Dog; Elder; Hand, Wayland D.; Healers; Native American tradition; Thomson, Samuel; Shakers, Sympathetic magic; Toads and frogs; Transference; Warts; Water.**

# Encyclopedia of Folk Medicine

# A

## Abortion

In this highly sensitive area, the folk medical practices are almost certainly underrepresented in the records. Religious, legal and ethical issues involved have led to secrecy. Such terms as "emmenagogue" (meaning an agent that provokes menstruation) are in many cases likely to be euphemisms for abortion. More picturesquely, in the eighteenth century, such remedies were employed to "bring down the flowers" (Leven and Melville Papers, SRO). Probably such remedies were used, as stated, to regulate menstruation, but probably also, at least unofficially, they were used to bring about abortions. Although these remedies are listed freely in the herbals from the sixteenth century onward, it is difficult to know what "the folk" actually did about such matters. It is not until we come to recent times, within living memory, that we can discover with any certainty the means used. Even within living memory, this has remained such a delicate matter that few people are ready to provide information.

Apart from purely mechanical means of destroying the fetus, in poor country areas of Britain girls "in trouble" would resort to strong laxatives or jumping off walls or stairs in an attempt to abort. If this failed, often gin was the next resort. Interestingly, gin is flavored with juniper (*Juniperus spp.*), one of the few plants that we know was al-

most universally used for abortion. In parts of Britain, the plant is known by the uncompromising name of "bastard killer" (Grigson 1955: 24). John Pechey, writing in 1694, says of this plant that it "forces the courses. . . . Upon which Account they are too well known, and too much used by wenches" (Pechey 1694: 164). Juniper was known by a number of names, including savin. Under this name it appears in the traditional ballad of the "Queen's Maries." When one of Mary Queen of Scot's ladies in waiting was found to be pregnant by the king, this, according to the ballads, was the plant she used to try to bring about an abortion (Child 1965: 379). Her attempts failed, and she was executed in the Tolbooth, Edinburgh.

Other plants used in British folk medicine as abortifacients include raspberry. Used in the later stages of pregnancy, a tea made from the leaves has been found to strengthen the uterine muscles and speed delivery, but in the early stages of pregnancy it has been used to procure an abortion. Another plant used similarly is pennyroyal, *Mentha pulegium*. This is native to Britain and has probably been one of the more secretive remedies handed down (usually by women) from one generation to the next. It has been used successfully as recently as twenty years ago in the United Kingdom (Hatfield MS). Actual records of its use are very rare, and it is still rarer to know the outcome. There is an oral history record of the use of houseleek (*Sempervivum tectorum*) in Ireland to procure abortion (Vickery 1995: 198). In this instance, the plant was apparently often used to cleanse cows of the afterbirth, a use that would have suggested the secondary use as an abortifacient. Three native plants that we know were used in the Scottish Highlands to procure abortions are meadow-rue (*Thalictrum minus*), fairy flax (*Linum catharticum*), and fir clubmoss (*Huperzia selago*). All were recorded in use in the seventeenth century in the western Highlands by James Robertson, who, as Beith points out, was unusual in apparently being able to gain women's confidence on such matters (Beith 1995: 96).

In general North American folk medicine it is equally difficult to find out about abortifacients, and for the same reasons. Collections of folk medical cures rarely address the subject at all. It is interesting that the UCLA folk medicine archive, so vast and extensive in many respects, has few records on this subject. This, of course, could reflect unwillingness on the part of recorders as well as of informants to discuss such matters. Meyer's collection of folk remedies for "suppressed menses" almost certainly includes some that were used to procure abortion (Meyer 1985: 171–173). For example, juniper appears here, more than once. It had official sanction as a menstrual regulator and was described by two nineteenth-century doctors as among the "best and most powerful medicines for the regulation of retained or obstructed menses," a medicine that "may be found upon almost any farm in New England" (Capron and Slack: 1848). Other plants recommended for regulation of menses are smartweed (*Polygonum* sp.) and seneca snakeroot (*Polygala senega*), as well as the herb called "female regulator" that Meyer identifies as *Senecio aureus* (Meyer 1985: 171–173).

European colonists to North America doubtless brought with them some knowledge of unofficial abortifacients, but their use is unlikely to have been recorded. Did their learning from Native Americans about unfamiliar plants, native to North America, include this subject? The plant called pennyroyal in North America is different from the British pennyroyal. American pennyroyal is *Hedeoma pulegioides,* also called squaw mint, and was used by the Native Americans, and perhaps by colonists too, to regulate the menstrual cycle and to procure abortions. The Cherokee, for example, are known to have used this plant as an abortifacient (Hamel and Chiltoskey 1975: 48). The amount of information about abortifacients used by Native Americans, as listed in Moerman's *Ethnobotany* (Moerman 1998), is truly amazing and suggests few of the taboos surrounding the subject that we have noted in Britain. More than a hundred genera are listed as abortifacients (Moerman 1998: 765–766). Among them are Juniper (*Juniperus virginiana*) and *Polygala seneca* (both used by the Cherokee [Hamel and Chiltoskey 1975: 55]). Species of *Artemisia* were used very widely, by nine different tribes (Moerman 1998: 765). This genus has been used all over the world as a "woman's herb," use that probably included contraception and sometimes abortion. *Artemisia franserioides* is used by New Mexico Spanish Americans for abortion (Kay 1996: 106).

Apart from plant remedies, there were other, ceremonial means of procuring abortions among the Native Americans. The medicine men of the Blackfoot claim to use the power of the moth for this (Wissler 1905: 260). An Ozark belief is that country women should never expose their naked bodies before a flowering hawthorn, or "redhaw" (*Crataegus* sp.), as this tree was associated with "rape, unfortunate pregnancies and disastrous abortions" (Randolph 1953: 336).

*See also* **Hawthorn, Houseleek.**

## References

Beith, Mary. *Healing Threads: Traditional Medicines of the Highlands and Islands*. Edinburgh: Polygon 1995.

Capron, George, and David Slack. *New England Popular Medicine*. 1848. Quoted in Meyer, 1985.

Child, F. J. *English and Scottish Popular Ballads*. Volume 3, *1882–1898*. New York: Dover Publications, 1965. Page 379.

Grigson, Geoffrey. *The Englishman's Flora*. London: Phoenix House, 1955.

Hamel, Paul B., and Mary U. Chiltoskey. *Cherokee Plants and Their Uses: A 400 Year History*. Sylva, NC: Herald, 1975.

Hatfield MSS. Manuscript notes in private possession of Gabrielle Hatfield.

Kay, Margarita Artschwager. *Healing with Plants in the American and Mexican West*. Tucson: University of Arizona Press, 1996.

Leven and Melville Papers. Scottish Records Office, Edinburgh. SRO GD 26.

Meyer, Clarence. *American Folk Medicine*. Glenwood, IL: Meyerbooks, 1985.

Moerman, Daniel E. *Native American Ethnobotany*. Portland, OR: Timber Press, 1998.

Pechey, John. *Compleat Herbal of Physical Plants*. London: 1694.

Randolph, Vance. "Nakedness in Ozark Folk Belief." *Journal of American Folklore* 66 (1953): 333–339.

Vickery, Roy. *A Dictionary of Plant Lore*. Oxford: Oxford University Press, 1995.

Wissler, Clark. "The Whirlwind and the Elk in the Mythology of the Dakota." *Journal of American Folklore* 18 (1905): 257–268.

# Abscesses

Many folk remedies for these were used in the form of poultices and depended on heat to bring the abscess to a head. Cow pats were used in this way in Britain as recently as the twentieth century, and their effectiveness has been vouched for in treating humans and animals (Hatfield 1994: 11; Beith 1995: 172–173). Less drastically, a bread poultice applied hot was often used, or a poultice made from flax seed. Alternatively, a glass bottle was filled with very hot water, emptied, and immediately applied to the abscess; the combination of heat and suction was apparently painful but often effective. Among plant poultices, common mallow *(Malva sylvestris)*, houseleek *(Sempervivum tectorum)*, and chickweed *(Stellaria media)* were some of the most frequently used in British folk medicine, but a large variety of other plants were also used, including vegetables such as onion, cabbage, and carrot.

In North American folk medicine poultices were used in a similar way, and again the use of bread or of cornmeal, or flaxseed was common. Nine bark *(Physocarpus opulifolius)* was a Native American remedy for abscesses, a decoction of the root being mixed with bran or Indian meal (Meyer 1985: 204). Sphagnum moss was also used as a poultice by the Native Americans (Souter 1995: 128) and was adopted as a remedy by settlers as well. North American folk medicine used a wide variety of plants for poulticing abscesses and these included cabbage, carrot, and houseleek (as in Britain), as well as fenugreek seed (a German remedy) and a wide variety of North American native plants not found in Britain, such as poke, slippery elm *(Ulmus fulva)*, smartweed *(Polygonum punctatum and P. hydopiper)*, catnip, and black alder *(Alnus glutinosa)*. Interestingly, many of these North American plants were imported into British and European herbalism in the nineteenth century (Meyer 1985: 200–205; Griggs 1997: 188 ff.).

*See also* **Boils, Catnip, Houseleek, Poke, Poultice, Sphagnum moss.**

### References

Beith, Mary. *Healing Threads: Traditional Medicines of the Highlands and Islands*. Edinburgh: Polygon, 1995.

Griggs, Barbara. *New Green Pharmacy*. London: Vermilion, 1997.

Hatfield, Gabrielle. *Country Remedies: Traditional East Anglian Plant Remedies in the Twentieth Century.* Woodbridge: Boydell, 1994.

Meyer, Clarence. *American Folk Medicine.* Glenwood, IL: Meyerbooks, 1985.

Souter, Keith. *Cure Craft: Traditional Folk Remedies and Treatment from Antiquity to the Present Day.* Saffron Walden: C. W. Daniel, 1995.

# Acne

In British folk medicine various plant infusions were drunk to improve the complexion. The commonest of these were an infusion of nettles and a decoction prepared by boiling the roots of burdock. In the Highlands of Scotland, dulse soup, prepared from seaweed, was recommended for skin disorders (Beith 1995: 240). External applications to clear spots include juice of marigold leaves *(Calendula officinalis)* (Hatfield 1994: 53); the crushed leaves of wood violet (*Viola* sp.), or of the juice of the ice plant, also called houseleek (Prince 1991: 93); a face pack made from oats and lemon (Souter 1995:131); and an ointment made from elder flowers *(Sambucus nigra)* boiled with almond oil and lard (Beith 1995: 215). Application of water from natural springs or simply drinking plenty of cold water was recommended in the Highlands (Beith 1995: 133); bathing the face in early-morning dew was held to be good for the complexion (Hatfield MS), as well as helping to remove freckles. Less pleasantly, urine was much used in folk medicine for treating and preventing acne (Souter 1995: 131). Rubbing the baby's face with a recently wet nappy was practiced in the Highlands of Scotland to prevent the child developing acne later and to give it a good complexion (Beith 1995: 188). A remedy from Norfolk was prepared from oak tree gall, strong vinegar, flowers of sulphur, and the root of Iris (Hatfield 1994: 53).

In North American folk practice, many similar remedies have been used. Among Native American remedies, burdock root was used for treating pimples, and one species of violet, *Viola pubescens,* has been used by the Iroquois to treat spots (Herrick 1977: 387, 474), both these remedies mirroring ones found in Britain. In addition, a huge number of other plant species have been used, including *Achillea* species (Densmore 1928: 350; Perry 1952: 40); *Alnus serrulata* (Hamel and Chiltoskey 1975: 22); various species of *Artemisia,* such as *A. ludoviciana,* used by the Paiute (Train, Henrichs and Archer 1941: 40–42); *A. tridentata,* used by Havasupai (Weber and Seaman 1985: 246). Other remedies featured in North American folk medicine include sulphur and molasses (UCLA Folklore Archives 15_5255), or water in which sulphur had been boiled (UCLA Folklore Archives 6_5446). Poultices of chamomile *(Chamaemelum nobile)* or of red clover (*Trifolium* sp.) were used by early settlers, also the juice of watermelons *(Citrullus lanatus).* Water that collected in old tree stumps was used to wash the face (Micheletti 1998: 21). Urine was widely recommended (UCLA Folklore Archives 8_8446).

Perhaps because acne is associated with puberty, there have been some strange ideas as to its cause. It has been suggested that masturbation (Cannon 1984: 91), or even thinking about sex (UCLA Folklore Archives 13_5255), causes acne; on the other hand, having sex has been claimed by one teenager in Arizona to clear up acne! (UCLA Folklore Archives 14_5255).

*See also* **Burdock, Dew, Freckles, Houseleek, Nettle.**

### References

Beith, Mary. *Healing Threads: Traditional Medicines of the Highlands and Islands.* Edinburgh: Polygon, 1995.

Cannon, Anthon S. *Popular Beliefs and Superstitions from Utah.* Edited by Wayland D.

Hand and Jeannine E. Talley. Salt Lake City: University of Utah Press, 1984.

Densmore, Frances. *Use of Plants by the Chippewa Indians.* Smithsonian Institution-Bureau of American Ethnology Annual Report 44, 1928.

Hamel, Paul B., and Mary U. Chiltoskey. *Cherokee Plants and Their Uses: A 400 Year History.* Sylva, NC: Herald, 1975.

Hatfield, Gabrielle. *Country Remedies: Traditional East Anglian Plant Remedies in the Twentieth Century.* Woodbridge: Boydell, 1994.

Herrick, James William. *Iroquois Medical Botany.* PhD thesis. Albany: State University of New York, 1977.

Micheletti, Enza (ed.). *North American Folk Healing: An A-Z Guide to Traditional Remedies.* New York and Montreal: Reader's Digest Association, 1998.

Perry, F. "Ethno-Botany of the Indians in the Interior of British Columbia." *Museum and Art Notes* 2(2), 1952.

Prince, Dennis. *Grandmother's Cures: An A-Z of Herbal Remedies.* London: Fontana, 1991.

Souter, Keith. *Cure Craft: Traditional Folk Remedies and Treatment from Antiquity to the Present Day.* Saffron Walden: C. W. Daniel, 1995.

Train, Percy, James R. Henrichs, and W. Andrew Archer. *Medicinal Uses of Plants by Indian Tribes of Nevada.* Washington, DC: US Department of Agriculture, 1941.

Weber, Steven A., and P. David Seaman. *Havasupai Habitat: A. F. Whiting's Ethnography of a Traditional Indian Culture.* Tucson: University of Arizona Press, 1985.

# African tradition

Every oral tradition is as extensive as its community. In the case of the many thousands of black African slaves imported from the seventeenth century onward into North America, these traditions were drawn from all over West Africa, and never represented a single tradition. Since emancipation of the slaves, all the fragmentary communities have become gradually absorbed into the wider patchwork of North American traditions, yet there still remain many distinctive features, and indeed today's folk medicine is indebted to African slaves for some of its remedies. At least one slave owed his freedom to imparting a remedy for gravel and stone to a white man.

As displaced people with no rights and no wealth, slaves must have been even more self-dependent than their forbears in times of illness. Although to their owners black slaves represented a valuable investment, which it was in their interest to keep well and working, plantation owners soon found that the remedies known to the slaves were at least as good as anything they could offer themselves.

Faced with a completely unfamiliar flora, it must have been a daunting task indeed for slaves to find their own remedies. Food items such as yams, okra, and kola imported to feed them cheaply were probably among the few familiar items, and it is not surprising, therefore, to find that some of their folk medical remedies were based on these. Pods of Okra *(Abelmoschus esculentus),* boiled, formed a nutritious broth for invalids (Heinerman 2001: 70), and kola nuts *(Cola acuminata)* were used to treat stomach pain (Sloane 1707–1725, 2: 61). Experimentation with the local flora led to use of a large number of native plant species, too. Pneumonia, to which the slaves of South Carolina were apparently particularly susceptible, was treated with snakeroot *(Aristolochia serpentaria).* Ringworm was treated with a wash prepared from the so-called ringworm bush *(Cassia alata).* The seeds of avocado *(Persea americana)* were ground to treat diarrhea, dysentery, and whitlows (Heinerman 2001: 72, 88).

Not only was the flora unfamiliar, but some of the diseases that afflicted the slaves were unfamiliar too. There were parasitic worms different from those in Africa. Barton in his early nineteenth-century journal recorded the use of persimmon fruit *(Dios-*

*pyros virginiana)* among the black African slaves (Barton 1802, 2: 52). Plantation owners sometimes dosed slave children with a plant called cowitch *(Macuna pruriens),* which, according to Bancroft in the eighteenth century, was remarkably successful in expelling worms (Bancroft 1769: 39). The disease known as yaws was especially prevalent among black slaves, and it seems that their own remedies for it were fairly effective. The roots of the lime *(Citrus aurantifolia)* were used in treating this condition, as described in an eighteenth-century account by Du Pratz (Du Pratz 1774: 378–380). An infusion of holly berries *(Ilex obcordata)* was successfully used as a wash for treating the sores of yaws (Heinerman 2001: 85). Lime was also used to treat scurvy and sores on the feet. The fruit of papaya *(Carica papaya)* was used to treat sores and stomach ache. Cayenne pepper was used to treat a condition described as "cachexia," characterized by weight loss, fall in body temperature, and, if untreated, death (Heinerman 2001: 74). Snake bite was treated with various plants, including so-called rattlesnake's master *(Aralia spinosa),* while it was claimed that "inoculation" with boneset *(Eupatorium perfoliatum)* could actually render a snake bite harmless (Descourtilz 1833, 3: 214). Barton records the cure of a black slave suffering from consumption. It consisted of the root of Indian turnip *(Arisaema triphyllum)* boiled in milk (Barton 2001, 1: 110).

Pregnancy among slaves represented another child born into slavery; this was of benefit to the slave owner, but women would often go to extreme lengths to avoid pregnancy and childbirth under these circumstances. It is ironic that the very plant, cotton *(Gossypium herbaceum),* for which their freedom had been sacrificed was in some cases able to afford relief from unwanted pregnancy (especially unwanted where this was a result of rape by the plan-

tation owner, anxious to see his human investment multiply). A decoction of the roots of the cotton plant was found to be an effective abortifacient, taken during the first two months of pregnancy. The planters, in their turn, tried to prevent the effects of this plant by forcibly administering black haw *(Viburnum prunifolium)* to their female slaves (King's American Dispensatory, 1898, quoted by Micheletti [ed.] 1998).

Apart from the empirical folk remedies they used, slaves have also bequeathed a legacy of their fundamentally different approach to illness, which was seen by them as caused by a loss of balance between forces for good and evil. Some illnesses were regarded as natural, others as having supernatural causes. For the latter category, it was necessary to have recourse to magical healing, administered usually by a respected voodoo healer. Indeed, these unnatural illnesses were often thought to be caused by an enemy, and they could be cured only by someone with magical powers. Some plants were directly associated with spiritual healing and magical powers. Among them the cotton tree *(Ceiba pentandra)* was regarded as consecrated to spirits. It was never cut down; religious ceremonies were often held under it. The overlook bean, or horse bean *(Canavalia ensiformis),* was regarded as a watchman and was planted around valuable crops to protect them from plunder (Macfadyen 1837, 1: 179). Remnants of these folk beliefs, mixed and modified by religious and Western medical systems, still persist among black Africans today (Matthews 1992: 68–98).

The extent to which there was an exchange of information between Native Americans and the black slaves is difficult to establish, but there are examples of remedies used in common. The Indian turnip *(Arisaema triphyllum),* for example, was used by the Cherokee as well as by slaves to treat consumption (Hamel and Chiltoskey

1975: 41), and papaya fruit were used to treat cuts by the Hawaii, in much the same way as the slaves used them (Akana 1922: 43). The snakeroot (*Aristolochia serpentaria*) was used among numerous Native American tribes to treat snake bite (Moerman 1998: 92). One healer who today combines the heritage of Native American, European, and African folk medicine is John Lee of Moncure, in the North Carolina Piedmont. He is of mixed Lumbee, Cherokee, African, Irish, and English descent. He combines empirical treatment with herbs with spiritual divination. He was born with a caul, a fact that has probably enhanced his reputation as a healer (Micheletti 1998: 179).

*See also* **Caul, Cayenne, Gravel and stone, Ringworm, Scurvy, Snake bite, Tuberculosis.**

### References

Akana, Akaiko. 1922. *Hawaiian Herbs of Medicinal Value.* Honolulu: Pacific Book House.

Bancroft, E. *Essay on the Natural History of Guiana in South America.* London: 1769.

Barton, B. S. *Journal of Benjamin Smith Barton on a Visit to Virginia in 1802.* Quoted in Heinerman 2001: 72.

Descourtilz, M. E. *Flore Pittoresque et Médical Des Antilles.* Paris, 1833.

Du Pratz, M. L. P. *History of Louisiana, or of the Western Parts of Virginia and Carolina.* London: T. Becket, 1774.

Hamel, Paul B., and Mary U. Chiltoskey. *Cherokee Plants and Their Uses: A 400 Year History.* Sylva, NC: Herald, 1975.

Heinerman, John. *Folk Medicine in America Today: A Guide for a New Generation of Folk Healers.* New York: Kensington, 2001.

Macfadyen, J. *Flora of Jamaica.* London: Longmans Green, 1837.

Matthews, Holly. "Doctors and Root Doctors: Patients Who Use Both." In *Herbal and Magical Medicine: Traditional Healing Today.* Edited by James Kirkland, Holly F. Matthews, C. W. Sullivan III and Karen Baldwin. Durham, NC: Duke University Press, 1992.

Micheletti, Enza (ed.). *North American Folk Healing: An A-Z Guide to Traditional Remedies.* New York and Montreal: Reader's Digest Association, 1998.

Moerman, Daniel E. *Native American Ethnobotany.* Portland, OR: Timber Press, 1998.

Sloane, H. *Natural History of Jamaica.* London. 1707–1725.

# Alder (*Alnus spp.*)

The British species of alder, *Alnus glutinosa,* has not been prominent in folk medicine. Its leaves have been placed in shoes to prevent tired, sore feet and also have been used in treating burns (Salhouse, Norfolk, pers. com. 1990). Parson Woodforde, in his diary for March 7, 1767, reported using alder bark steeped in water for his unspecified ailment (Woodforde Society 1985, 3, 71), and recommended it as a springtime tonic. There are reports of using alder cones boiled in water for the treatment of gout (Vickery 1995: 2), while in the nineteenth century a piece of alder wood was carried as a preventive against rheumatism (Gomme 1884: 134). Otherwise, British uses of alder are nonmedicinal.

In North America the picture is quite different. There are ten species of alder native to North America. The range of uses for them in folk medicine is wide. The use of the "tags" (conelike fruits) of tag alder, *Alnus serrulata,* for treating chills has been reported in Carolina (Brown 1952–1964, 6: 145). Alder bark ointment has been used for treating itching (Brendle and Unger 1935: 61) and burns (Bergen 1899: 110). In colonial days, alder bark was used to prevent scarring from smallpox (Lick and Brendle 1922: 233–234). The water in which alder buds have been steeped was drunk for rheumatism (Bergen 1899: 110). To help teething in children, a necklace was made from threaded pieces of alder twig (Browne 1958: 25). For coughs a tea was made from swamp alder bark (Brewster 1939: 35). Red alder bark is recorded as a treatment for leucorrhoea (Meyer 1985: 164). More generally, alders have had a reputation in North America as blood purifiers (Meyer 1985: 41), to be taken as a springtime tonic (Meyer 1985: 258). Alder bark has also been used, combined with elder bark and wild cherry bark, for eczema (Meyer 1985: 106).

In the Native American tradition, the uses of alder have been very numerous (Moerman 1998: 60–64). The bruised leaves of the tag alder are reported to have been used by Native Americans as a poultice on the breasts to stop the flow of milk (Meyer 1985: 47). Willard reports a wide range of uses in the Rockies and neighboring territories. The use by Native Americans of alder leaves for sore and aching feet echoes that in Britain. The leaves were placed by a wife under her husband's hat as a cure for grumpiness and hangover. As in Britain, alder leaves were used in treatment of burns. In addition, the alder tree in North America has yielded remedies for a very wide range of other complaints: the leaves were used to deter fleas, the fresh bark to treat rashes, including that from poison ivy; a decoction of the bark was used by the Kutenai Indians to regulate menstruation, and by the Blackfoot for treating tuberculosis; in addition it was used for constipation, jaundice and diarrhea. The inner bark was used for wounds and skin ulcers (Willard 1992: 67–69). Four different species of alder have been recorded in use for treating toothache and for cleaning teeth (Turner, Thompson, and Thompson et al. 1990: 188; Black 1980: 153; Hamel and Chiltoskey 1975: 22). Mixed with dried bumblebees, alder has been used to help childbirth (Densmore 1928: 358).

*See also* **Burns, Childbirth, Constipation, Coughs, Diarrhea, Jaundice, Poison ivy, Rheumatism, Smallpox, Sore feet, Teething, Tonic, Tuberculosis, Wounds.**

## References

Bergen, Fanny D. *Animal and Plant Lore Collected from the Oral Tradition of English Speaking Folk.* Boston and New York: Memoirs of the American Folk-Lore Society 7, 1899.

Black, Meredith Jean. *Algonquin Ethnobotany: An Interpretation of Aboriginal Adaptation in South Western Quebec.* Ottawa: National Museums of Canada. Mercury Series 65, 1980.

Brendle, Thomas R. and Claude W. Unger. "Folk Medicine of the Pennsylvania Germans. The Non-Occult Cures." *Proceedings of the Pennsylvania German Society* 45, 1935.

Brewster, Paul G. "Folk Cures and Preventatives from Southern Indiana." *Southern Folklore Quarterly* 3 (1939): 33–43.

Brown, Frank C. *Collection of North Carolina Folklore.* 7 vols. Durham, NC: Duke University Press, 1952–1964.

Browne, Ray B. *Popular Beliefs and Practices from Alabama.* Folklore Studies 9. Berkeley and Los Angeles: University of California Publications, 1958.

Densmore, Frances. "Uses of Plants by the Chippewa Indians." *Smithsonian Institution-Bureau of American Ethnology Annual Report* 44 (1928): 273–379.

Gomme, G. L. (ed.). *The Gentleman's Magazine Library: Popular Superstitions.* London, 1884.

Hamel, Paul B., and Mary U. Chiltoskey. *Cherokee Plants and Their Uses: A 400 Year History.* Sylva, NC: Herald, 1975.

Lick, David E., and Thomas R. Brendle. "Plant Names and Plant Lore among the Pennsylvania Germans." *Proceedings and Addresses of the Pennsylvania German Society* 33 (1922).

Meyer, Clarence. *American Folk Medicine.* Glenwood, IL: Meyerbooks, 1985.

Moerman, Daniel E. *Native American Ethnobotany.* Portland, OR: Timber Press, 1998.

Turner, Nancy J., Laurence C. Thompson, and M. Terry Thompson et al. *Thompson Ethnobotany: Knowledge and Usage of Plants by the Thompson Indians of British Columbia.* Victoria: Royal British Columbia Museum, 1990.

Vickery, Roy. *A Dictionary of Plant Lore.* Oxford: Oxford University Press, 1995.

Willard, Terry. *Edible and Medicinal Plants of the Rocky Mountains and Neighbouring Territories.* Calgary: Wild Rose College of Natural Healing, 1992.

Woodforde, Parson James. *Ansford Diary.* Edited by R. L. Winstanley, Parson Woodforde Society, 1985.

# Aloe vera

This is an African plant, used in official medicine by the ancient Egyptians as well as in classical Greek and ancient Chinese medicine. It was introduced into North America by missionaries and gradually became a familiar plant of domestic medicine throughout North and South America. Its main use in official medicine was as a purgative, but in folk medicine it has been used primarily as a skin healer, and its fame has spread for the treatment of burns (the gel from the scraped leaves is used). Along with many other people, Columbus confused aloe with the rather similar-looking but unrelated agave, which he found growing as a native in the New World. The true aloe reached Mexico shortly after the conquest (Valdés and Flores 1984: 86), when Hernandez reported that the Aztecs used it in treating various skin conditions. The aloe now thrives throughout North and South America. In modern times in the American and Mexican West it has been used for treating a variety of skin conditions, such as dermatitis and boils (Kay 1996: 91). It has even been used in the treatment of radiation burns (Meyer 1985: 54). As its popularity has increased, extravagant claims have been made for the plant as a panacea. At least some of these claims are justifiable in the light of modern research (Chevallier 1996: 57), and it is now widely used by herbalists and as an over-the-counter medication in

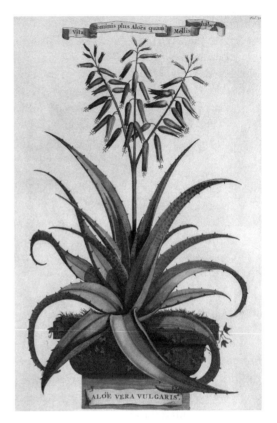

Claimed to be one of the most widely used healing plants in the world, *Aloe vera* has been used primarily to treat a variety of skin conditions, such as burns, dermatitis, and boils. (Historical Picture Archive/ CORBIS)

both North America and Britain. It has been claimed to be one of the most widely used healing plants in the world (Bloomfield 1985: 2). Although most of these uses belong to modern herbalism, the plant has been used to some extent in folk medicine too. It has been applied to rashes, burns, warts, insect stings, and taken internally for stomach ache (Anderson 1970: 70).

Recently Aloe vera has become a popular constituent of many cosmetic as well as herbal preparations in Britain as well as in North America. It is one of a number of plants to achieve fame in the modern secondary return to herbalism among the middle class.

## References

Anderson, John Q. *Texas Folk Medicine.* Austin: Encino Press, 1970.

Bloomfield, Frena. *Miracle Plants: Aloe Vera.* London: Century, 1985.

Chevallier, Andrew. *The Encyclopedia of Medicinal Plants.* London: Dorling Kindersley, 1996.

Kay, Margarita Artschwager. *Healing with Plants in the American and Mexican West.* Tucson: University of Arizona Press, 1996.

Meyer, Clarence. *American Folk Medicine.* Glenwood, IL: Meyerbooks, 1985.

Valdés, Javier, and Hilda Flores. *Comentarios a la Obra de Francisco Hernández.* Vol. 7 of *Obras Completas.* Mexico City: Universidad Nacional Autónoma de México, 1984.

# Amber

This is the translucent golden resin obtained from coniferous trees now largely extinct. It was credited with the power to ease depression, when worn next to the skin. It was also considered to be an aphrodisiac. In Scotland amber beads were a traditional gift by the parents to a bride, to make her irresistible to her new husband (Souter 1995: 176). Amber was also rubbed onto a stye to heal it (Souter 1995: 190). In England necklaces of amber beads were used as amulets to prevent whooping cough, croup, and asthma (Gardner 1942: 98).

In North American folk medicine amber beads were worn both to prevent and cure a range of ailments, especially goitre (Koch 1980: 94). Other ailments for which amber was used include asthma (Brown 1952–1964, 6: 119), croup (Whitney and Bullock 1925: 92), teething (Thomas and Thomas 1920: 118), and weak eyes (Hoke 1892: 117). In contrast to the belief in Scotland, it has been reported from Salt Lake City that an amber bead necklace will prevent desire (Cannon 1984: 158).

*See also* **Amulet, Asthma, Croup, Depression, Teething.**

## References

Brown, Frank C. *Collection of North Carolina Folklore.* 7 vols. Durham, NC: Duke University Press, 1952–1964.

Cannon, Anthon S. *Popular Beliefs and Superstitions from Utah.* Edited by Wayland D. Hand and Jeannine E. Talley. Salt Lake City: University of Utah Press, 1984.

Gardner, Gerald Brosseau. "British Charms, Amulets and Talismans." *Folk-Lore* 53 (1942): 95–103.

Hoke, N. C. "Folk Customs and Folk Belief in North Carolina." *Journal of American Folklore* 5 (1892): 113–120.

Koch, William E. *Folklore from Kansas: Beliefs and Customs.* Lawrence: Regent Press, 1980.

Souter, Keith. *Cure Craft: Traditional Folk Remedies and Treatment from Antiquity to the Present Day.* Saffron Walden: C. W. Daniel, 1995.

Thomas, Daniel Lindsay, and Lucy Blayney Thomas. *Kentucky Superstitions.* Princeton, NJ: Princeton University Press, 1920.

Whitney, Annie Weston, and Caroline Canfield Bullock. "Folk-Lore from Maryland." *Memoirs of the American Folklore Society* 18 (1925).

# Amulet

An object that is carried to avert illness or misfortune. In folk medicine it sometimes represents the vestiges of an earlier remedy. For instance, potatoes were carried in the pocket to ward off rheumatism in twentieth-century Norfolk (Hatfield 1994: 47); in the eighteenth century in Scotland the potato was used as an actual remedy for rheumatism. A necklace of horse chestnuts, made by a child who has never suffered from rheumatism, has been worn to prevent rheumatism (Mundford Primary School, Norfolk, unpub.), or an acorn has been carried (Hatfield 1994: 46). Rose hips were carried against piles (Hatfield 1994: 44). For toothache, carrying an amulet of a hazelnut with two kernels was recommended in Suffolk. A necklace of pieces of figwort (*Scrophularia* sp.) was worn by teething children in Essex (Hatfield MS). Nine pieces of elder cut from between two knots was used as an amulet against epilepsy (Black 1883: 120). Beads made from peony root were used in Sussex as an amulet against epilepsy and to help in teething (Thiselton Dyer 1889: 284).

In Cambridgeshire, carrying rabbit teeth or bones, or a hedgehog's skull, was practiced for toothache (Porter 1974: 46), while in Sussex, carrying a paw cut from a live mole was recommended (Black 1883: 161). Samuel Pepys reported in his diary for March 1665 the success of the hare's foot amulet he carried against cramp (Radford and Radford 1974: 183). Spiders were worn for ague (Black 1883: 59). In Sussex during the Great Plague, amulets of toad poison were carried (Souter 1995: 124). An alternative was to wear an arsenic-containing amulet around the neck (Miller 1933: 473). The stump of the umbilical cord was used in East Anglia as an amulet (Newman and Newman 1939: 185).

Colored threads served as amulets. For lumbago, red and white silk threads were recommended (Wright and Lovett 1908: 299, 302). An example from the 1960s of the use of the "cure of the threads" is cited by Beith (Beith 1995: 198). Black threads were used for treating sprains (Black 1883: 79).

Small stones credited with healing powers were handed down from one generation to another in Scotland. A stone was in some cases regarded as a specific cure for one ailment—for instance, the adder stones of the Scottish Highlands (Beith 1995: 152–155). A tooth-shaped stone might be valued as a cure for toothache (Guthrie 1945: Plate VI, opp. p. 13). In 1633 the countess of Newcastle was offered an aetites stone to wear to ease labor pains (Thomas 1973: 224). Birthstones have traditionally been given to a child according to its birth month to protect it against illness and other evil (Souter 1995: 37–38). A necklace of amber was

worn by a child to ward off croup, whooping cough, and asthma (Gardner 1942: 98). Stones with holes through them are widely regarded as "lucky" in general and as likely to avert misfortune; in this way they overlap with talismans. The concretions from goat intestine, known as bezoar, were prized until the late eighteenth century in official Western medicine as well as folk medicine. Eel-skin garters were regarded in Suffolk as a preventive and treatment for rheumatism (Porter 1974: 52); in Scotland, they were used as amulets against cramp (Black 1883: 161).

In North American folk medicine, to ward off illness in general, the wearing of a gold chain or a copper chain, a dime, or sow's teeth or owl's claws have all been recommended (Puckett 1981: 272). Other amulets worn to preserve health include a buckeye (chestnut, see entry) carried in a pocket (UCLA Folklore Archive 3_6345), an onion worn around the neck (UCLA Folklore Archives 8_6345), or a string of garlic (UCLA Folklore Archive 6_6345). An old lemon carried in the purse has also been suggested (UCLA Folklore Archive 7_6345). Asafoetida has been frequently used as an amulet, either to protect health in general (UCLA Folklore Archives 1_6344), or to help with a particular ailment. To bring on labor, a pregnant woman was advised to wear asafoetida around the neck and put rabbit's foot under the head when she slept (Brown 1952–1964 6: 7). Carrying a shell during labor was another recommendation (De Lys 1948: 92). Jasper has been worn as an amulet against drowning (UCLA Folklore Archives 14_7584). Copper amulets have been claimed to reduce blood pressure (UCLA Folklore Archives 17_5290). Teething children were given necklaces of the bean called Job's tears (*Coix lacryma-jobi*) (Meyer 1985: 248). Various amulets have been used against rheumatism. As in Britain, a potato carried in the pocket has been recommended (Wintemberg 1918: 137). In Newfoundland, a haddock fin has been used as a rheumatism amulet (English 1968: 443). In Lebanon County, the cents placed on the eyelids of the dead to keep them shut were subsequently used as amulets for rheumatism (Grumbine 1905–1906: 274–275). Amulets used for fevers include birch catkins (*Betula* sp.) (Brendle and Unger 1935: 83) and Solomon's seal (*Polygonatum* sp.) (UCLA Folklore Archive 11_6235).

In the Native American tradition, amulets made of bone and shell, or of maize, or of wood, were used by Shamans during healing ceremonies (Lyon 1996: 99, 175, 296). An ivory doll was held by Inuit women in labor (Micheletti 1998: 326). The Alasakan eskimo medicine man sometimes carried the soul of a sick child in an amulet for safekeeping (Frazer 1923: 679).

Examples of amulets still in use today are copper bracelets, worn against rheumatism, and hare's paws, made into costume jewelry, worn to protect against illness and evil.

*See also* **Amber, Caul, Elder, Epilepsy, Fevers, Plague, Rheumatism, Teething.**

### References

Beith, Mary. *Healing Threads: Traditional Medicines of the Highlands and Islands.* Edinburgh: Polygon, 1995.

Black, William George. *Folk-Medicine: A Chapter in the History of Culture.* London: Folklore Society, 1883.

Brendle, Thomas R., and Claude W. Unger. "Folk Medicine of the Pennsylvania Germans: The Non-Occult Cures." *Proceedings of the Pennsylvania German Society* 45, 1935.

Brown, Frank C. *Collection of North Carolina Folklore.* 7 vols. Durham, NC: Duke University Press, 1952–1964.

De Lys, Claudia. *A Treasury of American Superstitions.* New York: Philosophical Library, 1948.

English, L. E. F. *Historic Newfoundland.* St. John's: Newfoundland Tourist Development Division, 1968.

Frazer, Sir James George. *The Golden Bough: A Study in Magic and Religion.* London: Macmillan, 1923.

Gardner, Gerald Brosseau. "British Charms, Amulets and Talismans." *Folk-Lore* 53 (1942): 95–103.

Grumbine, E. "Folk-Lore and Superstitions Beliefs of Lebanon County." *Papers and Addresses of the Lebanon County Historical Society* 3 (1905–1906): 252–294.

Guthrie, Douglas. *A History of Medicine.* London: Thomas Nelson, 1945.

Hatfield, Gabrielle. *Country Remedies: Traditional East Anglian Plant Remedies in the Twentieth Century.* Woodbridge: Boydell, 1994.

Lyon, William S. *Encyclopedia of Native American Healing.* Denver and Oxford: ABC-CLIO, 1996.

Meyer, Clarence. *American Folk Medicine.* Glenwood, IL: Meyerbooks, 1985.

Micheletti, Enza (ed.). *North American Folk Healing: An A-Z Guide to Traditional Remedies.* New York and Montreal: Reader's Digest Association, 1998.

Miller, Joseph L. "The Healing Gods or Medical Superstitions." *West Virginia Medical Journal* 29 (1933): 465–478.

"Mundford Primary School Project," Norfolk, 1980, unpublished.

Newman, Barbara, and M. A. Newman. "Some Birth Customs in East Anglia." *Folklore* 50 (1939): 176–187.

Porter, Enid. *The Folklore of East Anglia.* London: Batsford, 1974.

Puckett, Newbell Niles. *Popular Beliefs and Superstitions: A Compendium of American Folklore from the Ohio Collection of Newbell Niles Puckett.* Edited by Wayland D. Hand, Anna Casetta, Sondra B. Thiederman. 3 vols. Boston: G. K. Hall, 1981.

Radford, E., and M. A. Radford, ed. "Christina Hole." *Encyclopaedia of Superstitions.* London: Book Club Associates, 1974.

Souter, Keith. Cure Craft. *Traditional Folk Remedies and Treatment from Antiquity to the Present Day.* Saffron Walden: C. W. Daniel, 1995.

Thiselton Dyer, T. F. *The Folk-Lore of Plants.* Facsimile reprint of 1889 edition by Llanerch, Dyfed, 1994.

Thomas, Keith. *Religion and the Decline of Magic: Studies in Popular Beliefs in Sixteenth- and Seventeenth-Century England.* Harmondsworth: Penguin, 1973.

Wintemberg, W. J. "Folk-Lore Collected in the Counties of Oxford and Waterloo, Ontario." *Journal of American Folklore* 31 (1918): 135–153.

Wright, A. R., and E. Lovett. "Specimens of Modern Mascots and Amulets of the British Isles." *Folk-Lore* 19 (1908): 288–302.

# Anemia

This was not always recognized as a distinct ailment but a number of remedies for blood disorders in general clearly involve anemia. Water from a so-called chalybeate well (rich in iron salts) was one such remedy. In Dumfriesshire, Scotland, for example, there is a well whose water was particularly recommended for "women's ailments" (Beith 1995: 132). In Ireland too, chalybeate waters were valued for anemia (Logan 1972: 142). Water from the forge, in which iron had been quenched was another folk remedy for anemia (Souter 1995: 132). One lady in Cambridgeshire made pills for anemia consisting of dust from the anvil and powdered dandelion root rolled in butter (Porter 1964: 9–11). Until fifty years ago, children suffering from what was then called pernicious anemia were given raw liver to eat (J.C., pers. com., 1960). This remedy can be traced back to the writings of Hippocrates (Raycroft 1940: 125–131). The most widely used plant remedy for anemia is nettle (Allen and Hatfield, in press), still recommended today by herbalists for its high iron content. Many of the tonics used in folk medicine were described as blood purifiers, and some of these too were probably useful in treating anemia. Into this category come burdock (*Arctium lappa*) and yarrow (*Achillea millefolium*). Dandelion tea (*Taraxacum officinale*), generally regarded as a tonic, was used in the East Anglian fens for anemia (Chamberlain 1981). Carrot has traditionally been recommended for anemia (Souter 1995: 132). In Sussex, beetroot was used to treat anemia (Brew, n.d.).

In North American folk medicine, some of the same remedies for anemia have been traced. Water out of a rusty can was recommended in New Mexico (Moya 1940: 74). Red beets were regarded in Pennsylvania as blood "makers" (Brendle and Unger 1935: 39) (compare with the remedy from Sussex, England, above). Dandelion leaf tea was used to treat anemia in West Virginia (Mason 1957: 29). Blackstrap molasses was held to be good for anemia (UCLA Folklore Archives 17_5461). A strange ritual of bleeding an anaemic child, diluting the blood with water, and giving it back as a drink, is reported by Brown (Brown 1952–1964, 6: 117).

In Native American practice, a large number of plants were used "for the blood" (Moerman 1998: 775–776). Some at least of these were targeted specifically at anemia. Dandelion tea, for example, was used widely (e.g. Herrick 1977: 478) for this purpose, as was sarsaparilla. Oregongrape *(Mahonia repens)* was taken to "enrich" (Hart 1992: 18) or "thicken" the blood (Nickerson 1966: 47).

*See also* **Burdock, Dandelion, Forge water, Sarsaparilla, Stinging nettle, Yarrow.**

### References

Allen, David E., and Gabrielle Hatfield. *Medicinal Plants in Folk Tradition: An Ethnobotany of Britain and Ireland.* Portland, OR: Timber Press, in press.

Beith, Mary. *Healing Threads Traditional Medicines of the Highlands and Islands.* Edinburgh: Polygon, 1995.

Brendle, Thomas R., and Claude W. Unger. "Folk Medicine of the Pennsylvania Germans: The Non-Occult Cures." *Proceedings of the Pennsylvania German Society* 45, 1935.

Brew, Barbara. *Grandmother's Remedies.* Privately published pamphlet, East Grinstead. Copy in Folklore Society archives, E30.

Brown, Frank C. *Collection of North Carolina Folklore.* 7 vols. Durham, NC: Duke University Press, 1952–1964.

Chamberlain, Mary. *Old Wives' Tales.* London: Virago, 1981.

Hart, Jeff. *Montana Native Plants and Early Peoples.* Helena: Montana Historical Society Press, 1992.

Herrick, James William. *Iroquois Medical Botany.* PhD thesis, State University of New York, Albany, 1977.

Logan, Patrick. *Making the Cure: A Look at Irish Folk Medicine.* Dublin: Talbot Press, 1972.

Mason, James. "Home Remedies in West Virginia." *West Virginia Folklore* 7 (1957): 27–32.

Moerman, Daniel E. *Native American Ethnobotany.* Portland, OR: Timber Press, 1998.

Moya, Benjamin S. *Superstitions and Beliefs among the Spanish-Speaking People of New Mexico.* Master's thesis, University of New Mexico, 1940.

Nickerson, Gifford S. "Some Data on Plains and Great Basin Indian Uses of Certain Native Plants." *Tebiwa* 9(1) (1966): 45–51.

Porter, Enid M. "Some Old Fenland Remedies." *Education Today* (July 1964).

Raycroft, Joseph E. "Old Wine in New Bottles." *Bulletin of the Medical Library Association* 28 (1940): 125–131.

Souter, Keith. *Cure Craft: Traditional Folk Remedies and Treatment from Antiquity to the Present Day.* Saffron Walden: C.W. Daniel. 1995.

# Apple

Folk medicine does not usually distinguish between different kinds of apple. Strictly speaking, only crab-apple (*Malus sylvestris*) is native to Britain; cultivated varieties of apple belong to a separate species *(Malus domestica)*. Emerson (1887: 15) reports the use in Suffolk of crab-apple juice for treating bruises. In general, though, the type of apple is not specified. In Britain raw apple has been rubbed on warts (Hatfield 1999: 148; Allen 1995: 179). In Lincolnshire the method was further refined: the

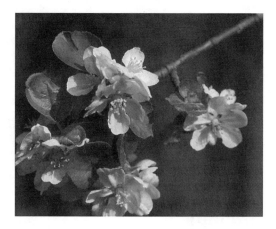

Apples have treated bruises, sprains, sores and warts. They have been found to regulate the bowels. Cider vinegar has many varied uses on both sides of the Atlantic. (Sarah Boait)

apple was cut into nine pieces and rubbed nine times over the warts (Black 1883: 42). Apple juice has been used to treat constipation (Mrs. B., Essex 1991). Rotten apples have been used to poultice sore eyes (Gunton Household Book), weak eyes (Black 1883: 201), and styes (Vickery 1995: 13), as well as chilblains (Vickery 1995: 13), boils (Gutch 1908: 69), or "any sore place" (Hatfield 1994: 52). Withering reported that apple juice, or "verjuice," was extensively used in England for treating sprains (Withering 1787–1792: 296). It was reported in Cambridgeshire that an apple was placed in the bedroom of a smallpox patient and that the disease then transferred to the apple (Vickery 1995: 13). Warts too have been "transferred" to an apple (Lafont 1984: 8).

In New England, the following remedy was reported in 1879 as a cure for an ague (fever): the patient should take a piece of yarn made of three colors and go by himself to an apple tree. Using his right hand, he should then tie his left hand loosely to the tree, then slip his hand out and run from the tree without looking back (Black 1883: 38). In the Appalachians, apple bark had a reputation for treating stomach ailments

(Crellin and Philpott 1990: 185). A "cure" for cancer has been recorded involving visiting an apple tree three mornings in succession and saying special words (Thomas and Thomas 1920: 98). A treatment for a drunkard is to eat an apple held by a dying man (Grumbine 1905–1906: 280).

Apple has been used in the treatment both of diarrhea and of constipation; it is claimed that apples regulate the bowels. In American folk medicine raw apple is recommended for diarrhea in older children and adults (Meyer 1985: 90). As in Britain, a rotten apple is recommended as treatment for sore eyes (Browne 1958: 61). This has also been a treatment for frostbite (cf. in Britain its use for chilblains, above) (UCLA Folklore Archives 5_6834). A poultice of rotten apples has been used to treat mumps (Parler 1962: 783). The same wart remedy using an apple reported from Britain figures in North American folk medicine too (Hyatt 1965: 291). Eating the core of a green apple has been recommended for arthritis (Puckett 1981: 309); an alternative has been the bark of the crabapple steeped in whisky (Meyer 1985: 212). An infusion prepared by pouring boiling water on apple slices has been drunk for asthma (UCLA Folklore Archives 5_5266).

Apple-cider vinegar has been regarded as a cure for a very wide variety of ailments. It has been used to staunch bleeding (Browne 1958: 500) and to treat the rash of poison ivy (UCLA Folklore Archive 4_5453). It has been made famous in particular by Jarvis, whose books on folk medicine in Vermont have run into numerous editions. Jarvis recommends apple-cider vinegar for diarrhea and vomiting, for kidney inflammation, as an aid to weight loss, to relieve lameness, and to treat poison ivy rash, shingles, night sweats, burns, varicose veins, impetigo and ringworm (Jarvis 1961). His books underline the old proverb that "An apple a day keeps the doctor away."

Various species of apple have been widely used in Native American medicine (Moerman 1998: 333–334). *Malus sylvestris* has been used for hoarseness (Taylor 1940: 29), earache, black eyes and bruises, and even for blindness (Herrick 1977: 350).

*See also* **Asthma, Bleeding, Boils, Cancer, Chilblains, Constipation, Eye problems, Poison ivy, Rheumatism, Smallpox, Transference, Warts.**

### References

Allen, Andrew. *A Dictionary of Sussex Folk Medicine.* Newbury: Countryside Books, 1995.

Black, William George. *Folk-Medicine: A Chapter in the History of Culture.* London: Folklore Society, 1883.

Browne, Ray B. *Popular Beliefs and Practices from Alabama.* Folklore Studies 9. Berkeley and Los Angeles: University of California Publications, 1958.

Crellin, John K., and Jane Philpott. *A Reference Guide to Medicinal Plants.* Durham, NC: Duke University Press, 1990.

Emerson, P. H. *Pictures of East Anglian Life.* London: Sampson Low, 1887.

Grumbine, E. "Folk-Lore and Superstitious Beliefs of Lebanon County." *Papers and Addresses of the Lebanon County Historical Society* 3 (1905–1906): 252–294.

Gunton Household Book. Seventeenth/eighteenth century manuscript in Church of St. Peter Mancroft, Norwich.

Gutch (Eliza), and Mabel Peacock. *County Folklore.* Vol. 5, *Lincolnshire.* London: Folk-lore Society, 1908.

Hatfield, Gabrielle. *Country Remedies: Traditional East Anglian Plant Remedies in the Twentieth Century.* Woodbridge: Boydell, 1994.

Hatfield, Gabrielle. *Memory, Wisdom, and Healing: The History of Domestic Plant Medicine.* Phoenix Mill: Sutton, 1999.

Herrick, James William. *Iroquois Medical Botany.* PhD thesis. Albany: State University of New York, 1977.

Hyatt, Harry Middleton. *Folklore from Adams County Illinois.* 2nd rev. ed. Memoirs of the Alma Egan Hyatt Foundation, 1965.

Jarvis, D. C. *Folk Medicine.* London: Pan Books, 1961.

Lafont, Anne-Marie. *A Herbal Folklore.* Bideford: Badger Books, 1984.

Meyer, Clarence. *American Folk Medicine.* Glenwood, IL: Meyerbooks, 1985.

Moerman, Daniel E. *Native American Ethnobotany.* Portland, OR: Timber Press, 1998.

Parler, Mary Celestia, and University Student Contributors. *Folk Beliefs from Arkansas.* 15 vols. Fayetteville: University of Arkansas, 1962.

Puckett, Newbell Niles. *Popular Beliefs and Superstitions: A Compendium of American Folklore from the Ohio Collection of Newbell Niles Puckett.* Edited by Wayland D. Hand, Anna Casetta, and Sondra B. Thiederman. 3 vols. Boston: G. K. Hall, 1981.

Taylor, Linda Averill. *Plants Used as Curatives by Certain Southeastern Tribes.* Cambridge, MA: Botanical Museum of Harvard University, 1940.

Thomas, Daniel Lindsay, and Lucy Blayney Thomas. *Kentucky Superstitions.* Princeton, NJ: Princeton University Press, 1920.

Vickery, Roy. *A Dictionary of Plant Lore.* Oxford: Oxford University Press, 1995.

Withering, William. *A Botanical Arrangement of British Plants.* 2nd ed. 3 vols. Birmingham: M. Swinney, 1787–1792.

# Arthritis

*See* **Rheumatism and arthritis.**

# Ash (*Fraxinus spp.*)

The British native species of ash, *Fraxinus excelsior* has had numerous uses in folk medicine and folklore. In the Scottish Highlands, ash sap was traditionally given to a newborn baby as its first nourishment (Beith 1995: 203)—a practice that it has been suggested, could originate in Persia, where the sweet sap of the so-called manna ash *(Fraxinus ornus)* was dried and eaten for its food value and its action as a gentle laxative. Ash sap has been used to treat earache in Ireland, and also in England right up to the present day (Hatfield MS). This remedy can be traced back to Saxon Britain (Black

1883: 197). In the Scottish Highlands, burned ash bark was used as a treatment for toothache (Beith 1995: 203). Other folk medicinal uses for the native British ash include a poultice of the leaves to treat snake bites (Beith 1995: 203). Both Pliny and Gerard claimed that there was such a strong antipathy between the ash and the snake that a snake would pass through fire to avoid the tree (Black 1883: 196). A Somerset proverb recorded in 1912 reflects this belief (Tongue 1965: 35). In West Somerset, there was a custom of hanging a wreath of flowers on an ash tree near a farm to protect the animals and people against snake bites (Tongue 1965: 28). Smoke from burning ash was used to treat ringworm (Vickery 1995: 20).

Folk uses of the ash involve some clear examples of the transference of disease. One custom, made famous by Gilbert White in the eighteenth century (White 1789–1822, 1: 344), was to make a so-called shrew-ash, by imprisoning a live shrew in a hole bored in an ash tree. This tree then maintained its medicinal virtue for its lifetime. Such trees were used as "cures" for a variety of ailments, including whooping cough (Vickery 1995: 19) and paralysis (Grieve 1931: 67). Warts were "transferred" to ash trees in a variety of ways. In one method, a pin was stuck in each wart and afterward in the ash tree, where it was left (Grieve 1931: 67). Hernia in children was thought to be curable by splitting open a growing ash sapling and passing the child through the opening. The tree was then bound up, and as it healed, so would the child. This custom has been recorded in use in Sussex as recently as the 1920s (Allen 1995: 162).

In North American folk medicine, as in British and Irish, ash sap was used to treat earache. Another use for the ash was as an aid to weight reduction; for this purpose, the dried leaves were used as a tea (Meyer 1985: 101, 265). A preparation of ash bark tea was used in the treatment of snake bite, again reflecting the claim of an antipathy between snakes and ash. There is an echo of the British folk remedy for hernia in a report from Burlington County, New Jersey, of children being treated for ruptures by being passed through a split in a tree, but the type of tree is not specified (Black 1883: 68). A child could be passed through a split holly, oak, or ash, for the cure of hernia (Puckett 1981: 396). Other uses of ash in North American folk medicine include wound treatment (Brendle and Unger 1935: 75). *Fraxinus americana* was also used as an emmenagogue (UCLA Folklore Archives 1_5605).

In Native American medicine there were numerous uses for various species of ash (Moerman 1998: 238–239). Ash sap was widely used to treat earache, and the method of obtaining the sap is identical to that described for Scotland (Black 1980: 218). White ash *(Fraxinus americana)* was used to provoke menstruation and as an abortifacient by the Abnaki (Rousseau 1947: 154, 172). Both roots and flowers of this species have been used in snake bite treatment (Moerman 1998: 238). Black ash *(Fraxinus nigra)* has been used as a tonic and an antirheumatic (Moerman 1998: 239).

*See also* **Earache, Ringworm, Snake bite, Toothache, Transference, Whooping cough.**

### References

Allen, Andrew. *A Dictionary of Sussex Folk Medicine.* Newbury: Countryside Books, 1995.

Beith, Mary. *Healing Threads: Traditional Medicines of the Highlands and Islands.* Edinburgh: Polygon, 1995.

Black, Meredith Jean. *Algonquin Ethnobotany: An Interpretation of Aboriginal Adaptation in South Western Quebec.* Mercury Series 65. Ottawa: National Museums of Canada, 1980.

Black, William George. *Folk-Medicine: A Chapter in the History of Culture.* London: Folklore Society, 1883.

Brendle, Thomas R., and Claude W. Unger. "Folk Medicine of the Pennsylvania Germans: The Non-Occult Cures." *Proceedings of the Pennsylvania German Society* 45 (1935).

Grieve, Mrs. M. *A Modern Herbal.* Edited by Mrs. C. F. Leyel. London: Jonathan Cape, 1931.

Meyer, Clarence. *American Folk Medicine.* Glenwood, IL: Meyerbooks, 1985.

Moerman, Daniel E. *Native American Ethnobotany.* Portland, OR: Timber Press, 1998.

Puckett, Newbell Niles. *Popular Beliefs and Superstitions: A Compendium of American Folklore from the Ohio Collection of Newbell Niles Puckett.* Edited by Wayland D. Hand, Anna Casetta, and Sondra B. Thiederman. 3 vols. Boston: G. K. Hall, 1981.

Rousseau, Jacques. "Ethnobotanique Abénakise." *Archives de Folklore* 11 (1947): 145–182.

Tongue, Ruth L. *Somerset Folklore.* Edited Katharine Briggs. County Folklore 8. London: Folklore Society, 1965.

Vickery, Roy. *A Dictionary of Plant Lore.* Oxford: Oxford University Press, 1995.

White, G. *The Natural History of Selbourne.* London, 1822. (First edition 1789).

## Asthma

In acute phases this can be life threatening, and as one would expect, folk medicine has over the centuries developed a large and miscellaneous range of remedies. One plant remedy stands out in recent times as being used in folk medicine on both sides of the Atlantic. This is the thornapple *(Datura stramonium),* also known in North America as Jamestown weed or Jimson Weed. In Britain, the dried leaves were smoked as a treatment for asthma (e.g., by the fishermen of the North Norfolk coast; T.E., pers. com., 1988). The plant is not native to Britain but turns up as a weed of recently disturbed land. Clearly the remedy was imported from North America, but it is unusual in that it was adopted not only by medical herbalists but by the folk tradition as well. Going back farther in time it becomes increasingly difficult to separate asthma remedies from those of bronchitis;

in folk medicine the two complaints seem to have been linked together. For example, coltsfoot *(Tussilago farfara)* was recommended by Pliny for the treatment of bronchitis and has continued in herbal and in folk medicine to be used for coughs ever since. This use has extended to asthma in the Scottish Highlands (Beith 1995: 212) and in England (Prince 1991: 11). In the English early twentieth-century use of honeysuckle for treating asthma (Miss N., Hampshire, pers. com., 1990) we have an early example of the now-popular complementary medicine of aromatherapy (Miss N., Hampshire, pers. com., 1980). A romantic-sounding remedy was recorded in the 1950s by Beith from Inverness-shire in Scotland. The sufferer had to row alone across a lake and back before sunrise (Beith 1995: 135). Also in the Scottish Highlands, dogfish oil was given to asthma sufferers (Beith 1995: 174). In some parts of Scotland, the skin of a hare, placed over the chest during sleep, was apparently used to ward off asthma attacks (Souter 1995: 136). Bogbean *(Menyanthes trifoliata)* was recommended in the Isle of Lewis (Beith 1995: 207). An infusion of bramble root *(Rubus fruticosus)* and pennyroyal *(Mentha pulegium),* wine made from elder berries *(Sambucus nigra),* snuff made from the dried leaves of ground ivy *(Glechoma hederacea),* an infusion of horehound *(Marrubium vulgare)* and a decoction of the roots and bark of the sloe *(Prunus spinosa)* have all been used in the Scottish Highlands for treating asthma (Beith 1995: 215, 221, 223, 232, 242). The story of a lifesaving poultice made from hot, cooked potatoes was told by a lady now in her nineties who has lived all her life in Norfolk, England (Hatfield 1994: 75).

In North American folk medicine the remedies used for asthma reflect those in Britain. The Inverness-shire method to relax the patient is echoed in a remedy from Rochester: the patient is advised to walk alone three times round the house at midnight when the moon is waning (Black 1883: 125). There are records for the use of oil from a goose and of the fat from a chicken, reminiscent of the Scottish use of dogfish oil, while the skin of a muskrat worn against the lungs echoes the British use of hareskin (Meyer 1985: 31). Among a large collection (almost eighty) of different asthma remedies in the UCLA Folk Medicine Archive there are several bizarre ones, such as a stew containing badger and jackdaw (Bourke 1894: 120). Miscellaneous remedies include drinking goat's milk (UCLA Folklore Archives 6_5263), swallowing a teaspoonful of sea sand (UCLA Folklore Archives 24_6175), or eating bees' honey and sulphur (Welsch 1966: 360).

A good example of transference comes from the African American tradition. Three nights in succession, the patient must find a frog by moonlight and spit into its throat (UCLA Folklore Archives 24_6176). Another transference remedy is to sleep with a chihuahua (UCLA Folklore Archives 1_6828). Some of the remedies are clearly related to the observation, or the hope, that children often "grow out of" asthma. Some of the child's hair is cut off and placed into a hole in a tree bored above the child's head. When he or she grows above the hole, the asthma will be cured (see e.g. Puckett 1981: 312). Ash, birch, willow, sugar maple, and hickory all feature in versions of this remedy. Amulets worn to prevent or to cure asthma include amber beads (Brown 1952_1964, 6: 119).

Among plant remedies used, the smoking of jimson weed has already been mentioned (UCLA Folklore Archives 1–5263). Other plants native to North America but not to Britain used in asthma treatment include Aloe vera, bloodroot, skunk cabbage *(Symplocarpus foetidus)* and licorice *(Glycyrrhiza glabra),* as well as so-called asthma weed *(Lobelia inflata)* (Meyer 1985: 32–35). This plant became celebrated for its fame in treating a wide range of conditions, after it was promoted by Samuel Thomson. However, long before that it was known to and used by the Native Americans (Grieve 1931: 495). Cottonseed water was a remedy from the African tradition (UCLA Folklore Archives 21_5263). Boiled chestnut leaves (*Castanea* sp.) have also been used (Browne 1958: 32).

Plants common to both Britain and North America that were used in American folk remedies for asthma include daisy (*Bellis perennis*), elecampane (*Inula helenium*), wild plum *(Prunus spinosa),* elder *(Sambucus nigra),* mullein (*Verbascum thapsus*), wild cherry (*Prunus* sp.), and horehound *(Marrubium vulgare)* (Meyer 1985: 31–35).

In the Native American tradition, willow bark *(Salix lucida)* was smoked for asthma (Speck 1917: 309). Among the Kwakiutl a recommendation for asthma was to eat part of the heart of a wolf (Boas 1932: 184).

*See also* **African tradition; Aloe vera; Amber; Amulet; Ash; Asthma; Birch; Bloodroot; Honey; Lobelia; Native American tradition; Thomson, Samuel; Transference; Willow.**

## References

Beith, Mary. *Healing Threads: Traditional Medicines of the Highlands and Islands.* Edinburgh: Polygon,1995.

Black, William George. *Folk-Medicine: A Chapter in the History of Culture.* London: Folklore Society, 1883.

Boas, Franz. "Current Beliefs of the Kwakiutl Indians." *Journal of American Folklore* 45 (1932): 177–260.

Bourke, John G. "Popular Medicine, Customs, and Superstitions of the Rio Grande." *Journal of American Folklore* 7 (1894): 119–146.

Brown, Frank C. *Collection of North Carolina Folklore.* 7 vols. Durham, NC: Duke University Press, 1952–1964.

Browne, Ray B. *Popular Beliefs and Practices from Alabama.* Folklore Studies 9. Berkeley and Los Angeles: University of California Publications, 1958.

Grieve, Mrs. M. *A Modern Herbal.* Edited by Mrs. C. F. Leyel. London: Jonathan Cape, 1931.

Hatfield, Gabrielle. *Country Remedies: Traditional East Anglian Plant Remedies in the Twentieth Century.* Woodbridge: Boydell, 1994.

Meyer, Clarence. *American Folk Medicine.* Glenwood, IL: Meyerbooks, 1985.

Prince, Dennis. *Grandmother's Cures: An A-Z of Herbal Remedies.* London: Fontana, 1991.

Puckett, Newbell Niles. "Popular Beliefs and Superstitions." *A Compendium of American Folklore from the Ohio Collection of Newbell Niles Puckett.* Edited by Wayland D. Hand, Anna Casetta, and Sondra B. Thiederman. 3 vols. Boston: G. K. Hall, 1981.

Souter, Keith. *Cure Craft: Traditional Folk Remedies and Treatment from Antiquity to the Present Day.* Saffron Walden: C. W. Daniel, 1995.

Speck, Frank G. "Medicine Practices of the Northeastern Algonquians." *Proceedings of the 19th International Congress of Americanists* (1917): 303–321.

Welsch, Roger L. *A Treasury of Nebraska Pioneer Folklore.* Lincoln: University of Nebraska Press, 1966.

# B

## Backache

Still one of the commonest causes of lost working days, backache has attracted a wide variety of folk remedies. For the lower-back pain often known as lumbago, ironing with a flat iron was a traditional if drastic treatment used in East Anglia until very recent times; the patient lay down, his back was covered with red flannel, and he was ironed! (D.T., Norfolk, pers. com., 1980). The comfort provided by heat is exploited in the use of various "rubs" that increase the local blood circulation and give rise to a feeling of warmth. Horse oils were often used by farm laborers in East Anglia before the advent of the National Health Service. These had a very wide variety of constituents but often contained turpentine. On St. Kilda the fat of black-throated divers was used to relieve sciatica (Beith 1995: 165). In Sussex, England, there was a belief that a person suffering from lumbago could be relieved by rolling on the ground when he heard the first cuckoo of the spring (Allen 1995: 42).

Another approach was to seek a cure from a local healer with a reputation for curing bad backs and other skeletal problems. The treatment sometimes involved the healer walking along the patient's spine. When the healer was a large man, as in the case of Neil in the Inner Hebrides, this must have been a heroic procedure! (Beith 1995: 168). Reputedly in the northeast of Scotland it was believed that a child born feet first had the power of healing lumbago, rheumatism, and sprains; the usual procedure again was to walk on the part afflicted. In Cornwall, this special power extended to the mother of a child born feet first (Black 1883: 137).

An intriguing cure for severe backache was related by a retired carpenter from Essex. His pain was so bad it made work almost impossible, and a painter working with him on a building site one day told him about "the potato cure." He was to lie in a warm bath and then rub the sorest part of his back with the newly cut surface of a raw potato. The other half of the potato was to be carried in his trouser pocket at all times. The man was cured of his pain and always carried the dried-up potato (A.G. S., Age Concern Essays, 1991). In the Highlands of Scotland potatoes carried in a pocket had a reputation for preventing rheumatism (Beith 1995: 235).

Other plants used in folk medicine for the treatment of back pain and sciatica include ground elder (*Aegopodium podagraria*), which was crushed and made into a poultice to treat sciatica in the Scottish Highlands (Beith 1995: 215). Plantain, used in healing at least since Anglo-Saxon times, was an East Anglian remedy for lumbago (Rider Haggard (ed.), 1974: 16). Oil of juniper (from *Juniperus* sp.) was used to

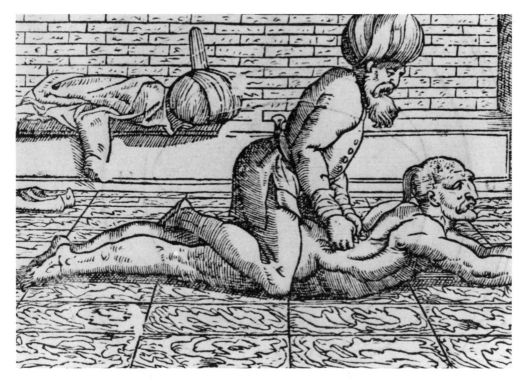

A treatment approach for backache was to seek a cure from a local healer with a reputation for curing bad backs. The treatment sometimes involved the healer walking along the patient's spine. (National Library of Medicine)

treat low back pain in humans and in animals (I. N. Norfolk, pers. com., 1980).

In North American folk medicine, a similar array of remedies for back pain exists. There is even an American counterpart for the Sussex remedy mentioned above. The sufferer is instructed to lie down and roll over three times when he hears the whippoorwill call! (Brown 1952–1964, 6: 120). Red flannel features, as in Britain, in backache cures. In one, a piece of red flannel with a hole in it is positioned so that the hole is on the small of the back. The evil spirit passes out through the hole (UCLA Folklore Archives 15_5273). Trampling on a sore back was also practiced in North America (Cannon 1984: 92). Other miscellaneous folk remedies for backache include wearing a snakeskin belt (Parler 1962, 3: 443a). Carrying a chestnut (buckeye) in the pocket was said to help backache

(Brown 1952–1964, 66: 121). Turpentine features in backache cures in North America as well as Britain. In New Mexico, it was combined in a poultice with rosemary *(Rosmarinus officinalis)* (Moya 1940: 47).

Various plants native to North America but not to Britain have been used to treat backache and sciatica. They include bugleweed *(Lycopus virginicus),* black cohosh, and bull thistle *(Carduus lanceolatus)* (Meyer 1985: 220). In addition, wintergreen, also known as checkerberry *(Gaultheria procumbens),* has been widely used, both by Native Americans and later by European settlers. Oil of wintergreen was adopted for use in domestic medicine both in North America and in Britain, and it still forms a constituent of some "rubs" for painful joints and backs. Other plants used by Native Americans in the treatment of backache include pipsissewa, confusingly also called wintergreen *(Chimaphila unbellata),* mannagrass *(Glyceria obtusa),* and horsemint *(Monarda punctata)* (Speck 1944: 41, 45).

*See also* **Amulet, Black cohosh, Plantain, Rheumatism, Snake.**

### References

Age Concern Essays. Held in Suffolk Record Office, England, 1991.

Allen, Andrew. *A Dictionary of Sussex Folk Medicine.* Newbury: Countryside Books, 1995.

Beith, Mary. *Healing Threads: Traditional Medicines of the Highlands and Islands.* Edinburgh: Polygon, 1995.

Black, William George. *Folk-Medicine: A Chapter in the History of Culture.* London: Folklore Society, 1883.

Brown, Frank C. *Collection of North Carolina Folklore.* 7 vols. Durham, NC: Duke University Press, 1952–1964.

Cannon, Anthon S. *Popular Beliefs and Superstitions from Utah.* Edited by Wayland D. Hand and Jeannine E. Talley. Salt Lake City: University of Utah Press, 1984.

Meyer, Clarence. *American Folk Medicine.* Glenwood, IL: Meyerbooks, 1985.

Moya, Benjamin S. *Superstitions and Beliefs among the Spanish-Speaking People of New Mexico.* Master's thesis, University of New Mexico, 1940.

Parler, Mary Celestia, and University Student Contributors. *Folk Beliefs from Arkansas.* 15 vols. Fayetteville: University of Arkansas, 1962.

Rider Haggard, Lilias (ed.). *I Walked by Night.* Woodbridge: Boydell Press, 1974.

Speck, Frank G. "Catawba Herbals and Curative Practices." *Journal of American Folklore* 57 (1944): 37–50.

# Bad breath

This must have been a common problem when teeth decayed and no dental treatment was available. One simple British folk remedy was to drink and gargle with a solution of salt (Prince 1991: 15). This remedy also appears in a book of North American household remedies first published in 1895 (Wilkes 1895: 94). Baking soda was used similarly (Micheletti 1998: 43). In both Britain and North America, a variety of cultivated plants were and are traditionally chewed to sweeten breath, including parsley *(Petroselinum crispum)* and cinnamon *(Cinnamomum verum)* (Souter 1995: 164). To remove the smell of garlic on the breath, chewing parsley is particularly recommended. Chewing spice from the spice wood tree (? *Styrax* sp.) is another suggestion (UCLA Folklore Archives 14_5299). Other plants used to sweeten the breath include peppermint *(Mentha piperita),* wintergreen *(Gaultheria procumbens),* myrrh *(Commiphora myrrha),* and fennel *(Foeniculum vulgare).* Both chamomile and raspberry *(Rubus idaeus)* tea were used in North American folk medicine. Chewing cloves (buds of *Syzygium aromaticum*), cardamom seeds *(Elettaria cardamomum),* or a cubeb *(Piper cubeba)* was also recommended (Meyer 1985: 177). The Cherokee Indians used a mouthwash made from foamflower *(Tiarella cordifolia)* to clean a coated tongue (Micheletti 1998: 42).

*See also* **Chamomile.**

### References

Meyer, Clarence. *American Folk Medicine.* Glenwood, IL: Meyerbooks, 1985.

Micheletti, Enza (ed.). *North American Folk Healing: An A-Z Guide to Traditional Remedies.* New York and Montreal: Reader's Digest Association, 1998.

Prince, Dennis. *Grandmother's Cures: An A-Z of Herbal Remedies.* London: Fontana, 1991.

Souter, Keith. *Cure Craft: Traditional Folk Remedies and Treatment from Antiquity to the Present Day.* Saffron Walden: C. W. Daniel, 1995.

*Wilkes' Priceless Recipes.* Compiled by Dr. N. T. Oliver. Stockton, Rugby: G. & F. Wilkes. Entered in Library of Congress, Washington, DC, 1895.

# Baldness

At a time when the human genome is being unraveled for the first time and the hunt for the gene controlling baldness is now possible, it is interesting to see the variety of weird and sometimes revolting home remedies tried for treating baldness. In Roman times, the ashes from the burned genitals of an ass were mixed with one's own urine and rubbed onto the scalp to prevent baldness (Souter 1995: 164). Rubbing on the dung of various animals was recommended not only in folk medicine but also in the official pharmacopoeia at least until the eighteenth century. As well as recommending hedgehog fat mixed with bear's grease as a baldness remedy, the physician William Salmon also lists a great variety of other animal products, including mouse dung and hedgehog dung, for the treatment of baldness (Salmon 1693: 356). In Sussex folk medicine, the hindquarters of hedgehogs were cooked and mixed with the inner fat of the pig to produce an ointment for baldness (Allen 1995: 81). Well-rotted mice were recommended by a healer in the Highlands of Scotland, but as Beith (1985) points out, one wonders how far such remedies were given tongue in cheek (Dewar MS, quoted in Beith 1995: 65). Bat's blood was recommended for treating baldness in both England and North Carolina (McCracken 1992: 14). Onion rubbed on the head was considered a cure for baldness in both England and Ireland (Vickery 1995: 267). Rosemary, nettle, and hedgehog fat were made into an ointment to rub into the scalp to stimulate hair growth (Souter 1995: 164). A "miracle ageing brew" recorded in the twentieth century from Shropshire claimed to restore hair. It was composed of nettle, dandelion flowers, and roots, red clover, sugar, honey, and lemon, fermented overnight with yeast (Prince 1991: 10). Drinking a decoction of burdock root was also claimed to be effective (Prince 1991: 31). More bizarrely, "gas-water" (the water through which coal gas is passed during purification) was rubbed into the scalp as a hair restorer (Prince 1991: 31).

In Native American practice, various species of Yucca have been used to produce a hair tonic to treat baldness (Kavasch and Baar 1999: 100). A recent compilation of folk remedies from North America includes the use of Aloe vera juice, onion juice, olive oil, lemon juice, burdock "oil," or vinegar to treat baldness. Eating kelp and horseradish is also recommended. Less pleasantly, a poultice on the scalp of chicken dung or cow manure is suggested (Trent 2000: 45, 46). Among a collection of "Old Settlers' Remedies" from Nova Scotia, there is one for increasing hair growth. It consists of hartshorn shavings mixed with oil (Robertson 1960: 6). Rubbing the scalp with the cut surface of an onion is recorded (UCLA Folklore Archives 13_5650). Bear's grease rubbed on the head is recorded from Alabama (Puckett 1981: 315) and rattlesnake oil from the central Midwest (UCLA Folklore Archives13_5277). Drinking very dark tea is said to prevent baldness, a remedy recorded from California but apparently originating in England (UCLA Folklore Archives 24_5579). A Mexican Native American remedy for baldness was to use greasewood root as a hair rinse. This plant, *Sarcobatus vermiculatus,* is a native of western North America and known mainly for its hard wood used as fuel and in tool making (Moerman 1998: 518).

*See also* **Hair problems.**

### References

Allen, Andrew. *A Dictionary of Sussex Folk Medicine.* Newbury: Countryside Books, 1995.

Beith, Mary. *Healing Threads: Traditional Medicines of the Highlands and Islands.* Edinburgh: Polygon, 1995.

Kavasch, E. Barrie, and Karen Baar. *American In-*

*dian Healing Arts.* New York: Bantam
Books, 1999.

McCracken, Gary. "Bats in Magic, Potions and
Medicinal Preparations." *Bats* 10(3) (1992).

Moerman, Daniel E. *Native American Ethnobotany.* Portland, OR: Timber Press. 1998.

Prince, Dennis. *Grandmother's Cures: An A-Z of
Herbal Remedies.* London: Fontana, 1991.

Puckett, Newbell Niles. *Popular Beliefs and Super-
stitions: A Compendium of American Folklore
from the Ohio Collection of Newbell Niles
Puckett.* Edited by Wayland D. Hand, Anna
Casetta, and Sondra B. Thiederman. 3 vols.
Boston: G. K. Hall, 1981.

Robertson, Marion. *Early Settlers' Remedies.* Barrington, NS: Cape Sable Historical Society,
1960.

Salmon, William. *The Compleat English Physician.*
London: 1693.

Souter, Keith. *Cure Craft: Traditional Folk Remedies and Treatment from Antiquity to the
Present Day.* Saffron Walden: C. W. Daniel,
1995.

Trent, Wendell Campbell. *Colossus of Folk Medicine: An Encyclopedia.* First Books Library,
2000.

Vickery, Roy. *A Dictionary of Plant Lore.* Oxford:
Oxford University Press, 1995.

# Balm of Gilead (*Populus balsamifera*)

This tree is native to North America, but not to Britain. The sticky resin from its buds has formed the basis for many home remedies. It was named after the balm of Gilead mentioned in the Bible, although that reference is to quite a different plant. It has been used in official medicine and herbalism in Britain (Chevallier 1996: 252) but not in traditional folk medicine there. It has, however, played a significant role in North American folk medicine. The sticky resin has been used as a basis for cough syrups (Meyer 1985: 82) and for treating colds (Browne 1958: 87) and earache (Dykeman 1955: 253). It was an ingredient of a tonic taken for "female weakness" (Meyer 1985:

124). It was used for a large range of skin conditions. Mixed with sheep's tallow and beeswax, it has formed an ointment for treating chapped hands (Meyer 1985: 225). Eczema has been treated with an ointment prepared from balm of Gilead and lard (UCLA Folklore Archives 17_5368). The resin has been used to treat burns (Clark 1970: 14), wrinkles (Oklahoma Folklore: 57), and boils (Ansell 1959: 9). Steeped in alcohol, the buds have provided a tincture for treating sores and ulcers (Meyer 1985: 229). It was an ingredient of a tonic for a weak stomach (Meyer 1985: 242) and has been used to treat piles (Brown 1952–1964: 249). The bark of the tree reputedly cures leprosy (Hatcher 1955: 150–155).

Along with other species of poplar, its uses in Native American practice have been very numerous and diverse (Moerman 1998: 427–429). The resinous buds have provided a cough medicine (Smith 1929: 54), a salve for wounds, sores (Black 1980: 148) and eczema (Smith 1933: 80), and a wash for sore eyes (Gunther 1973: 26) or sore throat (Train, Henrichs and Archer 1941: 210). These uses may have been passed on from Native Americans to the settlers. The bark of the balsam poplar and its root are also widely used in Native American practice, for uses ranging from rheumatism (Reagan 1928: 231), excessive bleeding during childbirth (Densmore 1928: 358), tuberculosis (Train, Henrichs and Archer 1941: 121), and worms (Herrick 1977: 291) to broken bones (Turner et al. 1990: 276).

*See also* **Colds, Coughs, Earache, Fractures, Piles, Rheumatism, Tuberculosis, Worms.**

## References
Ansell, Henry B. "Recollections of a Knotts Island
Boyhood." *North Carolina Folklore* 7(1)
(1959): 1–13.

Black, Meredith Jean. *Algonquin Ethnobotany: An
Interpretation of Aboriginal Adaptation in*

*South Western Quebec.* Mercury Series 65. Ottawa: National Museums of Canada, 1980.

Brown, Frank C. *Collection of North Carolina Folklore.* 7 vols. Durham, NC: Duke University Press, 1952–1964.

Browne, Ray B. *Popular Beliefs and Practices from Alabama.* Folklore Studies 9. Berkeley and Los Angeles: University of California Publications, 1958.

Chevallier, Andrew. *The Encyclopedia of Medicinal Plants.* London: Dorling Kindersley, 1996.

Clark, Joseph D. "North Carolina Popular Beliefs and Superstitions." *North Carolina Folklore* 18 (1970): 1–66.

Densmore, Frances. "Uses of Plants by the Chippewa Indians." *Smithsonian Institution-Bureau of American Ethnology Annual Report* 44 (1928): 273–379.

Dykeman, Wilma. *The French Broad (Rivers of America).* New York: Rinehart, 1955.

Gunther, Erna. *Ethnobotany of Western Washington.* Rev. ed. Seattle: University of Washington Press, 1973.

Hatcher, Mildred. "Superstitions in Middle Tennessee." *Southern Folklore Quarterly* 19 (1955): 150–155.

Herrick, James William. *Iroquois Medical Botany.* Ph.D. thesis, State University of New York, Albany, 1977.

Meyer, Clarence. *American Folk Medicine.* Glenwood, IL: Meyerbooks, 1985.

Moerman, Daniel E. *Native American Ethnobotany.* Portland, OR: Timber Press, 1998.

*Oklahoma Folklore.* Oklahoma Writers Project. UCLA Folklore Archives 21_3939.

Reagan, Albert B. "Plants Used by the Bois Fort Chippewa (Ojibwa) Indians of Minnesota." *Wisconsin Archaeologist* 7(4) (1928): 230–248.

Smith, Harlan I. "Materia Medica of the Bella Coola and Neighboring Tribes of British Columbia." *National Museum of Canada Bulletin* 56 (1929): 47–68.

Smith, Huron H. "Ethnobotany of the Forest Potawatomi Indians." *Bulletin of the Public Museum of the City of Milwaukee* 7 (1933): 1–230.

Train, Percy, James R. Henrichs, and W. Andrew Archer. *Medicinal Uses of Plants by Indian Tribes of Nevada.* Washington, DC: U.S. Department of Agriculture, 1941.

Turner, Nancy J., Laurence C. Thompson, M. Terry Thompson, and Annie Z. York. *Thompson Ethnobotany: Knowledge and Usage of Plants by the Thompson Indians of British Columbia.* Victoria: Royal British Columbia Museum, 1990.

# Bartram, John (1699–1777)

Descended from an English grandfather who went from Derbyshire to America in 1682, John Bartram received little formal education but became a very successful farmer. He bought a 102-acre plot of land near Philadelphia, and alongside conventional crops he grew numerous medicinal plants from both the Old World and the New. He corresponded with various plant collectors in Britain and at one stage of his life was supplying more than fifty individuals with plants. At a time when little information was available to European settlers about the medicinal uses of Native American plants, he provided some of the earliest printed information on the subject, publishing in 1751 an essay entitled *Description, virtues and uses of sundry plants of these northern parts of America, and particularly of the newly discovered Indian cure for the venereal disease.* In the same year, after a trip to Onondaga, he wrote *Observations on the inhabitants, Climate, soil, rivers, productions worthy of notice, made by John Bartram in his travels from Pennsylvania to Onadaga, Oswego and the Lake Ontario in Canada* (London: J. Whiston and B. White, 1751). Apart from the importance of the information he printed, during his lifetime he was highly respected and liked, and was able to assist others as a result of his knowledge of medicinal plants. Though he was self-taught as a botanist, the importance of his work was recognized by induction as one of the original members of the American Philosophical Society. He was appointed botanist to King George III, for which service he received an annual income of fifty pounds. His contribution both to knowledge of folk medicine during his lifetime and to subsequent botanical studies earned him the title of "father of American botany."

### Reference

Earnest, E. *John and William Bartram.* Philadelphia: University of Pennsylvania Press, 1940.

# Beans

The broad bean *(Vicia faba)* is not a native of Britain but has been grown in cultivation as a vegetable since the Iron Age (Harrison, Masefield and Wallis 1985: 40). In folk medicine in Britain its principal use has been in the treatment of warts. The wart is rubbed with the fluffy inside of the broad bean pod. This remedy is widespread throughout Britain and persisted well into the twentieth century (Hatfield 1999: 148; Vickery 1995: 50; Allen 1995: 176). In Devon, the same remedy is applied to chapped lips and to nettle stings (Lafont 1984: 13). Another folk use is for whooping cough; in Suffolk, a child suffering from this disorder was carried through a field of beans in flower, where inhaling the scent was thought to be helpful (Taylor MSS). A poultice of bean flowers was used in Ireland to reduce hard swellings (Radford and Radford 1961: 36). In some areas of Britain the scent of the broad bean flower was said to be powerfully aphrodisiac (Vickery 1995: 49–50). Worldwide, there is a general association between beans of various kinds and lust and fertility (Souter 1995: 106). In Vedic India, urd beans were associated particularly with conception of male offspring (Simoons 1999: 173).

Beans of various kinds were carried as amulets. Horse beans were used in this way in Lincolnshire within living memory (Taylor MSS), where, carried in the pocket, they were thought to prevent thirst. Exotic seeds, carried by the Gulf Stream, are sometimes washed up on the western coasts of Britain, and in Scotland especially these were valued as bringing good luck. Though described as "beans," many are not strictly beans in the botanical sense. They were also used as amulets to ease childbirth. Seeds of the genus *Merremia,* which have a crosslike marking, were especially valued in this way (W. B. Hemsley 1892: 371).

Beans of various kinds have been widely used in North American folk medicine in the treatment of warts. In most of these remedies, the wart is rubbed either with a bean (Brown 1952–1964, 66: 321) or with the leaves of a bean (Fentress 1934: 58). The beans are then disposed of by throwing them away, burying them, or planting them. In a wart cure recorded from Illinois, each of eight beans is named after a spiteful woman, rubbed on the wart, and then thrown in a well (Hyatt 1965: 295). Apart from treating warts, beans have been used in a wide variety of ailments in North America. As amulets red beans have been worn as a necklace to prevent rheumatism (Wheeler 1892–1893: 65) or smallpox (UCLA Folklore Archives 5_5472). Placed under the tongue or upper lip, a bean has been recommended for nosebleed (Wilson 1967: 302). As a dietary item, various kinds of beans have been recommended to treat indigestion (UCLA Folklore Archives 8_6473), alcoholism (UCLA Folklore Archives 4_7630), arthritis (UCLA Folklore Archives 1_6214), high blood pressure (UCLA Folklore Archives 24–5289), fevers (Puckett 1981: 376), bruises (UCLA Folklore Archives 21_6199), and dysentery (UCLA Folklore Archives 19_5362). Eating specially prepared black beans on New Year's Day is a Japanese folk tradition imported into North America; it is said to ensure good health for the following year

(UCLA Folklore Archives 6_6370). Beans have played a role in childbirth, too; eating pinto beans was believed to precipitate childbirth (Marquez and Pacheco 1964: 83), while eating green beans during pregnancy was held to ensure the offspring was male (UCLA Folklore Archives 22_6651). Poultices of cooked beans have been used in a wide variety of remedies, too—for treating freckles (UCLA Folklore Archives 2_6008), sore throat (Anonymous, 1939: 215), and lung congestion (Levine 1941: 488), and for drawing out poisons (Bergen 1899: 114), infections, and even tetanus (UCLA Folklore Archives 5_5292). Sitting over a pot of beans was believed by some to cure mumps (Puckett 1981: 417).

*See also* **Amulet, Bruises, Childbirth, Dysentery, Fevers, Freckles, Indigestion, Nosebleed, Pregnancy, Rheumatism, Smallpox, Sore throat, Warts, Whooping cough.**

## References

Allen, Andrew. *A Dictionary of Sussex Folk Medicine.* Newbury: Countryside Books, 1995.

Anonymous. *Idaho Lore.* Caldwell, ID: AMS Press Incorporated, 1939.

Bergen, Fanny D. "Animal and Plant Lore Collected from the Oral Tradition of English Speaking Folk." *Memoirs of the American Folklore Society, Boston and New York* 7 (1899).

Brown, Frank C. *Collection of North Carolina Folklore.* 7 vols. Durham, NC: Duke University Press, 1952–1964.

Fentress, Elza E. *Superstitions of Grayson County (Kentucky).* M.A. thesis, Western State Teachers College, 1934.

Harrison, S. G., G. B. Masefield, and Michael Wallis. *The Oxford Book of Food Plants.* London: Peerage Books, 1985.

Hatfield, Gabrielle. *Memory, Wisdom and Healing: The History of Domestic Plant Medicine.* Stroud: Sutton, 1999.

Hemsley, W. B. "A Drift-Seed (*Ipomoea tuberosa* L.)." *Annals of Botany* 6 (1892): 369–372.

Hyatt, Harry Middleton. *Folklore from Adams County Illinois.* 2nd rev. ed. New York: Memoirs of the Alma Egan Hyatt Foundation, 1965.

Lafont, Anne-Marie. *Herbal Folklore.* Bideford: Badger Books, 1984.

Levine, Harold D. "Folk Medicine in New Hampshire." *New England Journal of Medicine* 224 (1941): 487–492.

Marquez, May N., and Consuelo Pacheco. "Midwifery Lore in New Mexico." *American Journal of Nursing* 64(9) (1964): 81–84.

Puckett, Newbell Niles. *Popular Beliefs and Superstitions: A Compendium of American Folklore from the Ohio Collection of Newbell Niles Puckett.* Edited by Wayland D. Hand, Anna Casetta, Sondra B. Thiederman. 3 vols. Boston: G. K. Hall, 1981.

Radford, E., and M. A. Radford. *Encyclopedia of Superstitions.* Edited and revised by Christina Hole. London: Hutchinson, 1961.

Simoons, Frederick J. *Plants of Life, Plants of Death.* Madison: University of Wisconsin Press, 1999.

Souter, Keith. *Cure Craft: Traditional Folk Remedies and Treatment from Antiquity to the Present Day.* Saffron Walden: C. W. Daniel, 1995.

Taylor MSS. Manuscript notes of Mark R. Taylor, Norfolk Record Office, Norwich. MS4322.

Vickery, Roy *A Dictionary of Plant Lore.* Oxford: Oxford University Press, 1995.

Wheeler, Helen M. "Illinois Folk-Lore." *Folklorist* 1 (1892–1893): 55–68.

Wilson, Gordon W. "Swallow It or Rub It On: More Mammoth Cave Remedies." *Southern Folklore Quarterly* 31 (1967): 296–303.

# Bed-wetting

Mice, burned to a cinder, powdered and mixed with jam, were given to children in Sussex to cure them of bed-wetting (Allen 1995: 114). Honey is claimed to help prevent bed-wetting (Souter 1995: 138). Marjoram *(Origanum vulgare)* and sea lavender (*Limonium* spp.) have also been used to treat urinary incontinence (de Baïracli Levy 1974: 97, 131). St. John's wort (*Hypericum perforatum)* as an infusion has been used to treat enuresis in young and old alike (Quelch n.d.: 142).

In North American folk medicine, mice again feature in several remedies (see, for instance, UCLA Folklore Archives record number 4_5887). An alternative is the powder of a burned hog's bladder (Allen 1963: 85). A frog tied to the child's leg is another suggestion (Puckett 1981: 96). Breaking a twin loaf over a child's head is a curious remedy from Pennsylvania (Myers 1954: 10). Alternatively, the child can be stood in ice-cold water (Cannon 1984: 34). Other suggestions include placing hazel twigs under the sheets (UCLA Folklore Archives record number 1_5279) or giving pulverized toasted egg-shell (UCLA Folklore Archives record number 23_5277). Parched corn from a red ear of corn is an alternative (Puckett 1981: 97). Other plant preparations used to prevent bedwetting include mullein *(Verbascum thapsus),* St. John's wort *(Hypericum perforatum,* as in Britain), and red bark *(Cinchona officinalis).* Honey has also been used, as in Britain (Meyer 1985: 36). A tea made from pumpkin seeds has been used, for example in Saskatchewan (UCLA Folklore Archives 13_5867); one made from sumac berries *(Rhus* sp.) is reported from North Carolina (Walker 1955: 9). The red berries of sumac *(Rhus copallinum)* are chewed for bed-wetting among the Cherokee (Hamel and Chiltoskey 1975: 57).

Chewing pine gum has been encouraged to prevent bed-wetting (Baker and Wilcox 1948: 191). An African American suggestion is that if a newborn baby is marched around the house before it is washed, it will never get measles or wet the bed (Turner 1937: 147).

*See also* **Corn, Honey, Mouse.**

### References

Allen, Andrew. *A Dictionary of Sussex Folk Medicine.* Newbury: Countryside Books, 1995.
Allen, Jon W. *Legends and Lore of Southern Illinois.* Carbondale, IL: Southern Illinois University, 1963.
Baker, Pearl, and Ruth Wilcox. "Folk Remedies in Early Green River." *Utah Humanities Review* 2 (1948).
Cannon, Anthon S. *Popular Beliefs and Superstitions from Utah.* Edited by Wayland D. Hand and Jeannine E. Talley. Salt Lake City: University of Utah Press, 1984.
de Baïracli Levy, Juliette. *The Illustrated Herbal Handbook.* Devon: Reader's Union, 1974.
Hamel, Paul B., and Mary U. Chiltoskey. *Cherokee Plants and Their Uses: A 400 Year History.* Sylva, NC: Herald, 1975.
Meyer, Clarence. *American Folk Medicine.* Glenwood, IL: Meyerbooks, 1985.
Myers, George H. "Folk Cures." *Pennsylvania Dutchman* 5(9) (January 1, 1954).
Puckett, Newbell Niles. *Popular Beliefs and Superstitions: A Compendium of American Folklore from the Ohio Collection of Newbell Niles Puckett.* Edited by Wayland D. Hand, Anna Casetta, and Sondra B. Thiederman. 3 vols. Boston: G. K. Hall, 1981.
Quelch, Mary Thorne. *Herbs for Daily Use.* London: Faber and Faber, n.d.
Souter, Keith. *Cure Craft: Traditional Folk Remedies and Treatment from Antiquity to the Present Day.* Saffron Walden: C. W. Daniel, 1995.
Turner, Tressa. "The Human Comedy in Folk Superstitions." *Publications of the Texas Folklore Society* 13 (1937): 146–175.
Walker, Jon. "A Sampling of Folklore from Rutherford County." *North Carolina Folklore* 3(2) (December 1955).

# Bee

All the products of the bee have been used in folk medicine; honey, royal jelly, beeswax, propolis (the gluey substance used for filling in cracks within the beehive), and even bee venom have all found uses. Royal jelly, a rich food source, has been used as a tonic and propolis as a wound healer (Stein 1989: 25, 44). Bee stings have been used for rheumatism (Souter 1995: 86) and beeswax from local bees chewed to prevent hay fever (Hatfield, pers. com., 1980). Beeswax formed the basis for many healing salves. For example, an ointment for healing sores used in Badenoch in the Scottish Highlands was composed of beeswax, hog's lard, and pine resin (Beith 1995: 233).

The British folk remedies associated with bees have their counterparts in North American folk medicine. The honey bee *(Apis mellifera)* was introduced to North America in the early seventeenth century. The Native Americans termed honey bees "white man's flies," since their presence indicated a colonist settlement nearby (Micheletti 1998: 197). They had used wild bees and their products for many hundreds of years, and the Aztecs are known to have kept wild bees in captivity. There are more than two thousand species of wild bee in North America (Kavasch and Baar 1999: 19).

Honeycomb cappings are chewed in Vermont for colds and hay fever (Jarvis 1961: 110). Bee stings as a cure for rheumatism have been reported, for example in Pennsylvania (Brendle and Unger 1935: 206) and in Nebraska (Welsch 1966: 343). As in Britain, beeswax formed the basis for many healing ointments. A salve for chapped skin consisted of resin, sheep tallow, and beeswax (Browne 1958: 46); it was very similar to the one in Scotland above. Beeswax has been used to prevent a burn from blistering (UCLA Folklore Archives 5_5301). A quasi-magical cure for a swelling was to make a model of the swelling in beeswax and stand it in the sun; as the model melted, so the swelling would subside (Crosby 1927: 307). In Texas, "parched" bees have been used to treat hives (UCLA Folklore Archive 8_5415).

Dried bumblebees form part of several Native American remedies—for example, one for easing labor. The importance of beeswax in Native American medicine is indicated by the Navajo folktale of Bee Woman, who reveals that beeswax is good to take away the pain of scratches from eagle's claws and to heal the wound (Newcomb 1940: 66). Honey, propolis, and lemon are the components of a present-day Native American salve used for treating minor burns and scratches (Kavasch and Baar 1999: 22).

There is a widespread country tradition that a death in the family must immediately be reported to the bees (Radford and Radford 1974: 38).

*See also* **Childbirth, Hay fever, Hives, Honey, Rheumatism.**

### References

Beith, Mary. *Healing Threads: Traditional Medicines of the Highlands and Islands.* Edinburgh: Polygon, 1995.

Brendle, Thomas R., and Claude W. Unger. "Folk Medicine of the Pennsylvania Germans: The Non-Occult Cures." *Proceedings of the Pennsylvania German Society* 45 (1935).

Browne, Ray B. *Popular Beliefs and Practices from Alabama.* Folklore Studies 9. Berkeley and Los Angeles: University of California Publications, 1958.

Crosby, Rev. John R. "Modern Witches of Pennsylvania." *Journal of American Folklore* 40 (1927): 304–309.

Jarvis, D. C. *Folk Medicine.* London: Pan Books, 1961.

Kavasch, E. Barrie, and Karen Baar. *American Indian Healing Arts. Herbs, Rituals and Remedies for Every Season of Life.* New York: Bantam Books, 1999.

Micheletti, Enza (ed.). *North American Folk Healing: An A–Z Guide to Traditional Remedies.* New York and Montreal: Reader's Digest Association, 1998.

Newcomb, Franc J. "Origin Legend of the Navajo Eagle Chant." *Journal of American Folklore* 53 (1940): 50–77.

Radford, E., and M. A. Radford. *Encyclopaedia of Superstitions.* Edited by Christina Hole. London: Book Club Associates, 1974.

Souter, Keith. *Cure Craft: Traditional Folk Remedies and Treatment from Antiquity to the Present Day.* Saffron Walden: C. W. Daniel, 1995.

Stein, Irene. *Royal Jelly: The New Guide to Nature's Richest Food.* Wellingborough: Thorsons, 1989.

Welsch, Roger L. *A Treasury of Nebraska Pioneer Folklore.* Lincoln: University of Nebraska Press, 1966.

# Birch (*Betula spp.*)

In British folk medicine, birch has been employed as a pain killer. In Scotland, the leaves were made into an infusion for treating rheumatism. The bark of the tree as a decoction has been used for headache and rheumatism. The springtime sap was believed in the Scottish Highlands to be beneficial for the kidneys and bladder. It was also fermented and made into wine (Darwin 1996: 85). Resin from the buds has been used to form an oil rubbed into inflamed joints. Birch juice has been used in Sussex as a laxative (Allen 1995: 182).

In North America, birch has been used in innumerable ways, some of them medicinal. Birch bark has been used in Newfoundland for treating frostbite (Bergen 1899: 110). An infusion of the bark has been used to treat night sweats (Browne 1958: 105), and chewing a piece of bark has been recommended for hiccups (UCLA Folklore Archives 5_5404). Birch catkins have been worn as an amulet against inflammation (Brendle and Unger 1935: 83). The juice of various birches has, as in Britain, been used to treat pain. The oil of one species of birch, *Betula lenta,* was used for treating rheumatism and was marketed as "wintergreen" oil, presumably because of a similarity in its scent. Birch sap was used by the pioneers as a springtime tonic, as a gargle for sore throats, and a wash for skin conditions (Willard 1992: 70). The inner bark or the root of birch was cooked and eaten for a weak stomach (Meyer 1985: 242). Ground birch bark was said to get rid of intestinal worms (Meyer 1985: 268).

In the Native American tradition birch has been used extensively. The inner bark of the paper birch has been used by the Thompson Indians as a contraceptive (Turner et al. 1990: 189); the bark is very strong, pliable and waterproof, and squaws used it to make contraceptive diaphragms (Fischer 1989: 92). Birch bark has been used to splint fractures (Wells 1954: 282). A syrup has been made from birch buds and used for ringworm (Speck 1944: 43). Birch sap has been used in treatment of consumption (Vogel 1970: 95–96). (For the numerous other uses of birch by Native Americans see Moerman 1998: 122–125.)

*See also* **Contraception, Fractures, Frostbite, Headache, Hiccups, Native American tradition, Rheumatism, Tonic.**

## References

Allen, Andrew. *A Dictionary of Sussex Folk Medicine.* Newbury: Countryside Books, 1995.

Bergen, Fanny D. "Animal and Plant Lore Collected from the Oral Tradition of English Speaking Folk." *Memoirs of the American Folk-Lore Society* 7 (1899).

Brendle, Thomas R., and Claude W. Unger. "Folk Medicine of the Pennsylvania Germans: The Non-Occult Cures." *Proceedings of the Pennsylvania German Society* 45 (1935).

Browne, Ray B. *Popular Beliefs and Practices from Alabama.* Folklore Studies 9. Berkeley and Los Angeles: University of California Publications, 1958.

Darwin, Tess. *The Scots Herbal: The Plant Lore of Scotland.* Edinburgh: Mercat Press, 1996.

Fischer, David Hackett. *Albion's Seed.* Oxford: Oxford University Press, 1989.

Meyer, Clarence. *American Folk Medicine.* Glenwood, IL: Meyerbooks, 1985.

Moerman, Daniel E. *Native American Ethnobotany.* Portland, OR: Timber Press, 1998.

Speck, Frank G. "Catawba Herbals and Curative Practices." *Journal of American Folklore* 57 (1944): 37–50.

Turner, Nancy J., Laurence C. Thompson, M. Terry Thompson, and Annie Z. York. *Thompson Ethnobotany: Knowledge and Usage of Plants by the Thompson Indians of Brit-*

ish Columbia. Victoria: Royal British Columbia Museum, 1990.

Vogel, Virgil J. American Indian Medicine. Norman: University of Oklahoma Press, 1970.

Wells, Warner. "Surgical Practice in North Carolina: A Historical Commentary." North Carolina Medical Journal 15 (1954): 281–287.

Willard, Terry. Edible and Medicinal Plants of the Rocky Mountains and Neighbouring Territories. Calgary: Wild Rose College of Natural Healing, 1992.

# Bites and stings.

See **Insect bites and stings.**

# Black, William George

Black was born in 1857 and lived in Hillhead, Glasgow, Scotland. Trained as a lawyer, he wrote on a number of subjects and was the first to use the term "folk medicine" in print, first in newspaper articles and later in a paper published in 1878 by the British Archaeological Society (Black 1878). Here he defined folk medicine as "meant to comprehend the subjects of charms, incantations, and those habits related to the preservation of health, or the cure of disease, which were and are practiced by the more superstitious and old-fashioned." His definition reflects the patronizing attitude of folklorists of his time. His book Folk Medicine: A Chapter in the History of Culture was published by Elliot Stock for the Folklore Society in London in 1883. It was the first book on folk medicine to be published in Britain, and despite its emphasis on the bizarre and its strong flavor of social condescension, it contains a wealth of valuable information, gathered together for the first time. In Black's words, it did indeed serve to direct attention to "the important study which I have ventured to call Folk-Medicine" (Black 1878: 332). Black died in 1932.

### Reference
Black, William George. "Folk-Medicine." Journal of the British Archaeological Association 34 (1878): 327–332.

# Black cohosh (Cimicifuga racemosa)

Native to Canada and Eastern North America but not to Britain, this plant was used by Native Americans to treat rheumatic pain. Among the Iroquois, the affected limbs were held in the steam from a decoction of the plant (Herrick 1977: 320). The Cherokee used an infusion of the plant to treat rheumatism (Hamel and Chiltoskey 1975: 30). Its other principal uses were for amenorrhoea (Hamel and Chiltoskey 1975: 30) and to aid childbirth (Coffey 1993: 14); hence its alternative name of squaw root. (For other uses see Moerman 1998: 162–163.)

Among settlers in North America, it became a very fashionable and expensive medicine, in the seventeenth century reaching the price of three pounds sterling per pound (Hughes 1957). By the nineteenth and early twentieth centuries, partly owing to its promotion by the Eclectic school of herbalists, it was viewed as a panacea (Crellin and Philpott 1990: 166). The root was used, as a decoction, for treating rheumatism (Meyer 1985: 40, 214, 216, 217, 220). It was a constituent of an herbal mixture for treating bronchitis (Meyer 1985: 51). It was recommended for female "weakness" (Meyer 1985: 124, 125) and figured in a liver tonic (Meyer 1985: 168). Herbalists in Europe adopted the plant as part of their materia medica, and it is still used by them today for treating period pain, menopausal problems, and rheumatic complaints (Chevallier 1996: 78). It is currently the subject of studies in Germany for the treatment of menopausal symptoms (Micheletti 1998: 97).

*See also* **Childbirth, Rheumatism and arthritis.**

## References

Chevallier, Andrew. *The Encyclopedia of Medicinal Plants.* London: Dorling Kindersley, 1996.

Coffey, Timothy. *The History and Folklore of North American Wildflowers.* New York: Facts On File, 1993.

Crellin, John K., and Jane Philpott. *A Reference Guide to Medicinal Plants.* Durham, NC: Duke University Press, 1990.

Hamel, Paul B., and Mary U. Chiltoskey. *Cherokee Plants and Their Uses: A 400 Year History.* Sylva, NC: Herald, 1975.

Herrick, James William. *Iroquois Medical Botany.* Ph.D. thesis, State University of New York, Albany, 1977.

Hughes, Thomas P. *Medicine in Virginia 1607–1699.* Jamestown 350th Anniversary Historical Booklet 21. Williamsburg, VA: 1957.

Meyer, Clarence. *American Folk Medicine.* Glenwood, IL: Meyerbooks, 1985.

Micheletti, Enza (ed.). *North American Folk Healing: An A-Z Guide to Traditional Remedies.* New York and Montreal: Reader's Digest Association, 1998.

Moerman, Daniel E. *Native American Ethnobotany.* Portland, OR: Timber Press, 1998.

# Blackberry, Bramble (*Rubus fruticosus*)

In British folk medicine the bramble has had a reputation for curing and preventing a wide variety of ailments. The shoots have the unusual ability to root where they touch the ground, and sufferers from boils, rheumatism, and hernia were passed through the arch formed in this way (Grieve 1931: 109). A child suffering from whooping cough was sometimes passed under the arch seven times. The cough was then thought to leave the child and stay with the bramble, an example of transference (Black 1883: 70). To ward off evil spirits, the Scottish Highlanders used a length of bramble shoot entwined with ivy and rowan (Grigson 1955: 145). The blackberry has been used to treat diarrhea (Lafont 1984: 17). In Scotland, the roots of bramble were used with pennyroyal to treat bronchitis and asthma and the leaves were used to treat erysipelas (Beith 1995: 209). In Somerset, the sufferer from bronchitis was advised to carry a blackberry shoot and nibble it when the cough started (Tongue 1965: 37). In England, as well as Scotland, the leaves have been used to treat burns and swellings (Grigson 1955: 145). The leaves of the blackberry have been chewed for toothache (Hatfield 1994: 55) and the fruit in the form of a jelly used to treat sore throat, a use that can be traced back to Dioscorides (Chevallier 1996: 261). The first blackberry of the season was said in Cornwall to cure warts (Black 1883: 202). To eat blackberries after the first frost was considered unlucky, a belief widespread throughout Britain (Vickery 1995: 45).

The species of blackberry (*Rubus fruticosus*) most common in Britain is naturalized throughout most of the world, including North America. In folk medicinal records, it is often not possible to trace the actual species used in the past. Blackberry roots are one component of a decoction used to treat dysentery (Meyer 1985: 98). Blackberry root has been used to treat diarrhea (Cadwallader and Wilson 1965: 220) and thrush (Meyer 1985: 178). "Passing through" a blackberry bush has been used to treat whooping cough (Hohman 1904: 111) and pleurisy (Pickard and Buley 1945: 82). Blackberry juice has been recommended for colitis (Browne 1958: 52) and for nausea and vomiting (Parler 1962, 3: 980), while a tea made from the roots has been used for labor pain (Parler 1962, 3: 51) and as a wash for rheumatism (Cadwallader and Wilson 1965: 220), as well as a lotion for sore gums in teething babies (Parler 1962, 3: 287). Whereas in England blackberry leaves have been used to treat toothache, in Pennsylvania the gall growing on a blackberry has been carried as an amulet to protect against toothache (Brendle and Unger 1935: 116).

In Native American medicine at least three different species of Rubus have been recorded in use for diarrhea and four for sore throat (Hamel and Chiltoskey 1975: 26). The so-called Long Blackberry *(Rubus allegheniensis)* has been used by the Iroquois for treating coughs, colds, and tuberculosis (Herrick 1977: 357). Burns have been treated using the bark or leaves of the salmonberry, *Rubus spectabilis* (Gunther 1973: 35). Whooping cough has been treated with a decoction of the black raspberry *(Rubus occidentalis)* (Herrick 1977: 356). There was a Cherokee belief that a blackberry bramble pulled backward could cure blackheads (Mellinger 1967: 69).

*See also* **Amulet, Asthma, Burns, Erysipelas, Rheumatism, Transference.**

### References

Beith, Mary. *Healing Threads: Traditional Medicines of the Highlands and Islands.* Edinburgh: Polygon, 1995.

Black, William George. *Folk-Medicine: A Chapter in the History of Culture.* London: Folklore Society, 1883.

Brendle, Thomas R., and Claude W. Unger. "Folk Medicine of the Pennsylvania Germans: The Non-Occult Cures." *Proceedings of the Pennsylvania German Society* 45 (1935).

Browne, Ray B. *Popular Beliefs and Practices from Alabama.* Folklore Studies 9. Berkeley and Los Angeles: University of California Publications, 1958.

Cadwallader, D. E., and F. J. Wilson. "Folklore Medicine among Georgia's Piedmont Negroes after the Civil War." *Collections of the Georgia Historical Society* 49 (1965): 217–227.

Chevallier, Andrew. *The Encyclopedia of Medicinal Plants.* London: Dorling Kindersley, 1996.

Grieve, Mrs. M. *A Modern Herbal.* London: Jonathan Cape, 1931.

Grigson, Geoffrey. *The Englishman's Flora.* London: Phoenix House, 1955.

Gunther, Erna. *Ethnobotany of Western Washington.* Rev. ed. Seattle: Washington Press, 1973.

Hamel, Paul B., and Mary U. Chiltoskey. *Cherokee Plants and Their Uses: A 400 Year History.* Sylva, NC: Herald Publishing,1975.

Hatfield, Gabrielle. *Country Remedies: Traditional East Anglian Plant Remedies in the Twentieth Century.* Woodbridge: Boydell, 1994.

Herrick, James William. *Iroquois Medical Botany.* Ph.D. thesis, State University of New York, Albany, 1977.

Hohman, John George. "The Long Hidden Friend." *Journal of American Folklore* 17 (1904): 89–152.

Lafont, Anne-Marie. *Herbal Folklore.* Bideford: Badger Books, 1984.

Mellinger, Marie B. "Medicine of the Cherokees." *Foxfire* 1(3) (1967): 13–20, 65–72.

Meyer, Clarence. *American Folk Medicine.* Glenwood, IL: Meyerbooks, 1985.

Parler, Mary Celestia, and University Student Contributors. *Folk Beliefs from Arkansas.* 15 vols. Fayetteville: University of Arkansas, 1962.

Pickard, Madge E., and R. Carlyle Buley. *The Midwest Pioneer, His Ills, Cures and Doctors.* Crawfordsville, IN: R. E. Banta, 1945.

Tongue, Ruth L. *Somerset Folklore.* Edited by Katharine Briggs. County Folklore 8. London: Folklore Society, 1965.

Vickery, Roy. *A Dictionary of Plant Lore.* Oxford: Oxford University Press, 1995.

# Blacksmith

The Celtic smith-god Gobniu was associated with healing, which may explain the faith in the power of the blacksmith to treat a variety of illnesses. Blacksmiths were usually strong men, which would have added to the esteem in which they were held. Their association with fire and iron would have further strengthened this faith. Some of their "cures," such as one for depression reported by Martin in the seventeenth century from the Scottish Highlands, depended on terrifying the patient by almost striking them with a hammer (Beith 1995: 100). Blacksmiths were thought to have the power to arrest bleeding (Radford and Radford 1974: 56). As part of their treatment of patients, some blacksmiths in Scotland used bloodletting, a practice reported as recently as the 1930s (Beith 1995: 116). Others used herbal treatment, such as the nineteenth-century Mackintosh from Bohuntin in the Scottish Highlands (Beith 1995: 149). He pounded his herbs in the oil-lamp mold of his anvil, a practice that was probably thought to enhance the power of the herbs. The water in which the smith quenched his iron was in demand for folk medicine right up to the twentieth century, for healing sick children and strengthening the weak.

Some of these beliefs are also to be found in North American folk medicine. A twentieth-century Pennsylvania blacksmith cured people suffering from erysipelas (Shoemaker 1951: 2). By applying slake water from his forge and saying certain words, it was believed that a blacksmith could cure warts (Puckett 1981: 497). Whooping cough, poison ivy rash (Puckett 1981: 427, 500), and freckles (Brown 1952–1964, 66: 198) have all been treated with "slake" water.

See also **Bleeding, Erysipelas, Forge water, Warts.**

### References

Beith, Mary. *Healing Threads: Traditional Medicines of the Highlands and Islands.* Edinburgh: Polygon, 1995.

Brown, Frank C. *Collection of North Carolina Folklore.* 7 vols. Durham, NC: Duke University Press, 1952–1964.

Puckett, Newbell Niles. *Popular Beliefs and Superstitions: A Compendium of American Folklore from the Ohio Collection of Newbell Niles Puckett.* Edited by Wayland D. Hand, Anna Casetta, and Sondra B. Thiederman. 3 vols. Boston: G. K. Hall, 1981.

Radford, E., and M. A. Radford. *Encyclopaedia of Superstitions.* Edited and revised by Christina Hole. London: Book Club Associates, 1974.

Shoemaker, Alfred L. "Blacksmith Lore." *Pennsylvania Dutchman* 3(6) (August 1, 1951): 2.

# Blackthorn (*Prunus spinosa*)

This plant has been used for a wide range of conditions in British folk medicine, ranging from diarrhea to sore throat (Allen and Hatfield, in press) and the treatment of fevers (Beith 1995: 205). Particularly in southern Britain, the fruit, known as sloes, have been rubbed on warts. Though introduced in North America, blackthorn does not feature in folk medicine there; instead, other species of Prunus have been used.

See also **Cherry, Warts.**

### References

Allen, David E., and Gabrielle Hatfield. *Medicinal Plants in Folk Tradition.* Portland, OR: Timber Press, in press.

Beith, Mary. *Healing Threads: Traditional Medicines of the Highlands and Islands.* Edinburgh: Polygon, 1995.

# Bleeding

As one of the most obvious domestic emergencies, bleeding has attracted a wide range of home remedies. In British folk medicine, the simplest treatment has been cold water. Cobwebs were very widely used right up to the end of the twentieth century to treat serious cuts in humans and animals. In the Highlands of Scotland so-called toadstones (actually the teeth of fossil fish) were used to arrest bleeding (Beith 1995: 158). Ashes of a burned frog were reputedly used to stop bleeding (Beith 1995: 176). Pepper has been used as a styptic in both Scotland (Beith 1995: 232) and Northumberland (Prince 1991: 122). Also in the Highlands, individual healers had a reputation for treating bleeding, and their treatment included administering dried blood of the patient (Beith 1995: 165). Puffballs have been another source of emergency first aid. The spores have been sprinkled onto a wound to arrest bleeding, and the whole fungus has been chopped to provide a poultice. In barber shops and in farm sheds a dried puffball was kept throughout the year to use in emergencies. In Sussex, bracket fungus, known there as amadou, was used similarly (Allen 1995: 27).

A remedy common throughout Britain, but especially in Suffolk, was to preserve the petals of a lily (usually the Madonna lily) in brandy. The petals were then used to bandage cuts (Hatfield 1994: appendix). Also in East Anglia, the root of the horseradish *(Armoracia rusticana)* was used to treat deep cuts (Porter 1974: 43). Horsetail *(Equisetum* spp.) has been recommended by the ancients in official medicine but has also been used in folk medicine, for example on the Isle of Man, to stop bleeding (Quayle 1973: 70). Plantain leaves were used to stem the bleeding from minor wounds, in Scotland, England, and Ireland (Beith 1995: 233; Vickery 1995: 285; Westropp 1911: 449–456). In Somerset, bird's foot trefoil *(Lotus corniculatus)* has been used to staunch bleeding (Tongue 1965: 36). In the nineteenth century mistletoe *(Viscum album)* was reputedly chopped small and applied to injuries to stop the bleeding (Notes and Queries 1849: 325). The boiled plant of St. John's wort *(Hypericum perforatum)* was used in the Scottish Highlands to staunch bleeding (Beith 1995: 238), as were the leaves of tobacco or dried tobacco (Beith 1995: 246). Shepherd's purse *(Capsella bursa-pastoris)* was used to staunch bleeding (Beith 1995: 242). Yarrow *(Achillea millefolium)* was universally accepted as a styptic and formed a constituent of many healing ointments (Hatfield 1994: 33). Willow *(Salix* spp.) was used in Cumbria to arrest bleeding (Freethy 1985: 118). The blood-staunching properties of marsh woundwort *(Stachys palustris)* were drawn

to Gerard's attention in the sixteenth century when he witnessed their effectiveness on a man badly cut by a scythe. Gerard was so impressed that he adopted the plant in his own practice (Allen 1995: 184). Both the marsh and the hedge woundwort *(Stachys sylvatica)* have been used in this way. Also in Sussex, the leaves of woad plants *(Isatis tinctoria)* naturalized from cultivation for dye, have been used to stem the flow of blood (Allen 1995: 185). The resin from pine trees *(Pinus* spp.) has been used to staunch bleeding in both England and Scotland (Allen and Hatfield, in press). In the twentieth century, castor oil was used in Hampshire with great success to treat deep cuts (Prince 1991: 114).

In North America amulets worn to stop bleeding have included pieces of bloodroot worn as a necklace. In Georgia, a necklace of mulberry roots and buttons has been used (Waller and Killion 1972: 75). As in Britain, certain individuals have been credited with the power to stop bleeding. A woman born with a caul (Dorson 1952: 159) was thought to have this ability, also the seventh son of a seventh son (UCLA Folklore Archives record number 2_5287). It is claimed that people who have never seen their fathers have this power too (Brown 1952–1964: 6: 126). When the injury has been caused by a knife, a widespread belief goes, the knife should be thrust into the ground or into a tree (Randolph 1931: 103).

Recommended applications in North American folk medicine for bleeding include cobwebs, pepper, tobacco (all used in Britain as well), tea leaves, ashes of burned rags, a paste (made from flour, salt, and water), and wood soot, as well as powdered bone and powdered dried beef (Meyer 1985: 276–277). Powdered rice (Parler 1962: 450), coffee grounds (UCLA Folklore Archives 18_6287), corn silk (Koch 1980: 70), urine, bread, sugar (Puckett 1981: 318, 319), the lining of an eggshell

(Cannon 1984: 94), and bleeding chicken meat (Brown 1952–1964, 66: 123) have all been applied to bleeding injuries. For arterial bleeding in an arm, thrusting the arm into a sack of flour has been found to help (UCLA Folklore Archives 10_6287). Applying brown paper, as in the nursery rhyme of Jack and Jill, has also been used to stem bleeding (Secrest 1964: 481–482). The sap from a pine tree *(Pinus elliottii)* has been used in Florida to stem bleeding (as in Cumbria, England, where a different Pine species was used; see above) (Murphree 1965: 178). The sap of spruce trees *(Picea* sp.) has been used similarly (UCLA Folklore Archives 22_5286). Wild alum root *(Heuchera* sp.) has been used in the mountain South of the United States to stop bleeding (Long 1962: 5). A poultice of wolf's bane *(Arnica* sp.) was used in Mexico (UCLA Folklore Archives record number 3_6182). Other plant remedies include sumac *(Rhus* sp.) (Beck 1957: 45), witch hazel *(Hamamelis virginiana)* (UCLA Folklore Archives 19_6287), goldenrod *(Solidago* sp.) (Clark 1970: 13), and bloodweed blossoms *(Conyza canadensis)* (Creighton 1968: 199). Plant-derived remedies also include puffball spores, woundwort, yarrow, and woad, as used in Britain. In addition, the leaves of sunflower *(Helianthus annuus)* or peach *(Prunus persica),* as well as sassafras leaves *(Sassafras albidum),* chewed fine and applied, are recommended. Matico-leaf *(Piper angustifolium)* and bistort *(Polygonum bistorta)* have been used, also the leaves and bark of willow, as in Britain *(Salix* spp.) (Meyer 1985: 277). Green walnut juice *(Juglans* sp.) has been used in Tennessee (Parr 1962: 11). In Mexico, the organ pipe cactus *(Pachycereus* sp.) was particularly popular for healing cuts in the eighteenth century, and it is still used today to check bleeding after a tooth extraction (Kay 1996: 57). The crushed young leaves of Mexican elder *(Sambucus mexicana)* are used to poultice cuts (Kay 1996: 247).

In Native American medicine, plants belonging to nearly a hundred different genera have been used to staunch bleeding (Moerman 1998: 772). They include red willow *(Salix lucida)* (Wallis 1922: 26); wormwood leaves *(Artemisia* sp.) (Vogel 1970: 396), various species of juniper (for instance *Juniperus occidentalis,* used by the Paiute) (Train, Henrichs, and Archer 1941: 92), and the chewed leaves of pigeon berries or poke *(Phytolacca americana)* (Van Wart 1948: 577). Interestingly, both puffball spores and spider webs have been used—for example, by the Kwakiutl—to stem bleeding (Boas 1932: 188).

*See also* **Amulet, Bloodroot, Caul, Corn, Mistletoe, Nosebleed, Poke, Puffball, Seventh son, Spider, Sympathetic magic, Wounds, Yarrow.**

### References

Allen, Andrew. *A Dictionary of Sussex Folk Medicine.* Newbury: Countryside Books, 1995.
Beck, Horace P. *The Folklore of Maine.* Philadelphia and New York: J. B. Lippincott, 1957.
Beith, Mary. *Healing Threads: Traditional Medicines of the Highlands and Islands.* Edinburgh: Polygon 1995.
Boas, Franz. "Current Beliefs of the Kwakiutl Indians." *Journal of American Folklore* 45 (1932): 177–260.
Brown, Frank C. *Collection of North Carolina Folklore.* 7 vols. Durham, NC: Duke University Press 1952–64.
Cannon, Anthon S. *Popular Beliefs and Superstitions from Utah.* Edited by Wayland D. Hand and Jeannine E. Talley. Salt Lake City: University of Utah Press, 1984.
Clark, Joseph D. "North Carolina Popular Beliefs and Superstitions." *North Carolina Folklore* 18 (1970): 1–66.
Creighton, Helen. *Bluenose Magic, Popular Beliefs and Superstitions in Nova Scotia.* Toronto: Ryerson Press, 1968.
Dorson, Richard M. *Bloodstoppers and Bearwalkers: Folk Traditions of the Upper Peninsula.* Cambridge, MA: Harvard University Press, 1952.

Freethy, Ron. *From Agar to Zenry.* Marlborough: Crowood Press 1985.

Hatfield, Gabrielle. *Country Remedies: Traditional East Anglian Plant Remedies in the Twentieth Century.* Woodbridge: Boydell, 1994.

Kay, Margarita A. *Healing with Plants in the American and Mexican West.* Tucson: University of Arizona Press, 1996.

Koch, William E. *Folklore from Kansas. Beliefs and Customs.* Lawrence, KS: Regent Press, 1980.

Long, Grady M. "Folk Medicine in McMinn, Polk, Bradley, and Meigs Counties, Tennessee, 1910–1927." *Tennessee Folklore Society Bulletin* 28 (1962): 1–8.

Meyer, Clarence. *American Folk Medicine.* Glenwood, IL: Meyerbooks, 1985.

Moerman, Daniel E. *Native American Ethnobotany.* Portland, OR: Timber Press, 1998.

Murphree, Alice H. "Folk Medicine in Florida: Remedies Using Plants." *Florida Anthropologist* 18 (1965): 175–185.

Notes and Queries, London 1849 ff. Vol. 43, p. 325.

Parler, Mary Celestia, and University Student Contributors. *Folk Beliefs from Arkansas.* 15 vols. Fayetteville: University of Arkansas, 1962.

Parr, Jerry S. "Folk Cures of Middle Tennessee." *Tennessee Folklore Society Bulletin* 28 (1962): 8–12.

Porter, Enid. *The Folklore of East Anglia.* London: Batsford, 1974.

Prince, Dennis. *Grandmother's Cures: An A-Z of Herbal Remedies.* London: Fontana, 1991.

Puckett, Newbell Niles. *Popular Beliefs and Superstitions: A Compendium of American Folklore from the Ohio Collection of Newbell Niles Puckett.* Edited by Wayland D. Hand, Anna Casetta, and Sondra B. Thiederman. 3 vols. Boston: G. K. Hall, 1981.

Quayle, George. *Legends of a Lifetime: Manx Folklore.* Douglas: Courier Herald, 1973.

Randolph, Vance. *The Ozarks: An American Survival of Primitive Society.* New York: Vanguard Press, 1931.

Secrest, A. Jack. "Contemporary Folk Medicine." *Carolina Medical Journal* 25 (1964): 481–482.

Tongue, Ruth L. *Somerset Folklore.* Edited by K. M. Briggs. London: Folklore Society, 1965.

Train, Percy, James R. Henrichs, and W. Andrew Archer. *Medicinal Uses of Plants by Indian Tribes of Nevada.* Washington, DC: U. S. Department of Agriculture, 1941.

Van Wart, Arthur F. "The Indians of the Maritime Provinces, Their Diseases and Native Cures." *Canadian Medical Association Journal* 59(6) (1948): 573–577.

Vickery, Roy. *A Dictionary of Plant Lore.* Oxford: Oxford University Press, 1995.

Vogel, Virgil J. *American Indian Medicine.* Norman: University of Oklahoma Press, 1970.

Waller, Tom, and Gene Killion. "Georgia Folk Medicine." *Southern Folklore Quarterly* 36 (1972): 71–92.

Wallis, Wilson D. "Medicines Used by the Micmac Indians." *American Anthropologist* 24 (1922): 24–30.

Westropp, Thomas J. "A Folklore Survey of County Clare" (continued) XVIII "Animal and Plant Superstitions" (continued). *Folk-Lore* 22 (1911): 449–456.

# Blisters

Although medically trivial, foot blisters are sufficiently painful to have attracted a number of folk remedies. There have been conflicting fashions in the domestic treatment of blisters. Some have recommended preserving the blisters intact in order to avoid infection; others have advised puncturing the blister and applying surgical spirit to cleanse and harden the skin. Passing a needle and thread through the blister has been practiced (Harvey, pers. com., 1955). Soaked cabbage leaves have been used in treating blisters, while the leaves of greater plantain *(Plantago major)* have been used both to prevent and to treat blisters (Souter 1995: 138). In the west country of England, ashes of burned wood from the ash *(Fraxinus excelsior)* have been used to "draw" blisters (Hartland 1895: 29). In Ulster, poultices were made from bread or linseed meal (Foster 1951: 61, 261).

In North American folk medicine, many similar blister treatments were used.

It was suggested that blisters should be broken, but only after sunset (Anderson 1968: 313). Drawing a worsted thread through the blister to dry it up is a recommendation familiar from Britain also (Parler 1962: 456). It has been suggested in California that urinating on the hands toughens the skin and prevents blisters (UCLA Folklore Archives 4_6185). As in Britain, cabbage leaves were used throughout the United States for blister treatment (Bergen 1899: 110). Onions applied was another recommended treatment from California (UCLA Folklore Archives 3_5291). Both pepper and grease have been used to treat blisters (Woodhull 1930: 18, 19). Venison tallow has also been used (Yoder 1965: 23). A recommendation from China used in California is to rub the blisters with heated pieces of dried turnip (UCLA Folklore Archives 7_6185).

## References

Anderson, John Q. "Popular Beliefs in Texas, Louisiana and Arkansas." *Southern Folklore Quarterly* 32 (1968): 304–319.

Bergen, Fanny D. "Animal and Plant Lore Collected from the Oral Tradition of English Speaking Folk." *Memoirs of the American Folk-Lore Society* 7 (1899).

Foster, Jeanne Cooper. *Ulster Folklore.* Belfast: H. R. Carter, 1951.

Hartland, Edwin Sidney. *County Folklore: Gloucestershire.* Printed extract 1, vol. 37. London: Folklore Society, 1895.

Parler, Mary Celestia, and University Student Contributors. *Folk Beliefs from Arkansas.* 15 vols. Fayetteville: University of Arkansas, 1962.

Souter, Keith. *Cure Craft: Traditional Folk Remedies and Treatment from Antiquity to the Present Day.* Saffron Walden: C. W. Daniel, 1995.

Woodhull, Frost. "Ranch Remedios." *Publications of the Texas Folklore Society* 8 (1930): 9–73.

Yoder, Don. "The 'Domestic Encyclopaedia' of 1803–1804." *Pennsylvania Folklife* 14(3) (Spring 1965): 10–27.

# Blood

As a healing agent in folk medicine, blood has been widely used. In the Highlands of Scotland, administering the patient's own blood in dried form was held to cure a hemorrhage (Beith 1995: 94). In the seventeenth century, there was a belief that the blood of healthy people could cure bleeding (Wright 1912: 495–496). Human blood has been widely used to treat epilepsy. In Scotland, the patient's own blood was administered (Beith 1995: 101). The blood of a cat has been used since Anglo-Saxon times to treat epilepsy (Newman 1948: 135). In the Isle of Lewis the blood of a black cock, or of a person named Munro, was applied for treating shingles. Blood from a black cat was an alternative in the north of Scotland (Black 1883: 151). The blood of members of the clan Keogh was held to be effective in treating toothache in Ireland and was also used in the treatment of erysipelas (Black 1883: 140). In the Scottish Highlands, kidney and gallstones were treated with the blood of wild goats (Beith 1995: 177), while hare's blood was used to treat skin blemishes (Beith 1995: 177). The blood of numerous different animals has been used in wart treatment. In the north of England, eel blood was used (Black 1883: 162), while in East Anglia, the blood obtained by sharply tapping the nose of a live mole was applied to warts (Randell, pers. com., 1989). In Scotland pig's blood was used in wart treatment (Beith 1995: 180). Styes too were traditionally treated with either hair or blood from a black cat (Black 1883: 151). In Ireland, a black cat's blood was used to treat the itch (Jones 1908: 316–317).

In North American folk medicine blood has been used in most of these ways, and in others as well. For treatment of epilepsy, the blood of an executed criminal has been used (Hand 1970: 325). An alternative was the blood of a black hen (Wintemberg 1899:

47). The latter was also used to treat measles (Letcher 1910–1911: 172), rheumatism (Pickard and Buley 1945: 84), and sore gums (Brewster 1939: 39). The blood of a black cat was used for shingles (Roberts 1927: 167) and scarlet fever (Hyatt 1965: 218), as well as for warts (Cannon 1984: 130). Mole blood (UCLA Folklore Archives 1_6825) and bat's blood (Anderson 1970: 60) were both used in treating rheumatism. Drinking the hot blood from the heart of a heifer was considered a cure for consumption (Puckett 1926: 370), while a child suffering from asthma was stood in the warm blood of a newly killed animal (Creighton 1950: 85). Woodpecker blood was considered a cure for heart trouble (UCLA Folklore Archive 2_5404). A drop of blood from a "bessy" bug was used to treat earache (Norris 1958: 105).

For pneumonia, deer blood and wine were mixed and drunk among the Nahuatl (Madsen 1955: 135).

*See also* **Earache, Erysipelas, Heart trouble, Rheumatism, Shingles, Toothache, Tuberculosis.**

### References

Anderson, John. *Texas Folk Medicine.* Austin: Encino Press, 1970.

Beith, Mary. *Healing Threads: Traditional Medicines of the Highlands and Islands.* Edinburgh: Polygon, 1995.

Black, William George. *Folk-Medicine: A Chapter in the History of Culture.* London: Folklore Society, 1883.

Brewster, Paul G. "Folk Cures and Preventives from Southern Indiana." *Southern Folklore Quarterly* 3 (1939): 33–43.

Cannon, Anthon S. *Popular Beliefs and Superstitions from Utah.* Edited by Wayland D. Hand and Jeannine E. Talley. Salt Lake City: University of Utah Press, 1984.

Creighton, Helen. *Folklore from Lunenburg County, Nova Scotia.* National Museum of Canada Bulletin 117, Anthropological series 29. Ottawa: 1950.

Hand, Wayland D. "Hangmen, the Gallows, and the Dead Man's Hand in American Folk Medicine." In *Medieval Literature and Folklore Studies: Essays in Honor of Francis Lee Utley.* Edited by Jerome Mandell and Bruce A. Rosenberg. Pages 323–329, 381–387. New Brunswick, NJ: Rutgers University Press, 1970.

Hyatt, Harry Middleton. *Folklore from Adams County Illinois.* 2nd rev. ed. New York: Memoirs of the Alma Egan Hyatt Foundation, 1965.

Jones, B. H. "Folk Medicine." *Folk-Lore* 19 (1908): 315–319.

Letcher, James H. "The Treatment of Some Diseases by the 'Old Time' Negro." *Railway Surgical Journal* 17 (1910–1911): 170–175.

Madsen, William. "Hot and Cold in the Universe of San Francisco Tecospa, Valley of Mexico." *Journal of American Folklore* 68 (1955): 123–139.

Newman, Leslie F. "Some Notes on the Pharmacology and Therapeutic Value of Folk-Medicine." *Folk-Lore* 59 (1948): 118–135, 145–156.

Norris, Ruby R. "Folk Medicine of Cumberland County." *Kentucky Folklore Record* 4 (1958): 101–110.

Pickard, Madge E., and R. Carlyle Buley. *The Midwest Pioneer, His Ills, Cures and Doctors.* Crawfordsville, IN: R. E. Banta, 1945.

Puckett, Newbell Niles. *Folk Beliefs of the Southern Negro.* Chapel Hill, NC: Greenwood Press, 1926.

Roberts, Hilda. "Louisiana Superstitions." *Journal of American Folklore* 40 (1927): 144–208.

Wintemberg, W. J. "Items of German-Canadian Folklore." *Journal of American Folklore* 12 (1899): 45–86.

Wright, A. R. "Seventeenth Century Cures and Charms." *Folk-Lore* 23 (1912): 230–236, 490–497.

# Bloodroot (*Sanguinaria canadensis*)

This plant is not native in Britain, and has played no role in its folk medicine. In North American folk medicine it has been very widely used. In gin or whisky it has been recommended to sufferers from asthma (Meyer 1985: 32). Eating the root, or drinking an infusion made from it, was said to hasten menstruation (Puckett 1981: 414). A similar infusion has been used to treat coughs and colds, and to relieve the pain of burns (Mellinger 1968: 50). Combined with tormentil (*Potentilla erecta*), cinnamon (*Cinnamomum* sp.), and plantain (*Plantago* sp.), it has been used as a treatment for dysentery among the Pennsylvania Germans (Brendle and Unger 1935: 171). For "winter itch" the root has been steeped in strong pure apple vinegar and applied (Parler 1962: 731). Croup in children has been treated with a similar decoction of bloodroot in vinegar (Browne 1958: 18). The plant has been used, combined with scokeroot (*Phytolacca americana*), to treat nasal polyps (Browne 1964: 35–70). It has even been used to treat cancers, the powdered root being mixed to a paste with wheat flour and zinc chloride and applied (UCLA Folklore Archives 2_6285). It has been considered useful for liver troubles (Clark 1970: 25). A wash made from bloodroot has been used to treat poison oak rash (UCLA Folklore Archives 5_6462). Boiled in olive oil, the root has been used to treat sores (Street 1959: 81). It has been used by African Americans to treat tetters (? ringworm) (Cadwallader and Wilson 1965: 220, 224). A tea made from bloodroot has been drunk for rheumatism (Jack 1964: 36). In New England, a piece of bloodroot has been hung over the bed to prevent nosebleeds (Levine 1941: 489).

*See also* **Asthma, Burns, Cancer, Colds, Coughs, Nosebleed, Poison ivy, Rheumatism.**

### References
Brendle, Thomas R., and Claude W. Unger. "Folk Medicine of the Pennsylvania Germans: The Non-Occult Cures." *Proceedings of the Pennsylvania German Society* 45 (1935).
Browne, Ray B. *Popular Beliefs and Practices from Alabama.* Folklore Studies 9. Berkeley and Los Angeles: University of California Publications, 1958.
Browne, Ray B., (ed.). "The Indian Doctor." *Indiana History Bulletin* 41 (1964).
Cadwallader, D. E., and F. J. Wilson. "Folklore Medicine among Georgia's Piedmont Negroes after the Civil War." *Collections of the Georgia Historical Society* 49 (1965): 217–227.
Clark, Joseph D. "North Carolina Popular Beliefs and Superstitions." *North Carolina Folklore* 18 (1970): 1–66.
Jack, Phil R. "Folk Medicine from Western Pennsylvania." *Pennsylvania Folklife* 14(1) (October 1964): 35–37.
Levine, Harold D. "Folk Medicine in New Hampshire." *New England Journal of Medicine* 224 (1941): 487–492.
Mellinger, Marie B. "Sang Sign." *Foxfire* 2(2) (1968): 15, 47–52.
Meyer, Clarence. *American Folk Medicine.* Glenwood, IL: Meyerbooks, 1985.
Parler, Mary Celestia, and University Student Contributors. *Folk Beliefs from Arkansas.* 15 vols. Fayetteville: University of Arkansas, 1962.
Puckett, Newbell Niles. *Popular Beliefs and Superstitions: A Compendium of American Folklore from the Ohio Collection of Newbell Niles Puckett.* Edited by Wayland D. Hand, Anna Casetta, and Sondra B. Thiederman. 3 vols. Boston: G. K. Hall, 1981.
Street, Anne C. "Medicine Populaire des Isles Saint-Pierre et Miquelon." *Arts et Traditions Populaires* 7 (January–June 1959): 75–85.

# Bogbean (*Menyanthes trifoliata*)

This plant, widespread in the boggy places of the north and west of Britain and Ireland, has been valued in folk medicine as a tonic. In the Scottish Highlands an infusion of the shoots has been drunk for stomach pain, constipation, and skin complaints such as boils; the roots have been used for tuberculosis (Beith 1995: 206–207). The fresh leaves have been laid on cuts to promote healing and "draw out" infection (Beith 1995: 206). In Ireland, the plant has been highly valued not only as a tonic but also to treat kidney troubles (Allen and Hatfield, in press). In Wales it has been used for treating kidney and liver complaints, as well as treating wounds in humans and animals (Jones 1980: 59–60). In that country it has also been used particularly widely for treating rheumatism.

This plant is also native to North America, where it is known as buckbean. Its role in folk medicine has been a minor one. It has been used to soothe the stomach and as a general tonic (Meyer 1985: 59, 256). In Native American medicine it has been used for stomach pain, rheumatism, and tuberculosis (Moerman 1998: 342–343), a list strikingly similar to that for Celtic Britain.

*See also* **Boils, Constipation, Cuts, Rheumatism, Tonic, Tuberculosis, Wounds.**

### References

Allen, David E., and Gabrielle Hatfield. *Medicinal Plants in Folk Tradition.* Portland, OR: Timber Press, in press.

Beith, Mary. *Healing Threads: Traditional Medicines of the Highlands and Islands.* Edinburgh: Polygon, 1995.

Jones, Anne E. "Folk Medicine in Living Memory in Wales." *Folk Life* 18 (1980): 58–68.

Meyer, Clarence. *American Folk Medicine.* Glenwood, IL: Meyerbooks, 1985.

Moerman, Daniel E. *Native American Ethnobotany.* Portland, OR: Timber Press, 1998.

# Boils

This affliction seems to have been even more common in the recent past in Britain than it is today, and there was once a proportionately larger number of folk medical treatments for boils. In Ulster, the seventh son of a blacksmith could cure boils simply by opening and shutting tongs three times in front of the boil (Rolleston 1940: 74). In Cornwall, crawling through a loop of bramble rooted at both ends was one way of getting rid of boils. Another was to poultice the boils and then place the bandaging and poultice in the coffin of a corpse, to which the disease would be passed (Thiselton Dyer 1880: 171). Swallowing enough gunpowder to cover a sixpence, rolled into a pill with some butter, was a gypsy cure adopted in Essex (Prince 1991: 122). Nutmeg was a common treatment for boils; one suggestion was to eat ground nutmeg mixed with water (Prince 1991: 118); another version was to wear a nutmeg around the neck and nibble a bit every morning, fasting for nine days (Hawke 1973: 28).

A simple method of bringing boils to a head, used in twentieth-century Norfolk, was to fill a glass bottle with boiling water, empty it, and rapidly clamp the open end on the boil. The partial vacuum created "drew" the boil painfully but effectively (Hatfield MS). Bread poultices were widely used to treat boils (Hatfield 1994: 22). Drinking a mixture of soot and milk has been recommended for boils (EFS 111La). In Scotland, soap and sugar, or oatmeal and butter, were used to "draw" the pus from boils and infected wounds (Beith 1995: 174). In Suffolk, as recently as the twentieth century a poultice of cow-dung was used to treat boils (Rolleston 1940: 74). Herbal treatments were numerous. Among the most common were dock (*Rumex* sp.) roots or seeds, boiled, and the decoction drunk; a poultice of houseleek, or of mallow *(Malva sylvestris),* or of groundsel *(Senecio vulgaris)* and onions, either eaten or applied. Chickweed and woundwort (*Stachys sylvatica*) were also used (Hatfield 1994: 21–22). Poultices were made from both parsley and cabbage in East Anglia (Taylor MSS). Another commonly used poultice was linseed, prepared from flax (*Linum usitatissimum*) (Beith 1995: 218). Potato poultices were used in Wales (Jones 1980: 61). A large number of plants that have been used for healing infected wounds have been seen in a dual role: the lower, generally rougher, side of the leaf has been used to draw the pus, the upper side to heal the injury. This practice has been widespread throughout Britain. Examples of plants used in this way include bogbean *(Menyanthes trifoliata)* (Beith 1995: 206), madonna lily *(Lilium candidum)* (Fragments of Oxfordshire Plant Lore 1951), and plantain *(Plantago major)* (Allen and Hatfield, in press). Elder berries *(Sambucus nigra)* fried in mutton fat were a boil treatment in County Clare, Ireland (Vickery 1995: 124). A Dorset remedy was to find a place where a foot could cover seven or nine daisies *(Bellis perennis),* then pick and eat them (Rawlence 1914: 84). Other plants used in boil treatment include foxglove *(Digitalis purpurea),* figwort *(Scrophularia* sp.), burdock *(Arctium lappa),* dandelion *(Taraxacum officinale),* and comfrey *(Symphytum officinale)* (Allen and Hatfield, in press). In Gloucestershire, the buds of beech *(Fagus sylvatica)* were infused for treating boils (Palmer 1994: 122). Pineapple weed *(Matricaria discoidea)* has been used to treat boils in Wales (Plant Lore Notes and News 1999: 289). This is an unusual instance of a folk remedy of demonstrably recent origin. The plant is native to North America and was introduced to Britain in the mid-nineteenth century.

In North American folk medicine both gunpowder and nutmeg appear as frequent remedies, as in Britain. There were a number of other household remedies for treating boils. They were poulticed with salt pork, wrapped with the skin of a boiled egg, treated with cooked milk and salt, or bathed with vinegar. Among the herbal treatments used, flaxseed, elder, plantain, white lily, burdock, beech, onion, and cabbage are all familiar in British folk medicine too. In addition, poultices were made from ripe figs *(Ficus carica),* from the leaves of the dollar vine *(Rhynchosia tomentosa)* or of sea squill *(Urginea maritima),* from the bark of slip-

pery elm *(Ulmus fulva),* from black horehound *(Ballota nigra),* and from a mixture of chamomile *(Chamaemelum nobile),* yarrow *(Achillea millefolium),* and ground ivy *(Glechoma hederacea)* (Meyer 1985: 42–44). Prickly pear *(Opuntia* spp.) (Browne 1958: 380) and red oak *(Quercus rubra)* (Brown 1952–1964, 66: 132) were other plants widely used in boil treatment.

Some plant preparations were thought to prevent boils developing. These include burdock *(Arctium* sp.), sassafras *(Sassafras albidum),* St. John's wort *(Hypericum perforatum),* nutmeg *(Myristica fragrans),* horseradish *(Armoracia rusticana),* cone flower *(Echinacea angustifolia),* yellow dock *(Rumex crispus),* birch tree bark *(Betula* sp.), and boneset *(Eupatorium perfoliatum)* (Meyer 1985: 44).

In Native American practice, some of these same plants were used in the treatment of boils. Burdock *(Arctium minus),* for example, was used by the Micmac (Chandler, Freeman and Hooper 1979: 55). One species of cone flower *(Echinacea pallida)* was mixed with skunk oil and puffball spores and applied to boils by the Cheyenne (Hart 1992: 38), and slippery elm *(Ulmus rubra)* bark was used by the Potawatomi (Smith 1933: 86).

*See also* **Blackberry, Chickweed, Elder, Elm, Houseleek, Mallow, Seventh son, Transference.**

### References

Allen, David E., and Gabrielle Hatfield. *Medicinal Plants in Folk Tradition.* Portland, OR: Timber Press, in press.

Beith, Mary. *Healing Threads: Traditional Medicines of the Highlands and Islands.* Edinburgh: Polygon, 1995.

Brown, Frank C. *Collection of North Carolina Folklore.* 7 vols. Durham, NC: Duke University Press, 1952–1964.

Browne, Ray B. *Popular Beliefs and Practices from Alabama.* Folklore Studies 9. Berkeley and Los Angeles: University of California Publications, 1958.

Chandler, R. Frank, Lois Freeman, and Shirley N. Hooper. "Herbal Remedies of the Maritime Indians." *Journal of Ethnopharmacology* 1 (1979): 49–68.

EFS. English Folklore Survey. Manuscript notes in University College London.

*Fragments of Oxfordshire Plant Lore.* Oxford and District Folklore Society. Annual record 1951.

Hart, Jeff. *Montana Native Plants and Early Peoples.* Helena: Montana Historical Society Press, 1992.

Hatfield, Gabrielle. *Country Remedies: Traditional East Anglian Plant Remedies in the Twentieth Century.* Woodbridge: Boydell, 1994.

Hawke, Kathleen (comp.). *Cornish Sayings, Superstitions and Remedies.* Redruth: Dyllanson Truran, 1973.

Jones, Anne E. "Folk Medicine in Living Memory in Wales." *Folk Life* 18 (1980): 58–68.

Meyer, Clarence. *American Folk Medicine.* Glenwood, IL: Meyerbooks, 1985.

Palmer, R. *The Folklore of Gloucestershire.* Tiverton: Westcountry Books, 1994.

*Plant Lore Notes and News,* no. 6 (1999): 289.

Prince, Dennis. *Grandmother's Cures: An A-Z of Herbal Remedies.* London: Fontana, 1991.

Rawlence, E. A. "Folk-Lore and Superstitions Still Obtaining in Dorset." *Proceedings of the Dorset Natural History and Antiquarian Field Club* 35 (1914): 81–87.

Rolleston, J. D. "Dermatology and Folk-Lore." *The British Journal of Dermatology and Syphilis* 52 (March 1940): part 2, 74–86.

Smith, Huron H. "Ethnobotany of the Forest Potawatomi Indians." *Bulletin of the Public Museum of the City of Milwaukee* 7 (1933): 1–230.

Taylor MSS. Manuscript notes of Mark R. Taylor, in Norfolk Record Office, Norwich. MS4322.

Thiselton Dyer, T. F. *English Folk-Lore.* 2nd ed. London: Bogue, 1880.

Vickery, Roy. *A Dictionary of Plant Lore.* Oxford: Oxford University Press, 1995.

# Boneset (*Eupatorium* spp.)

The species of this genus most widely used in North American folk medicine is *Eupatorium perfoliatum.* The name "boneset" is thought to refer to its use in treating "breakbone," dengue fever, common in the nineteenth century in southern North America (Crellin and Philpott 1989: 107). Agueweed is another of its country names, and as both these names suggest, its main use in folk medicine was originally for treating fevers of all kinds. Another of its names, gravel-root, implies another of its uses, to treat kidney stones and gravel. In his collection of folk medicine, Meyer includes numerous references to this plant, which was used in remedies for colic, to prevent boils; for the treatment of bronchitis, chicken pox, coughs, diarrhea, erysipelas, and headache; to "restore the tone of the stomach" after intoxication; for jaundice, renal colic, and hoarseness; and as a tonic (Meyer 1985). It was widely used for colds (Barrick 1964: 104) and chills (Brown 1952–1964, 6: 145). It was also used as both an emetic and a purgative. When gathering the herb, the leaves were pulled upward to use as an emetic, downward to use as a purgative (Lick and Brendle 1922: 86). Boneset tea was drunk for a sick headache (Browne 1958: 70) and for treating gallstones (Browne 1958: 68) and indigestion (Puckett 1981: 403). There are records of its use in treating broken bones (Dober 1956: 17).

In the nineteenth century, Millspaugh suggested that in his time it was one of the most frequently used domestic remedies, and dried bunches of it were kept in most farmhouses (Millspaugh: 1892). Perhaps its reputation for treating fevers led to experiments with treating nearly everything else. On the other hand, its uses by Native American tribes are equally diverse. It was used by them to treat fevers, colds, coughs, sore throat, snakebite, broken bones, as an emetic and a purgative (Moerman 1998: 229). It was regarded by the Mohegan as a panacea (Tantaquidgeon 1928: 265). A related species, *Eupatorium purpureum,* is known as Joe-Pye Weed, a name of disputed origin. It could have been named after an individual of that name or could be taken from the Indian word *Jopi,* meaning fever (Micheletti 1998: 63). In Native American practice *Eupatorium purpureum* has been used to treat rheumatism, gout, dropsy, and kidney and gynaecological problems, as well as colds, constipation, and burns (Moerman 1998: 230). Joe-Pye weed is not a native of Britain and does not appear in the folk records there. However, a related species, *Eupatorium cannabinum,* is a native of Britain and was used in official medicine there. Its claims as a British folk herb are tenuous. In the eighteenth century, Lightfoot (Lightfoot 1777: 464) suggested it was used for gout and dropsy by the poorer people, but no convincing records of its folk usage have been traced.

*See also* **Boils, Colic, Coughs, Diarrhea, Dropsy, Erysipelas, Gout, Gravel and stone, Headache, Jaundice, Rheumatism, Tonic.**

### References

Barrick, Mac E. "Folk Medicine in Cumberland County." *Keystone Folklore Quarterly* 9 (1964): 100–110.

Brown, Frank C. *Collection of North Carolina Folklore.* 7 vols. Durham, NC: Duke University Press, 1952–1964.

Browne, Ray B. *Popular Beliefs and Practices from Alabama.* Folklore Studies 9. Berkeley and Los Angeles: University of California Publications, 1958.

Crellin, John K., and Jane Philpott. *A Reference Guide to Medicinal Plants.* Durham, NC: Duke University Press, 1989.

Dober, Virginia. "We'll Tell 'Em." *North Carolina Folklore* 4(1) (July 1956): 15–22.

Lick, David E., and Thomas R. Brendle. "Plant Names and Plant Lore among the Pennsylvania Germans." *Proceedings and Addresses of the Pennsylvania German Society* 33 (1922).

Lightfoot, John. *Flora Scotica.* 2 vols. London: Benjamin White, 1777.

Meyer, Clarence. *American Folk Medicine.* Glenwood, IL: Meyerbooks, 1985.

Micheletti, Enza (ed.). *North American Folk Healing: An A-Z Guide to Traditional Remedies.* New York and Montreal: Reader's Digest Association, 1998.

Millspaugh, Charles F. *American Medicinal Plants: An Illustrated and Descriptive Guide to Plants Indigenous to and Naturalized in the United States Which Are Used in Medicine.* 1892. Reprint, New York: Dover, 1974.

Moerman, Daniel E. *Native American Ethnobotany.* Portland, OR: Timber Press, 1998.

Puckett, Newbell Niles. *Popular Beliefs and Superstitions: A Compendium of American Folklore from the Ohio Collection of Newbell Niles Puckett.* Edited by Wayland D. Hand, Anna Casetta, and Sondra B. Thiederman. 3 vols. Boston: G. K. Hall, 1981.

Tantaquidgeon, Gladys. "Mohegan Medicinal Practices, Weather-Lore and Superstitions." *Smithsonian Institution-Bureau of American Ethnology Annual Report* 43 (1928): 264–270.

## Bread

Bread poultices have been much used in British folk medicine for swellings, boils, and sprains and for removing splinters (Prince 1991: 15, 52). Boiled bread and milk poultices were used for sore eyes (EFS 100Db). In East Anglia, so-called Good Friday bread was kept for first-aid purposes throughout the year. Baked on Good Friday, it had the reputation of healing any slight injury and was also considered good for fevers as well as indigestion, diarrhea and dysentery (Thiselton Dyer 1876: 149). Hot cross buns, again if baked on Good Friday, were similarly thought to bring good luck and were kept for many years, small pieces being grated off when needed for medicinal use (Porter 1974: 29). One nineteenth-century remedy prescribed burying a piece of bread in earth for three days. It was then dug up and given to a sufferer from whooping cough (Radford and Radford 1974: 66). Moldy bread has also been used for treating infected cuts and for preventing infection (Foster 1951: 62).

In North American folk medicine, bread poultices were similarly used. To "draw out" infection, a poultice of bread and milk was recommended (Brown 1952–1964, 6: 225). A similar poultice was used for treating boils (Koch 1980: 72), smallpox (Lathrop 1961: 14) and sore eyes (Hyatt 1965: 242). Bread dough has been used to treat sunburn (Levenson and Levenson 1960: 27), and a paste of chewed white bread has been used to treat a sty (UCLA Folklore Archives 4_5506), while as in Britain, wet bread has been used to poultice a splinter (UCLA Folklore Archives 5_6470). For diarrhea, the water in which burned bread has soaked has been given (UCLA Folklore Archives 4_6284). Moldy rye bread has treated sores (Puckett 1981: 449), while bread made from ground corn shucks has been a remedy for measles (Anderson 1970: 51). A remedy for whooping cough was for the parents each to have some bread, then give some to the child: however, the cure only worked in families where the parents shared the same surname (Puckett 1981: 121).

Bread has been widely used as a medium for transferring disease, as in the cure for toothache in which one gives a child a crust that a mouse has nibbled (Wintemberg 1899: 48). Numerous warts cures also employ bread as an agent of transference.

*See also* **Boils, Diarrhea, Dysentery, Eye problems, Indigestion, Molds, Smallpox, Sunburn, Transference, Warts.**

## References

Anderson, John. *Texas Folk Medicine.* Austin, TX: Encino Press, 1970.

Brown, Frank C. *Collection of North Carolina Folklore.* 7 vols. Durham, NC: Duke University Press, 1952–1964.

EFS. English Folklore Survey. Manuscript notes at University College London.

Foster, Jeanne Cooper. *Ulster Folklore.* Belfast: H. R. Carter, 1951.

Hyatt, Harry Middleton. *Folklore from Adams County Illinois.* 2nd rev. ed. New York: Memoirs of the Alma Egan Hyatt Foundation, 1965.

Koch, William E. *Folklore from Kansas: Beliefs and Customs.* Lawrence, KS: Regent Press, 1980.

Lathrop, Amy. "Pioneer Remedies from Western Kansas." *Western Folklore* 20 (1961): 1–22.

Levenson, Beverly, and Myron H. Levenson. "Some Southern Folk Remedies and Related Beliefs." *North Carolina Folklore* 8(2) (1960): 26–31.

Porter, Enid. *The Folklore of East Anglia.* London: Batsford, 1974.

Prince, Dennis. *Grandmother's Cures: An A-Z of Herbal Remedies.* London: Fontana, 1991.

Puckett, Newbell Niles. *Popular Beliefs and Superstitions: A Compendium of American Folklore from the Ohio Collection of Newbell Niles Puckett.* Edited by Wayland D. Hand, Anna Casetta, and Sondra B. Thiederman. 3 vols. Boston: G. K. Hall, 1981.

Radford, E., and M. A. Radford. *Encyclopaedia of Superstitions.* Edited and revised by Christina Hole. London: Book Club Associates 1974.

Thiselton Dyer, T. F. *British Popular Customs, Present and Past.* London, 1876.

Wintemberg, W. J. "Items of German-Canadian Folklore." *Journal of American Folklore* 12 (1899): 45–86.

# Breast problems

The embarrassment surrounding this subject, together with the fact that the majority of books are written by men, has led to a scarcity of written information concerning folk medicine in this field, at least in Britain. Advice concerning breast feeding was handed down orally, and once official medicine took over antenatal and postnatal care, much of this oral tradition was lost. There are occasional clues—for instance, in the names of plants. Two Gaelic names for

*Lapsana communis* translate as "good leaf" and "breast leaf"; the plant was used in the Scottish Highlands for sore nipples in nursing mothers (MacFarlane 1929: 1–48). Parkinson learned of a similar use in Prussia (Britten and Holland 1878–1886: 354) and coined the English name of "nipplewort" for the plant. In Ireland the heath speedwell *(Veronica officinalis),* again judging by its Gaelic name, was used similarly (Moloney: 1919).

For treating breast abscesses, a large warmed cabbage leaf, with the main vein removed, has been used in England within living memory (Hatfield MS). To dry up the milk supply at weaning, there is a record from the Forest of Dean of the large leaves of foxglove *(Digitalis purpurea)* being used to poultice the breasts (Hatfield MS). Swollen breasts were treated in the Scottish Highlands with a poultice of groundsel *(Senecio vulgaris)* or with the roots of celandine *(Chelidonium majus),* applied under the armpits. A hot compress of peppermint leaves *(Mentha* sp.*)* was used in Somerset (Tongue 1965: 41). A less attractive remedy for swollen and engorged breasts was to poultice them with fresh cowdung (Beith 1995: 210, 221, 172).

In the Western Isles of Scotland, a broth made from limpets was used to increase the milk supply in poorly nourished nursing mothers (Martin 1716: 146). In both the Highlands of Scotland and in Wales there are records of limpet shells being collected and used as nipple shields for nursing mothers (Jones 1980: 63). Their name in Caernarvonshire translates as "breast shell." These shells can often be found with a circular hole; failing this, the center was knocked out.

Books on midwifery, such as Jane Sharp's book (Sharp 1724), contain a large number of prescriptions for increasing the milk supply; whether these can really be regarded as folk medicine in Britain is doubtful, but printed sources such as these doubtless were

used by European settlers in North America and became a part of folk medicine there.

An account is on record of a woman taken captive shortly after giving birth by Canadian Indians in the seventeenth century. Her newborn baby's life was saved by ice-cold water from a brook, a broth made from beaver entrails, and finally by a friendly squaw who showed her how to make a nourishing broth with walnut kernels and fine cornmeal (Ulrich 1991: 231).

Poultices of cow dung were used, as in Britain, to treat inflamed breasts (Black 1935: 99). For engorged breasts it was recommended to let a puppy suckle (Puckett 1981: 124). The skin of either a mole (Hyatt 1965: 154) or a weasel (Waugh 1918: 22) has been placed over the breast to relieve "caked" breasts. Poulticing the breast with clay was an alternative (Hyatt 1965: 154), as was poulticing with cornstarch (Lathrop 1961: 6). Massaging the caked breasts with goat's milk was also tried (Hyatt 1965: 154). There was a belief that placing a broad axe under the mother's bed was a remedy for caked breasts (Rogers 1941: 41). Sore nipples at the time of delivery were sometimes relieved by rubbing with the afterbirth (Hyatt 1965: 154).

For sore and swollen breasts, poultices were made from hot pancakes, or baked potatoes, roasted turnips, whisky and soap, chamomile *(Chamaemelum nobile),* mallows *(Malva* sp.*),* peach leaves *(Prunus persica)* or wild indigo *(Baptisia* sp.*).* An ointment made from elderflowers *(Sambucus canadensis)* fried in lard was also used. For treating sore nipples, clear molasses was recommended, or brandy and water, starch powder, or mutton tallow. Herbal salves for sore nipples were prepared from bayberry *(Myrica* sp.*),* comfrey *(Symphytum officinale),* quince seed *(Cydonia oblonga),* and false bittersweet *(Celastrus scandens).* An application of fir balsam *(Abies* sp.*)* or of the oil from butternuts *(Juglans cinerea)* has also been used (Meyer 1985: 46–50). Herbal

applications for caked breasts included jimson weed (*Datura stramonium*) (Browne
1958: 42) and tobacco (Free 1962: 10). To
relieve sore or inflamed breasts during nursing, collard leaves were sometimes used
(reminiscent of the cabbage leaf remedy in
Britain) (Parler 1962: 65), an ointment
made from male fern buds (*Dryopteris filix-
mas*) (Fosbroke 1835: 165), or a poultice
made from queen-of-the-meadow roots
(*Eupatorium purpureum*) (Jack 1964: 36).

In North American folk medicine a
number of herbs were used to increase milk
supply, such as fennel (*Foeniculum vulgare*),
anise seeds (*Pimpinella anisum*), and rosemary (*Rosmarinus officinalis*), all of which
appear in Sharp's Manual of Midwifery
mentioned above, as well as the plant
named squaw weed (*Senecio aureus*): the last
named clearly borrowed from the Native
American tradition. A gruel made from
powdered mulberry twigs (*Morus* sp.) was
thought to boost milk production (Bourke
1849: 123). Another recommendation was
to scrape elm bark (*Ulmus* sp.) upward on
the east side of the tree and drink an infusion of the scrapings (Marie-Ursule 1951:
177).

To dry up the milk supply at weaning
sage tea (*Salvia* sp.) was given, or an ointment made from smartweed (*Polygonum*
sp.) was applied, or the fresh leaves of tag
alder (*Alnus serrulata*) were bruised and applied, the latter a remedy said to be of Native American origin (Meyer 1985: 47).
Another suggestion was to rub the breasts
with soot for three days (Hyatt 1965: 156).

For helping breast development at puberty, there are a number of herbal suggestions, including goat's rue (*Galega
officinalis*) (Meyer 1985: 46), bananas
(*Musa* spp.) (UCLA Folklore Archives
3_5664), and rubbing with cocoa butter
(UCLA Folklore Archives 4_5664). For
sore, tender breasts during puberty, drinking an infusion of pigweed (*Amaranthus*

sp.) or the juice from milkweed (*Asclepias*
sp.) was recommended in Ontario (UCLA
Folklore Archives 12_6187). Rubbing with
camphor and cabbage leaves was believed to
shrink breasts that are too large (UCLA
Folklore Archives 2_5972).

In Native American medicine, the
downy white pea (*Galactia volubilis*) was
used by the Seminole to treat babies who
were unwilling to suckle (Sturtevant 1955:
255). Various plants were used to increase
the mother's milk supply; for instance, *Betula papyrifera* was used by the Woodlands
Cree (Leighton 1985: 32) and skeleton-
plant (*Lygodesmia juncea*) by the Cheyenne
(Grinnell 1905: 41). Various species of lettuce are used to ease lactation—for example, *Lactuca biennis*, used by the Ojibwa
(Smith 1932: 364). *Salix tristis* was used to
prepare a wash for sore nipples (Vogel
1970: 55). Red baneberry (*Actaea rubra*)
and puffball poultices (*Lycoperdon* sp.), or a
preparation of elder roots (*Sambucus* sp.)
were used to relieve sore and inflamed
breasts (Vogel 1970: 235, 301). Reputedly
a live duck or goose cut open was sometimes applied to inflamed breasts (Hyatt
1965: 154).

From Alabama, the belief has been reported that holding a live mole above one's
head for an hour will cure sore breasts
(Browne 1958: 42).

*See also* **Jimson weed, Poultice, Puffball.**

## References
Beith, Mary. *Healing Threads: Traditional Medicines of the Highlands and Islands.* Edinburgh: Polygon, 1995.
Black, Pauline Monette. *Nebraska Folk Cures.*
University of Nebraska Studies in Language, Literature, and Criticism 15. Lincoln, NE: University of Nebraska Press,
1935.
Bourke, John G. "Popular Medicine, Customs
and Superstitions of the Rio Grande." *Journal of American Folklore* 7 (1849): 119–146.
Britten, James, and Holland, Robert. *A Dictionary*

*of English Plant Names.* London: Trübner for English Dialect Society, 1878–1886.

Browne, Ray B. *Popular Beliefs and Practices from Alabama.* Folklore Studies 9. Berkeley and Los Angeles: University of California Publications, 1958.

Fosbroke, John, M.D. "On the Effects of Male Fern Buds, in Cases of Worms." *Boston Medical and Surgical Journal* 13(11) (1835): 165–168.

Free, William Joseph. "A Note on Tobacco Magic." *North Carolina Folklore* 10 (1962): 2, 9–10.

Grinnell, George Bird. "Some Cheyenne Plant Medicines." *American Anthropologist* 7 (1905): 37–43.

Hyatt, Harry Middleton. *Folklore from Adams County Illinois.* 2nd rev. ed. New York: Memoirs of the Alma Egan Hyatt Foundation, 1965.

Jack, Phil R. "Folk Medicine from Western Pennsylvania." *Pennsylvania Folklife* 14(1) (October 1964): 35–37.

Jones, Anne E. "Folk Medicine in Living Memory in Wales." *Folk Life* 18 (1980): 58–68.

Lathrop, Amy. "Pioneer Remedies from Western Kansas." *Western Folklore* 20 (1961): 1–22.

Leighton, Anna L. *Wild Plant Uses by the Woods Cree (Nihithawak) of East-Central Saskatchewan.* Mercury Series 101. Ottawa: National Museums of Canada, 1985.

MacFarlane, A. M. "Gaelic Names of Plants: Study of their Uses and Lore." *Transactions of the Gaelic Society of Inverness* 32 (1929): 1–48.

Marie-Ursule, Soeur. "Civilisation traditionelle des Lavalois." *Les Archives de Folklore* 5–6 (1951): 1–403.

Martin, M. *A Description of the Western Islands of Scotland.* 2nd ed. London, 1716 (facsimile, James Thin 1976).

Meyer, Clarence. *American Folk Medicine.* Glenwood, IL: Meyerbooks, 1985.

Moloney, Michael F. *Irish Ethnobotany and the Evolution of Medicine in Ireland.* Dublin: M. H. Gill and Son, 1919.

Parler, Mary Celestia, and University Student Contributors. *Folk Beliefs from Arkansas.* Vol. 3. Fayetteville: University of Arkansas, 1962.

Puckett, Newbell Niles. *Popular Belief and Superstitions: A Compendium of American Folklore from the Ohio Collection of Newbell Niles Puckett.* Edited by Wayland D. Hand, Anna Casetta, Sondra B. Thiederman. 3 vols. Boston: G. K. Hall, 1981.

Rogers, E. G. *Early Folk Medical Practices in Tennessee.* Murfreesboro, TN: Mid-South, 1941.

Sharp, Jane. *The Compleat Midwife's Companion.* London, 1724.

Smith, Huron H. "Ethnobotany of the Ojibwe Indians." *Bulletin of the Public Museum of Milwaukee* 4 (1932): 327–525.

Sturtevant, William Curtis. *The Mikasuki Seminole: Medical Beliefs and Practices.* Ph.D. thesis, Yale University, New Haven, Connecticut. Ann Arbor, MI: University Microfilms, 1955.

Tongue, Ruth L. *Somerset Folklore.* In *County Folklore,* edited by K.M. Briggs. Vol. 8. London: Folk-Lore Society, 1965.

Ulrich, Laurel Thatcher. *Good Wives: Image and Reality in the Lives of Women in Northern New England 1650–1750.* New York: Vintage Books, 1991.

Vogel, Virgil J. *American Indian Medicine.* Norman: University of Oklahoma Press, 1970.

Waugh, F. W. "Canadian Folk-Lore from Ontario." *Journal of American Folklore* 31 (1918): 4–82.

# Bruises

In British folk medicine there were a number of first-aid measures for bruising. Cold water or a cold compress has often been used. In Wales, a poultice of vinegar was employed (Jones 1980: 66). A slice of raw potato was applied to a black eye in the Scottish Highlands (Beith 1995: 235). Other plant remedies used have included black bryony *(Tamus communis)* (Bromfield 1856), yellow-horned poppy *Glaucium flavum* (one country name for which is brusewort, another being "squatmore"—"squat" in west country dialect means bruise) (Aubrey 1881: 254), soapwort *Saponaria officinalis* (Vesey-Fitzgerald 1944: 28), comfrey *(Symphytum officinale)* (EFS Card Index No. 277), and kidney vetch *(Anthyllis vulneraria)* (Beith 1995: 247). Solomon's seal *(Polygonatum multiflorum)* was used both in official medicine (it was recommended by Gerard in his sixteenth-century herbal) and in folk medicine to treat bruising (Porter 1974: 43). Crushed mallow leaves (*Malva* spp.) have been used to treat bruising (Hawke 1973: 28). Crab-apple juice has been used to treat bruises (Emerson 1887). Rubbing with a raw onion *(Allium cepa)* was recently reported from Manchester as a cure for bruises (Vickery 1995: 267). Lily leaves steeped in brandy, a cure widely used in England for treating cuts, has also been applied to bruises (Allen 1995: 45). In recent times, arnica *(Arnica montana)* has been widely used. This is not native to Britain, but its fame in treating bruises has spread from continental Europe, and it is now a worldwide remedy (Souter 1995: 141).

In North American folk medicine, first aid for bruises included application of cold metal, such as the flat surface of a knife (Koch 1980: 132). Epsom salts have been used (Cannon 1984: 96), or a poultice made from soap (Frazier 1936: 34). Eggs have been used to treat bruising (McGlasson 1941: 17). Animal fat in various forms has also been used: unsalted butter (Koch 1980: 133), raw pork (UCLA Folklore Archives 1_5495), or hog's grease (Beck 1957: 77). Unwashed sheep's wool (which contains lanolin) has similarly been used (UCLA Folklore Archives 5_5578). In a curious example of transference, stone bruises have been treated by placing them in contact with a live toad (Brewster 1939: 39) or frog (Farr 1935: 34). As the animal dies, the bruise disappears. Cutting the turf from around a bruised foot and reversing the turf, soil upward, is an unusual remedy suggested from Virginia. As the grass dies, the bruise will heal (UCLA Folklore Archives 25_5495). Other miscellaneous cures for bruising include human urine (UCLA Folklore Archives 12_6188), wood ashes (Puckett 1981: 332), and rendered jellyfish (Bergen 1899: no. 828). Cow manure has been used as a poultice for bruising (UCLA Folklore Archives 6_5295).

Plant remedies for bruises used in North American folk medicine are numerous. Green tobacco leaves have been used (Clark 1970: 19), or tansy leaves bruised in vinegar (Bergen 1899: 1323). A salve has been prepared from self-heal *(Prunella vulgaris)* (Lick and Brendle 1922: 63) or from the stalk of evening primrose *(Oenothera biennis)* (Lick and Brendle 1922: 155). Crushed plantain leaves (*Plantago* sp.) have been used (Matschat 1938: 88), or a poultice made from wheat bran (Frazier 1936: 34) or from the inner bark of black oak (*Quercus* sp.) (Randolph 1947: 100), or from sumac bark (*Rhus* sp.) and wheat bran (Browne 1958: 104). A poultice of cornmeal and salt has been used (Wilson 1968: 61). Other plant remedies include witch hazel bark *(Hamamelis virginica)* (Wintemberg 1925: 621), or the bark of slippery elm *(Ulmus rubra)* (McGlasson 1941: 17) or of elder (*Sambucus* sp.) (Fogel 1915: 131). Poultices have been prepared from prickly pear (Michael and Barrow 1967: 781), from the leaves of mullein *(Verbascum thapsus)* (Clark 1970: 14), or of peach (Browne 1958: 43), or of wild sage (UCLA Folklore Archives 24_6746) or burdock (Puckett 1981: 454). A lotion prepared from daisies *(?Bellis perennis)* was reputedly used by colonists to treat bruising (Kell 1956: 371). Arnica is native to North America and both has been and continues to be used to treat bruises (Peattie 1943: 118). Not only the species *Arnica montana* but also *Arnica fulgens* is used in this way (Chevallier 1996: 170). As in Britain, both raw onion (Koch 1980: 133) and raw potato (Waller and Killion 1972: 76), as well as white lily steeped in whisky (Lick and Brendle 1922: 97), have been used in treatment of bruises. A

Mexican American remedy is to apply the juice of Aloe vera (UCLA Folklore Archives 14_5592). Balm of Gilead has been used to cure bruising (Beck 1957: 78). Pine tar has been applied to bruises (Wilson 1968: 324). The Jack and Jill remedy of vinegar and brown paper has also been employed in recent times for bruising (Wilson Sr. 1968: 79). Interestingly, brown paper used to be made from pine wood; vinegar would extract some of the pine tar (Howkins, pers. com., 2001). Poultices have been prepared from turpentine and sugar (UCLA Folklore Archives 4_5300), or from a mixture of turpentine, coal oil, camphor, gum, and lard (Trice 1956: 91). Finally, eating radishes is held to prevent bruising (UCLA Folklore Archives 9_5303).

In Native American treatment of bruises, spermaceti, from stranded whales, was used in the seventeenth century, as was sassafras ointment. The root of sunflower (*Helianthus* sp.) or of jimson weed was also used (Vogel 1970: 42, 83, 230). In eastern Canada, ground hemlock (*Taxus* sp.) was used to treat bruising (MacDonald 1959: 223). Many of the plants mentioned above were also used in Native American practice, such as arnica, self-heal (Hamel and Chiltoskey 1975: 54, 58), and witch hazel (Herrick 1977: 347), as well as various species of pine (e.g., Pinus virginiana [Hamel and Chiltoskey 1975: 49]) and of sumac (Herrick 1977: 372).

*See also* **Aloe vera, Balm of Gilead, Burdock, Earth, Elm, Jimson weed, Mullein, Sassafras, Thornapple, Tobacco, Transference.**

## References

Allen, Andrew. *A Dictionary of Sussex Folk Medicine.* Newbury: Countryside Books, 1995.

Aubrey, John. *Remaines of Gentilisme and Judaisme.* Edited by James Britten. London, 1881.

Beck, Horace P. *The Folklore of Maine.* Philadelphia and New York: J.B. Lippincott, 1957.

Beith, Mary. *Healing Threads: Traditional Medicines of the Highlands and Islands.* Edinburgh: Polygon, 1995.

Bergen, Fanny D. "Animal and Plant Lore Collected from the Oral Tradition of English Speaking Folk." *Memoirs of the American Folk-Lore Society* 7 (1899).

Brewster, Paul G. "Folk Cures and Preventives from Southern Indiana." *Southern Folklore Quarterly* 3 (1939): 33–43.

Bromfield, William Arthur. *Flora Vectensis.* Edited by Sir William Jackson Hooker and Thomas Bell Salter. London: Pamplin, 1856.

Browne, Ray B. *Popular Beliefs and Practices from Alabama.* Folklore Studies 9. Berkeley and Los Angeles: University of California Publications, 1958.

Cannon, Anthon S. *Popular Beliefs and Superstitions from Utah.* Edited by Wayland D. Hand and Jeannine E. Talley. Salt Lake City: University of Utah Press, 1984.

Chevallier, Andrew. *The Encyclopedia of Medicinal Plants.* London: Dorling Kindersley, 1996.

Clark, Joseph D. "North Carolina Popular Beliefs and Superstitions." *North Carolina Folklore* 18 (1970): 1–66.

EFS. English Folklore Survey. Manuscript notes at University College London.

Emerson, P. H. *Pictures of East Anglian Life.* London: Sampson Low, 1887.

Farr, T. J. "Riddles and Superstitions of Middle Tennessee." *Journal of American Folklore* 48 (1935): 318–336.

Fogel, Edwin Miller. "Beliefs and Superstitions of the Pennsylvania Germans." *Americana Germanica* 18 (1915).

Frazier, Neal. "A Collection of Middle Tennessee Superstitions." *Tennessee Folklore Society Bulletin* 2 (1936): 33–48.

Hamel, Paul B., and Mary U. Chiltoskey. *Cherokee Plants and Their Uses: A 400 Year History.* Sylva, NC: Herald, 1975.

Hawke, Kathleen. *Cornish Sayings, Superstitions and Remedies.* Redruth: Dyllanson Truro, 1973.

Herrick, James William. *Iroquois Medical Botany.* Ph.D. thesis, State University of New York, Albany, 1977.

Jones, Anne E. "Folk Medicine in Living Memory in Wales." *Folk Life* 18 (1980): 58–68.

Kell, Katherine T. "The Folklore of the Daisy."

*Journal of American Folklore* 69 (1956): 369–376.

Koch, William E. *Folklore from Kansas: Beliefs and Customs.* Lawrence, KS: Regent Press, 1980.

Lick, David E., and Thomas R. Brendle. "Plant Names and Plant Lore among the Pennsylvania Germans." *Proceedings and Addresses of the Pennsylvania German Society* 33 (1922).

MacDonald, Elizabeth. "Indian Medicine in New Brunswick." *Canadian Medical Association Journal* 80(3) (1959): 220–224.

Matschat, Cecile Hulse. *Suwannee River* (Rivers of America). New York: Rinehart and Company, 1938.

McGlasson, Cleo. "Superstitions and Folk Beliefs of Overton County Tennessee." *Folklore Society Bulletin* 7 (1941): 13–27.

Michael, Max, Jr., and Mark V. Barrow. "'Old Timey' Remedies of Yesterday and Today." *Journal of the Florida Medical Association* 54(8) (August 1967): 778–784.

Peattie, Roderick (ed.). *The Great Smokies and the Blue Ridge.* New York: Vanguard Press, 1943.

Porter, Enid. *The Folklore of East Anglia.* London: Batsford, 1974.

Puckett, Newbell Niles. *Popular Beliefs and Superstitions: A Compendium of American Folklore from the Ohio Collection of Newbell Niles Puckett.* Edited by Wayland D. Hand, Anna Casetta, and Sondra B. Thiederman. 3 vols. Boston: G. K. Hall, 1981.

Randolph, Vance. *Ozark Superstitions.* New York: Columbia University Press, 1947.

Souter, Keith. *Cure Craft: Traditional Folk Remedies and Treatment from Antiquity to the Present Day.* Saffron Walden: C. W. Daniel, 1995.

Trice, Henry L. "The Lore of the Hopkins-Webster Line." *Kentucky Folklore Record* 2 (1956): 91–97.

Vesey-Fitzgerald, B. "Gypsy Medicine." *Journal of the Gypsy Lore Society* 23 (1944): 21–33.

Vickery, Roy. *A Dictionary of Plant Lore.* Oxford: Oxford University Press, 1995.

Vogel, Virgil J. *American Indian Medicine.* Norman: University of Oklahoma Press, 1970.

Waller, Tom, and Gene Killion. "Georgia Folk Medicine." *Southern Folklore Quarterly* 36 (1972): 71–92.

Wilson, Gordon, Sr. *Folklore of the Mammoth Cave Region.* Kentucky Folklore Series 4. Bowling Green, KY: Kentucky Folklore Society, 1968.

Wilson, Gordon. "Local Plants in Folk Remedies in the Mammoth Cave Region." *Southern Folklore Quarterly* 32 (1968): 320–327.

———. "'Store-Bought' Remedies in the Mammoth Cave Region." *North Carolina Folklore* 16 (1968): 58–62.

Wintemberg, W. J. "Some Items of Negro-Canadian Folk-Lore." *Journal of American Folklore* 38 (1925): 621.

# Bryony *(Bryonia dioica)*

This plant has had a role in magical medicine and in purely practical folk medicine too. The plant is poisonous, and most remedies employ it externally, as in the remedy from Essex for chilblains, which uses the crushed berries rubbed on. For rheumatism the roots were scraped and applied (Pratt 1898, 1: 70), or a piece was carried in the pocket (Taylor 1929: 117). Its roots were made into a tea for promoting fertility (Porter 1974: 21)—a remedy where the plant was being used as a native substitute for mandrake, with its associated aphrodisiac and magical powers. It has been the subject of "gender pairing," being regarded as the female plant of a pair, with the in fact unrelated black bryony *(Tamus communis)* as the male. This notion occurs in British folk medicine for a number of species, but in this instance the idea was reinforced by the official herbals. The plant is not native to North America and does not have a significant role there in folk medicine.

*See also* **Chilblains, Mandrake.**

### References
Porter, Enid. *The Folklore of East Anglia.* London: Batsford, 1974.

Pratt, A. *Wild Flowers.* 2 vols. London: Society for Promoting Christian Knowledge, 1898.

Taylor, Mark R. Norfolk Folklore. *Folk-Lore* 40 (1929): 113–133.

# Burdock (*Arctium lappa, Arctium minus*)

Native to Britain and Ireland, this plant has been extensively used in folk medicine as a tonic and a "blood purifier." Specifically, it has been used for treating skin complaints such as boils and acne, and for the treatment of rheumatism (Deane and Shaw 1975). The seeds were carried by gypsies as an amulet against rheumatism (Vesey-Fitzgerald, 1944: 23). In addition, the plant has been used to treat a wide and miscellaneous group of ailments, including urinary complaints (Johnston 1853: 129) and nervous disorders (Johnson 1862), as well as burns (McClafferty 1979).

The plant was introduced into North America and has been used very similarly there. It formed an ingredient of many preparations for treating rheumatism, being combined, for example, with dandelion and Virginia snakeroot (*Aristolochia serpentaria*) or with white pine bark and seneca snakeroot (*Polygala senega*) (Meyer 1985: 213, 216). Meyer reports its use in the treatment of boils, and, combined with dandelion, as a liver tonic (Meyer 1985: 44, 167). The mashed fresh leaves have been used to treat burns (Meyer 1985: 54). For diarrhea in babies, the seed or the root has been mixed with yeast and bandaged on to the navel (Meyer 1985: 90), and for severe dysentery in adults the seeds have been ground and infused like coffee (Meyer 1985: 97). A large leaf with the rough veins removed was warmed on a shovel and rolled up to fit in the hollow of a sore foot (Meyer 1985: 120). Mixed with white mustard, horseradish and cider the seed was used for treating headache (Meyer 1985: 137). An infusion of the seed treated sleeplessness and teething in infants (Meyer 1985: 146, 249), while a stronger decoction of the seed treated kidney pain (Meyer 1985: 159) and neuralgia (Meyer 1985: 186), as well as asthma (Puckett 1981: 311). The leaves were applied to piles (Meyer 1985: 193) and were worn in the hat to prevent sunstroke (Wilson 1968: 199) and for headache (Lick and Brendle 1922: 124). The root boiled in vinegar was used as a wash for ringworm (Meyer 1985: 221). For warts, the leaf was rubbed on and then buried; as it decayed, the wart would go (UCLA Folklore Archives 20_5521). Quinsy was treated with burdock (Browne 1958: 87). A teething necklace was made from pieces of burdock root. These varied and extensive uses of burdock in North America are perhaps surprising in view of the fact that neither species is native there. However, similar uses have been recorded among Native Americans. The species *Arctium lappa* has been used to treat rheumatism (Hamel and Chiltoskey 1975: 27). *Arctium minus* has been used as a tonic (Smith 1933: 49) for the relief of pain (Tantaquidgeon 1942: 66, 82) and for the treatment of boils (Herrick 1977: 474). For other Native American uses of burdock, see Moerman 1998: 84–85.

*See also* **Acne, Amulet, Asthma, Boils, Burns, Dandelion, Headache, Piles, Quinsy, Rheumatism, Teething, Tonic, Warts.**

## References

Browne, Ray B. *Popular Beliefs and Practices from Alabama.* Folklore Studies 9. Berkeley and Los Angeles: University of California Publications, 1958.

Deane, Tony, and Tony Shaw. *The Folklore of Cornwall.* London: Batsford, 1975.

Hamel, Paul B., and Mary U. Chiltoskey. *Cherokee Plants and Their Uses: A 400 Year History.* Sylva, NC: Herald, 1975.

Herrick, James William. *Iroquois Medical Botany.* Ph.D. thesis, State University of New York, Albany, 1977.

Johnson, C. Pierpoint. *The Useful Plants of Great Britain: A Treatise.* London: William Kent, 1862.

Johnston, George. *The Natural History of the East-*

*ern Borders.* Vol. 1, *The Botany.* London: Van Voorst, 1853.

Lick, David E., and Thomas R. Brendle. "Plant Names and Plant Lore among the Pennsylvania Germans." *Proceedings and Addresses of the Pennsylvania German Society* 33 (1922).

McClafferty, George. *The Folk Medicine of Co. Wicklow.* Master's thesis, National University of Ireland, 1979.

Meyer, Clarence. *American Folk Medicine.* Glenwood, IL: Meyerbooks, 1985.

Moerman, Daniel E. *Native American Ethnobotany.* Portland, OR: Timber Press, 1998.

Puckett, Newbell Niles. *Popular Beliefs and Superstitions: A Compendium of American Folklore from the Ohio Collection of Newbell Niles Puckett.* Edited by Wayland D. Hand, Anna Casetta, and Sondra B. Thiederman. 3 vols. Boston: G. K. Hall, 1981.

Smith, Huron H. "Ethnobotany of the Forest Potawatomi Indians." *Bulletin of the Public Museum of the City of Milwaukee* 7 (1933): 1–230.

Tantaquidgeon, Gladys. *A Study of Delaware Indian Medicine Practice and Folk Beliefs.* Harrisburg: Pennsylvania Historical Commission, 1942.

Vesey-Fitzgerald, B. "Gypsy Medicine." *Journal of the Gypsy Lore Society* 23 (1944): 21–33.

Wilson, Gordon, Sr. *Folklore of the Mammoth Cave Region.* Kentucky Folklore Series 4. Bowling Green, KY: Kentucky Folklore Society, 1968.

# Burns

There seems to have been a widespread tradition throughout Britain that certain individuals could cure burns. In Scotland a belief existed that anyone licking the liver of a newly killed otter would receive the power to soothe burns by licking them (Beith 1995: 180–181). In Ireland it was suggested that licking a newt conferred the same power (Jones 1908: 317). Various charms were recited to draw the fire out of a burn (Black 1883: 80–81). Sometimes they accompanied a healing ointment (Porter 1974: 44–45). In Worcestershire it is

reported that a cure for a burned finger was to keep it secret, spit on it, and press it behind the left ear (Black 1883: 189). It is a reflection of the importance of immediate treatment for burns that a very wide variety of mineral, plant, and animal products have been used in folk medicine. Cold water is one of the simplest treatments, still used for minor burns. In Norfolk, the water from melted snow was particularly recommended (Mundford Primary School project 1980, unpub.).

In Britain native plants used include alder. The leaves were lightly crushed and placed on the burn (Hatfield 1994: 23). Chickweed was used for burn treatment in Scotland (Vickery 1995: 65), and so was ivy *(Hedera helix).* The leaves were crushed with vinegar and olive oil and applied to the burn (Hatfield 1994: 24). The leaves of elder were crushed in an ointment for burns, used particularly in Scotland (Beith 1995: 215) and Ireland (Allen and Hatfield, in press). Primrose *(Primula vulgaris)* leaves crushed in oil were used to treat burns in Norfolk (Taylor 1929: 118). Hart's-tongue fern *(Phyllitis scolopendrium)* was also made into a burn ointment in Scotland (Beith 1995: 216). An ointment made from marshmallow *(Malva* sp.) was used in the Cambridgeshire fens (Porter 1974: 44), and in Somerset a burn was crossed with spittle, and then mallow leaves were laid on (Tongue 1965: 37). In that same county, a burn ointment was prepared from fat and St. John's wort (Tongue 1965: 38). In Ireland, the boiled bark of elm was used to treat burns (Vickery 1995: 127). Houseleek and navelwort *(Umbilicus rupestris)* were both widely used in the treatment of burns (Allen and Hatfield, in press). Plantain leaves were used in burn treatment in England, Scotland and Ireland (Allen and Hatfield, in press). Blackberry leaves were used for treating burns, for instance in Cornwall (Hunt 1871: 413). A particularly interesting burn remedy has been recorded from

Norfolk. It involves boiling the prickly fruit of thornapple in pork fat to make a salve. The self-same remedy is recorded by Gerard in his herbal of 1597, where the author tells us that he had learned the remedy from a lady in Ipswich, Suffolk. Here, then, is a remedy that has passed into official medicine from folk medicine and then reappeared in folk medicine. Whether the twentieth-century lady in Norfolk learned the remedy from Gerard or from the oral folk tradition, we will probably never know (Hatfield 1994: 23). Potato was used in burn treatment: raw scraped potato was laid on burns in Norfolk (Taylor MSS) and raw onion was used "to take the fire out" (Hatfield 1994: 23).

For trawler men in the days of steam, burns were a regular risk of the trade. In Suffolk, many relied on an ointment made from the liver of a fish (Hatfield MS). Goose grease was considered excellent for treating burns (Prince 1991: 121). Oil prepared from seal-liver was similarly used in the Highlands of Scotland. Boiled cream was used as a burn salve in Scotland. Egg white was found helpful in reducing the pain of burns (Prince 1991: 17). Cold tea was another pain-relieving application, used in Cambridgeshire (Porter 1974: 44). Baking soda solution was used to bathe burns and scalds (Hatfield MS). Human excrement was apparently used in Ireland (Logan 1972: 154). A more pleasant-sounding Irish remedy was to rub the burns with wax candles that had been used at a wake (Wilde 1919: 82). In Sussex moldy bread was used as a burn treatment (Allen 1995: 116).

As in Britain, there has been a belief in North America that burns could be treated by certain individuals. A seventh son was believed to have the power to cure burns by breathing over them (Puckett 1981: 336). A woman who has never known her father has also been credited with this power (Musick 1947: 48). Sometimes an incantation accompanied the process of taking the fire

out of a burn (Rogers 1968: 50). In a study of burn healers in North Carolina it has been shown that these individuals relied more on the incantation used, which usually had religious overtones, than on the accompanying physical agent (Kirkland 1992: 41–51).

Some of the plant remedies noted above have also been used in North American folk treatment of burns. Boiled elm bark has been used, as has raw potato. Crushed plantain leaves were found helpful. Tea has also been used, as in Britain (Brown 1952–1964, 66: 137). The bark of alder was mixed with suet to form a burn salve in New Brunswick (Bergen 1899: 110). In addition, numerous plants native to North America but not to Britain have been employed in burn treatment. They include sweet gum leaves and balsam juice (Brown 1952–1964, 6: 136–137), a salve made from "live forever" (Sedum purpureum) and lard (Bergen 1899: 110), the rootstock of bloodroot (Mellinger 1968: 50), golden seal root (UCLA Folklore Archives 9_62216), peach tree leaves (UCLA Folklore Archives 13_6216), poke berries (Pickard and Buley 1945: 334), and a poultice of prickly pear (Roberts 1927: 170). Particularly in Mexico, Aloe vera gel has been used in the treatment of burns. Although this plant is not native to North America, it has become naturalized. The gel scraped from its fleshy leaves has even been used to treat radiation burns. Pine pitch has also been used (UCLA Folklore Archive 5_7611).

As in Britain, cold water has been recommended (UCLA Folklore Archive 3_6589). Also as in Britain, a number of types of fat have been applied to burns and scalds. They include linseed oil, butter, lard, and kerosene oil. Miscellaneous substances used to relieve burns include mud, soap, ditch water, charcoal, and freshly killed chicken flesh (Brown 1952–1964, 6: 136–137). Vanilla flavoring has been recommended (Puckett 1981: 334). Bread baked with worms inside has been used in Alabama (Browne 1958: 45). Bicarbonate of soda has been used (UCLA Folklore Archives 25_5300), and honey (UCLA Folklore Archives 9_6202), a use vindicated by its present employment in some Western hospitals (Root-Bernstein and Root-Bernstein 2000: 185). Egg white has been used, as in Britain (UCLA Folklore Archives 1_7591). Less pleasantly, the excrement of hens (Hyatt 1965: 231), or of geese (De Lys 1948: 26) or cows (Harris 1968: 41), has been applied.

More than a hundred different genera of plants have been used by Native Americans as burn dressings (Moerman 1998: 776–777). Among them are alder, pine and plantain, all of them in use in general North American folk medicine too. Elder bark simmered in lard has produced an ointment for burns much like that used in Ireland (Vogel 1970: 302). A poultice of "Indian meal" has also been used (Vogel 1970: 128). Ashes of the cedar whips used in the Navajo fire ceremony have been used as a good burn medicine (New Mexico Folklore Record 1948: 8).

*See also* **Alder, Aloe vera, Blackberry, Bloodroot, Chickweed, Elder, Elm, Golden seal, Honey, Houseleek, Ivy, Mallow, Peach, Pine, Plantain, Poke, Potato, St. John's wort, Seventh son, Thornapple.**

## References

Allen, Andrew. *A Dictionary of Sussex Folk Medicine.* Newbury: Countryside Books, 1995.

Allen, David E., and Gabrielle Hatfield. *Medicinal Plants in Folk Tradition.* Portland, OR: Timber Press, in press.

Beith, Mary. *Healing Threads: Traditional Medicines of the Highlands and Islands.* Edinburgh: Polygon, 1995.

Bergen, Fanny D. "Animal and Plant Lore Collected from the Oral Tradition of English Speaking Folk." *Memoirs of the American Folk-Lore Society* 7 (1899).

Black, William George. *Folk-Medicine: A Chapter in the History of Culture.* London: Folklore Society, 1883.

Brown, Frank C. *Collection of North Carolina Folklore.* 7 vols. Durham, NC: Duke University Press, 1952–1964.

Browne, Ray B. *Popular Beliefs and Practices from Alabama.* Folklore Studies 9. Berkeley and Los Angeles: University of California Publications, 1958.

De Lys, Claudia. *A Treasury of American Superstitions.* New York: Philosophical Library, 1948.

Harris, Bernice Kelly (ed.). *Southern Home Remedies.* Murfreesboro, NC: Johnson, 1968.

Hatfield, Gabrielle. *Country Remedies: Traditional East Anglian Plant Remedies in the Twentieth Century.* Woodbridge: Boydell, 1994.

Hunt, Robert (ed.). *Popular Romances of the West of England.* London: J. C. Hotten, 1871.

Hyatt, Harry Middleton. *Folklore from Adams County Illinois.* 2nd rev. ed. New York: Memoirs of the Alma Egan Hyatt Foundation, 1965.

Jones, B. H. "Folk Medicine." *Folk-Lore* 19 (1908): 315–319.

Kirkland, James. "Talking Fire Out of Burns: A Magico-Religious Healing Tradition." In *Herbal and Magical Medicine. Traditional Healing Today,* edited by James Kirkland, Holly F. Matthews, C. W. Sullivan III, and Karen Baldwin. Durham, NC: Duke University Press, 1992.

Logan, Patrick. *Making the Cure: A Look at Irish Folk Medicine.* Dublin: Talbot Press, 1972.

Mellinger, Marie B. "Sang Sign." *Foxfire* 2(2) (1968): 15, 47–52.

Moerman, Daniel E. *Native American Ethnobotany.* Portland, OR: Timber Press, 1998.

Musick, Ruth Ann. "Folklore from West Virginia." *Hoosier Folklore* 6 (1947): 41–49.

*New Mexico Folklore Record.* 10 vols. Albuquerque, NM: 1946–1956.

Pickard, Madge E., and R. Carlyle Buley. *The Midwest Pioneer, His Ills, Cures and Doctors.* Crawfordsville, IN: R. E. Banta, 1945.

Porter, Enid. *The Folklore of East Anglia.* London: Batsford, 1974.

Prince, Dennis. *Grandmother's Cures: An A-Z of Herbal Remedies.* London: Fontana, 1991.

Puckett, Newbell Niles. *Popular Beliefs and Superstitions: A Compendium of American Folklore* from the *Ohio Collection of Newbell Niles Puckett.* Edited by Wayland D. Hand, Anna Casetta, and Sondra B. Thiederman. 3 vols. Boston: G. K. Hall, 1981.

Roberts, Hilda. Louisiana Superstitions. *Journal of American Folklore* 40 (1927) 144–208.

Rogers, James C. "Talking Out Fire." *North Carolina Folklore* 16 (1968); 46–52.

Root-Bernstein, Robert, and Michèle Root-Bernstein. *Honey, Mud Maggots and other Medical Marvels: The Science behind Folk Remedies and Old Wives' Tales.* London: Pan Books, 2000.

Taylor, Mark R. "Norfolk Folklore." *Folklore* 40 (1929): 113–133.

Taylor MSS. Manuscript notes of Mark R. Taylor in the Norfolk Record Office, Norwich MS 4322.

Tongue, Ruth L. *Somerset Folklore.* Edited Katharine Briggs. County Folklore 8. London: Folklore Society, 1965.

Vickery, Roy. *A Dictionary of Plant Lore.* Oxford: Oxford University Press, 1995.

Vogel, Virgil J. *American Indian Medicine.* Norman: University of Oklahoma Press, 1970.

Wilde, Lady. *Ancient Legends, Mystic Charms and Superstitions of Ireland.* London: Chatto and Windus, 1919.

# Buttercups (*Ranunculus acris, Ranunculus bulbosus, Ranunculus repens*)

These grassland species have been used in British folk medicine mainly to raise blisters, a technique popular in official medicine for many centuries as a way of ridding the system of impurities. It was applied to rheumatism in particular (Vickery 1995: 55). In addition, the flowers of buttercups were used to make a skin ointment, and they were also used to treat eye ulcers (termed "kennings"). In Cornwall *Ranunculus repens* was known as kenning herb (Davey 1909: 10, 23). Warts have been treated with buttercup juice (Tongue 1965: 43). In Ireland there have been additional folk uses for buttercups. They have treated jaundice, hydrophobia, swellings, tuberculosis, toothache, and headache, as well as the ailments mentioned (Allen and Hatfield, in press).

None of these species is native to North America, and not surprisingly their role in folk medicine there has been minor. Among the Native Americans these three *Ranunculus* species have been used in ways similar to those of Ireland—for headache, toothache, swellings, rheumatism, as well as for diarrhea, a use not recorded in Britain (Moerman 1998: 467–469).

*See also* **Headache; Jaundice; Mad dog, bite of; Toothache; Tuberculosis.**

## References

Allen, David E., and Gabrielle Hatfield. *Medicinal Plants in Folk Tradition.* Portland, OR: Timber Press, in press.

Davey, F. Hamilton. *Flora of Cornwall.* Penryn: F. Clegwidden, 1909.

Moerman, Daniel E. *Native American Ethnobotany.* Portland, OR: Timber Press, 1998.

Tongue, Ruth L. *Somerset Folklore.* Edited Katharine Briggs. County Folklore 8. London: Folklore Society, 1965.

Vickery, Roy. *A Dictionary of Plant Lore.* Oxford: Oxford University Press, 1995.

# Button snakeroot (*Eryngium yuccifolium*)

This and a related species of Eryngium (*Eryngium aquaticum*) have been used as diuretics in North American folk medicine and to treat sexual exhaustion (Coffey 1993: 158–159). Interestingly, the British native species of this genus, *Eryngium maritimum,* also has a reputation as an aphrodisiac. *E. aquaticum* has been used to treat women after childbirth (Meyer 1985: 210). In Native American practice these plants were used to treat a wide variety of ailments, including stomach trouble, snake bite, kidney problems and whooping cough (Moerman 1998: 225–226). *E. yuccifolium* was used by the Seminole Indians ceremonially as well as to treat loneliness after bereavement (Snow and Stans 2001: 90–91 and plate 19).

*See also* **Eryngo, Snake bite, Whooping cough.**

## References

Coffey, Timothy. *The History and Folklore of North American Wildflowers.* Facts On File, New York, 1993.

Meyer, Clarence. *American Folk Medicine.* Glenwood, IL: Meyerbooks, 1985.

Moerman, Daniel E. *Native American Ethnobotany.* Portland, OR: Timber Press, 1998.

Snow, Alice, and Susan Enns Stans. *Healing Plants: Medicine of the Florida Seminole Indians.* Gainesville: University Press of Florida, 2001.

# C

## Cabbage (*Brassica oleracea*)

Wild cabbage is native to parts of Britain and the Mediterranean, and cabbage has also been grown in cultivation at least since the time of the ancient Greeks (Harrison et al. 1985: 156). Pliny ascribed great healing powers to the cabbage. His influence on subsequent written works in official medicine has probably spread over the centuries to folk medicine too. He particularly recommended it for drunkenness. This use in folk medicine is widespread, described in the European literature from the sixteenth century onward, and recorded in Britain as recently as the 1940s (Vickery 1995: 58). Many of the other British folk uses of cabbage relate to its large cooling leaves. These have been used as a compress for breast abscesses and ulcers, as well as (in Ireland) for reducing fever (Vickery 1995: 58). During World War I they were similarly used to treat "trench foot" (Hatfield MS). In Wales, they have been used for a great variety of ailments, including the treatment of sprains (Hatfield MS). The water in which cabbage leaves have been cooked has been used to treat rheumatism. In Ireland, burns have been treated with fresh macerated cabbage leaves (Logan 1972: 105), and cabbage leaves tied around the throat have been recommended for a sore throat (Black 1883: 192). Hoarseness has been treated in En-

gland with a mixture of cabbage juice and honey (Black 1883: 193). Cabbage cooked with honey and salt has been recommended for colic and melancholy (Prince 1991: 106).

In folk medicine in the southern United States the cabbage has a reputation for helping to cure a hangover (Crellin and Philpott 1990: 129), just as in Britain. The use of a young cabbage leaf warmed and applied as a treatment for an abscess is among a collection of early settlers' remedies from Shelburne County (Robertson 1960: 30). Sprains have been treated in New Mexico, as in Wales, with cabbage leaves soaked in vinegar (Moya 1940: 70). The cooling leaves were tied around the neck, wrists, and ankles for typhoid fever (Brown 1952–1964, 6: 308), or bound on the forehead for a fever (Hyatt 1965: 216). For a headache, cabbage leaves were applied to the forehead (Puckett 1981: 390). For preventing sunstroke, wearing a damp cabbage leaf on the head is suggested (UCLA Folklore Archives 12_5505). The leaves have formed dressings for blisters (Bergen 1899: 110) and chilblains (Parler 1962, 3: 511). For croup, a cabbage leaf was bound round a child's throat with a black thread (Fife 1957: 157). Other folk uses in North America are described by Meyer: the large leaves of cabbage, with their midribs removed, have been used in the same way as burdock for soothing sore feet (Meyer

1985: 120); mashed, they have formed the basis of healing poultices (Meyer 1985: 205). Cabbage poultices have been used to "draw" boils (Redfield 1937: 19). Hot leaves have been used for pneumonia (Baughman 1954–1955: 25) and appendicitis (Doering and Doering 1936: 64). Cabbage juice has been taken for ulcers (Puckett 1981: 468) and for dysentery (Parler 1962: 10), as well as dripped into the ears for deafness (Clark 1970: 19). Even the stump of an old cabbage has found a use in folk medicine; ground in vinegar, it has been used to treat warts (Dieffenbach 1952: 2). The urine of a cabbage eater is credited with healing and strengthening powers (UCLA Folklore Archives 5_6153).

In Native American practice, the Cherokee used wilted cabbage leaves as a poultice for boils (Hamel and Chiltoskey 1975: 28), and the Rappahannock bound the leaves on to an aching head (Speck, Hassrick and Carpenter 1942: 25).

This enormously variable species has given us vegetables as diverse as cauliflower, Brussels sprouts, sprouting broccoli, and kohl rabi. Recent interest in the possible anti-cancer properties of various forms of *Brassica oleracea* may mean that it will in the future be regarded as an important medicinal as well as a nourishing vegetable.

The so-called Skunk cabbage *(Symplocarpus foetidus)*, used by Native Americans for treating scurvy and as a sedative, is botanically unrelated.

*See also* **Abscesses, Blisters, Boils, Breast problems, Burdock, Chilblains, Colic, Croup, Deafness, Depression, Honey, Rheumatism, Sprains, Warts.**

## References

Baughman, Ernest Warren. "Folk Sayings and Beliefs." *New Mexico Folklore Record* 9 (1954–1955): 23–27.

Bergen, Fanny D. "Animal and Plant Lore Collected from the Oral Tradition of English Speaking Folk." *Memoirs of the American Folk-Lore Society* 7 (1899).

Black, William George. *Folk-Medicine: A Chapter in the History of Culture.* London: Folklore Society, 1883.

Brown, Frank C. *Collection of North Carolina Folklore.* 7 vols. Durham, NC: Duke University Press, 1952–1964.

Clark, Joseph D. "North Carolina Popular Beliefs and Superstitions." *North Carolina Folklore* 18 (1970): 1–66.

Crellin, John K., and Jane Philpott. *A Reference Guide to Medicinal Plants.* Durham, NC: Duke University Press, 1990.

Dieffenbach, Victor C. "Cabbage in the Folk Culture of My Pennsylvania Elders." *Pennsylvania Dutchman* 3(22) (April 15, 1952): 1–2.

Doering, John Frederick, and Eileen Elita Doering. "Some Western Ontario Folk Beliefs and Practices." *Journal of American Folklore* 51 (1936): 60–68.

Fife, Austin E. "Pioneer Mormon Remedies." *Western Folklore* 16 (1957): 153–162.

Hamel, Paul B., and Mary U. Chiltoskey. *Cherokee Plants and Their Uses: A 400 Year History.* Sylva, NC: Herald, 1975.

Harrison, S. G., G. B. Masefield, and Michael Wallis. *The Oxford Book of Food Plants.* Oxford: Oxford University Press, 1985.

Hyatt, Harry Middleton. *Folklore from Adams County Illinois.* 2nd rev. ed. New York: Memoirs of the Alma Egan Hyatt Foundation, 1965.

Logan, Patrick. *Making the Cure: A Look at Irish Folk Medicine.* Dublin: Talbot Press, 1972.

Meyer, Clarence. *American Folk Medicine.* Glenwood, IL: Meyerbooks, 1985.

Moya, Benjamin S. *Superstitions and Beliefs among the Spanish-Speaking People of New Mexico.* Master's thesis, University of New Mexico, 1940.

Parler, Mary Celestia, and University Student Contributors. *Folk Beliefs from Arkansas.* 15 vols. Fayetteville: University of Arkansas, 1962.

Prince, Dennis. *Grandmother's Cures: An A-Z of Herbal Remedies.* London: Fontana, 1991.

Puckett, Newbell Niles. *Popular Beliefs and Superstitions. A Compendium of American Folklore* from the Ohio Collection of Newbell Niles Puckett. Edited by Wayland D. Hand, Anna Casetta, and Sondra B. Thiederman. 3 vols. Boston: G. K. Hall, 1981.

Redfield, W. Adelbert. "Superstitions and Folk Beliefs." *Tennessee Folklore Society Bulletin* 3 (1937): 11–40.

Robertson, Marion. *Old Settlers' Remedies.* Barrington, NS: Cape Sable Historical Society, 1960.

Speck, Frank G., R. B. Hassrick, and E. S. Carpenter. "Rappahannock Herbals, Folk-Lore and Science of Cures." *Proceedings of the Delaware County Institute of Science* 10 (1942): 7–55.

Vickery, Roy. *A Dictionary of Plant Lore.* Oxford: Oxford University Press, 1995.

# Cancer

In the past in both folk and official medicine the diagnosis and definition of cancer was far from clear. Folk remedies for cancer therefore have to be viewed with some caution: some of them were probably used to treat conditions that we would not today regard as cancerous. Conversely, some illnesses treated in folk medicine may, by today's definition, have been malignant but were not recognized as such. In this account, the term "cancer" is used where the informants of remedies have used it, and this ambiguity needs to be borne in mind.

There is a widespread idea that the hand of a corpse has the power to cure cancer. This belief lingered in East Anglia up to the twentieth century (Rider Haggard, ed. 1974: 17). Toads were reputed to have the power to "suck the poison" from cancers (Thiselton Dyer 1878: 151). For breast cancer, a west country remedy used in the nineteenth century was to take mud from the puddles formed by hoof prints of cattle and apply this as a plaster (Aubrey 1881: 255). In Lincolnshire, the same cancer was treated with an infusion of horse spurs in ale (Gutch and Peacock 1908: 115). Woodlice in wine was another East Anglian

folk remedy for breast cancer (Newman 1945: 353). In the Scottish Highlands, it was once believed that the bite of a pig could cause cancer; on the other hand, a legend there suggests that the eating of a magical pigskin will cure all diseases and prevent them in the future (Beith 1995: 180, 181).

In British folk medicine a number of plant remedies were used to treat cancers. Carrot *(Daucus carota)* poultices were used both in the Highlands of Scotland (Beith 1995: 210) and in England (Taylor MSS); both wild carrot and cultivated have been used for this purpose. In the seventeenth century, ground ivy *(Glechoma hederacea)* was used for cancer treatment (Wright 1912: 493). Violet *(Viola sp.)* leaf poultices were used throughout Britain, particularly for treating skin cancers (Tongue 1965: 38). This remedy has been used in Norfolk as recently as the mid-twentieth century (Hatfield 1994: 26). Herb Robert *(Geranium robertianum)* had a reputation in the Scottish Highlands for treating skin cancer (Beith 1995: 222). There is an isolated record of the stems of thistles being used in the Scottish Highlands for cancer treatment (Prince 1991: 126–127). Narrow-leaved dock *(Rumex sp.)* was used to poultice tumors in East Anglia (Taylor MSS) and celandine, probably greater celandine *(Chelidonium majus)* was used internally to treat liver cancer (Taylor MSS). In Essex, a poultice of houseleeks has been used to treat "cancerous growths." Dandelion *(Taraxacum officinale)* has been used to treat a cancer on the lip, while in recent times a facial cancer has been treated using banana skin (Hatfield 1994: 25). Red clover tops infused have been used in Ireland for cancer treatment (McClafferty 1979). Woodsorrel *(Oxalis acetosella)* has also provided an Irish folk treatment for cancer (Egan 1887). A poultice of hemlock *(Conium maculatum)* has been used to treat cancer in Suffolk (Taylor MSS). More drastically, a plaster of hemlock has been used both in the Isle of Man (Gill 1932: 188) and in the Scottish Highlands (Carmichael 1900–1971: 2, 257, 266; 4: 201) to tear out a tumor by its roots. Hemlock was used by the ancients in cancer treatment and was promoted by a Viennese physician, Van Storck, in the eighteenth century; this may be a folk remedy borrowed from official medicine. Other plants too were used in plaster form. A particularly detailed account comes from County Tyrone, Ireland, where creeping buttercup *(Ranunculus repens)* leaves were dried and powdered and mixed with arsenic. White silk was coated with egg white and the mixture was sprinkled on. The plaster was applied to the cancer and remained in place for three to six weeks (Dickie and Hughes 1961: 99, 100).

Cancer treatment in North American folk medicine has been even more diverse. Visiting an apple tree at daybreak on three successive mornings was recommended in Kentucky (Thomas and Thomas 1920: 98). Allowing the sun to shine through a knothole onto a mouth cancer for nine mornings (with prayer) was another recommendation, this one from the African American tradition (Hyatt 1965: 286). As in Britain, there is an association of cancer cures with the dead. Rubbing a tumor with a human bone from a graveyard was suggested in Illinois (Hyatt 1965: 286). Touching the tumor with a dead hand was also recommended (Cannon 1984: 98). A variation was to tie a string around a corpse's finger, transfer the string to a tumor, and replace it in the coffin (Hyatt 1965: 286). The same belief in the efficacy of toads found in Britain is recorded from Illinois (Kimmerle and Gelber 1976: 11), while swallowing young frogs was recommended in Ohio (Puckett 1981: 336). Numerous other cures involve animal flesh, blood, or fat. Laying on the teats of a cow was recorded from Ohio (Puckett 1981: 336). A freshly killed cat, opened and laid

on the tumor, has also been suggested (Puckett 1981: 336). A chicken has been used similarly in Iowa (Stout 1936: 186), or a piece of beefsteak in California (UCLA Folklore Archives 10_6285). The blood of a buzzard was recommended in Arkansas (Parler 1962: 496). Sheep's fat bound on for more than a week will reputedly remove a tumor with it when taken off (UCLA Folklore Archives 20_5306). Alligator fat had a reputation for curing cancer (Brown 1952–1964, 6: 139). An ointment prepared from fishing worms and tallow was described in Ohio (Puckett 1981: 336). The tea made from horse-hoof scrapings in Illinois (Hyatt 1965: 286) recalls the remedy above used in Britain's west country. Eating or applying marrow from the jawbone of a pig is an interesting remedy recorded from Michigan (UCLA Folklore Archives 13_7609); this could tie in with the British belief that cancer can be caused by the bite of a pig (see above). In the Ozark mountains, a moleskin was worn between the breasts as an amulet to protect against breast cancer (Randolph 1947: 155). Other animal products used in folk treatment of cancer include cobwebs (UCLA Folklore Archives 9_5307), rattlesnake rattles in whisky (Thompson 1959: 101), and the oil from egg yolks (UCLA Folklore Archives 7_5309). Animal excreta were also employed: for rectal cancer, hog manure fried with lard and turpentine and applied as an ointment was recommended (Hyatt 1965: 286), and goose droppings boiled in water were given internally for cancers (Hyatt 1965: 286).

Among the plethora of plant remedies used in North American folk medicine for cancer treatment, some are recognizably the same as ones used in Britain. Thus an infusion of violet *(Viola* sp.) leaves was used (De Lys 1948: 316), as was a poultice of narrow-leaved dock (Pickard and Buley 1945: 42). Red clover was widely used (Browne 1958: 45). As in Britain, hemlock has been used in cancer treatment (Peattie 1943: 118), as have the blossoms of thistles (UCLA Folklore Archives 16_7610). Sheep shower, or sheep sorrel (*Oxalis* sp.), was widely used. The juice was beaten on a metal plate and combined with other constituents into an ointment (Clark 1970: 14).

However, many of the plants used in North American folk medical treatment of cancers are not native to Britain and not used in folk medicine there. Poke root was used as a poultice in the Native American tradition (Vogel 1970: 351). Ashes of prickly pear were sprinkled on cancers (Rogers 1941: 28). Bloodroot was made into a plaster, with zinc chloride and flour, and left on a tumor for twenty-four hours, at the end of which time it could be torn out bodily (cf. the plaster prepared in Ireland, above) (UCLA Folklore Archives 2_6285). Cancer weed (*Salvia lyrata*), as its name suggests, was crushed, both stem and roots, and rubbed on cancerous sores (Clark 1970: 14). A poultice of fresh cranberries *(Vaccinium vitis-idaea)* was suggested (UCLA Folklore Archives 6_5308), or a salve prepared from spikenard (? *Aralia* sp.) tallow, and beeswax (Puckett 1981: 336). A tea prepared from the roots of yerba mansa *(Anemopsis californica)* was drunk in the Mexican west (Kay 1996: 95), while one prepared from beech tree *(Fagus grandifolia)* sprouts has been used in Ohio (Puckett 1981: 337). Indian hemp *(Cannabis sativa)* in a sulphur bag is a cancer treatment reported from Ohio (Puckett 1981: 337). Various fruit and vegetables have been used in folk medical treatment of cancer. These include a poultice of raw grated potatoes for skin cancer (UCLA Folklore Archives 12_6189), a grapefruit rubbed on (UCLA Folklore Archives 12_6749), raisins soaked in whisky, eaten two a day (Hendricks 1966: 31), and a poultice of turkey figs (UCLA Folklore Archives 10_6189). Stolen musty corn (infected with the smut fungus)

has been claimed to cure a cancer when rubbed onto it (Hyatt 1965: 286). In addition to all these relatively simple plant remedies, a large number of complex ointments were prepared, often including tree barks of various kinds. One such ointment, used in Kentucky, included the barks of red oak (*Quercus* sp.), persimmon (*Diospyros* sp.), dogwood (*Cornus* sp.), and the roots of sassafras and dewberry (*Rubus* sp.). The barks were to be gathered from the north side (Thomas and Thomas 1920: 98). Wood ashes were also used to prepare a caustic treatment for tumors (Creighton 1950: 89).

Folk medicine has dietary recommendations for cancer. Drinking large volumes of carrot juice (UCLA Folklore Archives 11_6749) (cf. use of carrots in Britain) has been claimed to cure cancer, as has a diet of grapes (UCLA Folklore Archives 9_6189), lemon juice (UCLA Folklore Archives 13_6749), figs (Browne 1958: 45), or almonds (UCLA Folklore Archives 1_6285). Eating raw onions has been claimed to prevent cancer (UCLA Folklore Archives 11_6189). Even more simply, keeping a plant of live-forever *(Sedum telephium)* in the room wards off cancer (Stout 1936: 189).

Native American treatments of cancer are numerous. As well as numerous plants (Moerman 1998: 777), wood ashes were used (Vogel 1970: 137). The juice of ash that emerges from the ends of burning ash twigs (*Fraxinus* sp.) was claimed to cure cancerous sores (which may or may not have been malignant) (Vogel 1970: 276). Ash sap has been prized in the Scottish Highlands and was the first drink traditionally given to a newborn child there.

*See also* **African tradition, Amulet, Ash, Bloodroot, Excreta, Houseleek, Poke, Potato, Sassafras.**

### References

Aubrey, John. *Remaines of Gentilisme and Judaisme.* Edited by James Britten. London, 1881.

Beith, Mary. *Healing Threads: Traditional Medicines of the Highlands and Islands.* Edinburgh: Polygon, 1995.

Brown, Frank C. *Collection of North Carolina Folklore.* 7 vols. Durham, NC: Duke University Press, 1952–1964.

Browne, Ray B. *Popular Beliefs and Practices from Alabama.* Folklore Studies 9. Berkeley and Los Angeles: University of California Press, 1958.

Cannon, Anthon S. *Popular Beliefs and Superstitions from Utah.* Edited by Wayland D. Hand and Jeannine E. Talley. Salt Lake City: University of Utah Press, 1984.

Carmichael, Alexander (1900–1971). *Carmina Gadelica: Hymns and Incantations.* 6 vols. (3 and 4 edited by J. Carmichael Watson, 5 and 6 by Angus Matheson). Edinburgh: Constable (1900); Oliver and Boyd (1940–54); Scottish Academic Press, 1971.

Clark, Joseph D. "North Carolina Popular Beliefs and Superstitions." *North Carolina Folklore* 18 (1970): 1–66.

Creighton, Helen. *Folklore from Lunenburg County, Nova Scotia.* Ottawa: National Museum of Canada Bulletin 117, Anthropological Series 29, 1950.

De Lys, Claudia. *A Treasury of American Superstitions.* New York: Philosophical Library, 1948.

Dickie, W. R., and N. C. Hughes. "Caustic Pastes: Their Survival as Quack Cancer Remedies." *British Journal of Plastic Surgery* 14(2), (1961): 97–109.

Egan, F. W. "Irish Folk-lore: Medical Plants." *Folk-lore Journal* 5 (1887): 11–13.

Gill, W. Walter. *A Second Manx Scrapbook.* London and Bristol: Arrowsmith, 1932.

Gutch, Mrs., and Mabel G. W. Peacock. *Examples of Printed Folk-Lore Concerning Lincolnshire.* Publications of the Folk-Lore Society 63. London: Nutt, 1908.

Hatfield, Gabrielle. *Country Remedies: Traditional East Anglian Plant Remedies in the Twentieth Century.* Woodbridge: Boydell, 1994.

Hendricks, George D. *Mirrors, Mice and Mustaches: A Sampling of Superstitions and Popular Beliefs in Texas.* Austin: Texas Folklore Society, 1966.

Hyatt, Harry Middleton. *Folklore from Adams County Illinois.* 2nd rev. ed. New York: Memoirs of the Alma Egan Hyatt Foundation, 1965.

Kay, Margarita Artschwager. *Healing with Plants in the American and Mexican West.* Tucson: University of Arizona Press, 1996.

Kimmerle, Marjorie, and Mark Gelber. *Popular Beliefs and Superstitions from Colorado.* Boulder, Colorado, 1976, unpublished.

McClafferty, George. *The Folk Medicine of Co. Wicklow.* Master's thesis, National University of Ireland, 1979.

Moerman, Daniel E. *Native American Ethnobotany.* Portland, OR: Timber Press, 1998.

Newman, Leslie F. "Some Notes on Folk Medicine in the Eastern Counties." *Folk-Lore* 56 (1945): 349–360.

Parler, Mary Celestia, and University Student Contributors. *Folk Beliefs from Arkansas.* 15 vols. Fayetteville: University of Arkansas, 1962.

Peattie, Roderick (ed.). *The Great Smokies and the Blue Ridge.* New York: Vanguard Press, 1943.

Pickard, Madge E., and R. Carlyle Buley. *The Midwest Pioneer, His Ills, Cures and Doctors.* Crawfordsville, IN: R. E. Banta, 1945.

Prince, Dennis. *Grandmother's Cures: An A–Z of Herbal Remedies.* London: Fontana, 1991.

Puckett, Newbell Niles. *Popular Beliefs and Superstitions: A Compendium of American Folklore from the Ohio Collection of Newbell Niles Puckett.* Edited by Wayland D. Hand, Anna Casetta, and Sondra B. Thiederman. 3 vols. Boston: G. K. Hall, 1981.

Randolph, Vance. *Ozark Superstitions.* New York: Columbia University Press, 1947.

Rider Haggard, Lilias (ed.). *I Walked by Night.* Woodbridge: Boydell Press, 1974.

Rogers, E. G. *Early Folk Medical Practices in Tennessee.* Murfreesboro, TN: Mid-South, 1941.

Stout, Earl J. "Folklore from Iowa." *Memoirs of the American Folklore Society* 29 (1936).

Taylor MSS. Manuscript Notes of Mark R. Taylor in the Norfolk Record Office, Norwich. MS4322.

Thiselton Dyer, T. F. *English Folk-Lore.* London: Hardwick and Bogue, 1878.

Thomas, Daniel Lindsay, and Lucy Blayney Thomas. *Kentucky Superstitions.* Princeton, NJ: Princeton University Press, 1920.

Thompson, Lawrence S. "A Vanishing Science." *Kentucky Folklore Quarterly* 5 (1959): 95–105.

Tongue, Ruth L. *Somerset Folklore.* Edited Katharine Briggs. County Folklore 8. London: Folklore Society, 1965.

Vogel, Virgil J. *American Indian Medicine.* Norman: University of Oklahoma Press, 1970.

Wright, A. R. "Seventeenth Century Cures and Charms." *Folk-Lore* 23 (1912): 490–497.

# Catnip (*Nepeta cataria*)

This plant is not native to North America, but was introduced by the settlers, promoted by the Shakers, and now has a wide variety of uses in folk medicine in North America. It is used for colic, in babies and adults, as an infusion of the leaves (Micheletti 1998: 76), as well as for coughs, colds and asthma. In Britain it does not appear to have played a significant role in folk medicine. There are records of its use as an aromatic and medicinal infusion in England and France (Grieve 1931: 174), where it was generally drunk before the introduction of tea. Perhaps it was as a mildly stimulating alternative to tea that it was introduced by colonists. It has also been used to provoke menstruation, and perhaps also to procure abortions. In general North American folk medicine, Meyer (Meyer: 1985) records its use in treating asthma, chicken pox, chest colds, colic, erysipelas, nettle rash, urinary incontinence, as a gentle sedative, for pleurisy, for treating the rash of poison ivy, for boils, and mixed with unsalted butter and sugar for treating fresh wounds. In nineteenth-century Pennsylvania, catnip is described as being "highly popular among the good ladies who deal in simples" (Darlington 1847). The wide popularity of catnip in folk medicine is reflected in the numerous records (more than 350) for its use in the UCLA Folklore Archives. Many of these are for infant colic, as well as the ailments mentioned by Meyer. One record from Nova Scotia recommends the use of catnip under the pillow to help a child sleep (Creighton 1968: 219). Another, from the Smoky Mountains, includes catnip in a poultice to treat blood poisoning (Hall 1960: 50).

In Native American practice, there are records for use of this plant from thirteen different tribes (Moerman 1998: 353–354). Again, the variety of uses is wide. Rheumatism, boils, diarrhea, colic, stomach ache, headache, colds, pneumonia, and worms have all been treated with catnip. There is an emphasis on its use for treating children. The plant has also been used to procure abortions (Hamel and Chiltoskey 1975: 28).

*See also* **Abortion, Asthma, Colds, Colic, Coughs, Erysipelas, Shakers.**

### References
Creighton, Helen. *Bluenose Magic, Popular Beliefs and Superstitions in Nova Scotia.* Toronto: Ryerson Press, 1968.

Darlington, William. *Agricultural Botany: An Enumeration and Description of Useful Plants and Weeds.* Philadelphia: 1847.

Grieve, Mrs. M. *A Modern Herbal.* Edited by Mrs. C. F. Leyel. London: Jonathan Cape, 1931.

Hall, Joseph S. *Smoky Mountain Folks and Their Lore.* Gatlinburg, TN: Great Smoky Mountains Natural History Association, 1960.

Hamel, Paul B., and Mary U. Chiltoskey. *Cherokee Plants and Their Uses: A 400 Year History.* Sylva, NC: Herald, 1975.

Meyer, Clarence. *American Folk Medicine.* Glenwood, IL: Meyerbooks, 1985.

Micheletti, Enza (ed.). *North American Folk Healing: An A-Z Guide to Traditional Remedies.* New York and Montreal: Reader's Digest Association, 1998.

Moerman, Daniel E. *Native American Ethnobotany.* Portland, OR: Timber Press, 1998.

# Caul

Occasionally a baby is born with its head partially covered by fetal membrane. This membrane has been called a caul, and it has attracted a number of superstitions and folk remedies. In the north of England, the caul was called "sillyhow," meaning blessed hood (Radford and Radford 1974: 92). Fishermen carried a caul as an amulet while at sea to protect them from drowning, and also from seasickness and scurvy (Souter 1995: 40). In Scotland it was believed that a person born with a caul had special healing powers (Beith 1995: 94). A man from the Isle of Eigg in the Inner Hebrides, who died in the 1960s, was born with a caul. He came of a line of hereditary healers, famous for curing bad backs by walking on them. The fact that he had been born with a caul was thought to have added to his powers (Beith 1995: 169). If a caul was given away, its condition was believed to indicate the state of health of the owner: if it was dry, the owner was in good health, if moist, the converse. If it was lost or thrown away, the owner could die (Buchan, ed.: 1994, 91).

In North American folklore the belief similarly exists that a person born with a caul will have healing powers. The caul is considered generally lucky for the child, and it is also thought to confer special powers of seeing the supernatural (Brown 1952–1964, 6: 41). Mexican Native Americans preserved the caul as an amulet for the child to bring luck throughout life (Madsen 1955: 127).

*See also* **Amulet, Backache.**

**References**

Beith, Mary. *Healing Threads: Traditional Medicines of the Highlands and Islands*. Edinburgh: Polygon, 1995.

Brown, Frank C. *Collection of North Carolina Folklore*. 7 vols. Durham, NC: Duke University Press, 1952–1964.

Buchan, David (ed.). *Folk Tradition and Folk Medicine in Scotland: The Writings of David Rorie*. Edinburgh: Canongate Academic, 1994.

Madsen, William. "Hot and Cold in the Universe of San Francisco Tecospa, Valley of Mexico." *Journal of American Folklore* 68 (1955): 127.

Radford, E., and M. A. Radford. *Encyclopedia of Superstitions*. Edited by Christina Hole. London: Book Club Associates, 1974.

Souter, Keith. *Cure Craft: Traditional Folk Remedies and Treatment from Antiquity to the Present Day*. Saffron Walden: C.W. Daniel, 1995.

# Cayenne (*Capsicum annuum*)

Botanically, all the wide variety of red peppers belong to this species. This plant, a native of tropical America, has been widely used as a condiment but has also been used in folk medicine, particularly as a stimulant. The important role it has played in food culture as well as medicine is outlined in Wilson and Gillespie's recent book (Wilson and Gillespie (eds.). 1999: 89–119). In folk medicine it has been used for nausea, nosebleed, pain relief, rheumatism, sprains, stomach upsets, toothache, sore throat and tonsillitis (Meyer 1985: 184, 191, 219, 232, 236, 247, 250, 251). Samuel Thomson used cayenne as one of the main plants in his materia medica (Chevallier 1996: 25), along with lobelia. For colds, the ground pepper has been used with water and honey (Long 1962: 5). For coughs, it has been mixed with vinegar and butter (Fife 1957: 161). For earache, a pepper without its seeds is wrapped in cotton and applied to the sore ear (Browne 1958: 59). The ground pepper has been sprinkled on cuts to stop the bleeding (Cannon 1984: 93). A tea of ground cayenne has been drunk for nosebleed (UCLA Folklore Archives 16_6429) and for ulcers, as well as for yellow fever (Long 1962: 6). For typhoid, cayenne and vodka has been administered (UCLA Folklore Archive 10_6543). Cayenne in cold water has been given for a heart attack (Cannon 1984: 111).

In Native American medicine, the plant has been used by the Cherokee for fevers, colic, gangrene and as a stimulant (Hamel and Chiltoskey 1975: 48).

In Britain the plant has not been used in folk medicine, although it has been used in official herbalism (Chevallier 1996: 70). Interestingly, its analgesic properties have now been recognized by orthodox medicine, and the chemical capsaicin forms part of a preparation used for pain relief in rheumatism and headaches.

*See also* **Colds; Coughs; Cuts; Earache; Lobelia; Nosebleed; Rheumatism; Thomson, Samuel; Toothache.**

### References

Browne, Ray B. *Popular Beliefs and Practices from Alabama.* Folklore Studies 9. Berkeley and Los Angeles: University of California Publications, 1958.

Cannon, Anthon S. *Popular Beliefs and Superstitions from Utah.* Edited by Wayland D. Hand and Jeannine E. Talley. Salt Lake City: University of Utah Press, 1984.

Chevallier, Andrew. *The Encyclopedia of Medicinal Plants.* London: Dorling Kindersley, 1996.

Fife, Austin E. Pioneer Mormon Remedies. *Folklore* 16 (1957): 153–162.

Hamel, Paul B., and Mary U. Chiltoskey. *Cherokee Plants and Their Uses: A 400 Year History.* Sylva, NC: Herald, 1975.

Long, Grady M. "Folk Medicine in McMinn, Polk, Bradley and Meigs Counties, Tennessee 1910–1927." *Tennessee Folklore Society Bulletin* 28 (1962): 1–8.

Meyer, Clarence. *American Folk Medicine.* Glenwood, IL: Meyerbooks, 1985.

Wilson, David Scofield, and Angus Kress Gillespie (eds.). *Rooted in America.* Knoxville: University of Tennessee Press, 1999.

# Celtic tradition

Folk medicine in the Celtic areas of Britain (the Scottish Highlands and Wales) and Ireland differs in some respects from that of the rest of Britain. There is greater continuity with early pre-Christian traditions, and this has lasted right up to the present day in some areas. Many of the Christian saints were seamlessly incorporated into the religious traditions of the Celts (Souter 1995: 32). There has been less impact from outside sources than in England, where a great mixture of influences from outside sources has infiltrated folk medicine. The survival until relatively recent times of the Gaelic language has served to emphasize and preserve the isolation of the Celtic tradition. These remarks hold true also for the so-called Celtic fringe, which includes Cornwall, the Isle of Man, and Wales. The Isle of Man has maintained, along with its governmental autonomy, a number of unique folklore traditions. On Tynwald Day, when the island's parliament convenes, it was customary to wear a sprig of mugwort, a practice that was revived in the 1920s. This plant symbolizes the power to avert evil; it is also used in practical folk medicine.

The manufacture of amulets was a well-developed Celtic art from long before the Romans brought Christianity to the British Isles. Many of these amulets, designed to avert the evil eye, have survived, some of them in Christianized form. Similarly, some pre-Christian beliefs, such as the use of salt to avert the evil eye, have survived right through to the present day (Buchan 1994: 202). The Gaelic-speaking areas of Scotland remained free from the witchhunts in much of Britain during the sixteenth and seventeenth centuries, another reason that many of the ancient traditions were left untouched (Beith 1995: 84). An intimate blend of poetry, myth, and religion with a knowledge of the indigenous plants has led to a tradition that in some ways resembles that of the Native Americans. There has been a strong tradition of healers, often successive generations of one family. Some of these healing dynasties were learned doctors; others had no medical education but were valued nevertheless for their healing powers. Many blacksmiths were in this category. The Beaton dynasty yielded several generations of famous healers in Scotland, the more recent of whom incorporated many of the contemporary official medical ideas into their practice (Comrie 1927). This development was also seen in Wales, where in the thirteenth century the famous Physicians of Myddvai practiced a system of medicine which was a blend of folk tradition and official learned medicine (Williams ab Ithel 1861).

Although the Celtic tradition of folk medicine is now largely incorporated into that of the rest of Britain, differences do still remain. One informant in Ireland was asked whether folk medicine was enjoying a revival: "No," he said, "it has never gone away" (Nolan 1988: 55). This cannot be said of much of mainland Britain.

*See also* **Amulet, Evil eye, Mugwort, Native American tradition.**

### References

Beith, Mary. *Healing Threads: Traditional Medicines of the Highlands and Islands.* Edinburgh: Polygon, 1995.

Buchan, David (ed.). *Folk Tradition and Folk Medicine in Scotland: The Writings of David Rorie.* Edinburgh: Canongate Academic, 1994.

Comrie, John D. *History of Scottish Medicine to 1860.* London: Baillière, Tindall and Cox, 1927.

Nolan, Peter W. "Folk Medicine in Rural Ireland." *Folk Life* 27 (1988–1989): 44–56.

Souter, Keith. *Cure Craft. Traditional Folk Remedies and Treatment from Antiquity to the Present Day.* Saffron Walden: C. W. Daniel, 1995.

Williams ab Ithel, John (ed.). *The Physicians of Myddvai.* Llanodovery: D. J. Roderic; London: Longman, 1861.

# Chamomile
## (*Chamaemelum nobile*)

Throughout Britain and Ireland, this native plant has been used in folk medicine to relieve pain, including stomach pain (a use immortalized by Beatrix Potter in the "Tale of the Flopsy Bunnies"!), toothache (Allen 1995: 45), sore eyes, (Hatfield 1994: 37), neuralgia (Vickery 1995: 63), "stitches" (Beith 1995: 209), and as a general mild sedative. It is sometimes known as Roman chamomile or English chamomile, and it was introduced to North America by early British settlers. However, its place there in folk medicine was usurped by the German chamomile, *Matricaria recutita.*

German chamomile is estimated to be the most popular herb in use among Mexicans (Kay 1996: 192). It was introduced there, as *manzanilla,* by the Spanish in the eighteenth century. In other regions in the North American folk records it is difficult to know which chamomile is referred to. Meyer (1985), for example, gives more than thirty folk medical uses for chamomile. Probably most of these refer to the German chamomile. They include relief of asthma and croup; teething in infants; indigestion, nausea and bad breath, menstrual pain, sore or weeping eyes, headache, measles, mumps, bites and stings, piles and rheumatism. The UCLA folklore archive reveals a variety of uses for chamomile, including stomach pain (UCLA Folklore Archives 20_5582) and colds (UCLA Folklore Archives 4_5318). The Native Americans used chamomile for abortions, ulcers, and unsettled stomachs (Moerman 1998: 152).

The related pineapple weed (*Matricaria discoidea*), native to North America but not to Britain, was used by the Eskimo for colds and indigestion (Oswalt 1957: 22, 23), by the Costanoan Indians for stomach pain and fever (Boceck 1984: 27), and by the Shuswap Indians for colds and the heart

(Palmer 1975: 59). For other uses in the Native American tradition, see Moerman 1998: 337.

Pineapple weed became naturalized in Britain in the nineteenth century, and there is a single record of its use in folk medicine in Wales, where it was used to treat boils (*Plant Lore Notes and News,* no. 6 [1999], 289).

*See also* **Abortion, Asthma, Bad breath, Colds, Croup, Eye problems, Headache, Indigestion, Insect bites and stings, Menstrual problems, Nausea, Piles, Rheumatism, Teething, Toothache.**

### References

Allen, Andrew. *A Dictionary of Sussex Folk Medicine.* Newbury: Countryside Books, 1995.

Beith, Mary. *Healing Threads: Traditional Medicines of the Highlands and Islands.* Edinburgh: Polygon, 1995.

Boceck, Barbara R. "Ethnobotany of Costanoan Indians, California. Based on Collections by John P. Harrington." *Economic Botany* 38(2) (1984): 240–255.

Hatfield, Gabrielle. *Country Remedies: Traditional East Anglian Plant Remedies in the Twentieth Century.* Woodbridge: Boydell, 1994.

Kay, Margarita Artschwager. *Healing with Plants in the American and Mexican West.* Tucson: University of Arizona Press, 1996.

Meyer, Clarence. *American Folk Medicine.* Glenwood, IL: Meyerbooks, 1985.

Moerman, Daniel E. *Native American Ethnobotany.* Portland, OR: Timber Press, 1998.

Oswalt, W. H. "A Western Eskimo Ethnobotany." *Anthropological Papers of the University of Alaska* 6 (1957): 17–36.

Palmer, Gary. "Shuswap Indian Ethnobotany." *Syesis* 8 (1975): 29–51.

*Plant Lore Notes and News,* no. 6 (1999): 289.

Vickery, Roy. *A Dictionary of Plant Lore.* Oxford: Oxford University Press, 1995.

# Chapped skin

Working for long hours out of doors in the British winter and returning home to an inadequately heated house meant that many agricultural workers until the recent past suffered from chapped skin as well as chilblains. It was widely believed that one's own urine was a good lotion for chapped skin, applied night and morning. In Yorkshire, goose grease was considered an excellent ointment for chapped hands (Souter 1995: 142). Glycerine was widely used to treat chapped skin: badly chapped hands were thickly coated with glycerine and cotton gloves were worn during the night (MH pers. com., 1955). A mixture of mutton fat and caster sugar was another recommendation (Prince 1991: 32). Honey and lard made another hand cream for chapped skin (EFS 2441). In the Scottish Highlands, deer tallow was used on chapped skin, or the resin normally used to sew leather. Alternatively, a poultice of oatmeal and butter was applied (Beith 1995: 174).

Traditional plant remedies include the outer papery skin of an onion, applied to a sore chapped lip and the use of large dock leaves (*Rumex* sp.) wrapped around sore chapped legs in the winter (Hatfield 1994: 48). In North Norfolk, where marsh samphire (*Salicornia* sp.) is locally abundant, an ointment was made from it for treating cracked and chapped skin. Houseleek juice was another application used. Elder flowers (*Sambucus nigra*) were made into an ointment for treating various skin complaints, including chapped skin (Hatfield 1994: 48–49). An ointment was made from chicken fat and parsley (*Petroselinum crispum*) in the East Anglian fens (Porter 1964: 9). Alternatively, in the same area, bran and water was applied, or the water in which potato had been cooked (Chamberlain 1981, chap. 8). The water in which chickweed has been boiled was used for treating chapped skin (Prince 1991: 32). The fishermen of Whitby in Yorkshire used a salve made from gorse (*Ulex europaeus*) flowers and lard to heal cracked skin (Sekers 1980: 147). In the Scottish Highlands an infusion of groundsel (*Senecio vulgaris*) was employed, and in the island of Uist tormentil *(Potentilla erecta)* was used to treat a sore lip. In Suffolk, blackcurrant leaves *(Ribes nigrum)* served the same purpose (Emerson 1887: 15). Black records the use of leek juice and cream for chapped hands (Black 1883: 203).

In North American folk medicine, some of the same ingredients were employed to treat chapped skin. Salt and water (Welsch 1966: 361) or Epsom salts and water (Browne 1958: 46) were used to bathe the skin. Urine was widely used too. In Kansas a cloth soaked in urine was applied (Koch 1980: 110). In New Mexico, the urine of a male child was stipulated (Espinosa 1910: 410). Ointments were prepared from sugar and soap (Moya 1940: 73), or cider vinegar and glycerine (Gruber 1878: 25), or vaseline and oatmeal (Welsch 1966: 361). Fats of various kinds were used—pure cream (UCLA Folklore Archives 6–6192), or butter from grass-fed cows in May (Mississippi State Guide 1938: 14), or lard (Stout 1936: 186), mutton tallow and rosewater (Puckett 1981: 339), buffalo tallow (UCLA Folklore Archives 2_6751), or possum fat (Parler 1962: 501). Beeswax was mixed with resin and sheep tallow, or with turpentine and sweet oil, to form a soothing ointment (Browne 1958: 46). Plant remedies used include the sap of balm of Gilead (UCLA Folklore Archives 25_7595), fir balsam *(Abies* sp.) (used in Newfoundland) (Bergen 1899: 111), a lotion prepared from soaking the seeds of quince *(Cydonia oblonga)* (Meyer 1985: 224), and an ointment prepared from equal parts of yellowroot *(Xanthorhiza simplicissima),* goldenseal *(Hydrastis canadensis),* and elder bark *(Sambucus* sp.), simmered in lard (Browne 1958: 46). Sore lips were treated with a decoction of white oak *(Quercus alba)* (Meyer 1985: 180).

There has been a widespread belief that washing hands in the first snow of the season will prevent them from becoming chapped (UCLA Folklore Archives 1_6750). A cure for chapped lips is to kiss the middle bar of a five-rail fence (Cannon 1984: 98).

In Native American practice an enormous number of plants have been used for skin conditions (Moerman 1998: 783–788). Of those used in general North American folk medicine, golden seal was used by the Micmac for chapped lips (Chandler, Freeman, and Hooper 1979: 57), and white oak was used for sore chapped skin by the Cherokee (Hamel and Chiltoskey 1975: 46), suggesting that these two remedies may be of Native American origin.

*See also* **Balm of Gilead, Chickweed, Chilblains, Dock, Houseleek.**

### References

Beith, Mary. *Healing Threads: Traditional Medicines of the Highlands and Islands.* Edinburgh: Polygon, 1995.

Bergen, Fanny D. "Animal and Plant Lore Collected from the Oral Tradition of English Speaking Folk." *Memoirs of the American Folk-Lore Society* 7 (1899).

Black, William George. *Folk-Medicine: A Chapter in the History of Culture.* London: Folklore Society, 1883.

Browne, Ray B. *Popular Beliefs and Practices from Alabama.* Folklore Studies 9. Berkeley and Los Angeles: University of California Press, 1958.

Cannon, Anthon S. *Popular Beliefs and Superstitions from Utah.* Edited by Wayland D. Hand and Jeannine E. Talley. Salt Lake City: University of Utah Press, 1984.

Chamberlain, Mary. *Old Wives Tales.* London: Virago, 1981.

Chandler, R. Frank, Lois Freeman, and Shirley N. Hooper. "Herbal Remedies of the Maritime Indians." *Journal of Ethnopharmacology* 1 (1979): 49–68.

EFS. English Folklore Survey. Manuscript notes compiled in the 1960s by the Department of English, University College London.

Emerson, P. H. *Pictures of East Anglian Life.* London: Sampson Low, 1887.

Espinosa, Aurelio M. "New Mexican Spanish Folk-Lore." *Journal of American Folklore* 23 (1910): 395–418.

Gruber, John. Hagerstown, MD: *Hagerstown Town and Country Almanac,* 1852–1914.

Hamel, Paul B., and Mary U. Chiltoskey. *Cherokee Plants and Their Uses: A 400 Year History.* Sylva, NC: Herald, 1975.

Hatfield, Gabrielle. *Country Remedies: Traditional East Anglian Plant Remedies in the Twentieth Century.* Woodbridge: Boydell, 1994.

Koch, William E. *Folklore from Kansas: Beliefs and Customs.* Lawrence: Regent Press, 1980.

Meyer, Clarence. *American Folk Medicine.* Glenwood, IL: Meyerbooks, 1985.

*Mississippi State Guide.* Federal Writers Project. New York, 1938.

Moerman, Daniel E. *Native American Ethnobotany.* Portland, OR: Timber Press, 1998.

Moya, Benjamin S. *Superstitions and Beliefs among the Spanish-Speaking People of New Mexico.* Master's thesis, University of New Mexico, 1940.

Parler, Mary Celestia, and University Student Contributors. *Folk Beliefs from Arkansas.* 15 vols. Fayetteville: University of Arkansas, 1962.

Porter, Enid M. "Some Old Fenland Remedies." *Education Today* (July 1964): 9–11.

Prince, Dennis. *Grandmother's Cures: An A-Z of Herbal Remedies.* London: Fontana, 1991.

Puckett, Newbell Niles. *Popular Beliefs and Superstitions: A Compendium of American Folklore from the Ohio Collection of Newbell Niles Puckett.* Edited by Wayland D. Hand, Anna Casetta, and Sondra B. Thiederman. 3 vols. Boston: G. K. Hall, 1981.

Sekers, Simone. *Grandmother's Lore. A Collection of Household Hints from Past and Present.* London: Hodder and Stoughton, 1980.

Souter, Keith. *Cure Craft: Traditional Folk Remedies and Treatment from Antiquity to the Present Day.* Saffron Walden: C.W. Daniel, 1995.

Stout, Earl J. "Folklore from Iowa." *Memoirs of the American Folklore Society* 29 (1936).

Welsch, Roger. *A Treasury of Nebraska Pioneer Folklore.* Lincoln: University of Nebraska Press, 1966.

# Cherry *(Prunus avium)*

In British folk medicine this plant has provided a cough and cold remedy, prepared from the bark (Hatfield 1994: 30), the gum, or the fruit stalks (Beith 1995: 219). A similar infusion has also been used to treat bladder inflammation (Vickery 1995: 64).

In North America, wild cherry has been widely used in folk medicine, but another species *(Prunus serotina)* has mainly been used. Like its equivalent in Britain, it has largely been used for treating coughs (Crellin and Philpott 1990: 153). However, in combination with other herbs, wild cherry has treated a wide range of other conditions, including colic, jaundice, kidney complaints, and rheumatism (Meyer 1985: 70, 151, 156–157, 212). It has also been used as a blood tonic (Meyer 1985: 41). Native American uses of *Prunus serotina* have been extensive. In addition to all the uses mentioned, the plant has been used for indigestion, worms, burns, labor pains, diarrhea, headache, bronchitis, and tuberculosis (Moerman 1998: 443–444). Another species, *Prunus virginiana,* known as chokecherry, has been even more extensively used (Moerman 1998: 444–448).

*See also* **Colds, Colic, Coughs, Jaundice, Rheumatism.**

### References

Beith, Mary. *Healing Threads: Traditional Medicines of the Highlands and Islands.* Edinburgh: Polygon, 1995.

Crellin, John K., and Jane Philpott. *A Reference Guide to Medicinal Plants.* Durham, NC: Duke University Press, 1990.

Hatfield, Gabrielle. *Country Remedies: Traditional East Anglian Plant Remedies in the Twentieth Century.* Woodbridge: Boydell, 1994.

Meyer, Clarence. *American Folk Medicine.* Glenwood, IL: Meyerbooks, 1985.

Moerman, Daniel E. *Native American Ethnobotany.* Portland, OR: Timber Press, 1998.

Vickery, Roy. *A Dictionary of Plant Lore.* Oxford: Oxford University Press, 1995.

# Chickweed (*Stellaria media*)

This juicy plant common in the wild and as a weed of cultivated land has been used in British folk medicine, above all else, as a poultice for healing all kinds of skin ailments. In the Scottish Highlands it was used to heal cuts and grazes, abscesses, and inflammation of the breasts (Beith 1995: 211). It was also used to induce a refreshing sleep after a fever and was used generally to treat insomnia (Beith 1995: 211). An infusion of chickweed was used in the Scottish Highlands as an aid to slimming (Beith 1995: 211). Throughout Britain the plant has been eaten (and still is) in salad, and fed to chickens and caged birds, as its name suggests. In East Anglia it has been used to treat eczema and skin rashes (Hatfield 1994: 49), as well as boils and abscesses (Hatfield 1994: 21), rheumatism (Newman and Wilson 1951), and (mixed with saffron), jaundice (Newman 1945: 354). In the northeast of England it has been applied to bee stings (Johnston 1853: 43). In Somerset, the plant has been used, together with rose leaves, to form an eye lotion. It has also been used there for treating external ulcers and swellings (Tongue 1965: 39, 42). In Ireland the plant has been used for a very wide range of additional ailments, including headache (Barbour 1897: 389), coughs and sore throat, burns, and jaundice, as well as for treating the swellings of sprains and of mumps (Allen and Hatfield, in press).

This plant is not native in North America but has become naturalized. It does not appear to have been as widely used in folk medicine as in Britain, although it has been used as a salad (Long 1962: 5). As in Brit-ain, the plant was used in Newfoundland for treating boils (Bergen 1899: 111); in Ontario, this extended to wound treatment, and even to hydrophobia (Wintemberg 1950: 13, 15). The Shakers promoted its use in a number of conditions, mainly for skin troubles, much as in Britain (Crellin and Philpott 1990: 156). Meyer reports the use of an ointment prepared by boiling the plant in lard for treating piles and external sores and ulcers (Meyer 1985: 193, 230), while the water in which the plant has been boiled was used for treating freckles (Meyer 1985: 225). This same infusion had a reputation for aiding weight reduction (Puckett 1981: 224), as it had in the Highlands of Scotland.

*See also* **Abscesses, Boils, Burns, Coughs, Eczema, Freckles, Headache, Jaundice, Piles, Poultice, Rheumatism, Shakers, Sleeplessness, Sore throat.**

## References

Allen, David E., and Gabrielle Hatfield. *Medicinal Plants in Folk Tradition.* Portland, OR: Timber Press, in press.

Barbour, John H. "Some Country Remedies and Their Uses. *Folk-Lore* 8 (1897): 386–390.

Beith, Mary. *Healing Threads: Traditional Medicines of the Highlands and Islands.* Edinburgh: Polygon, 1995.

Bergen, Fanny D. "Animal and Plant Lore Collected from the Oral Tradition of English Speaking Folk." *Memoirs of the American Folk-Lore Society* 7 (1899).

Crellin, John K., and Jane Philpott. *A Reference Guide to Medicinal Plants.* Durham, NC: Duke University Press, 1990.

Hatfield, Gabrielle. *Country Remedies: Traditional East Anglian Plant Remedies in the Twentieth Century.* Woodbridge: Boydell, 1994.

Johnston, George. *The Natural History of the Eastern Borders.* Vol. 1, *The Botany.* London: Van Voorst, 1853.

Long, Grady M. "Folk Medicine in McMinn, Polk, Bradley, and Meigs Counties, Tennessee, 1910–1927." *Tennessee Folklore Society Bulletin* 28 (1962): 1–8.

Meyer, Clarence. *American Folk Medicine.* Glenwood, IL: Meyerbooks, 1985.

Newman, L. F. "Some Notes on Folk Medicine the Eastern Counties." *Folk-Lore* 56 (1945): 349–360.

Newman, L. F., and E. M. Wilson. "Folk-Lore Survivals in the Southern 'Lake Counties' and in Essex: A Comparison and Contrast. Part I." *Folk-Lore* 62 (1951): 252–266.

Puckett, Newbell Niles. *Popular Beliefs and Superstitions: A Compendium of American Folklore from the Ohio Collection of Newbell Niles Puckett.* Edited by Wayland D. Hand, Anna Casetta, and Sondra B. Thiederman. 3 vols. Boston: G. K. Hall, 1981.

Tongue, Ruth L. *Somerset Folklore.* Edited by Katharine Briggs. County Folklore 8. London: Folklore Society, 1965.

Wintemberg, W. J. *Folk-Lore of Waterloo County, Ontario.* Ontario: National Museum of Canada, Bulletin 116. Anthropological Series 28, 1950.

# Chilblains

These were a common affliction in Britain until cars replaced winter walking and houses were centrally heated. Folk remedies were varied. Walking in the snow, dipping them in one's own urine, and beating with holly sprigs until blood was drawn are among the remedies used within living memory in East Anglia (Hatfield 1994: 26). In another version of the holly remedy, the berries were crushed with lard to make an ointment (Whitlock, 1976: 167). The berries of bryony were crushed and rubbed on chilblains in Essex (Hatfield 1994: appendix). In the Highlands of Scotland, deer tallow was rubbed on chilblains (Beith 1995: 170). Dipping in urine was used here too, or in a solution of washing soda and hot water (Beith 1995: 187). An ointment made from pig's fat, flowers of sulphur, and olive oil was a traditional remedy of Romany origin but used in Scotland, and an oil prepared from fat and the leaves of adder's tongue fern *(Ophioglossum vulgare)* was also

used (Souter 1995: 142–143). Chickweed boiled in lard made a healing ointment for chilblains in Inverness-shire, Scotland (Vickery 1995: 65). Berries of bittersweet or woody nightshade *(Solanum dulcamara)* were used in the Cotswolds (Bloom 1930: 25), and the berries of black bryony *(Tamus communis)* were used in the Isle of Wight (Bromfield 1856: 507). Poultices were prepared from various fruits and vegetables. Rotten apples were used to treat chilblains in County Antrim, Ireland; beetroot wine was used in Devon; onion was rubbed onto chilblains in Wales; potato was used similarly in County Dublin (Vickery 1995: 13, 29, 267, 292). In Essex, a slice of raw salted potato was rubbed on (E.M., Barking, Essex, 1985, pers. com.). The celebrated Mrs. Beeton recommended the inner flesh of turnip mixed with mustard and grated horseradish, as an application for chilblains (Souter 1995: 143). Leek juice mixed with cream was another suggestion (Black 1883: 203).

In North American folk medicine, as one would expect given the harsher extremes of climate, there is a wealth of remedies for chilblains. In a collection of early settler remedies, there are several recommendations taken from Wesley's *Primitive Physic,* and also two domestic remedies of unknown origin. One consists of chalk dipped in vinegar and rubbed on the surface of the chilblain; the other of a hog's bladder dipped in spirits of turpentine and applied (Robertson 1960: 9). Meyer in his collection of American folk remedies gives recipes including turnip, parsnip juice, potato, onion, pine tar, and sassafras, as well as solutions containing vinegar, or ammonia, or iodine, or alum, potassium permanganate, or "muriatic acid." A salt solution and a mixture of brandy and salt are also given. The berries of poke could be rubbed on to chilblains, or twigs of hemlock spruce *(Tsuga canadensis)* pounded in lard to form an ointment (Meyer 1985: 60–62). Walking in snow is another recommendation, as are applying lard and gunpowder, and immersing them in water and horse dung (Brown 1952–1964, 6: 143).

*See also* **Bryony, Chickweed, Holly, Poke, Sassafras, Snow, Urine.**

### References

Beith, Mary. *Healing Threads: Traditional Medicines of the Highlands and Islands.* Edinburgh: Polygon,1995.

Black, William George. *Folk-Medicine: A Chapter in the History of Culture.* London: Folklore Society, 1883.

Bloom, J. Harvey. *Folk Lore, Old Customs and Superstitions in Shakespeare Land.* London: Mitchell, Hughes, and Clark, 1930.

Bromfield, William Arthur. *Flora Vectensis.* Edited by Sir William Jackson Hooker and Thomas Bell Salter. London: Pamplin, 1856.

Brown, Frank C. *Collection of North Carolina Folklore.* 7 vols. Durham, NC: Duke University Press, 1952–1964.

Hatfield, Gabrielle. *Country Remedies: Traditional East Anglian Plant Remedies in the Twentieth Century.* Woodbridge: Boydell, 1994.

Meyer, Clarence. *American Folk Medicine.* Glenwood, IL: Meyerbooks, 1985.

Robertson, Marion. *Old Settlers' Remedies.* Barrington, NS: Cape Sable Historical Society, 1960.

Souter, Keith. *Cure Craft: Traditional Folk Remedies and Treatment from Antiquity to the Present Day.* Saffron Walden: C.W. Daniel, 1995.

Vickery, Roy. *A Dictionary of Plant Lore.* Oxford: Oxford University Press, 1995.

Whitlock, Ralph. *The Folklore of Wiltshire.* London: Batsford, 1976.

# Childbirth

In all sections of British society until the nineteenth century, and long after that in rural communities, childbirth was an ordeal in which the mother was supported and treated by her fellow women. As a result, we have little written evidence of what actually happened. Printed books, such as Sharp's *Midwives Book,* 1671, reveal a plethora of ordinary and extraordinary agents used during childbirth, but to what extent these were really used we shall probably never know. Likewise, the recommendations of the herbals may or may not have influenced the village midwife. Most women living in the countryside would have had some knowledge of herbal healing. The living memories of twentieth-century elderly people showed that the local midwife was a trusted and respected figure in the village, often doubling as layer-out of the dead. What medicines, if any, did she use for a woman in labor? The "wise wife" of Keith was burned at the stake in 1560 for using herbs to ease another's labor pains (Beith 1985: 85). The witch-hunt spread, with Calvinism, to the New World. In Massachusetts in the mid-seventeenth century three midwives who used medicines were accused of witchcraft. In 1648 a midwife was hanged for witchcraft in Charlestown (Donnison 1988: 17). It is hardly surprising that women who used herbs did not broadcast the fact.

There were a large number of superstitions surrounding pregnancy. The mother-to-be and her unborn child were clearly recognized as vulnerable. Any shock to the system could endanger the development of the child, and as recently as the twentieth century in parts of Britain it was considered dangerous for a pregnant woman to meet a toad. Developmental abnormalities were often ascribed to such bad luck during pregnancy (Marshall 1967: 172).

Nowhere is the link between the magical and medicinal use of healing agents clearer than in the folk medicine associated with childbirth. At this time of obvious peril to mother and child, it was necessary to harness all the help possible. Pre-Christian charms and rituals survived the advent of Christianity in many places. In the Scottish

Highlands a woman in labor was recommended to have a piece of cold iron in her bed and a Bible under the pillow. Near Braemar in the Scottish Highlands, pregnant women used to visit the "wife stone" to ensure an easy time during labor. On the island of Rona, there was a series of stones kept in a small chapel. One of them was valued by pregnant women as a means of ensuring easy labor (Beith 1995: 98, 147, 151).

Otter skin was used as an amulet for protection in childbirth in the Scottish Highlands (Beith 1995: 180). Another birth amulet was provided by the "sea beans," the fruit of tropical species washed ashore on the western coasts of Britain by the Gulf Stream. These were considered lucky in many respects and were especially valued during childbirth. The kidney-shaped seeds of *Entada* spp. were noted by Carew at the beginning of the seventeenth century to have a reputation for easing childbirth (Carew 1602: 27). The so-called Bonduc bean was used in Uist in the Hebrides as recently as the twentieth century to speed delivery; the mother-to-be took the bean in her right hand and prayed (Beith 1995: 208). Higher up in society, charms were also used in labor; the aetites stone was recommended to the Countess of Newcastle in 1633 (Thomas 1973: 224).

We do know that some plants were used during pregnancy to minimize the pain of labor, and of these the most widespread in Britain, right up to the present time, is raspberry *(Rubus idaeus)*. In early pregnancy it was used (unofficially) to procure abortions, but taken throughout the last three months it has been found to speed and ease delivery. An infusion of the dried leaves is drunk like tea. In East Anglia, an infusion of hawthorn leaves was used similarly (Newman and Wilson 1951). In the Norfolk fens, some midwives used to make a special pain-killing cake from whole-meal flour, hemp seed *(Cannabis sativa)*, rhubarb root *(Rheum* sp.), grated dandelion root, egg yolks, milk, and gin. This was given not only to the mother in labor but also to the father! (Porter 1974: 20). Henbane *(Hyoscyamus niger)* was used to procure "twilight sleep" during labor (Whitlock 1992: 109).

Warm fomentations were used to ease the pain of delivery. In the seventeenth-century kitchen book of the Gunton household there is a remedy "For a poor country woman in labor to hasten their birth." It consists of mugwort boiled with cloves in white wine. The footnote to this recipe reads, "You may gather mugwort and dry it in a chamber and soe keep it all the year which is as usefull as the green is." Although such kitchen books largely contain remedies copied from official, learned sources and are therefore not strictly folk medicine, this detail suggests that the writer had some experience of actually using the plant for her social inferiors and perhaps for her own family too (Gunton Household Book).

In the Scottish Highlands, a poultice of the seaweed called dulse *(Laminaria palmata)* was applied to the belly to help expel the afterbirth (Beith 1995: 241). Also in the Scottish Highlands, fairy flax *(Linum catharticum)* was placed under the soles of the feet to bring about an easy delivery (Carmichael 1900: 5: 125). To nourish the newly delivered mother, one twentieth-century country midwife made up a gruel of sifted bran, oats, and skimmed milk (Rigby, pers. com.). In the Scottish Highlands there was a tradition that the first liquid tasted by a newborn child should be the sap of the ash *(Fraxinus excelsior)*. The midwife therefore put one end of an ash twig into the fire and gathered the drops of sap that oozed from the other end. It has been suggested (Kelly 1863: 145) that this tradition might go back to Persian origins, where the sap of another ash species, *Fraxinus ornus,* was fed to children as a divine food.

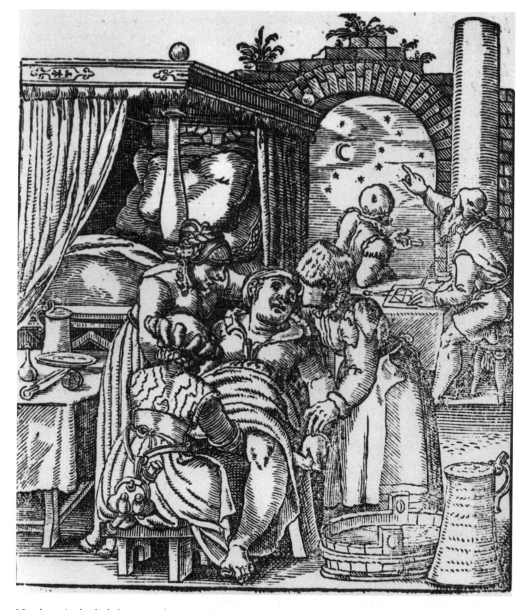

Nowhere is the link between the magical and medicinal use of healing agents clearer than in the folk medicine associated with childbirth. At this time of obvious peril to mother and child, it was necessary to harness all the help possible. (National Library of Medicine)

Colonial women in North America must have had an even harder time than their European counterparts when it came to surviving pregnancy and childbirth. Thousands of miles from their extended families and divorced even from the familiar plant remedies they might have used, they must have had to depend on any printed books they had and on a newly acquired knowledge of the local flora. There is occasional, incidental, information about plants used during labor, such as the reference in an eighteenth-century diary in New Hampshire to a husband gathering betony for his wife (Ulrich 1991: 128). However, without further detail we cannot know whether this was the betony used as a sedative by the Californian Indians (*Pedicularis* spp.) or the unrelated English plant known as betony (*Betonica officinalis*), which was a plant regarded as sacred from the time of Dioscorides and used for a huge variety of ailments.

Folk medical recommendations for bringing on labor include eating a red onion, sniffing up red pepper, taking quinine or gunpowder, and wearing asafoetida around the neck and a rabbit's paw under the pillow (Brown 1952–1964, 6: 7–8). During labor, a stone with a hole in it hung above the head, or an axe or knife under the bed, were suggested; tansy tea *(Tanacetum vulgare)* might be given (Brown 1952–1964, 6: 10, 11).

In contrast with this fragmentary information, there is a wealth of information for the Native American usage of plants during pregnancy and childbirth. *Artemisia* is a genus that has been associated worldwide with women's ailments since the time of Pliny. The British species *A. vulgaris* (mugwort) is not native to North America, but various other species in the genus have been used by Native Americans to facilitate childbirth (Lévi-Strauss 1966: 46). Forty-four plant genera are recorded as in use in the American and Mexican West for easing delivery (Kay 1996: 69) These included plants such as sage (*Salvia* sp.) and chamomile (*Chamaemelum* sp.), familiar to the European herbalist, as well as many local indigenous species, such as the star thistle, cardo santo (*Centaurea* sp.), the flowers of which are chewed during labor by Spanish American women in New Mexico (Kay 1996:17). Among the Catawba, plants used in childbirth include poplar *(Populus deltoides)*, dogwood *(Cornus florida)*, and squaw weed *(Senecio aureus)* (Speck 1944: 41, 42, 44). Another plant still used today by Native Americans to speed delivery is blue cohosh *(Caulophyllum thalictroides)* (Kavasch and

Barr 1999: 4). This use was adopted by settlers in North America and during the nineteenth century became increasingly well known among herbalists. Raspberry was used in just the same way by the Cherokee Indians (Hamel and Chiltoskey 1975: 52) as it was by the East Anglians (see above).

*See also* **Amulet, Ash, Dandelion, Hawthorn, Midwife, Mugwort, Pregnancy, Toads and frogs.**

## References

Beith, Mary. *Healing Threads: Traditional Medicines of the Highlands and Islands.* Edinburgh: Polygon, 1995.

Brown, Frank C. *Collection of North Carolina Folklore.* 7 vols. Durham, NC: Duke University Press, 1952–1964.

Carew, R. *The Survey of Cornwall.* London, 1602.

Carmichael, Alexander. *Carmina Gadelica: Hymns and Incantations.* 6 vols. (3 and 4 edited by J. Carmichael Watson, 5 and 6 by Angus Matheson). Edinburgh: Constable, 1900; Oliver and Boyd, 1940–54; Scottish Academic Press, 1971.

Donnison, Jean. *Midwives and Medical Men: A History of the Struggle for Control of Childbirth.* London: Historical Publications, 1988.

*Gunton Household Book.* Suffolk. Church of St. Peter Mancroft, Norwich.

Hamel, Paul B., and Mary U. Chiltoskey. *Cherokee Plants and Their Uses: A 400 Year History.* Sylva, NC: Herald, 1975.

Kavasch, E. Barrie and Karen Baar. *American Indian Healing Arts: Herbs, Rituals and Remedies for Every Season of Life.* New York: Bantam Books, 1999.

Kay, Margarita Artschwager. *Healing with Plants in the American and Mexican West.* Tucson: University of Arizona Press, 1996.

Kelly, Walter Keating. *Curiosities of Indo-European Tradition and Folk-lore.* London: Chapman and Hall, 1863.

Lévi Strauss, Claude. *The Savage Mind.* London: Weidenfeld and Nicolson, 1966.

Marshall, Sybil. *Fenland Chronicle.* Cambridge: Cambridge University Press, 1967.

Newman, L. F., and E. M. Wilson. "Folk-Lore

Survivals in the Southern 'Lake Counties' and in Essex: A Comparison and Contrast. Part I." *Folk-Lore* 62 (1951): 252–266.

Porter, Enid. *The Folklore of East Anglia.* London: Batsford, 1974.

Sharp, Jane. *The Midwives Book.* London: 1671.

Speck, Frank G. "Catawba Herbals and Curative Practices." *Journal of American Folklore* 57 (1944): 37–50.

Thomas, Keith. *Religion and the Decline of Magic.* Harmondsworth: Penguin, 1973.

Ulrich, Laurel Thatcher. *Good Wives: Image and Reality in the Lives of Women in Northern New England 1650–1750.* New York: Vintage Books, 1991.

Whitlock, Ralph. *Wiltshire Folklore and Legends.* London: Robert Hale, 1992.

# Colds

In British folk medicine one of the commonest remedies, and preventatives, for colds in children was to coat brown paper in goose grease or tallow and wrap it round the child's chest. A Yorkshire version of this remedy was to sprinkle brown sugar onto the bacon fat from a frying pan, coat a piece of brown paper with the mixture, and apply it as a poultice around the child's chest (Souter 1995: 146). In the Scottish Highlands, seal oil was used similarly, rubbed on the chest for a cough and taken internally to prevent or cure colds (Beith 1995: 181). An alternative was camphorated oil rubbed into the chest, or a small bag of camphor worn around the neck (Beith 1995: 91). A hot footbath in which mustard seeds have been steeped was another recommendation. In contrast, a popular cold cure in the Scottish Highlands was to run fully clad into the sea, then go home, go to bed and sleep, still in the sea-soaked clothes (Beith 1995: 135). "Sweating" a patient by lighting a fire on the earthen floor, removing the fire, strewing the floor with straw and watering the straw, then laying the patient on the steaming straw, was another Highland cure for a cold (Beith 1995: 137). For a feverish cold, elder flower infusion, or elderberry wine was much used for children and adults. Whisky with hot water, lemon, and honey was a favorite remedy, especially in Scotland. Horehound, or "haryhound," tea was also very commonly used, prepared usually from white horehound (*Marrubium vulgare*). An infusion of yarrow was used to treat bronchitis and colds (Taylor MSS; Hatfield MS). Ground-ivy (*Glechoma hederacea*) was dried during the summer months and kept for winter use against colds (Taylor MSS). Infusions of various species of mint (*Mentha* spp.) were also widely used. Elecampane infusion (*Inula helenium*) was used, for instance in Sussex, for colds and coughs (Allen 1995: 66). In the Scottish Highlands, snuff prepared from the helleborine (*Epipactis latifolia*) or from the root of yellow flag (*Iris pseudacorus*) was used to treat a cold (Beith 1995: 217, 222). Also in Scotland, the gum of the wild cherry, known there as "gean" (*Prunus avium*), was dissolved in wine to treat colds (Beith 1995: 219). An infusion of thyme (*Thymus* spp.) was used especially for "bronchial" colds in Devon (Vickery 1995: 371).

Onions stewed in milk were recommended as a diet during a cold. In Scotland, water gruel, made from unsalted oatmeal, sweetened with honey, was given as nourishment during a cold (Beith 1995: 231). The bulbs of ramsons (*Allium ursinum*) were preserved in rum and brown sugar and kept to treat heavy, chesty colds in the Isle of Man (Vickery 1995: 306). Teas made from rosemary (*Rosmarinus officinalis*), sage (*Salvia officinalis*), chamomile (*Chamaemelum nobile*), or balm (*Melissa officinalis*) were also used. Blackcurrant tea (*Ribes nigrum*), usually made from hot water and blackcurrant jam, was another soothing drink used both to prevent and to treat a cold. For a heavy cold, the vapor from grated horse-radish (*Armoracia rusticana*) was inhaled (Vickery 1995: 197; EFS 195Bd).

In North American folk medicine, colds were treated in many similar ways. Among chest poultices used were a flannel wrung out in boiling water and then sprinkled with turpentine. Tar or mustard plasters (Brown 1952–1964, 6: 154) or red flannel coated with oils (Brown 1952–1964, 6: 155) were applied. Poultices of onion or of flaxseed, of hot hops or of catnip were also used (Meyer 1985: 67). Rubbing the chest with skunk oil was also recommended. For a baby congested with a cold, rubbing the hands and soles of the feet with pure lard was suggested. For a head cold, snuffing up the powdered flowers of sneezeweed *(Helenium autumnale)* or powdered borax could help congestion. Smoking rabbit-tobacco *(Gnaphalium* sp.) in a corn cob pipe was a remedy for a head cold from the African American tradition. Smoking crushed cubeb berries *(Piper cubeba)* was also considered good to clear congestion. Hot drinks to help a cold included lemon and ginger; milk and molasses; hot water, brown sugar, and rum; black tea; honey; brandy; and nutmeg. Herbal infusions included mayweed tea *(Anthemis cotula)*, an infusion of white pine needles sweetened with sugar, peppermint tea alone or mixed with elder blossoms and yarrow, horsemint *(Monarda punctata)*, pennyroyal *(Hedeoma pulegioides)*, boneset, dittany *(Cunila origanoides)*, or horehound. Camphorated oil was used, rubbed onto the nostrils—or oil of marjoram *(Origanum vulgare)*, or a spray of witch hazel *(Hamamelis virginiana)* (Meyer 1985: 64–68). Bark of wild cherry was another cold remedy (Brown 1952–1964, 6: 148).

There are more than fifteen hundred records of cold treatments in the UCLA Folklore Archives. One common treatment, which stands out as different from anything used in Britain, is asafoetida. This evil-smelling plant *(Ferula assafoetida)* is a native of Asia and some parts of Europe. It became fashionable in the eighteenth and nineteenth centuries in official European medicine, and it has evidently persisted in use in North American folk medicine. Sometimes it is worn in a bag around the neck: in this case it probably acted not simply as an amulet, but also as an inhalant, since the fumes are very penetrating. Other amulets used include a string of amber beads (Cannon 1984: 101), a sowbug, and a wet cotton string (Brown 1952–1964, 6: 149, 155).

There are occasional examples of transference of a cold, for example to a spider or a woodlouse sewn up in a bag and kept around the neck until it dies, or to a live fish thrust into the throat and then returned to the water (Pickard and Buley 1945: 81). Another example of transference is to bury a piece of hair or toenail from the cold sufferer in a hole in a tree (Brown 1952–1964, 6: 155). In Maine, a child with a cold could be passed three times under the belly of a horse (Beck 1957: 78).

Breaking open a blister on a balsam tree at the time of a full moon is another suggestion for a cold (Relihan 1947: 82). Catching a falling leaf in the autumn is said to ensure no colds during the winter (Kimmerle 1976: 22). Moustaches and beards are claimed to protect against colds (Masterson 1940: 45). Walking barefoot around the house or eating the first snow of the winter are other cold precautions reported from Illinois (Hyatt 1965: 278). Rolling children naked in the first snow of the season was claimed to protect them from colds (Parler 1962: 524).

Miscellaneous substances recommended for a cold include chicken soup (also recommended for flu) (UCLA Folklore Archive record number 2_5318) or, less pleasantly, the urine of a polecat (Puckett 1981: 344). A tea made from a hornet's nest was a remedy collected from Pennsylvania (Brendle and Unger 1935: 132). Using leeches has been suggested to draw off blood during a bad cold (Puckett 1981: 344).

Among the very numerous herbs used in cold treatment by the Native Americans are species of fir (*Abies* spp.), yarrow (*Achillea* spp.), sweet flag *(Acorus calamus),* sagebrush (*Artemisia* spp.), dogwood (*Cornus* spp.) and juniper (*Juniperus* spp.) (Moerman 1998: 780–782).

*See also* **African tradition, Amber, Amulet, Boneset, Catnip, Cherry, Elder, Flax, Hops, Horehound, Onion, Pine, Snow, Transference, Yarrow.**

### References

Allen, Andrew. *A Dictionary of Sussex Folk Medicine.* Newbury: Countryside Books, 1995.

Beck, Horace P. *The Folklore of Maine.* Philadelphia and New York: J. B. Lippincott, 1957.

Beith, Mary. *Healing Threads: Traditional Medicines of the Highlands and Islands.* Edinburgh: Polygon, 1995.

Brendle, Thomas R., and Claude W. Unger. "Folk Medicine of the Pennsylvania Germans: The Non-Occult Cures." *Proceedings of the Pennsylvania and German Society* 45 (1935).

Brown, Frank C. *Collection of North Carolina Folklore.* 7 vols. Durham, NC: Duke University Press, 1952–1964.

Cannon, Anthon S. *Popular Beliefs and Superstitions from Utah.* Edited by Wayland D. Hand and Jeannine E. Talley. Salt Lake City: University of Utah Press, 1984.

EFS. English Folklore Survey. Manuscript notes at University College London., EFS 195Bd.

Hyatt, Harry Middleton. *Folklore from Adams County Illinois.* 2nd rev. ed. New York: Memoirs of the Alma Egan Hyatt Foundation, 1965.

Kimmerle, Marjorie, and Mark Gelber. *Popular Beliefs and Superstitions from Colorado.* Boulder: University of Colorado, 1976 (unpublished).

Masterson, James R. "The Arkansas Doctor." *Annals of Medical History.* Series 3, no. 2 (1940): 30–51.

Meyer, Clarence. *American Folk Medicine.* Glenwood, IL: Meyerbooks, 1985.

Moerman, Daniel E. *Native American Ethnobotany.* Portland, OR: Timber Press, 1998.

Parler, Mary Celestia, and University of Arkansas Student Contributors. *Folk Beliefs from Arkansas.* 15 vols. Fayetteville: University of Arkansas, 1962.

Pickard, Madge E., and R. Carlyle Buley. *The Midwest Pioneer, His Ills, Cures and Doctors.* Crawfordsville, IN: R. E. Banta, 1945.

Puckett, Newbell Niles. *Popular Beliefs and Superstitions: A Compendium of American Folklore from the Ohio Collection of Newbell Niles Puckett.* Edited by Wayland D. Hand, Anna Casetta, Sondra B. Thiederman. 3 vols. Boston: G. K. Hall, 1981.

Relihan, Catherine M. "Folk Remedies." *New York Folklore Quarterly* 3 (1947): 81–84.

Souter, Keith. *Cure Craft: Traditional Folk Remedies and Treatment from Antiquity to the Present Day.* Saffron Walden: C. W. Daniel, 1995.

Speck, Frank G. "Medicine Practices of the Northeastern Algonquians." *Proceedings of the Nineteenth International Congress of Americanists,* 1917, 303–321.

Taylor MSS. Manuscript notes of Mark R. Taylor in the Norfolk Record Office, Norwich MS4322.

Vickery, Roy. *A Dictionary of Plant Lore.* Oxford: Oxford University Press, 1995.

# Colic

In folk medicine the different types of colic distinguished today (renal, biliary, etc.) were often not clearly distinguished in the records of treatment. Although gravel and stone were clearly recognized, renal colic was sometimes referred to simply as colic. An example of this is the "colickwort" *(Aphanes arvensis)* reported in use by Johnson in the seventeenth century (Johnson 1633, preface). This plant, also known as parsley piert, was definitely known for its use in treating gravel and stone. However, it is likely that many of the folk records for colic treatment are referring to the more common griping pain in infants and adults caused by trapped wind.

There were some mechanical suggestions in folk medicine for relieving this. Standing on one's head for a quarter of an hour was a suggestion from Cornwall (Black 1883: 183). In the Scottish Highlands the drastic suggestion of swallowing a bullet was thought to relieve colic (Beith 1995: 158). For infant colic, rubbing the baby's stomach, or rocking the child, will sometimes help it to pass wind and bring relief. Poulticing with turf is a novel cure for colic.

Plants used in folk medical treatment of colic include chickweed, used in Ireland, centaury (*Centaurium erythraea*) and dulse (*Palmaria palmata*) used in Scotland, sloe wine (from the fruit of *Prunus spinosa*) suggested in Suffolk (Allen and Hatfield, in press). Pepper saxifrage (*Silaum silaus*) was reported by Parkinson to soothe "frets" in infants (Parkinson 1640: 908). Nowadays in domestic medicine, dill water from the related plant *Anethum graveolens* is often used to treat infant colic (Lafont 1984: 34).

In North American folk medicine similar groups of colic remedies are to be found. For infant colic, rocking the baby, hanging it upside down, or rubbing its back are mechanical suggestions (Brown 1952–1964, 6: 48–49). Hanging round its neck a newly killed mouse is another suggestion. Catnip tea was a favorite remedy for colic in sufferers of all ages. An infusion of calamus root (*Acorus calamus*) or of ground ivy (*Glechoma hederacea*) were other herbal suggestions for infant colic, or blowing tobacco through the baby's milk (Brown 1952–1964, 6: 49). Preparations of aniseed (*Pimpinella anisum*), fennel seed (*Foeniculum vulgare*), or caraway seed (*Carum carvi*) have all been used, especially for infants. For patients of all ages peppermint (*Mentha* sp.), wild ginger (*Asarum canadense*), ginseng and yarrow have all been used (Meyer 1985: 69–71). Lobelia has been called colic weed in New England.

A suggestion for colic in adults is to stand the person on his head and shake him (cf. the Cornish recommendation above). Rubbing the back has also been suggested, or "cupping" over the abdomen (Brown 1952–1964, 6: 155–156). Warm water, soda, salt water, or application of hot poultices are other practical suggestions (Brown 1952–1964, 6: 157–158). Dog dung (Hyatt 1965: 246) or wolf dung are less appealing remedies. Alternatively, colic can be transferred to a duck. Among plants used by Native Americans to treat colic, catnip was used by the Cherokee (Hamel and Chiltoskey 1975: 28) and mint (*Mentha canadensis*) by several tribes, including the Okanagon (Perry 1952: 42). Garlic and onion have also been used, as has rattlesnake venom.

*See also* **Catnip, Earth, Excreta, Garlic, Ginseng, Gravel and stone, Lobelia, Mouse, Onion, Snake, Soda, Transference, Yarrow.**

## References
Allen, David E., and Gabrielle Hatfield. *Medicinal Plants in Folk Traditions.* Portland, OR: Timber Press, in press.

Beith, Mary. *Healing Threads: Traditional Medicines of the Highlands and Islands.* Edinburgh: Polygon, 1995.

Black, William George. *Folk-Medicine: A Chapter in the History of Culture.* London: Folklore Society, 1883.

Brown, Frank C. *Collection of North Carolina Folklore.* 7 vols. Durham, NC: Duke University Press, 1952–1964.

Hamel, Paul B., and Mary U. Chiltoskey. *Cherokee Plants and Their Uses: A 400 Year History.* Sylva, NC: Herald, 1975.

Hyatt, Harry Middleton. *Folklore from Adams County Illinois.* 2nd rev. ed. New York: Memoirs of the Alma Egan Hyatt Foundation 1965.

Johnson, Thomas (ed.). *The Herball or Generall Historie of Plantes.* London: Islip, Norton and Whitakers, 1633.

Lafont, Anne-Marie. *Herbal Folklore.* Bideford: Badger Books, 1984.

Meyer, Clarence. *American Folk Medicine.* Glenwood, IL: Meyerbooks, 1985.

Parkinson, John. *Theatrum Botanicum.* London: Thomas Cotes, 1640.

Perry, F. "Ethnobotany of the Indians in the Interior of British Columbia." *Museum and Art Notes* 2(2) (1952): 36–43.

# Colonists

Forced to be self-reliant in times of illness, the early European settlers of North America brought with them their inherited knowledge of their own folk medicine and their few medical books, such as Thomas Phaire's *The Boke of Chyldren* (London, 1553) and later John Wesley's *Primitive Physic; or an Easy and Natural Method of Curing Most Diseases* (London, 1747). Other medical texts available from Europe and known to have been owned by early settlers include William Buchan's *Domestic Medicine,* first published in 1772 and running into numerous editions into the nineteenth century. In the nineteenth century various North American publications became available, such as the two herbals written by Catherine Parr Traill in Canada (*The Canadian Settler's Guide,* 1855, and *Studies of Plant-Life in Canada*, 1885) and Charles Millspaugh's book *American Medicinal Plants* (1852), as well as Samuel Thomson's *New Guide to Health; or, Botanic Family Physician* (1831). The Tennessee physician Dr. John Gunn published in 1857 his *New Domestic Medicine or Family Physician,* which became enormously popular, reaching its 213th edition in 1885.

To what extent such texts were actually used in times of illness is impossible to know. Faced with a lack of some of the plants that they normally used at home, and presented with a whole new and unfamiliar flora, early European settlers must have been forced to experiment, and many were willing to learn from Native American healers. Groups such as the Shakers developed their own, largely home-grown, pharmacopoeia. At a time when orthodox medicine relied heavily on such drastic measures as bleeding, purging, and "chemical medicine," this self-reliance might ironically have been good for the health of the community. Newspaper articles and "almanacks" published medical advice, and some individuals set themselves up as healers and as herbalists (for example, Samuel Thomson). However, the basic first aid for most early European settlers, whether French, German, Dutch, or English, must have been the knowledge of the women of the households, brought from their native countries and supplemented by any local sources they could find. This was largely oral knowledge, handed down from one generation to the next, so that by definition there is a very incomplete record in the literature. As Ulrich has put it, remedies came from the barnyard and the forest (Ulrich 1991: 128). The types of remedy brought from home would depend on the social background of the immigrants (Fischer 1989). During the long journeys made across the North American continent by many settlers, a basic medicine chest was the only source of medical help, other than local remedies. Immigrants sometimes received advice from earlier pioneers. Emergency medical supplies often included castor oil and peppermint essence; by the eighteen hundreds, purpose-built kits of dried herbs were available (Micheletti 1998: 297).

Some householders kept kitchen books, collections of household recipes, and remedies. Those that have survived indicate a reliance initially on remedies brought from home, together with medical texts and newspapers (see, for example, Robertson 1960). The few "orthodox" Western doctors among the settlers were influenced by the existing medical knowledge of the Native Americans, especially by their treatment of wounds, treatments that appeared often to be much more successful than their own. Some individuals exploited the appeal to the new arrivals of the native medicine and even set themselves up as quasi-Native American healers. Lighthall, for example, published in 1883 a book entitled *The Indian Folk Medicine Guide.* He was of only one-eighth Indian descent but is described in the book as "The Great Indian Medicine Man."

What was mainstream medicine for the Native Americans therefore became partially incorporated, with modifications and in some cases distortions, into American folk medicine. Colonists adopted, for example, the Native American use of sweat tents (Hanzlik 1936: 276). There was undoubtedly some exchange between Native Americans and the colonists of New England, New France, New Netherlands, and New Sweden, though it is hard to know to what extent remedies were shared (Fenton 1942: 514). Vogel cites the examples of goldthread (*Coptis* spp.), used for a sore mouth by both Native Americans and colonists, and skunk cabbage (*Symplocarpus foetidus*) roots used for itch (Vogel 1970: 310, 367). The dogwood (*Cornus* spp.), used by early colonists for treatment of malaria (Brewster 1969: 39), might be another example of a remedy learnt from Native American practice; species of dogwood were certainly used by various Native American tribes to treat fevers (Moerman 1998: 176–179). There are numerous examples of contemporary remedies used by both general North American folk medicine and by Native Americans, but whether they all represent direct "borrowing" in colonial times from the Native American tradition is difficult to establish. Systematic studies of the medicinal plants used by Native Americans began in earnest in the nineteenth century (Croom 1992: 138), and at least some present-day uses of Native American rem-

edies by the general population of North America probably postdate these works.

*See also* **Shakers; Thomson, Samuel; Traill, Catherine Parr; Wounds.**

### References
Brewster, Paul G. "The Myth of Modernity." *Tennessee Folklore Bulletin* 35 (1969): 37–40.
Croom, Edward M., Jr. "Herbal Medicine among the Lumbee Indians." In *Herbal and Magical Medicine: Traditional Healing Today.* Edited by James Kirkland, Holly F. Matthews, C. W. Sullivan III, and Karen Baldwin. Durham, NC: Duke University Press, 1992.
Fenton, William N. *Contacts between Iroquois Herbalism and Colonial Medicine.* Annual Report of the Smithsonian Institution 1941. Washington, D.C., 1942, 503–527.
Fischer, David Hackett. *Albion's Seed.* Oxford: Oxford University Press, 1989.
Hanzlik, Harold. "Medical Conditions, Practices and Foundations in the Continental Colonies." *California and Western Medicine* 45 (1936): 275–278.
Lighthall, J. I. *The Indian Folk Medicine Guide.* New York: Popular Library Edition, n.d.
Micheletti, Enza (ed.). *North American Folk Healing.* New York and Montreal: Reader's Digest Association, 1998.
Moerman, Daniel E. *Native American Ethnobotany.* Portland, OR: Timber Press, 1998.
Robertson, Marion. *Old Settlers' Remedies.* Barrington, NS: Cape Sable Historical Society, 1960.
Ulrich, Laurel Thatcher. *Good Wives: Image and Reality in the Lives of Women in Northern New England 1650–1750.* New York: Vintage, 1991.
Vogel, Virgil J. *American Indian Medicine.* Norman: University of Oklahoma Press, 1970.

# Color

Certain colors are associated in folk medicine with healing. Red is one such color, perhaps because it is associated with heat (Black 1883: 108). Red threads are tied around parts of the body—for instance, to prevent nosebleeds. Red is the preferred color for flannel to wrap around an injury. Backache was in the recent past treated by "ironing" with a flat iron, over a piece of red flannel. Patients suffering from smallpox were given red bed coverings to draw out the pustules (Black 1883: 108). Red flannel worn around the neck was used to ward off whooping cough in the west of Scotland (Black 1883: 111). In the nineteenth century "tongues" of red flannel were sold in London to be worn around the necks of patients suffering from scarlet fever (Notes and Queries, 5th series, vol. xi, 166). In fourteenth-century Ireland in sacrificial ceremonies associated with healing, a red cock was specified as the sacrificial victim (Black 1883: 112). Black suggests that as well as its association with heat, red was thought to ward off evil spirits and quotes the example of cattle in nineteenth-century Aberdeenshire having a red thread tied around their tails before going out to pasture for the first time (Black 1883: 112). A healing charm known as the "cure of the threads" is still practiced on one of the Scottish islands. It is known there as *bàrr a' chinn* (the top of head). Red threads are wound around the neck while reciting a charm to drive evil spirits out through the top of the head (Beith 1995: 198).

Blue is another color that figures frequently in folk medical cures. A necklace of blue beads was worn in Norfolk as a cure for bronchitis (Porter 1974: 43). This color is associated in Christian, and particularly Catholic, belief with the Virgin Mary. This may explain its use for "evil" purposes in the Orkneys, where anything that smacked of popery was abhorred. In 1635 a man in Orkney was ruined by a blue necklace given to his sister (Black 1883: 112). By contrast, a blue thread was treasured and handed down the female line in families in the Scottish borders. It was worn to prevent fevers at the time of weaning (Black 1883: 113).

Black is another color associated with folk cures. The tail of a black cat was recommended for curing styes, and the blood of a black cat for shingles. Black wool has been recommended for deafness. Black snails were used in wart treatment.

Very similar color associations are to be found in North American folk medicine. Again, red has the dual significance of warmth and blood. As a symbol of warmth, red flannel or red thread was recommended for rheumatism (Brown 1952–1964, 6: 264), sore throat (Black 1935: 13), and colds (Morgan 1934: 669). Red ribbon was said to protect a baby from the evil eye (Puckett 1981: 131). Red thread was used to stop hiccups (UCLA Folklore Archives 2_5411). Warm milk from a red cow was recommended for tuberculosis (Hyatt 1965: 252). Examples of the association between red and blood include red beads worn for nosebleed (Bergen 1896: 94) or a red bean worn around the neck (Brown 1952–1964, 6: 241). To trigger periods, red food should be eaten (Hyatt 1965: 219). For palpitations of the heart, a red tape was worn around the chest (Riddell 1934: 262). To arrest bleeding, the sufferer should be wrapped in a red cloak (UCLA Folklore Archives 2_6287).

As in Britain, blue seems to have been associated with chest ailments. For whooping cough, wearing stolen blue ribbon (Aurand 1929: 71), or eating from a blue dish (Fogel 1915: 339) is suggested. Perhaps because of an association with coolness, pale blue stones were worn for headache (Cannon 1984: 111) and blue string for cramp (Brown 1952–1964, 6: 164); wearing a blue sweater was a suggestion for a high fever (UCLA Folklore Archives 2_5377). Blue was also recommended as protection against the evil eye (Puckett 1981: 1080).

As in Britain, black cats were chosen in folk medicine. Again, the tail of a black cat was used as a cure for styes (Brown 1952–1964, 6: 294), and blood from a black cat for shingles (Roberts 1927: 167). Black snails were rubbed on warts (Wintemberg 1918: 127). Black threads were used in wart treatment (Cannon 1984: 134), backache (Puckett 1981: 313), and croup (Whitney and Bullock 1925: 92).

The color of plants used in folk medicine is discussed under doctrine of signatures.

*See also* **Backache, Bleeding, Colds, Cramp, Croup, Deafness, Evil eye, Eye problems, Fevers, Headache, Heart trouble, Nosebleed, Rheumatism, Shingles, Smallpox, Sore throat, Tuberculosis, Warts, Whooping cough.**

### References

Aurand, A. Monroe, Jr. *The Pow-Wow Book: A Treatise on the Art of "Healing by Prayer" and "Laying on of Hands." etc., Practised by the Pennsylvania Germans and others.* Harrisburg: Aurand Press, 1929.

Beith, Mary. *Healing Threads: Traditional Medicines of the Highlands and Islands.* Edinburgh: Polygon, 1995.

Bergen, Fanny D. "Animal and Plant Lore Collected from the Oral Tradition of English Speaking Folk." *Memoirs of the American Folk-Lore Society* 4 (1896).

Black, Pauline Monette. *Nebraska Folk Cures. Studies in Language, Literature, and Criticism* 15. Lincoln, Nebraska: University of Nebraska, 1935.

Black, William George. *Folk-Medicine: A Chapter in the History of Culture.* London: Folklore Society, 1883.

Brown, Frank C. *Collection of North Carolina Folklore.* 7 vols. Durham, NC: Duke University Press, 1952–1964.

Cannon, Anthon S. *Popular Beliefs and Superstitions from Utah.* Edited by Wayland D. Hand and Jeannine E. Talley. Salt Lake City: University of Utah Press, 1984.

Fogel, Edwin Miller. "Beliefs and Superstitions of the Pennsylvania Germans." *Americana Germanica* 18 (1915).

Hyatt, Harry Middleton. *Folklore from Adams County Illinois.* 2nd rev. ed. New York: Memoirs of the Alma Egan Hyatt Foundation, 1965.

Morgan, Edward A. "Some Traditional Beliefs Encountered in the Practice of Pediatrics." *Canadian Medical Association Journal* 31 (December 1934): 666–669.

*Notes and Queries* 5th Series, Vol. xi, p. 166. London, 1849.

Porter, Enid. *The Folklore of East Anglia.* London: Batsford, 1974.

Puckett, Newbell Niles. *Popular Beliefs and Superstitions: A Compendium of American Folklore from the Ohio Collection of Newbell Niles Puckett.* Edited by Wayland D. Hand, Anna Casetta, and Sondra B. Thiederman. 3 vols. Boston: G. K. Hall, 1981.

Riddell, William Renwick. "Some Old Canadian Folk Medicine." *Medical Record* 140 (1934): 262.

Roberts, Hilda. "Louisiana Superstitions." *Journal of American Folklore* 40 (1927): 144–208.

Whitney, Annie Weston, and Caroline Canfield Bullock. "Folk-Lore from Maryland." *Memoirs of the American Folklore Society* 18 (1925).

Wintemberg, W. J. "Folk-Lore Collected in Toronto and Vicinity." *Journal of American Folklore* 31 (1918): 125–134.

# Columbo (*Frasera caroliniensis*)

This plant is not native to Britain, and is unused there in folk medicine.

In North American folk medicine, it has been used for stomach trouble and vomiting caused by teething in infants or by pregnancy (Meyer 1985: 242, 248, 262). It has been a constituent of many tonics (Coffey 1993: 168) and has treated worms and constipation in children (Meyer 1985: 208, 271). In Native American medicine, the Cherokee used it to treat gastrointestinal disorders of all kinds and used it as a tonic (Hamel and Chiltoskey 1975: 30).

*See also* **Constipation, Pregnancy, Teething, Tonic, Worms.**

### References

Coffey, Timothy. *The History and Folklore of North American Wildflowers.* New York: Facts On File, 1993.

Hamel, Paul B., and Mary U. Chiltoskey. *Cherokee Plants and Their Uses: A 400 Year History.* Sylva, NC: Herald, 1975.

Meyer, Clarence. *American Folk Medicine.* Glenwood, IL: Meyerbooks, 1985.

# Comfrey (*Symphytum officinale*)

From the Highlands of Scotland (Beith 1995: 212) to the southwest of England (Lafont 1984: 26), comfrey has been used in British folk medicine for treating sprains and fractures. There are innumerable stories of the dramatic healing power that the plant appears to have (Hatfield 1994: 5; Lafont 1984: 26). It has also been used for healing wounds and for treating the pain of arthritis. In Ireland comfrey root has been used for treating boils, and the juice of the root has been considered good for the complexion (Logan 1972: 61, 77). Early writers identified the plant with the "sumphuton" of Dioscorides, hence its botanical name Symphytum, the "grow-together" plant (Grigson 1955: 281). Interestingly, it has been used in the western parts of Britain, where it is abundant in much the same way as houseleek (*Sempervivum tectorum*) has been used in the rest of Britain, where comfrey is relatively scarce (Allen and Hatfield, in press). Despite recent scares over the hepatotoxicity of some of its alkaloids, the plant is still widely used by herbalists, especially as an external treatment. It has been referred to as "nature's putty," and the root when scraped and soaked does indeed make a thick healing sludge. The plant has two forms, a red-flowered and a white-flowered; in some areas, such as Dorset (FLR 6 (1888); 116), there was a belief that the red-flowered form should be used for treating men, the white-flowered reserved for women.

The plant is not native to North America but has become naturalized there, and its popularity in folk medicine is again striking. Meyer records uses for treatment of sore breasts and nipples, cough medicine, diarrhea, "female weakness," liver complaints, as a soothing poultice, for sores and surface ulcers, for hoarseness, and for cuts and wounds (Meyer 1985: 48, 50, 51, 81, 87, 91, 124, 125, 168, 202, 254, 276). It has been used to treat crush injuries (Puckett 1981: 373), dysentery (Browne 1958: 40), and asthma (Cannon 1984: 92), as well as being used as a boost to virility (Peattie 1943: 190). Some of these uses are also recorded among the Cherokee (Hamel and Chiltoskey 1975: 30), by whom it is also taken for constipation and heartburn during pregnancy.

*See also* **Arthritis, Asthma, Boils, Dysentery, Houseleek, Pregnancy, Rheumatism, Wounds.**

## References

Allen, David E., and G. V. Hatfield. *Medicinal Plants in Folk Tradition.* Portland, OR: Timber Press, in press.

Beith, Mary. *Healing Threads: Traditional Medicines of the Highlands and Islands.* Edinburgh: Polygon 1995.

Browne, Ray B. *Popular Beliefs and Practices from Alabama.* Folklore Studies 9. Berkeley and Los Angeles: University of California Publications, 1958.

Cannon, Anthon S. *Popular Beliefs and Superstitions from Utah.* Edited by Wayland D. Hand and Jeannine E. Talley. Salt Lake City: University of Utah Press, 1984.

FLR. *Folk Lore Record* 6 (1888): 116.

Grigson, Geoffrey. *The Englishman's Flora.* London: Phoenix House, 1955.

Hamel, Paul B., and Mary U. Chiltoskey. *Cherokee Plants and Their Uses: A 400 Year History.* Sylva, NC: Herald, 1975.

Hatfield, Gabrielle. *Country Remedies: Traditional East Anglian Plant Remedies in the Twentieth Century.* Woodbridge: Boydell, 1994.

Lafont, Anne-Marie. *Herbal Folklore.* Bideford: Badger Books, 1984.

Logan, Patrick. *Making the Cure: A Look at Irish Folk Medicine.* Dublin: Talbot Press, 1972.

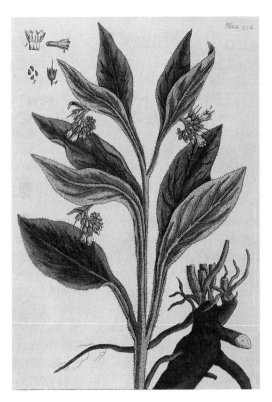

Comfrey has been used in British folk medicine for treating sprains, fractures, and arthritic pain. It has also been used for healing wounds. The juice of the root is considered good for the complexion. (Stapleton Collection/CORBIS)

Meyer, Clarence. *American Folk Medicine.* Glenwood, IL: Meyerbooks, 1985.

Peattie, Roderick (ed.). *The Great Smokies and the Blue Ridge.* New York: Vanguard Press, 1943.

Puckett, Newbell Niles. *Popular Beliefs and Superstitions: A Compendium of American Folklore from the Ohio Collection of Newbell Niles Puckett.* Edited by Wayland D. Hand, Anna Casetta, and Sondra B. Thiederman. 3 vols. Boston: G. K. Hall, 1981.

# Concepts of disease

By definition, folk medicine was primarily a practical response to illness by those too poor to afford official medical aid. Much of British folk medicine has been do-it-yourself practical treatment of illness within a family or small group. A system of beliefs has developed only when there is an established group of healers within a tradition (see, for example, the Celtic tradition). On the whole, theories of disease were a luxury for the more educated. However, glimpses are to be found of some folk ideas about the causation of disease. In British folk medicine, certain ailments were in the past ascribed to witchcraft. They include epilepsy, drastic weight loss, and loss of appetite (Porter 1974: 51). The devil, in Britain a personification of old paganism, was blamed for many illnesses but was also credited with the power to cure them. Black quotes a witch in Scotland famous for her cures of children who would apply the remedy saying it was given in God's name "but the devil give thee good of it" (Black 1883: 14). In Scotland Rorie comments that disease is regarded as an entity that can be "drawn" from the body—for example by means of poultices, which should then be burned (Buchan 1994: 239). Warts were said to be caused by a host of external sources, including sea foam (Black 1883: 30), the water in which eggs have been boiled, touching a frog or toad, etc. Birthmarks and congenital abnormalities were frequently attributed to shock sustained by the mother during pregnancy.

Contagious magic has seeped into folk medicine, giving rise not only to the like-curing-like principle but also to practices involving transference of disease to plants or animals. Ideas concerning infectious diseases were inconsistent. Long before the discovery of bacteria and viruses, the air was blamed for spreading contagion, such as the plague, and efforts were made to purify the air by carrying highly scented herbs or by the use of onion left lying in a sick chamber or around the house. In more recent times, "bad air" was often seen as a cause of disease. In some parts of England country people wore pieces of tansy in their boots to protect themselves from the "miasma" rising from the ground, which was seen there as a cause of ague (Quelch 1941: 153). The night air of the fens was blamed for the prevalence there of fevers and rheumatism (Porter 1974: 48). Conversely, some air was valued as "healthy." In Wales there is a place in Parc Llewelyn where it is supposed that four winds meet; sufferers from tuberculosis were recommended to walk to this spot (Jones 1980: 63–64). In Norfolk there was a curious belief that tuberculosis could only be spread within a family between members of the same sex. Also in East Anglia, it was believed that bringing wild arum into a house could cause tuberculosis and that eating kernels of wheat could cause scarlet fever (Porter 1974: 48). In Fife, Scotland, it was believed that an infectious disease did not pass from a young person to an older one, also that if a person was unafraid of infection he would not catch it (Buchan 1994: 240).

The picture in North American folk medicine is different. Here folk medicine is a much broader-based conglomerate of ideas drawn from the oral folk traditions of many different countries, but also in part from their medical literature (see introduction). It follows that not only is North American folk medicine richer in theories of disease but that it shows more overlap with official medical ideas and with the concepts of healers within any one community. No generalizations are meaningful in this context, and attempts to produce an overview must remain, as Hufford puts it, "an intellectual device" (Hufford 1992: 24).

Supernatural causes for disease have been invoked by many different traditions. As in Britain, so in Mexico, witchcraft has been regarded as a significant cause of disease (Holland 1963: 93). In the Native American tradition the role of spirits is central in affecting man's welfare (Lyon 1996: 60–61). In the past, five causes of disease were recognized by the Seminole Indians: soul

loss, external agents, sorcery, intrusion of foreign objects, and wounds (Snow and Stans 2001: 29). Among the external agents were animals, seen as causes of disease, while plants were seen as providing remedies (Lévi-Strauss 1966: 164–165). In the African tradition, "natural" illness is seen as a punishment for sin, "unnatural" illness as the work of malevolent forces (Micheletti 1998: 176). Alongside influences from cultural and religious beliefs there are to be found vestiges of official medical concepts. An example is the belief in heat or cold as the cause of disease among Spanish-Americans (Foster 1953: 205).

In North America, as in Britain, birthmarks and deformities of all kinds are attributed to events during the mother's pregnancy, including fear, shock, or cravings (Brown 1952–1964, 6: 18–24). Some illnesses are thought to be caused by animals, in which case the remedy will be from something related to the same animal (Brown 1952–1964, 6: 107). Eating the first snow of the season is thought to cause sickness (Brown 1952–1964, 6: 108). On the other hand, cold air is sometimes regarded as healthy (Brown 1952–1964, 6: 99). Blindness is said by some to be caused by sleeping in moonlight (Brown 1952–1964, 4: 126). Eye ailments can be "caught" simply by looking at a person suffering from them (Brown 1952–1964, 6: 293). Living on recently cleared land is thought by some to be a cause of typhoid fever (Brown 1952–1964, 6: 308). As in Britain, handling frogs is thought to cause warts; other supposed causes are handling jellyfish and washing hands in water in which eggs have been boiled (Brown 1952–1964, 6: 310).

*See also* **African tradition, Celtic tradition, Doctrine of signatures, Fevers, Onion, Plague, Pregnancy, Rheumatism, Transference, Tuberculosis, Warts.**

## References

Black, William George. *Folk-Medicine: A Chapter in the History of Culture.* London: Folklore Society, 1883.

Brown, Frank C. *Collection of North Carolina Folklore.* 7 vols. Durham, NC: Duke University Press, 1952–1964.

Buchan, David (ed.). *Folk Tradition and Folk Medicine in Scotland: The Writings of David Rorie.* Edinburgh: Canongate Academic, 1994.

Foster, George M. "Relationships between Spanish and Spanish-American Folk Medicine." *Journal of American Folklore* 66 (1953): 201–217.

Holland, William R. "Mexican-American Medical Beliefs: Science or Magic?" *Arizona Medicine* 20(5) (May 1963): 89–101.

Hufford, David J. "Folk Medicine in Contemporary America." In *Herbal and Magical Medicine: Traditional Healing Today,* edited by James Kirkland, Holly F. Matthews, C. W. Sullivan III, and Karen Baldwin. Durham, NC: Duke University Press, 1992.

Jones, Anne E. "Folk Medicine in Living Memory in Wales." *Folk Life* 18 (1980): 58–68.

Lévi-Strauss, Claude. *The Savage Mind.* London: Weidenfeld and Nicolson, 1966.

Lyon, William S. *Encyclopedia of Native American Healing.* Santa Barbara: ABC-CLIO, 1996.

Micheletti, Enza (ed.). *North American Folk Healing: An A–Z Guide to Traditional Remedies.* New York and Montreal: Reader's Digest Association, 1998.

Porter, Enid. *The Folklore of East Anglia.* London: Batsford, 1974.

Quelch, Mary Thorne. *Herbs for Daily Use.* London: Faber, 1941.

Snow, Alice Micco, and Susan Enns Stans. *Healing Plants: Medicine of the Florida Seminole Indians.* Gainesville: University Press of Florida, 2001.

# Constipation

Recommendations in British folk medicine for constipation include drinking plenty of water, eating prunes or rhubarb or orange juice, chewing the fruit of mallow, and eating molasses and flowers of sulphur, or castor oil. Woodlice have been used to treat constipation in Norfolk (Taylor MSS). More pleasantly, ripe blackberries *(Rubus fruticosus)* have been eaten for their laxative effect in Devon (Lafont 1984: 17). Herbal treatments include groundsel *(Senecio vulgaris)* boiled in milk, used in Ireland for constipated babies (Moloney 1919: 30). In Scotland fairy flax *(Linum catharticum)* has been used as a purgative (McNeill 1910: 108). Cloves soaked in boiling water overnight have been used in Suffolk (Taylor MSS). Bogbean has been used in Scotland to treat constipation (Beith 1995: 207). In the Western Isles of Scotland the seaweed known as dulse *(Rhodymenia palmata)* was eaten raw to relieve constipation (Beith 1995: 241). Chamomile tea, or a tea made from rice and raisins, or eating boiled onions, were all recommendations in Norfolk in the twentieth century (Hatfield 1994: 28). The rhizomes of the stinking iris *(Iris foetidissima)* have been famous as a purge since Anglo-Saxon times. Gerard writing in the sixteenth century records the use of stinking iris root as a purge by the country people in Somerset (Gerard 1597: 54), and Parkinson records its use in the seventeenth century (Parkinson 1640: 259). By the nineteenth century, the milder leaves were being used (Pratt 1855). Seeds of various species of plantain *(Plantago spp.)* have also been used to treat constipation (Newman 1948: 150).

In North American folk medicine, household remedies for constipation again include hot water. Other suggestions are a well-beaten fresh hen's egg with cold water or a pinch of salt in water. Olive oil has been recommended. In Canada, bear's grease has been similarly used (Tantaquidgeon 1932: 266). In New Mexico, an egg broken against a child's stomach is a remedy for constipation (Espinosa 1910: 410). A strange idea reported from Utah and elsewhere is that sewing a piece of sheep's intestine to the shirttail helps constipation (UCLA Folklore Archives 5_6797). Soup made from a totally black chicken, cooked whole with its feathers on, is another surprising remedy (Rupp 1946: 254). Molasses and honey make up a more prosaic remedy from Utah (UCLA Folklore Archives 4_6797). A recommendation from California is to boil almonds until their skins come off, then insert them into the rectum (UCLA Folklore Archives 17_6276).

Dietary suggestions to help constipation are similar to those in Britain; eating apples (UCLA Folklore Archives 16_7612), rhubarb, celery, parsley, asparagus, and watercress (Lathrop 1961: 16). The use of the seaweed dulse *(Rhodymenia palmata),* under the name "varette," is reported in the Maritime Provinces as a purgative, just as in Scotland (UCLA Folklore Archives 4_5341). Both the berries and the bark of elder (*Sambucus* sp.) have been used to treat constipation (Browne, Ray B. 1958: 390). It is reported that if the bark is scraped downward it acts as a laxative, upward as an emetic, a belief reported for a number of different plants in Native American practice (Black 1935: 37). This belief evidently extends to general North American folklore, too; boneset is used as a purge, but in this instance it is the leaves that are stripped upward to provide an emetic, downward for a purge (Fogel 1915: 278).

Other herbal recommendations include tea made from the roots of queen's delight *(Stillingia sylvatica)* (Hendricks 1980: 97). Wild cherry bark has been used in Kentucky (Wilson 1968: 326). An infusion of weeping willow tree leaves *(Salix babylonica)* has been reported in Arkansas (Parler 1962: 554). Life everlasting tea *(Gnaphalium obtusifolium)* was used to cure constipation in Virginia (UCLA Folklore Archives 5_5341). Roots of silkweed *(Asclepias syriaca)* have been used in Alabama to treat constipation (Browne, Ray B. 1958:

400). Flaxseed has been widely used. Other native plants used to treat constipation are butternut *(Juglans cinerea),* sweet flag *(Acorus calamus),* mayapple *(Podophyllum peltatum),* alder bark *(Alnus* spp.), bark of white ash *(Fraxinus americana),* and buckthorn (*Rhamnus* spp.). Manna from another type of ash, *Fraxinus ornus,* has been used especially for children, as it acts gently (Meyer 1985: 71–75). Tobacco and water have been used as an enema for severe constipation (UCLA Folklore Archives 1_1346). The use of alfalfa *(Medicago sativa)* leaves has been recorded from California (UCLA Folklore Archives 1_6276). In Mexico, a tea has been made for constipation from the seeds of ripe apricots (Madsen 1955: 133). Senna (*Senna* spp.) and prunes as well as orange juice have been used both in Britain and in North America, and they continue in use today.

All these plants, and many more besides, have been used in Native American practice to treat constipation. Moerman lists more than 150 different genera used by different tribes as laxatives (Moerman 1998: 805–806). Of these, the most widely used are elder and alder. Two Native American species of Senna are used as laxatives, *Senna hebecarpa* and *Senna marilandica.* The senna used in commercial preparations in Britain is derived from an African species, *Cassia senna* (formerly known as *Senna alexandrina*).

*See also* **Alder, Bogbean, Boneset, Chamomile, Cherry, Elder, Flax.**

### References

Beith, Mary. *Healing Threads: Traditional Medicines of the Highlands and Islands.* Edinburgh: Polygon, 1995.

Black, Pauline Monette. *Nebraska Folk Cures.* Studies in Language, Literature, and Criticism 15. Lincoln: University of Nebraska, 1935.

Browne, Ray B. *Popular Beliefs and Practices from Alabama.* Folklore Studies 9. Berkeley and

Los Angeles: University of California Publications, 1958.

Espinosa, Aurelio M. "New Mexican Spanish Folk-Lore." *Journal of American Folklore* 23 (1910): 395–418.

Fogel, Edwin Miller. "Beliefs and Superstitions of the Pennsylvania Germans." *Americana Germanica* 18 (1915).

Gerard, John. *The Herball or General Historie of Plantes.* London: John Norton, 1597.

Hatfield, Gabrielle. *Country Remedies: Traditional East Anglian Plant Remedies in the Twentieth Century.* Woodbridge: Boydell, 1994.

Hendricks, George D. *Roosters, Rhymes and Railroad Tracks: A Second Sampling of Superstitions and Popular Beliefs in Texas.* Dallas: Southern Methodist University Press, 1980.

Lafont, Anne-Marie. *Herbal Folklore.* Bideford: Badger Books, 1984.

Lathrop, Amy. "Pioneer Remedies from Western Kansas." *Western Folklore* 20 (1961): 1–22.

Madsen, William. "Hot and Cold in the Universe of San Francisco Tecospa, Valley of Mexico." *Journal of American Folklore* 68 (1955): 123–139.

McNeill, Murdoch. *Colonsay: One of the Hebrides.* Edinburgh: David Douglas, 1910.

Meyer, Clarence. *American Folk Medicine.* Glenwood, IL: Meyerbooks, 1985.

Moerman, Daniel E. *Native American Ethnobotany.* Portland, OR: Timber Press, 1998.

Moloney, Michael F. *Irish Ethno-botany and the Evolution of Medicine in Ireland.* Dublin: M. H. Gill & Son, 1919.

Newman, Leslie F. "Some Notes on the Pharmacology and Therapeutic Value of Folk-Medicine." 2 parts. *Folk-Lore* 59 (1948): 118–156.

Parkinson, John. *Theatrum Botanicum.* London: Thomas Cote, 1640.

Parler, Mary Celestia, and University Student Contributors. *Folk Beliefs from Arkansas.* 15 vols. Fayetteville: University of Arkansas, 1962.

Pratt, Anne. *The Flowering Plants and Ferns of Great Britain.* London: Society for Promoting Christian Knowledge, 1855.

Rupp, William J. "Bird Names and Bird Lore of the Pennsylvania Germans." *Pennsylvania German Society Proceedings and Addresses* 52 (1946).

Tantaquidgeon, Gladys. "Notes on the Origin and Uses of Plants of the Lake St. John Montagnais." *Journal of American Folklore* 45 (1932): 265–267.

Taylor MSS. Manuscript notes of Mark R. Taylor in the Norfolk Record Office, Norwich. MS4322.

Wilson, Gordon. "Local Plants in Folk Remedies in the Mammoth Cave Region." *Southern Folklore Quarterly* 32 (1968): 320–327.

# Consumption

*See* **Tuberculosis.**

# Contraception

This is probably the most sensitive area for enquiry within folk medicine, and the relative paucity of records probably reflects this fact rather than the absence of suggested methods within folklore. In British folk medicine, one of the simplest contraceptive agents, known to have been widely used up to the present day, is vinegar, used as a spermicidal douche (Unpublished Age Concern Essay 1991). Breast feeding was widely believed to at least delay the next pregnancy, though it must have been realized that it offered no real guarantee. Explicit herbal records of contraceptives are rare, and one has to read between the lines to recognize what is probably a contraceptive remedy. In Cambridgeshire in the twentieth century a strong infusion of white horehound *(Marrubium vulgare)* and rue *(Ruta graveolens)* was taken "to delay childbirth." In Yorkshire, at the same time, rue was given forcibly to women who had "been on the razzle" to "reduce the activity of the ova" (EFS 100Db). It seems highly likely that in these instances the rue was acting as an abortifacient, and indeed until very recently abortion was probably the only effective means of limiting family size for a large number of country women in Britain. Remedies such as raspberry tea and rye mouldy with ergot were used for procuring abortion, and in effect were also used as contraceptives. The same was probably true of juniper (*Juniperus* spp.) and pennyroyal *(Mentha pulegium)*. Taken at the time when a period is due, the woman would probably never know whether or not she was pregnant.

Riddle (Riddle 1992: 155) suggests that women in the past had some control over their own fertility by dietary methods, and instances pot herbs such as rue and pennyroyal, which possibly doubled as food and contraception. Such assertions are, of course, hard to prove, but the idea is at least plausible and may well have applied all over the world. This whole area must have been kept necessarily even more secret than most plant remedies, since at least in post-Christian times the penalty for abortion was heavy.

For European colonial women in North America the situation was similar; there was no simple and effective means of limiting family size, and indeed in many colonial circles a large family was seen as a blessing, particularly when infant mortality was high. Breast feeding, whether it was the intention or not, may have helped space children within a family (Ulrich 1991: 139), a belief that has survived to recent times (Parler 1962, 3: 65). Such simple means as the vinegar douche used in Britain may well have been used by them as well. Certainly in present-day America women are still aware of this method, and in a survey done by a magazine in 1980 the belief was recorded that a white vinegar douche would lead to conception of a girl (Sullivan 1992: 179). Eating starch has been practiced as a contraceptive measure, and carrying a buckeye has been suggested too (Parler 1962, 3; 14, 16, 17). In the African tradition, eating heart ventricles has been claimed to prevent conception (Brown 1952–1964, 6: 5). In the same tradition, jimson weed has been

used for contraception and abortion (Peavy 1966: 446).

To what extent colonial women supplemented their knowledge of contraceptive means from Native American knowledge is difficult to know for certain. The Native American knowledge in this field is enormous, and the wealth of records suggest few or no inhibitions associated with the subject. Some plants familiar to British folk medicine in this context were also used by Native Americans, such as tansy (*Tanacetum parthenium),* used for example by the Micmac (Chandler, Freeman and Hooper 1979: 62) and juniper species, used widely by, for example, the Zuni (Camazine and Bye 1980: 373). Many other non-British native American plants were also used, such as *Viburnum* sp., used by the Iroquois (Herrick 1977: 445); *Senecio aureus,* used by the Cherokee (Hamel and Chiltoskey 1975: 52); *Cornus sericea* by the Okanagan-Colville (Turner, Bouchard and Kennedy 1980: 96); *Prunus emarginata* by the Lummi (Gunther 1973: 37); and *Maianthemum stellatum* by the Shoshoni (Train, Henrichs and Archer 1941: 139). The Navajo used *Rhus trilobata* to induce impotence as a means of contraception (Vestal 1952: 35), while *Gaultheria shallon* was recommended among the Nitinaht to be taken by both newlyweds to ensure a male as their firstborn (Turner, Thomas, Carlson and Ogilvie 1983: 102). The Native Americans made contraceptive diaphragms from birch bark (Fischer 1989: 92).

*See also* **Abortion, Birch, Thornapple.**

### References

Age Concern Essay, 1991. Average Age of Informants 80 years. Unpublished: in Suffolk Record Office.

Brown, Frank C. *Collection of North Carolina Folklore.* 7 vols. Durham, NC: Duke University Press, 1952–1964.

Camazine, Scott, and Robert A. Bye. "A Study of the Medical Ethnobotany of the Zuni Indians of New Mexico." *Journal of Ethno-pharmacology* 2 (1980): 365–388.

Chandler, R. Frank, Lois Freeman, and Shirley N. Hooper. "Herbal Remedies of the Maritime Indians." *Journal of Ethnopharmacology* 1 (1979): 49–68.

EFS. English Folklore Survey. Unpublished notes at University College London.

Fischer, David Hackett. *Albion's Seed*. Oxford: Oxford University Press, 1989.

Gunther, Erna. *Ethnobotany of Western Washington*. Rev. ed. Seattle: University of Washington Press, 1973.

Hamel, Paul B., and Mary U. Chiltoskey. *Cherokee Plants and Their Uses: A 400 Year History*. Sylva, NC: Herald, 1975.

Herrick, James William. *Iroquois Medical Botany*. PhD thesis. State University of New York, Albany, 1977.

Parler, Mary Celestia, and University Student Contributors. *Folk Beliefs from Arkansas*. 15 vols. Fayetteville: University of Arkansas, 1962.

Peavy, Charles D. "Faulkner's Use of Folklore in *The Sound and the Fury*." *Journal of American Folklore* 79 (1966): 437–447.

Riddle, John M. *Contraception and Abortion from the Ancient World to the Renaissance*. Cambridge, Mass.: Harvard University Press, 1992.

Sullivan, C. W. "Childbirth Education and Traditional Beliefs." In *Herbal and Magical Medicine*, ed. Kirkland et al. Durham, NC: Duke University Press, 1992.

Train, Percy, James R. Henrichs, and W. Andrew Archer. *Medicinal Uses of Plants by Indian Tribes of Nevada*. Washington, D.C.: U.S. Department of Agriculture, 1941.

Turner, Nancy J., R. Bouchard, and Dorothy I. D. Kennedy. *Ethnobotany of the Okanagan-Colville Indians of British Columbia*. Victoria: British Columbia Provincial Museum, 1980.

Turner, Nancy J., John Thomas, Barry F. Carlson, and Robert T. Ogilvie. *Ethnobotany of the Nitinaht Indians of Vancouver Island*. Victoria: British Columbia Provincial Museum, 1983.

Ulrich, Laurel Thatcher. *Good Wives: Image and Reality in the Lives of Women in Northern New England 1650–1750*. New York: Vintage, 1991.

Vestal, Paul A. "The Ethnobotany of the Ramah Navaho." *Papers of the Peabody Museum of American Archaeology and Ethnology* 40(4) (1952): 1–94.

# Corn (*Zea mays*)

Maize was domesticated by Native Americans in about 5000 B.C. and since then has occupied a central role in their nutrition, religion, and ritual (Meléndez, in Wilson and Gillespie [eds.], 1999: 48). Different Native American tribes have developed different medicinal uses for the plant. Fresh corn silk quickly grows molds, and these were used medicinally for aiding labor (Kavasch and Baar 1999: 11). Corn meal was used as the basis for poultices, as well as being infused and drunk for stomach problems. Corn pollen was important in Navajo ritual (Lyon 1999: 54) but was also eaten by the Keres for "almost any kind of medicine" (Swank 1932: 77). A gruel made from cornmeal is used by the Mayo for treating diarrhea (Kay 1996: 269). Other Native American uses for corn include the treatment of gravel among the Cherokee (Hamel and Chiltoskey 1975: 30), of poison ivy rash among the Mohegan (Tantaquidgeon 1972: 77), and sore throat among the Navajo (Elmore 1944: 27).

The European settlers in North America must have been extremely grateful for this plant, which grew where their own crops failed. Apart from its food value, corn meal quickly became a familiar medicinal item used as the basis of poultices. A collection of settlers' remedies from Shelburne County includes a poultice, applied between the shoulder blades for a cough. It is composed of vinegar, mustard, and "Indian Meal" (Robertson 1960: 12). Medicinal uses for corn multiplied; the oil was used for treating dandruff (UCLA Folklore Archives 9_5357). Corn meal formed a poultice for a headache (Thomas and Thomas 1920: 105)

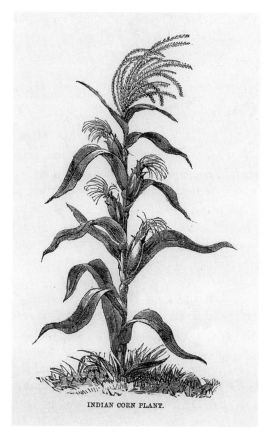

INDIAN CORN PLANT.

Maize was domesticated by Native Americans in about 5000 B.C. and since then has occupied a central role in their nutrition, religion and rituals. Corn meal quickly became a familiar medicinal item used as the basis of poultices. (North Wind Picture Archive)

and, mixed with onion, for pneumonia (Brown 1952–1964, 6: 250). Corn starch was used for chapped skin and for bee stings (UCLA Folklore Archive 7_6192, 7_5281). The "silk" of the corn (its threadlike stigmas) was dried and made into a tea that was used in particular for complaints of the urinary tract, such as kidney stones (Campa 1950: 341) and bedwetting (Clark 1970: 9). In a curious extension of its medicinal use for urinary complaints, a child was laid on a bed of corn shucks to cure bedwetting (UCLA Folklore Archives 22_5281).

Cornmeal gruel combined with cinnamon is used by Mexican Americans for diarrhea in infants (Kay 1996: 269). Corn starch was rubbed onto the blisters of poison ivy (UCLA Folklore Archives 8_5453), used to treat nappy rash (Cannon 1984: 37) and, mixed with peach leaves, formed a poultice for boils (UCLA Folklore Archives 3_5299). "Parched" corn was ground and boiled in sweetened milk and used to treat diarrhea and dysentery in children. It was also dusted onto the rash of prickly heat (Meyer 1985: 90, 227). Tea made from corn shucks was used to bring out the rash of measles (Puckett 1926: 387). Warm corn whiskey was drunk for colds (Bryant 1949: 139). Corn seems to have been a favorite remedy for the treatment of warts and corns. In many of these, the affected skin was rubbed with corn kernels, which were then fed to chickens (Anderson 1970: 82) or otherwise disposed of; such remedies are good examples of transference.

Nosebleeds could be prevented by wearing a necklace of red corn kernels as an amulet (Miller 1933: 474).

*See also* **Amulet, Bed-wetting, Boils, Chapped skin, Childbirth, Colds, Coughs, Diarrhea, Dysentery, Gravel and stone, Headache, Nosebleed, Poison ivy, Poultice, Sore throat, Transference, Warts.**

## References

Anderson, John. *Texas Folk Medicine.* Austin, TX: Encino Press, 1970.

Brown, Frank C. *Collection of North Carolina Folklore.* 7 vols. Durham, NC: Duke University Press, 1952–1964.

Bryant, Margaret M. "Folklore from Edgefield County, South Carolina: Beliefs, Superstitions, Dreams." *Southern Folklore Quarterly* 13 (1949): 136–148.

Campa, Arthur L. "Some Herbs and Plants of Early California." *Western Folklore* 9 (1950): 338–347.

Cannon, Anthon S. *Popular Beliefs and Superstitions from Utah.* Edited by Wayland D. Hand and Jeannine E. Talley. Salt Lake City: University of Utah Press, 1984.

Clark, Joseph D. "North Carolina Popular Beliefs and Superstitions." *North Carolina Folklore* 18 (1970): 1–66.

Elmore, Francis H. *Ethnobotany of the Navajo.* Santa Fe, New Mexico: School of American Research, 1944.

Hamel, Paul B., and Mary U. Chiltoskey. *Cherokee Plants and Their Uses: A 400 Year History.* Sylva, NC: Herald, 1975.

Kavasch, E. Barrie, and Karen Baar. *American Indian Healing Arts: Herbs, Rituals and Remedies for Every Season of Life.* New York: Bantam Books, 1999.

Kay, Margarita Artschwager. *Healing with Plants in the American and Mexican West.* Tucson: University of Arizona Press, 1996.

Lyon, William S. *Encyclopedia of Native American Healing.* Santa Barbara: ABC-Clio, 1999.

Meléndez, Theresa. "Corn." In *Rooted in America,* edited by David Scofield Wilson and Angus Kress Gillespie. Knoxville: University of Tennessee Press, 1999.

Meyer, Clarence. *American Folk Medicine.* Glenwood, IL: Meyerbooks, 1985.

Miller, Joseph L. "The Healing Gods or Medical Superstition." *West Virginia Medical Journal* 29 (1933): 465–478.

Puckett, Newbell Niles. *Folk Beliefs of the Southern Negro.* Chapel Hill, NC: Greenwood Press 1926.

Robertson, Marion. *Old Settlers' Remedies.* Barrington, NS: Cape Sable Historical Society, 1960.

Swank, George R. *The Ethnobotany of the Acoma and Laguna Indians.* M.A. thesis, Albuquerque, University of New Mexico, 1932.

Tantaquidgeon, Gladys. "Folk Medicine of the Delaware and Related Algonkian Indians." *Pennsylvania Historical Commission Anthropological Papers,* no. 3 (1972).

Thomas, Daniel Lindsay, and Lucy Blayney Thomas. *Kentucky Superstitions.* Princeton, N.J.: Princeton University Press, 1920.

# Corns

There are a large number of folk treatments for corns. Corns were often removed by cutting; in folk belief, this should be done on the first Friday after a full moon (Salisbury 1894: 71). Simple measures include soaking in a solution of soda, or applying a mixture of potash and gum arabic (Prince 1991: 20). A pearl button dissolved in lemon juice was a cure recommended in Lincolnshire (Notes and Queries 1849: 550). A variety of plant remedies have been recorded. The juice of red campion *(Silene dioica)* has been used in Somerset (Tongue 1965: 38). Dried and crumbled elder leaves have been soaked in water and used as a corn treatment (Prince 1991: 26). Ivy leaves have been widely used for corn treatment; in the simplest version of the remedy, the leaf was bound to the corn (Taylor MSS). Alternatively, it could be crushed in vinegar and applied, a remedy used in Essex (Hatfield 1994: 53) and Somerset (Tongue 1965: 38). The ivy was thought to be particularly effective if taken from an ash tree (Taylor MSS). Ground-ivy *(Glechoma hederacea)* was mixed with lard to form an ointment for corns in East Anglia (Taylor MSS). A poultice of houseleek has been used in Cornwall (Davey 1909: 193). The roots of celandine *(Ranunculus ficaria),* better known for their treatment of piles, have been used on the Isle of Colonsay to treat corns as well (McNeill 1910: 96). Pennywort *(Umbilicus rupestris)* has been used in Ireland to treat corns (Vickery 1995: 280). In Derbyshire hot boiled potato has been applied to corns (Black 1883: 193).

In North American folk medicine, a wide variety of corn remedies were used. Corns should traditionally be cut in the wane of the moon (Aurand 1941: 24). Simply walking barefoot in the morning dew was recommended in West Virginia (Musick 1964: 38). Another simple treatment was to throw beans into the fire and run away before they popped (Puckett 1981: 352). A mustard plaster and soaking in salt water were measures recommended in Kansas (UCLA Folklore Archives 8_5347). Various caustic solutions were used to soften the corn; pearl buttons dissolved in lemon juice have been used in Kentucky (Norris 1958: 103), as in Britain. Binding on a piece of lemon was an alternative (UCLA Folklore Archives 7_5343). Wood ashes in hot water were used in Nebraska (Welsch 1966: 362). Other applications include vinegar and breadcrumbs (Puckett 1981: 352), cow's urine (Cannon 1984: 102), or the "lye" from human urine (the deposit left on a chamber pot) (Riddell 1934: 41). Walking in fresh animal droppings was successfully tried in Illinois (Hyatt 1965: 225).

Covering corns with chewing gum was tried in California (UCLA Folklore Archives 4_6278).

Several remedies employ fat of various types. Rattlesnake oil was used in Texas (Hendricks 1966: 39), and fatty salt pork in Colorado (Kimmerle and Gelber 1976: 16). Castor oil was used in Utah (UCLA Folklore Archives 1_6797) and ear wax in Arkansas (Parler 1962: 563).

A variety of plants or plant products have been employed to treat corns. Soaking the feet in sauerkraut was recommended in Utah (Cannon 1984: 102). Rubbing the corns with cedar wax (Norris 1958: 103) or bathing them with turpentine (Browne 1958: 53) or with vanilla (UCLA Folklore Archives 2_6278) were alternatives. As in Britain, houseleek had a reputation for curing corns (Baker 1969: 191). In Pennsylvania, cabbage stumps and vinegar were applied to corns (Dieffenbach 1952: 2).

Corns have been subjected to some of the same cures used for warts, including some of the quasi-magical ones. In Utah, the advice was to steal a piece of beef and bury it; as the meat rots, the corn will disappear (UCLA Folklore Archives 2_6798). Burying corn kernels in the ground is another remedy using a time factor: as the corn sprouts, the corns will disappear (UCLA Folklore Archives 11_6278). Various remedies involve transference. In North Carolina, corns have been rubbed with a snail

(Clark 1970: 17). In California, rubbing them with a wooden peg, which is then driven into a tree, has been suggested (UCLA Folklore Archives 9_6278). Rubbing a piece of cotton onto a corn and then burying it alongside a corpse is another suggestion (Hoffman 1889: 31). A candle rubbed on a corpse and then on a corn was another cure from Pennsylvania (Fogel 1915: 274). Paring corns with the razor of a dead man is another version of this remedy (Hyatt 1965: 226).

*See also* **Ash, Dew, Elder, Houseleek, Ivy, Snail, Soda, Transference, Warts.**

### References

Aurand, A. Monroe, Jr. *Popular Home Remedies and Superstitions of the Pennsylvania Germans.* Harrisburg, PA: The Aurand Press, 1941.

Baker, Ronald L. "Folk Medicine in the Writings of Rowland E. Robinson." *Vermont History* 37 (1969): 184–193.

Black, William George. *Folk-Medicine: A Chapter in the History of Culture.* London: Folklore Society, 1883.

Browne, Ray B. *Popular Beliefs and Practices from Alabama.* Folklore Studies 9. Berkeley and Los Angeles: University of California Publications, 1958.

Cannon, Anthon S. *Popular Beliefs and Superstitions from Utah.* Edited by Wayland D. Hand and Jeannine E. Talley. Salt Lake City: University of Utah Press, 1984.

Clark, Joseph D. "North Carolina Popular Beliefs and Superstitions." *North Carolina Folklore* 18 (1970): 1–66.

Davey, F. Hamilton. *Flora of Cornwall.* Penryn: F. Clegwidden, 1909.

Dieffenbach, Victor C. "Cabbage in the Folk-Culture of My Pennsylvania Dutch Elders." *Pennsylvania Dutchman* 3(22) (April 15, 1952): 1–2.

Fogel, Edwin Miller. "Beliefs and Superstitions of the Pennsylvania Germans." *Americana Germanica* 18 (1915).

Hatfield, Gabrielle. *Country Remedies: Traditional*

*East Anglian Plant Remedies in the Twentieth Century.* Woodbridge: Boydell, 1994.

Hendricks, George D. *Mirrors, Mice and Mustaches: A Sampling of Superstitions and Popular Beliefs in Texas.* Austin: Texas Folklore Society, 1966.

Hoffman, W. J. "Folk-Lore of the Pennsylvania Germans." *Journal of American Folklore* 2 (1889): 23–35.

Hyatt, Harry Middleton. *Folklore from Adams County Illinois.* 2nd rev. ed. New York: Memoirs of the Alma Egan Hyatt Foundation, 1965.

Kimmerle, Marjorie, and Mark Gelber. Popular Beliefs and Superstitions from Colorado, unpublished manuscript, University of Colorado, Boulder, 1976.

McNeill, Murdoch. *Colonsay: One of the Hebrides.* Edinburgh: David Douglas, 1910.

Musick, Ruth Ann (ed.) "Superstitions." *West Virginia Folklore* 14 (1964): 38–52.

Norris, Ruby R. "Folk Medicine of Cumberland County." *Kentucky Folklore Record* 4 (1958): 101–110.

*Notes and Queries* 41, p. 550. London, 1849.

Parler, Mary Celestia, and University Student Contributors. *Folk Beliefs from Arkansas.* 15 vols. Fayetteville: University of Arkansas, 1962

Prince, Dennis. *Grandmother's Cures: An A–Z of Herbal Remedies.* London: Fontana, 1991.

Puckett, Newbell Niles. *Popular Beliefs and Superstitions: A Compendium of American Folklore from the Ohio Collection of Newbell Niles Puckett.* Edited by Wayland D. Hand, Anna Casetta, and Sondra B. Thiederman. 3 vols. Boston: G. K. Hall, 1981.

Riddell, William Renwick. "Some Old Canadian Folk Medicine." *The Canada Lancet and Practitioner* 83 (August 1934): 41–44.

Salisbury, Jesse. *A Glossary of Words and Phrases Used in South East Worcestershire.* London: English Dialect Society, Series C. Original Glossaries, no. 72, 1894.

Taylor MSS. Manuscript notes of Mark R. Taylor, in the Norfolk Record Office, Norwich. MS 4322.

Tongue, Ruth L. *Somerset Folklore.* Edited by Katharine Briggs. County Folklore 8. London: Folklore Society, 1965.

Vickery, Roy. *A Dictionary of Plant Lore.* Oxford: Oxford University Press, 1995.

Welsch, Roger L. *A Treasury of Nebraska Pioneer Folklore.* Lincoln: University of Nebraska Press, 1966.

# Coughs

Though the causes of coughs, in medical terms, are diverse, in folk medicine this has been treated as a single ailment and over the centuries has attracted a great variety of folk remedies. Even today many people resort to homely remedies, when the cause of the cough is often viral and antibiotics are irrelevant. In British folk medicine, a large number of cough treatments have been used, ranging from very simple measures, such as chewing a leaf, to more complex preparations involving different mixtures of plant and animal and mineral ingredients. In Norfolk, it was maintained that wearing a necklace of blue beads would cure bronchitis (Mundford Primary School project 1980, unpub.). Among native British plants, black-currant *(Ribes nigrum)* has been widely used in cough remedies. It is arguably native in Britain, but since it has been grown as a fruit-crop, there has been a ready supply from plants in cultivation as well. An infusion of the berries, or jam made from them, has been used to soothe coughs. Blackberries *(Rubus fruticosus)* were used similarly, in both England and Scotland. Honey has been a common ingredient in numerous cough mixtures, valued for its soothing nature (Beith 1995: 213; Allen and Hatfield, in press). Recent studies have vindicated its use in this way, showing it to be antibiotic and antiviral as well as simply soothing (Root-Bernstein 1997).

There is, of course, an overlap between cough and cold remedies. Lemon juice and honey, for example, have provided a remedy for both; in Scotland, whisky has been added. Elderberries have formed a cough medicine throughout much of Britain.

Coltsfoot *(Tussilago farafara)* has been used in cough preparations at least since the time of Pliny, and probably for far longer than that. Other native British plants used to treat coughs include horehound, both the white horehound, *Marrubium vulgare* and black horehound *(Ballota nigra),* as well as thyme *(Thymus serpyllum),* wild cherry *(Prunus avium),* mullein, and cowslip. Elecampane *(Inula helenium),* though not a native plant in Britain, has been cultivated as an herb and vegetable since Roman times and now exists in scattered parts of the British isles semiwild (Allen and Hatfield, in press). As well as being used in official medicine, it has been used in folk remedies, such as the cough treatment recorded from Suffolk in the 1920s, where the grated root was mixed with sugar, raisins, and the dried root of marshmallow *(Malva officinalis)* (Taylor MSS).

Vegetables have been widely used in cough preparations. Sliced onion, alone or mixed with grated carrot, has been sprinkled with brown sugar and left to stand overnight. The resulting syrup was a cheap cough medicine (Prince 1991: 108). Turnip was used similarly (Hatfield 1994: 30).

Animal ingredients used in cough remedies include the solan goose (gannet) used on the island of Kilda. Martin Martin in his travels in the late seventeenth century was told by the inhabitants of St. Kilda of a disease they termed "boat cough," since it always appeared after outsiders visited the island. He was sceptical until he witnessed for himself an outbreak after one such visit. The local remedy was to melt the fat of a "solan goose" and eat it with oatmeal (Beith 1995: 79–80). This is an unusual instance of early recognition of the infectious agent in coughs, and interesting also in that it shows lack of resistance of an isolated population to what was probably an everyday ailment on the mainland.

Cough cures made from snails were used in rural Britain as recently as the early twentieth century. Either the snails were crushed and the liquid drunk, or the snails were impaled above a bowl, which caught their juice, and this juice was used. Its primary use was in consumption, but it was also used for ordinary coughs and bronchitis (Allen 1995: 149).

In his collection of North American folk remedies for coughs, Meyer includes many variants on the lemon and honey mixture mentioned for Britain. The honey in some cases is replaced with molasses; glycerine, olive oil, or egg may be added. There is an interesting cough mixture prepared by dissolving an egg, including the shell, in vinegar and adding sugar (Meyer 1985: 77). Exactly the same remedy was used in Britain for treating whooping cough (Prince 1991:115). The onion remedy was evidently as popular in North America as in Britain, and again there are several variations. Beetroot and turnip were used similarly to produce a cough syrup. Syrup of blackberries was used, as in Britain. The blackberry is not native to North America but is naturalized there; presumably this remedy arrived with European settlers.

A remedy used by early settlers in Shelburne County was to mix marshmallow root with poppy heads and add conserve of roses (Robertson 1960: 12). Prominent among plants used in cough mixtures is pine, all the parts of which have been used medicinally. The simplest pine-based cough mixture consisted of the inner bark, steeped in water, simmered with honey to form a syrup. Other native herbs used to treat coughs include many of those already mentioned for Britain: horehound, mullein, coltsfoot (or coughwort, as it is often called), wild cherry *(Prunus* spp.), and elecampane *(Inula helenium).* In addition, many plants native to North America but not to Britain were used in cough treatment. They include skunk cabbage *(Symplocarpus foetidus),* wild Indian turnip *(Arisaema triphyllum),* and balm of Gilead, slippery elm and flaxseed *(Linum usitatissi-mum)* (Meyer 1985: 76–84). Feverfew *(Tanacetum parthenium),* today better known for its treatment of migraine, was used on both sides of the Atlantic to treat coughs (Hatfield 1994: appendix; Meyer 1985: 83), as was ground ivy *(Glechoma hederacea)* (Taylor MSS: Meyer 1985: 83). Inhaling the fumes from smoking fresh ground coffee mixed with pine sawdust sounds like an original cough treatment (Meyer 1985: 84). Ironically, tobacco smoke was also tried as a cough remedy (McCullen 1962: 34).

Some at least of these remedies that have found their way into general North American folk medicine are perhaps attributable to Native American knowledge. Various species of pine were extensively used, such as *Pinus strobus* by the Abnaki (Rousseau 1947: 163), the Iroquois (Herrick 1977: 264), the Micmac (Chandler, Freeman, and Hooper 1979: 59), and the Shinnecock (Carr and Westey 1945: 121). The Alaska Eskimos used juice of *Pinus contorta* to treat coughs (Smith 1973: 331). The Kwakiutl used a decoction of the buds and pitch of this species (Turner and Bell 1973: 269), the Shushwap used an infusion of the inner bark (Palmer 1975: 51), and the Sikani chewed the pitch and swallowed the saliva for a cough (Smith 1929: 49, 50), while the Thompson chewed the gum for the same purpose (Perry 1952: 40). Various other species of Pinus were similarly used, and other coniferous trees were sources of cough medicines as well, notably *Picea* (used by thirteen different tribes) and Juniperus (used by eighteen tribes) (Moerman 1998: 782–783).

Another plant very widely used for coughs among Native Americans is *Prunus.* The Cherokee used an infusion of the bark of *Prunus cerasus* for coughs (Hamel and Chiltoskey 1975: 28); *Prunus pennsylvanica* was used by the Algonquin (Black 1980: 184) and the Cherokee (Hamel and Chil-

toskey 1975: 28), *Prunus serotina* by the Cherokee (Hamel and Chiltoskey 1975: 28) and the Delaware (Tantaquidgeon 1972: 27) and the Iroquois (Herrick 1977: 360). Other very widely used plant genera include *Acorus* (used by thirteen tribes) and *Artemisia* (used by fifteen tribes) (Moerman 1998: 782). Slippery elm *(Ulmus rubra)* is used for cough treatment by the Cherokee (Hamel and Chiltoskey 1975: 33) and the Mohegan (Tantaquidgeon 1972: 132). El-ecampane *(Inula helenium)* is used by the Cherokee (Hamel and Chiltoskey 1975: 33) and the Iroquois (Herrick 1977: 466). *Polypodium,* used in Ireland for treating coughs (Hart 1873: 339), has also been used in North America—for example, the rhizomes of *P. glycirrhiza* are eaten by the Hesquiat for coughs (Turner and Efrat 1982: 30). The buds of balsam poplar were used by the Southern Carrier (Smith, H. I. 1929: 54) and the Upper Tanana (Kari 1985: 4).

*See also* **Asthma, Balm of Gilead, Colds, Cowslip, Elder, Elm, Honey, Migraine, Mullein, Pine, Snail, Tuberculosis, Whooping cough.**

### References

Allen, Andrew. *A Dictionary of Sussex Folk Medicine.* Newbury: Countryside Books, 1995.

Allen, David E., and Gabrielle Hatfield. *Medicinal Plants in Folk Tradition.* Portland, OR: Timber Press (in press).

Beith, Mary. *Healing Threads: Traditional Medicines of the Highlands and Islands.* Edinburgh: Polygon, 1995.

Black, Meredith Jean. *Algonquin Ethnobotany: An Interpretation of Aboriginal Adaptation in South Western Quebec.* Mercury Series 25. Ottawa: National Museums of Canada, 1980.

Carr, Lloyd G., and Carlos Westey. "Surviving Folktales and Herbal Lore among the Shinnecock Indians." *Journal of American Folklore* 58 (1945): 113–123.

Chandler, R. Frank, Lois Freeman, and Shirley N. Hooper. "Herbal Remedies of the Maritime

Indians." *Journal of Ethnopharmacology* 1 (1979): 49–69.

Hamel, Paul B., and Mary U. Chiltoskey. *Cherokee Plants and Their Uses: A 400 Year History.* Sylva, NC: Herald, 1975.

Hart, H. C. "Euphorbia hyberna, Equisetum trachyodon, etc. in County Galway." H. C. *Journal of Botany* 11 (1873): 338–339.

Hatfield, Gabrielle. *Country Remedies: Traditional East Anglian Plant Remedies in the Twentieth Century.* Woodbridge: Boydell, 1994.

Herrick, James William. *Iroquois Medical Botany.* Ph.D. thesis, State University of New York, Albany, 1977.

Kari, Priscilla Russe. *Upper Tanana Ethnobotany.* Anchorage: Alaska Historical Commission, 1985.

McCullen, J. T. "The Tobacco Controversy, 1571–1961." *North Carolina Folklore* 10(1) (1962): 30–35.

Meyer, Clarence. *American Folk Medicine.* Glenwood, IL: Meyerbooks, 1985.

Moerman, Daniel E. *Native American Ethnobotany.* Portland, OR: Timber Press, 1998.

Mundford Primary School, Norfolk. School project, 1980, unpublished.

Palmer, Gary. Shuswap Indian Ethnobotany. *Syesis* 8 (1975): 29–51.

Perry, F. "Ethno-Botany of the Indians in the Interior of British Columbia." *Museum and Art Notes* 2(2) (1952): 36–43.

Prince, Dennis. *Grandmother's Cures: An A–Z of Herbal Remedies.* London: Fontana, 1991.

Robertson, Marion. *Old Settlers' Remedies.* Barrington, NS: Cape Sable Historical Society, 1960.

Root-Bernstein, Robert, and Michèle Root-Bernstein. *Honey, Mud and Maggots and Other Medical Marvels: The Science behind Folk Remedies and Old Wives' Tales.* London: Pan, 1997.

Rousseau, Jacques. "Ethnobotanique Abénakise." *Archives de Folklore* 11 (1947): 145–182.

Smith, G. Warren. "Arctic Pharmacognosia." *Arctic* 26 (1973): 324–333.

Smith, Harlan I. "Materia Medica of the Bella Coola and Neighbouring Tribes of British Columbia." *National Museum of Canada Bulletin* 56 (1929): 47–68.

Tantaquidgeon, Gladys. *A Study of the Delaware Indian Medicine Practice and Folk Beliefs.* Harrisburg: Pennsylvania Historical Commission, 1942.

Tantaquidgeon, Gladys. "Folk Medicine of the Delaware and Related Algonkian Indians." *Pennsylvania Historical Commission Anthropological Papers,* no. 3 (1972).

Taylor MSS. Manuscript notes of Mark R. Taylor, in Norfolk Record Office, Norwich.

Turner, Nancy Chapman, and Marcus A. M. Bell. "The Ethnobotany of the Southern Kwakiutl Indians of British Columbia." *Economic Botany* 27 (1973): 257–310.

Turner, Nancy J., and Barbara S. Efrat. *Ethnobotany of the Hesquiat Indians of Vancouver Island.* Victoria: British Columbia Provincial Museum, 1982.

# Cowslip (*Primula veris*)

In British folk medicine this plant has been valued as a cosmetic (Lafont 1984: 29), as a mild sedative for treating coughs (Hatfield 1994: 30), and for promoting sleep. It has also been used to treat jaundice. In Ireland especially it has been used for treating insomnia, and there it has also been used to treat dropsy and deafness, as well as palsy (it is sometimes known as palsywort) (Allen and Hatfield, in press). In Wales, the plant has been used to treat "the decline" (?tuberculosis) and also to strengthen the senses (Trevelyan 1909: 91, 97).

The plant is an introduction to North America and has been used to a relatively slight extent in folk medicine there. An ointment has been used to treat eczema, and it has been recommended as a bedtime drink for insomnia (Meyer 1985: 106, 145). There has been little or no usage of the plant by Native Americans.

*See also* **Coughs, Deafness, Dropsy, Jaundice, Palsy, Sleeplessness**.

**References**
Allen, David and Gabrielle Hatfield. *Medicinal Plants in Folk Tradition.* Portland, OR: Timber Press, in press.
Hatfield, Gabrielle. *Country Remedies: Traditional East Anglian Plant Remedies in the Twentieth Century.* Woodbridge: Boydell, 1994.
Lafont, Anne-Marie. *Herbal Folklore.* Bideford: Badger Books, 1984.
Meyer, Clarence. *American Folk Medicine.* Glenwood, IL: Meyerbooks, 1985.
Trevelyan, Marie. *Folk-lore and Folk-stories of Wales.* London: Elliot Stock, 1909.

# Cramp

There is a small but strange collection of British folk remedies for cramp. Cork features in several of them; keeping a piece of cork in the pocket, or under the pillow, or under the bed is said to prevent cramp. Even standing on a cork bath mat is said to help (Porter 1969: 78). Sometimes the cork was sewn between silk ribbons and made into garters, worn to avoid cramp (Black 1883: 199). In Norfolk, tying a flint with a large hole in it under the bed was said to cure cramp, as was a potato under the bed (Mundford Primary School project, 1980, unpub.) or a bowl of water (Taylor 1929: 119). Carrying the fore feet of a mole in the pocket is recorded as an East Anglian preventative. In Suffolk it was common practice to place shoes "one coming and one going" at the foot of the bed (Rider Haggard [ed.] 1974: 164). Cramp bones were another type of amulet. The ankle bone of the hare is reputedly good against cramp. In Northamptonshire, the patella of a sheep was worn, as near to the skin as possible, to cure cramp; at night, it was placed under the pillow (Black 1883: 154, 156, 182). Brass, especially the brass from coffin handles, again kept under the bed, is recommended (Hatfield MS). Sometimes "cramp rings" were made from these handles (Sou-

ter 1995: 35); in Devonshire, England, such rings were also made from nails or screws that had been used to fasten a coffin (Black 1883: 175). In Somerset, rubbing the feet with Jack by the hedge *(Alliaria petiolata)* or wearing yarrow leaves in the shoes were both thought to help (Tongue 1965: 38). Among other plants used to treat cramp in British folk medicine, chamomile is one of the commonest. Scurvy grass *(Cochlearia officinalis)* was made into a poultice and used to treat cramp in the Highlands of Scotland (Beith 1995: 239).

Some of these folk practices are also found in North America. In New Jersey, it was believed that walking over a grave caused cramp (Black 1883: 27). Perhaps this belief was at one time widespread and led to the use of coffin handles as preventatives.

The idea of positioning shoes in a particular way under the bed (with toes pointing outward, or upside down) seems to have been particularly common in North American folk medicine (see, e.g., Brown 1952–1964, 6: 165). Twentieth-century remedies include putting the feet in hot ashes (Black 1935: 36). As in Britain, putting a bowl of water under the bed at night was also suggested (Thomas and Thomas 1920: 101). Alternatively, a buckeye (chestnut) could be carried in the pocket to ward off cramp (Browne 1958: 55), or a thread could be tied around the leg (Brown 1952–1964, 6: 164). Eelskin (Brown 1952–1964, 6: 163) or snakeskin worn (Bergen 1899: 76) was thought to protect against cramp. A fishbone was another amulet used for cramp (Brown 1952–1964, 6: 163–164), and wearing a brass ring was recommended, as in Britain (Brown 1952–196, 6: 165).

Rubs for treating cramp have included a decoction of cranberry bush bark (Meyer 1985: 182) (probably a species of *Viburnum* [Willard 1992: 194]), as well as various oils that doubled as rheumatism treatments, such as oil of wintergreen, camphorated oil.

*See also* **Amulet, Chamomile, Rheumatism, Yarrow.**

### References

Beith, Mary. *Healing Threads: Traditional Medicines of the Highlands and Islands.* Edinburgh: Polygon, 1995.

Bergen, Fanny D. "Animal and Plant Lore Collected from the Oral Tradition of English Speaking Folk." *Memoirs of the American Folk-Lore Society* 7 (1899).

Black, Pauline Monette. *Nebraska Folk Cures.* Studies in Language, Literature, and Criticism 15, Lincoln: University of Nebraska, 1935.

Black, William George. *Folk-Medicine: A Chapter in the History of Culture.* London: Folklore Society, 1883.

Brown, Frank C. *Collection of North Carolina Folklore.* 7 vols. Durham, NC: Duke University Press, 1952–1964.

Browne, Ray B. *Popular Beliefs and Practices from Alabama.* Folklore Studies 9. Berkeley and Los Angeles: University of California Publications, 1958.

Meyer, Clarence. *American Folk Medicine.* Glenwood, IL: Meyerbooks, 1985.

Mundford Primary School, Norfolk. School project, 1980 (unpublished).

Porter, Enid. *Cambridgeshire Customs and Folklore.* London: Routledge, 1969.

Rider Haggard, Lilias (ed.). *I Walked by Night.* Woodbridge: Boydell Press, 1974.

Souter, Keith. *Cure Craft: Traditional Folk Remedies and Treatment from Antiquity to the Present Day.* Saffron Walden: C. W. Daniel, 1995.

Taylor, Mark R. "Norfolk Folklore." *Folk-Lore* 40 (1929): 113–133.

Thomas, Daniel Lindsay, and Lucy Blayney Thomas. *Kentucky Superstitions.* Princeton, N.J.: Princeton University Press, 1920.

Tongue, Ruth L. *Somerset Folklore.* Edited by Katharine Briggs. County Folklore 8. London: Folklore Society, 1965.

Willard, Terry. *Edible and Medicinal Plants of the Rocky Mountains and Neighbouring Territories.* Calgary: Wild Rose College of Natural Healing, 1992.

# Cricket

In European folk medicine, the cricket has been used to nibble off warts. In North American folk medicine there is a similar tradition. Crickets have been used to either eat the center out of a wart (Wilson 1965: 39) or to suck the blood from a pricked wart (Parler 1962, 3: 1038). Grasshoppers have been used similarly (UCLA Folklore Archives 14_5532), and "grasshopper's molasses" has also been recommended (Brown 1952–1964, 6: 317). In a variation of this remedy, the left hind leg of a frog and the right hind leg of a cricket were placed under the pillow of the person suffering from warts (Anderson 1970: 81). Crickets have also been used to treat hives.

*See also* **Hives, Warts.**

### References

Anderson, John. *Texas Folk Medicine.* Austin, TX: Encino Press, 1970.

Brown, Frank C. *Collection of North Carolina Folklore.* 7 vols. Durham, North Carolina, 1952–1964.

Parler, Mary Celestia, and University Student Contributors. *Folk Beliefs from Arkansas.* 15 vols. Fayetteville: University of Arkansas, 1962.

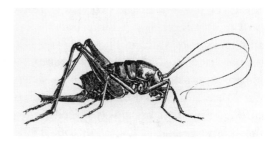

In European folk medicine, the cricket has been used to nibble off warts. In North American folk medicine, there is a similar tradition. Crickets have also been used to treat hives. (North Wind Picture Archive)

Wilson, Gordon. "Studying Folklore in a Small Region. VI: Folk Remedies." *Tennessee Folklore Society Bulletin* 31 (1965): 33–41.

# Croup

A common method of treatment, still in use today, is to boil water in the room where the child is, so that the patient inhales steamy air. This is done either by simmering a kettle in the bedroom or encouraging the child to inhale steam from a bowl of water held under the chin, with a towel over the head (Hatfield MS, schools survey Norfolk, 1980). A hot flannel around the neck was another version (Terrington St. Clement, Norfolk, 1980, schools survey). A remedy from Derbyshire, used as recently as 1959, was to fry currants and spread them on fat bacon, which is then applied as a poultice (EFS 305). In Norfolk, balls of sugar and butter were given for croup (Schools survey, Alderman Peel High School, 1980). Another treatment was to place a pot of tar under the bed (Porter 1974: 50). Smelling tar was another suggestion (Schools survey, Toftwood, Norfolk, 1980). In Suffolk houseleek was used in the treatment of croup (Taylor 1929: 119).

In North American folk medicine onions mixed with sugar or honey are used for croup, or vinegar and molasses. Vinegar boiled in the bedroom is recommended: an alternative was to hang a vinegar-soaked sheet in the room (Brown 1952–1964, 6: 166–167). A cold or a warm-water compress was used (Meyer 1985: 84–85). Inhaling night air was recommended (Cannon 1984: 103). To dip one baby sock in holy water and have the sufferer wear it was another croup treatment (Hyatt 1965: 279). Various fats were used to rub into the throat and chest. Lard, hog's foot oil, goose grease, and olive oil have all been used, both rubbed into the chest and sometimes given internally too. Sometimes an oil was given

as an emetic (Meyer 1985: 85–86). A soothing mixture was made from molasses and soda (Puckett 1981: 356). A thick "stew" made from apple cider vinegar, sugar, water, and butter was sometimes given (Pope 1965: 444) (a remedy reminiscent of the East Anglian butter balls, above).

Sulphur, or alum, was administered (Meyer 1985: 85–86), or a mixture of alcohol and water. Urine was given (Parler 1962, 3: 582), or ground deer antler (Brown 1952–1964, 6: 166). A tea made from the white portion of chicken droppings (Puckett 1981: 356) or a poultice of cow manure on the chest (Smith, Stewart, and Kyger 1962: 133) were other recommendations. Dried bumblebees in molasses (Levine 1941: 487) or tea made from a hornet's nest (Letcher 1910–1911: 171) were alternatives, or the hair from a donkey's flank chopped and given with treacle (UCLA Folklore Archives 5_6271). Plugging some hair from the sufferer into a tree was a remedy involving transference (Puckett 1926: 370).

Plant remedies administered for croup include a cabbage leaf, tied with a black thread around the neck (Fife 1957: 147). Beet juice was given in small quantities, or powdered bloodroot in molasses, or a mixture of chamomile and false saffron flowers *(Carthamus tinctorius)* fried in butter (Meyer 1985: 85–86). A tea made from mullein or horehound was sometimes given (Rogers 1941: 18). Infusions of pine-tops *(Pinus* sp.) (Browne 1958: 18), red clover roots *(Trifolium pratense)* (Lick and Brendle 1922: 113), tobacco *(Nicotiana* sp.) (Gardner 1937: 263), or leaves of black walnut *(Juglans nigra)* (Parler 1962: 582) have all been used.

Folk medicine provided suggestions for avoiding croup. A newborn child should be held so that its feet make tracks in new snow; this would ensure it would never suffer from cramp (Parler 1962, 3: 582). Amulets worn to prevent croup include a penny with a hole in it worn around the neck, and a black thread tied around the neck (Brown 1952–1964, 6: 166–167). Amber beads were also worn to protect against croup (Killion and Waller 1972: 108), or beads made from the rattan vine (*Berchemia scandens*) (Parler 1962: 586). It was believed that a person born after the death of his or her father had the ability to cure croup by blowing into the sufferer's mouth (Randolph 1947: 136).

Bloodroot was used also in the Native American tradition for treating croup (Hamel and Chiltoskey 1975: 26).

*See also* **Amber, Bloodroot, Chamomile, Horehound, Houseleek, Mullein, Onion, Poultice, Transference.**

## References

Brown, Frank C. *Collection of North Carolina Folklore.* 7 vols. Durham, NC: Duke University Press, 1952–1964.

Browne, Ray B. *Popular Beliefs and Practices from Alabama.* Folklore Studies 9. Berkeley and Los Angeles: University of California Publications, 1958.

Cannon, Anthon S. *Popular Beliefs and Superstitions from Utah.* Edited by Wayland D. Hand and Jeannine E. Talley. Salt Lake City: University of Utah Press, 1984.

EFS. English Folklore Survey. Manuscript notes at University College London.

Fife, Austin W. "Pioneer Mormon Remedies." *Western Folklore* 16 (1957): 153–162.

Gardner, Emelyn Elizabeth. *Folklore from the Schoharie Hills, New York.* Ann Arbor: University of Michigan Press, 1937.

Hamel, Paul B., and Mary U. Chiltoskey. *Cherokee Plants and Their Uses: A 400 Year History.* Sylva, NC: Herald, 1975.

Hyatt, Harry Middleton. *Folklore from Adams County Illinois.* 2nd rev. ed. New York: Memoirs of the Alma Egan Hyatt Foundation, 1965.

Killion, Ronald G., and Charles T. Waller. *A Treasury of Georgia Folklore.* Atlanta: Cherokee, 1972.

Letcher, James H. "The Treatment of Some Diseases by the 'Old Time' Negro." *The Railway Surgical Journal* 17 (1910–1911): 17–175.

Levine, Harold D. "Folk Medicine in New Hampshire." *New England Journal of Medicine* 224 (1941): 487–492.

Lick, David E., and Thomas R. Brendle. "Plant Names and Plant Lore among the Pennsylvania Germans." *Proceedings and Addresses of the Pennsylvania German Society* 33 (1922).

Meyer, Clarence. *American Folk Medicine.* Glenwood, IL: Meyerbooks, 1985.

Parler, Mary Celestia, and University Student Contributors. *Folk Beliefs from Arkansas.* 15 vols. Fayetteville: University of Arkansas, 1962.

Pope, Genevieve. "Superstitions and Beliefs of Fleming County." *Kentucky Folklore Record* 11 (1965): 41–51.

Porter, Enid. *The Folklore of East Anglia.* London: Batsford, 1974.

Puckett, Newbell Niles. *Folk Beliefs of the Southern Negro.* Chapel Hill, NC: Greenwood Press, 1926.

Puckett, Newbell Niles. *Popular Beliefs and Superstitions: A Compendium of American Folklore from the Ohio Collection of Newbell Niles Puckett.* Edited by Wayland D. Hand, Anna Casetta, and Sondra B. Thiederman. 3 vols. Boston: G. K. Hall, 1981.

Randolph, Vance. *Ozark Superstitions.* New York: Columbia University Press, 1947.

Rogers, E. G. *Early Folk Medical Practices in Tennessee.* Murfreesboro, TN: 1941.

Schools survey. Manuscript notes from survey of Norfolk schools, 1980, unpublished.

Smith, Elmer Lewis, John G. Stewart, and M. Ellsworth Kyger. "The Pennsylvania Germans of the Shenandoah Valley." *Publications of the Pennsylvania German Folklore Society* 25 (1962): 1–278.

Taylor, Mark R. "Norfolk Folklore." *Folk-Lore* 40 (1929): 113–133.

# Cuts

As an obvious domestic emergency, cuts have attracted a number of folk remedies. Cold water and bandaging was one basic treatment. In Norfolk one lady recalls how when she cut herself, she had to "swish it around in a bucket of cold water, until it was all red" (V.W., Halvergate, Norfolk, 1988 pers. com.). Salt water was sometimes preferred (Toftwood, Norfolk, 1980: schools survey, unpub.). The inner membrane of an egg was used as a natural plaster (B.G., Cambridgeshire, pers. com., June 2002). Cobwebs were widely used, as they were for more serious wounds. Shag tobacco was used to stop the bleeding (Alderman Peel school, Norfolk: schools survey, unpub.). Pepper was also used as a styptic (Taylor MSS). Moulds of various kinds were used to heal cuts. Moldy cheese was used in Sussex (Candlin 1987), as was moldy jam (Prince 1991: 113). In Yorkshire, moldy curd tarts have been used on cuts (Prince 1991: 95). In Sussex, moldy bacon fat has been used (Allen 1995: 118). The shed skin of an adder was sometimes used to heal deep cuts (Tongue 1965: 35; Prince 1991: 101). Dog's spit was considered beneficial by some (Simpkins 1914: 403).

Plant remedies include the root of horseradish (Armoracia rusticana), thick slices of which were bound onto cuts (Porter 1974: 44). Alternatives include the bruised leaves of geranium or an ointment made from comfrey (Schools survey, Norfolk 1980, unpub.). St. John's wort (Hypericum perforatum) was used to stem bleeding (Beith 1995: 238), and the bruised leaves of a related species, tutsan (Hypericum androsaemum), were used in Buckinghamshire (Science Gossip [1866]: 83). Primrose (Primula vulgaris) and tormentil (Potentilla erecta) were both used in Cumbria (Freethy 1985: 87, 127). Periwinkle, also known as cutfinger, was used in Devon for treating cuts (Baker 1980: 52).

In recent times, the large leaves of dock (Rumex sp.) have been crushed and laid on cuts (Vickery 1995: 108). Mallow has been used for cuts (Vickery 1995: 229). The inner layer of an onion skin was used as a natural plaster (Vickery 1995: 267). Valerian (Valeriana sp.) was called cut-leaf in Sussex, and its leaves were rubbed onto cuts (Vickery 1995: 379). Water betony, also known as water figwort (Scrophularia auriculata), was used to treat cuts (Vickery 1995: 385). Lily leaves preserved in brandy were a country standby for treating cuts, used all over Britain, but especially commonly in Suffolk (Taylor MSS). Castor oil (from Ricinus communis), more commonly used as a treatment for constipation, has also been used to treat cuts (Prince 1991: 114). A slice of bracket fungus was used in Sussex to stem bleeding from a cut (Allen 1995: 27). Woundwort (Stachys spp.) was another plant used to treat cuts (Allen 1995: 184). Leaves of ribwort plantain (Plantago lanceolata) have been used to treat cuts (Beith 1995: 233). Self-heal (Prunella vulgaris), as its name suggests, has been used to treat cuts; its use was reported in the Weald of Kent as recently as the 1940s (Mabey 1996: 317). Cleavers (Galium aparine) has been used for cuts and grazes (Hatfield 1994: 33, 88). The related species, woodruff (Asperula odorata), was reported by Parkinson in the seventeenth century in use for treating cuts (Parkinson 1640: 563). In Norfolk, it was still being used in the twentieth century (Bardswell 1911: 111). Rose leaves (Rosa canina) have been crushed and laid on cuts (Hatfield 1994: 32). Comfrey was used for treating cuts and wounds (Killip 1975: 135). Yarrow has been widely used to heal minor injuries both in Scotland (Beith 1995: 252) and in England (Tongue 1965: 36). In Scotland, an ointment made from daisies (Bellis perennis) was applied to cuts (Beith 1995: 213).

To this list could be added a large number of plants used in Ireland for treating cuts. They included chickweed, watercress (Rorippa nasturtium-aquaticum), blackberry, ivy, lady's mantle (Alchemilla vulgaris), hazel (Corylus avellana), and dandelion (Allen and Hatfield, in press).

Puffballs were important in first aid and were often kept dried in a shed for year-round use. The spores were sprinkled on to cuts, and the "body" of the puffball was used to poultice severe cuts (Hatfield 1994: 32).

In North American folk medicine there is an even greater array of remedies for cuts. Some of these are recognizably the same as in Britain—for instance the use of spider webs (Brown 1952–1964 6: 168) and of the inner membrane of an egg (UCLA Folklore Archives 18_6257). Sugar and flour, sheep's wool (Puckett 1981: 358), mud (UCLA Folklore Archives 20_6256), soot (Brown 1952–1964, 6: 168) or glue (Puckett 1981: 359) are other recommendations. Chicken manure and lard (Hyatt 1965: 207) or fresh horse manure (Brown 1952–1964, 6: 168) have been suggested. As in Britain, various molds have been used in treatment of cuts. Moldy bread and moldy orange peel have both been used (Parler 1962, 3: 591), as well as rotted wood (UCLA Folklore Archives 16_6259). Spit has been used on cuts (Brown 1952–1964, 6: 168). Spitting on a cut and then holding it against the bark of a tree is a variant of this (Cannon 1984: 104). Coon fat (Parler 1962, 3: 587) and bacon fat (UCLA Folklore Archives 4_6591) have both been rubbed on cuts. Tea leaves (UCLA Folklore Archives 19_6259) or coffee grains mixed with kerosene (Anderson 1970: 25) have also been used.

Among the plant remedies used in North American folk medicine, some are recognizably the same as ones used in Britain. A salve made from houseleek and lard has been used (UCLA Folklore Archives 9_6259), as has one made from elder bark (Puckett 1981: 358). Plantain leaves have been used (Hand 1958: 66), and horseradish leaves crushed in vinegar (Pickard and Buley 1945: 42). Geranium leaves have been bruised and laid on cuts (Puckett 1981: 358). White lilies in whisky, used in

Pennsylvania (Lick and Brendle 1922: 97), mirror the lilies in brandy used in Suffolk, England. The daisy lotion used by colonists (Kell 1956: 371) may have been brought with them from Scotland. Where East Anglians used the bruised leaves of rose, in North America the dried stems of roses have been powdered and applied (Clark 1970: 19). A salve has been made from watercress (Puckett 1981: 358). Puffball spores have been used (Clark 1970: 19) just as in Britain.

This is an impressive overlap between British and American plant remedies, but in addition to these a large number of plants not native to Britain have been used in North American folk treatment of cuts. Pine extracts, resin, and turpentine (Brown 1952–1964, 6: 168), or pitch (UCLA Folklore Archives 5_7611), have been widely used. A poultice of prickly pear has been used (Murphree 1965: 179). Crushed squash seeds (*Cucurbita* sp.) have been applied (Clark 1970: 19), or the liquid from balsam blisters (*Abies balsamea*) (Clark 1970: 18). Green tobacco leaves (*Nicotiana* sp.) have been used to dress cuts (Clark 1970: 19). An ointment has been prepared from pokeberry roots (Pickard and Buley 1945: 42). Spruce juice (*Picea* sp.) has been used (Brown 1952–1964, 6: 168), or the juice of milkweed (*Asclepias* sp.) (Woodhull 1930: 53). A salve has been made from devil's bush (? *Aralia spinosa*) and lard (Miller 1958: 64).

In the Native American tradition many of these plant remedies have been used to treat cuts. In particular, the gum of many coniferous trees has been used. Juniper gum has been used (Van Wart 1948: 576), as well as the gum or pitch derived from numerous species of pine (Moerman 1998: 409–413) and fir (Moerman 1998: 33–36). Basswood bark (*Tilia americana*) has been used (Carmer 1940: 366). Apart from plant remedies, mutton tallow has been used by the Shinnecock Indians (Carr and Westey

1945: 122), and the bodies of snails have been applied to cuts by the Kwakiutl (Boas 1932: 193).

*See also* **Blackberry, Bleeding, Chickweed, Comfrey, Dandelion, Elder, Houseleek, Ivy, Mallow, Molds, Plantain, Poke, Puffball, Snail, Wounds, Yarrow.**

## References

Allen, Andrew. *A Dictionary of Sussex Folk Medicine.* Newbury: Countryside Books, 1995.

Allen, David E., and Gabrielle Hatfield. *Medicinal Plants in Folk Tradition.* Portland, OR: Timber Press, in press.

Anderson, John. *Texas Folk Medicine.* Austin, TX: Encino Press, 1970.

Baker, Margaret. *Discovering the Folklore of Plants.* 2nd ed. Aylesbury: Shire, 1980.

Bardswell, Frances A. *The Herb Garden.* London: Adam and Charles Black, 1911.

Beith, Mary. *Healing Threads: Traditional Medicines of the Highlands and Islands.* Edinburgh: Polygon, 1995.

Boas, Franz. "Current Beliefs of the Kwakiutl Indians." *Journal of American Folklore* 45 (1932) 177–260.

Brown, Frank C. *Collection of North Carolina Folklore.* 7 vols. Durham, NC: Duke University Press, 1952–1964.

Candlin, Lillian. *Memories of Old Sussex.* Countryside Books, 1987.

Cannon, Anthon S. *Popular Beliefs and Superstitions from Utah.* Edited by Wayland D. Hand and Jeannine E. Talley. Salt Lake City: University of Utah Press, 1984.

Carmer, Carl. *Listen for the Lonesome Drum.* New York: Blue Ribbon Books 1940.

Carr, Lloyd G., and Carlos Westey. "Surviving Folktales and Herbal Lore among the Shinnecock Indians of Long Island." *Journal of American Folklore* 58 (1945): 113–123.

Clark, Joseph D. "North Carolina Popular Beliefs and Superstitions." *North Carolina Folklore* 18 (1970): 1–66.

Freethy, Ron. *From Agar to Zenry.* Marlborough: Crowood Press, 1985.

Hand, Wayland D. "Popular Beliefs and Superstitions from Pennsylvania." *Keystone Folklore Quarterly* 3 (1958): 61–74.

Hatfield, Gabrielle. *Country Remedies: Traditional East Anglian Plant Remedies in the Twentieth Century.* Woodbridge: Boydell, 1994.

Hyatt, Harry Middleton. *Folklore from Adams County Illinois.* 2nd rev. ed. New York: Memoirs of the Alma Egan Hyatt Foundation, 1965.

Kell, Katherine T. "The Folklore of the Daisy." *Journal of American Folklore* 69 (1956): 369–376.

Killip, Margaret. *The Folklore of the Isle of Man.* London: Batsford, 1975.

Lick, David E., and Thomas R. Brendle. "Plant Names and Plant Lore among the Pennsylvania Germans." *Proceedings and Addresses of the Pennsylvania German Society* 33 (1922).

Mabey, Richard. *Flora Britannica.* London: Sinclair Stevenson 1996.

Miller, Mary E. "A Folklore Survey of Dickson County, Tennessee." *Tennessee Folklore Society Bulletin* 24 (1958): 57–71.

Moerman, Daniel E. *Native American Ethnobotany.* Portland, OR: Timber Press, 1998.

Murphree, Alice H. "Folk Medicine in Florida: Remedies using Plants." *Florida Anthropologist* 18 (1965): 175–185.

Parkinson, John. *Theatrum Botanicum.* London: Thomas Cotes, 1640.

Parler, Mary Celestia, and University Student Contributors. *Folk Beliefs from Arkansas.* 15 vols. Fayetteville: University of Arkansas, 1962.

Pickard, Madge E., and R. Carlyle Buley. *The Midwest Pioneer, His Ills, Cures and Doctors.* Crawfordsville, IN: R. E. Banta, 1945.

Porter, Enid. *The Folklore of East Anglia.* London: Batsford, 1974.

Prince, Dennis. *Grandmother's Cures: An A–Z of Herbal Remedies.* London: Fontana, 1991.

Puckett, Newbell Niles. *Popular Beliefs and Superstitions: A Compendium of American Folklore from the Ohio Collection of Newbell Niles Puckett.* Edited by Wayland D. Hand, Anna Casetta, and Sondra B. Thiederman. 3 vols. Boston: G. K. Hall, 1981.

Simpkins, John Ewart. *Examples of Printed Folklore Concerning Fife, with Some Notes on Clackmannan and Kinross-Shires.* County Folklore 7. London: Publications of the Folklore Society, 1914.

Taylor MSS. Manuscript Notes of Mark R. Taylor in the Norfolk Record Office, Norwich. MS 4322.

Tongue, Ruth L. *Somerset Folklore.* Edited by Katharine Briggs. County Folklore 8. London: Folklore Society, 1965.

Van Wart, Arthur F. "The Indians of the Maritime Provinces, Their Diseases and Native Cures." *The Canadian Medical Association Journal* 59(6) (1948): 573–577.

Vickery, Roy. *A Dictionary of Plant Lore.* Oxford: Oxford University Press, 1995.

Woodhull, Frost. "Ranch Remedios." *Publications of the Texas Folklore Society* 8 (1930): 9–73.

# D

## Dandelion (*Taraxacum officinale*)

This is one of the most widely used plants in British folk medicine. The white latex present in all parts of the plant has been used to treat warts. The root contains powerful diuretics and has been used as a kidney tonic. This has earned the plant the name of "piss-a-bed" and has given rise to a widespread idea that touching the plant, or picking bunches of the flowers, will make a child wet the bed (Vickery 1995: 102–103). Dandelion has been regarded as a general tonic. It has been used in the treatment of jaundice and other liver troubles, and it has formed a common cure for coughs and colds. The leaves are eaten in salads. In addition to these common uses, there are a large number of minor ones. The leaves were used in both Scotland and Ireland to treat stings (Vickery 1995: 105), in much the same way that dock leaves were used. In the Scottish Highlands, the plant was particularly valued for promoting the appetite of sufferers from tuberculosis. Eaten in a bread and butter sandwich, the leaves were regarded as an ulcer cure in Glencoe (Beith 1995: 213–214). Other minor British uses include the treatment of indigestion, of corns, of scarlet fever, and even of lip cancer (Allen and Hatfield, in press).

It is from Ireland that the widest ranges of folk medical uses of dandelion have been

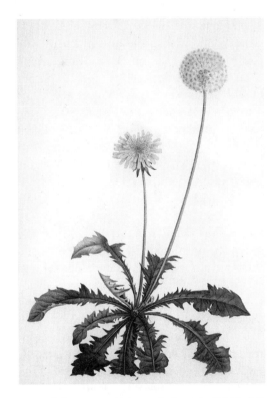

One of the most widely used plants in British folk medicine, dandelion has been used to treat jaundice and other liver troubles and has formed a common cure for coughs and colds. In Ireland dandelion has been used for a large number of other ailments (Library of Congress)

recorded. A wise woman from Donegal recommended three leaves on three successive mornings eaten for heart trouble (Black 1883: 199). The plant was called by her "heart fever grass." Such use of the dandelion for treating heart problems is exclusive to Ireland. In Ireland it has been used for a large number of other ailments too, including cuts, sprains, fractures, sore eyes, diabetes, headache, toothache and anemia, and stys (Logan 1972: 59). In Donegal it is described as being used for "every disease" (Allen and Hatfield, in press). There is an interesting belief recorded from Limerick that when used as a tonic, the white-veined leaves should be eaten by a man, the red-veined ones by a woman (Allen and Hatfield, in press).

Though not native to North America, dandelion is widespread and much used in folk medicine there too. As in Britain, it has been used as a tonic, for jaundice, kidney complaints, rheumatism (Meyer 1985: 37, 150, 157, 213–216) and the sap has been used to treat nettle stings (UCLA Folklore Archives 2_5442). Also similar to the British use is the common employment of the plant juice to treat warts (see, for example, Puckett 1981: 475). Dandelion wine, drunk hot, has been used as a cold cure ("Folklore Fragments" 1964: 118). A cough syrup has been made in Pennsylvania from the blossoms, with lemon and sugar (Fogel 1915: 131), while for cataract, pieces of the root have been worn as an amulet around the neck (Brendle and Unger 1935: 124). A tea made from the root has been recommended for the nerves (Lick and Brendle 1922: 73) and for dyspepsia, dropsy, and edema (Harris 1968: 99). Dandelion leaves have been suggested for insomnia (UCLA Folklore Archives 10_6769) and to increase virility (UCLA Folklore Archives 8_6386). In Pennsylvania there is a custom of eating dandelion leaves on Green Thursday (Maundy Thursday), as a health promoter, and to prevent the itch (Brendle 1951: 7). Echoing the Irish belief mentioned above, dandelions are regarded as a cure-all (UCLA Folklore Archive 6_6446).

The uses of dandelion by Native Americans are very wide (Moerman 1998: 550–551) and include many familiar in Britain, such as kidney complaints, toothache, tonic. In addition, they have been used to treat gynecological troubles. The flowers are eaten for menstrual cramps—for instance, by the Papago (Castetter and Underhill 1935: 65); the Navajo have used an infusion of the plant to speed delivery (Vestal 1952: 53). The Meskwaki took dandelion root for chest pain when other remedies failed (Vogel 1970: 298–299).

*See also* **Amulet, Anemia, Bed-wetting, Colds, Corns, Coughs, Cuts, Diabetes, Dock, Dropsy, Eye problems, Fractures, Headache, Heart trouble, Indigestion, Jaundice, Sleeplessness, Sprains, Tonic, Toothache, Tuberculosis, Warts.**

## References

Allen, David E., and Gabrielle Hatfield. *Medicinal Plants in Folk Tradition*. Portland, OR: Timber Press, in press.

Beith, Mary. *Healing Threads: Traditional Medicines of the Highlands and Islands*. Edinburgh: Polygon, 1995.

Black, William George. *Folk-Medicine: A Chapter in the History of Culture*. London: Folklore Society, 1883.

Brendle, Rev. Thomas R. "Customs of the Year in the Dutch Country." *Pennsylvania Dutchman* 3 (November 15, 1951): 12.

Brendle, Thomas R., and Claude W. Unger. "Folk Medicine on the Pennsylvania Germans: The Non-Occult Cures." *Proceedings of the Pennsylvania German Society* 45 (1935).

Castetter, Edward E., and Ruth M. Underhill. "Ethnobiological Studies in the American Southwest II. The Ethnobiology of the Papago Indians." *University of New Mexico Bulletin* 4(3) 1935: 1–84.

Fogel, Edwin Miller. "Beliefs and Superstitions of the Pennsylvania Germans." *Americana Germanica* 18 (1915).

Folklore Fragments. *Keystone Folklore Quarterly* 9 (1964).

Harris, Bernice Kelly (ed.). *Southern Home Remedies*. Murfreesboro, NC: Johnson, 1968.

Lick, David E., and Thomas R. Brendle. "Plant Names and Plant Lore among the Pennsylvania Germans." *Proceedings and Addresses* of the *Pennsylvania German Society* 33 (1922).

Logan, Patrick. *Making the Cure: A Look at Irish Folk Medicine.* Dublin: Talbot Press, 1972.

Meyer, Clarence. *American Folk Medicine.* Glenwood, IL: Meyerbooks, 1985.

Moerman, Daniel E. *Native American Ethnobotany.* Portland, OR: Timber Press, 1998.

Puckett, Newbell Niles. *Popular Beliefs and Superstitions: A Compendium of American Folklore from the Ohio Collection of Newbell Niles Puckett.* Edited by Wayland D. Hand, Anna Casetta, and Sondra B. Thiederman. 3 vols. Boston: G. K. Hall, 1981.

Vestal, Paul A. "The Ethnobotany of the Ramah Navaho." *Papers of the Peabody Museum of American Archaeology and Ethnology* 40(4) (1952): 1–94.

Vickery, Roy. *A Dictionary of Plant Lore.* Oxford: Oxford University Press, 1995.

Vogel, Virgil J. *American Indian Medicine.* Norman: University of Oklahoma Press, 1970.

# Dead man's hand

In British folk medicine, the touch of a dead man's hand was used as a cure for various kinds of swelling, especially goiter. In Cambridgeshire in the 1940s this was still being practiced (Porter 1974: 47). That the method involved the idea of transference is confirmed by the story of a man who placed his dead grandfather's hand on his warts, asking his grandfather to "take them with you" (Porter 1974: 51). "Wens," a folk medical term for a swelling, including sebaceous cysts as well as goiter, were sometimes so treated (Radford and Radford 1974: 125). Sometimes people attended an execution so that they could be cured in this way; the hangman charged the sufferer a fee (Black 1883: 100–101). Sometimes it was specified that the corpse must be of the opposite sex to the sufferer (Taylor 1929: 119). The touch of a suicide's hand was considered effective against the King's Evil (Black 1883: 101).

In North American folk medicine, the same treatment for goiter was practiced un-

til the twentieth century (Wintemberg 1918: 137). In the Carolinas, wens were likewise treated by the touch of a dead man's hand (Hand 1970: 327). The "cure" extended to cancer as well (Cannon 1984: 98).

*See also* **Transference, Tuberculosis.**

### References

Black, William George. *Folk-Medicine: A Chapter in the History of Culture.* London: Folklore Society, 1883.

Cannon, Anthon S. *Popular Beliefs and Superstitions from Utah.* Edited by Wayland D. Hand and Jeannine E. Talley. Salt Lake City: University of Utah Press, 1984.

Hand, Wayland D. "Hangman, the Gallows, and the Dead Man's Hand in American Folk Medicine." In *Medieval Literature and Folklore Studies. Essays in Honor of Francis Lee Utley.* Edited by J. Mandel and B. A. Rosenberg. New Brunswick, NJ: Rutgers University Press, 1970, 323–330.

Porter, Enid. *The Folklore of East Anglia.* London: Batsford, 1974.

Radford, E., and M. A. Radford. *Encyclopaedia of Superstitions.* Edited and revised by Christina Hole. London: Book Club Associates 1974.

Taylor, Mark R. "Norfolk Folklore." *Folk-Lore* 50 (1929): 113–133.

Wintemberg, W. J. "Folk-Lore Collected in the Counties of Oxford and Waterloo, Ontario." *Journal of American Folklore* 31 (1918): 135–153.

# Deafness

The water of a particular healing well was sometimes believed to help deafness. For example, on the remote island of St. Kilda there is a well named, in Gaelic, the Well of the Special Powers (Beith 1995: 142). Hedgehog oil was widely used to treat deafness; this is a remedy reputedly of gipsy origin (Taylor MSS, Norfolk). The oil is prepared by baking the hedgehog, whole, in a clay covering. The flesh could be eaten. Melted-down fat from the adder was used to treat deafness and earache in Sussex as recently as the 1920s (Allen 1995: 164). Ants' eggs mixed with onion juice was another remedy for deafness from Scotland (Black 1883: 161). More prosaic remedies for deafness include juice of the houseleek. The Gaelic name for this plant translates as "ear plant." It was used for both earache and deafness (Beith 1995: 224).

An Irish remedy for earache was recorded by Oscar Wilde's mother at the end of the nineteenth century. The flowers, leaves and roots of the cowslip were crushed and the resulting juice mixed with honey. This mixture was dripped into the nostrils and ears of the prone patient. After a few minutes, when the patient turned over, the juice flowed out, and, one hoped, the deafness was improved (Wilde 1898: 42). Mint juice (*Mentha* sp.), squeezed from nine plants, was another Irish remedy (Allen and Hatfield, in press). Wearing black wool in the ears was considered in nineteenth-century Scotland to be a preservative against deafness (Dalyell 1835: 116).

North American folk medicine for deafness includes an analogous assortment of animal oils and plant remedies. Meyer in his collection (Meyer 1985: 102–103) includes hedgehog oil, skunk oil, pickerel oil, eel oil, goose fat, and civet. He mentions a mid-nineteenth-century recipe calling for black wool (as in Scotland, see above) to be dipped in civet and placed in the ears. A remarkably similar recipe appears in a late seventeenth-century recipe from Staffordshire, England (Smith and Randall 1987: 25). Powdered earwig is another recommendation (Brown 1952–1964, 6: 169).

Plant remedies include sow-thistle juice, houseleek (as in Britain), sassafras oil, and oil of bitter almonds (Meyer 1985: 102–103). The juice of black radish has also been suggested (Brown 1952–1964, 6: 169).

At least some of the folk remedies listed here may be an inheritance from official "book" medicine. Innumerable animal ingredients in official medicine at the end of the seventeenth century include civet for deafness, as well as spirit of ants (Salmon 1693: 328, 680).

Native American remedies for ear "disorders," presumably including deafness, include the use of wintergreen (*Pyrola* sp.) by the Blackfoot (Hellson 1974: 82). The same tribe used the juice of the berries of *Amelanchier alnifolia* as eardrops (Hellson 1974:80). The Tarahumara use the pincushion cactus (*Mamillaria heyderi*) to treat earache and deafness (Kay 1996: 190).

*See also* **Cowslip, Earache, Houseleek, Sassafras.**

## References

Allen, Andrew. *A Dictionary of Sussex Folk Medicine.* Newbury: Countryside Books, 1995.

Allen, David E., and Gabrielle Hatfield. *Medicinal Plants in Folk Tradition.* Portland, OR: Timber Press (in press).

Beith, Mary. *Healing Threads: Traditional Medicines of the Highlands and Islands.* Edinburgh: Polygon, 1995.

Black, William George. *Folk-Medicine: A Chapter in the History of Culture.* London: Folklore Society, London, 1883.

Brown, Frank C. *Collection of North Carolina Folklore.* 7 vols. Durham, NC: Duke University Press, 1952–1964.

Dalyell, John Graham. *The Darker Superstitions of Scotland.* Glasgow: Griffin, 1835.

Hellson, Jon C. *Ethnobotany of the Blackfoot Indians.* Mercury Series 19. Ottawa: National Museums of Canada, 1974.

Kay, Margarita Artschwager. *Healing with Plants in the American and Mexican West.* Tucson: University of Arizona Press, 1996.

Meyer, Clarence. *American Folk Medicine.* Glenwood, IL: Meyerbooks, 1985.

Salmon, William, M.D. *The Compleat English Physician.* London, 1693.

Smith, Janet, and Thea Randall, eds. *Kill or Cure. Medical Remedies from the Staffordshire Records Office.* Staffordshire Record Office, 1987.

Taylor MSS. Manuscript notes of Mark R. Taylor in Norfolk Record Office, Norwich. MS4322.

Wilde, Lady Jane. *Ancient Cures, Charms and Us-*

*ages of Ireland.* London: Ward and Downey, 1898.

# Depression

Under varying names, this condition must be as old as mankind. Simply because it is less tangible than many afflictions, we have probably even less written evidence of folk treatments for depression than of other more obvious physical illnesses. The term "melancholy" is a learned rather than a folk one, meaning literally "black-humored," reflecting the official medical humoral theory. In folk medicine among the less educated there would have been many ways of describing what we would call depression, ranging from "possessed by evil spirits," cast down, to simply bad tempered. Wearing as jewelry carnelian, amber, garnet or jasper was thought to ease depression (Souter 1995: 152). In the Highlands of Scotland in the seventeenth century a heroic cure for "faintness of the spirits" was recorded by Martin Martin from the Isle of Skye. The healer was a smith, the thirteenth generation in his family to practice this treatment. The cure consisted of laying the patient on the anvil and bringing down a huge hammer, as if to strike him. This, they say, "has always the design'd effect" (Martin 1716: 183). Perhaps more acceptably, whisky was regarded in the Scottish Highlands as a cure for most things, including melancholia, having the power to "make the sad man into a happy man" (National Library of Scotland Advocates MS 72.1.2).

Some plants thought to protect against evil spirits were also thought to prevent depression, for example ivy, which was grown on Roman houses for these purposes (Souter 1995: 41). Of the plants mentioned in the herbals, lemon balm *(Melissa officinalis)* and *Rosa gallica* would probably have been available only to those wealthy enough to afford physicians or a physic garden at least, so it seems unlikely that these nonnative

plants would have featured in British folk medicine. The proverb "I borage bring always courage" is quoted by Gerard in his herbal. Perhaps this plant, *Borago officinalis,* a native of the Mediterranean but naturalized in Britain, may have been used in British folk medicine. A rare glimpse of an eighteenth-century treatment for bad moods is given in the *Diary of a Farmer's Wife* 1796–1797. The recipe is given for violet pudding, "a good sure cure for cross husbands" (*The Diary of a Farmer's Wife 1796–1797:* 104). A twentieth-century cure for "sour nature" is recorded from Hampshire, consisting of eating cabbage cooked with honey and salt (Prince 1991: 106). There is a fascinating legend from the Highlands of Scotland involving the plant St. John's wort, which has recently sprung to fame throughout the Western world as an antidepressant. The story tells of Calum Cille treating a young herd boy whose mind had been disturbed by long lonely nights on the hills. St. John's wort was placed in the boy's armpit, and he recovered. The Gaelic name for the plant translates as "St. Columba's oxterful," which suggests that treating with plants in the groin or armpit may have been regularly practiced (Beith 1995: 40). Apart from this allusion, the plant has not figured widely in the British folk medical literature as a treatment for depression, though it has had a wide variety of other uses. A late-nineteenth-century book refers to its use in the Isle of Man for treating lowness of spirits (Moore 1898). Otherwise, this use seems to have been confined to the herbals and official medicine. In the Scottish Highlands, a tea made from thistles was used to treat depression (Beith 1995: 246). In very recent times, a mixture of chamomile flowers and angelica leaves (*Angelica* sp.) has been successfully used to treat depression (P.S., Nottingham, 1985, pers. com.).

In North America, a number of native plants not found in Britain have been used to treat depression. In Mexico, the Mayo treat depression using "brasil" *(Haematoxylon brasiletto)* (Kay 1996: 159). Lady's slipper *(Cypripedium* spp.) is also known as nerve root and has been used in the Rocky Mountains for depression (Willard 1992: 61), and by the Iroquois as a nerve medicine (Herrick 1977: 289). It was apparently widely used as a sedative in domestic practice (Meyer 1985: 146). According to Rafinesque it is used by the Indians "in all nervous disorders" (Rafinesque 1828–1830). Asafoetida *(Ferula asafoetida)* had a reputation for treating nervous disorders, both in the medical literature and to some extent in folk practice (McWhorter 1966: 13). A tea made from tansy *(Tanacetum vulgare)* has been used to treat melancholy (UCLA Folklore Archives 11_5398). Rhubarb *(Rheum* spp.) and senna leaves *(Senna* spp.) have likewise been used (UCLA Folklore Archives 24_6394). An American folk remedy of German origin for treating "melancholy" uses elecampane *(Inula helenium)* combined either with yarrow and sassafras or with wine heated with red-hot steel (Wilson 1908: 71). Both onions (Puckett 1981: 292) and turnips (Gruber 1902: 15) have been recommended for depression and nervous disorders. Motherwort *(Leonurus cardiaca)* was recommended for nervous disorders and to "raise the drooping spirits" (Meyer 1985: 185). St. John's wort, although used in North American folk medicine for a number of disorders, does not seem to have been used in folk medicine in the past for its antidepressant properties. Pine trees have been said to comfort a diseased mind (Brown 1952–1964, 6: 357).

In the Native American tradition, numerous plants have been used for psychological disturbances (Moerman 1998: 816), though few seem to have been singled out for treating what in the modern West is termed depression. Mental, psychological and physical symptoms were not separated as they are in orthodox modern Western medicine, and many plants used ceremonially by the Native Americans may well have treated what we would call depression. James's buckwheat *(Eriogonum jamesii)* was used by the Western Keres to treat despondency (Swank 1932: 43). A modern Native American herbal mixture recommended for its cheering qualities includes the flowers of St. John's wort and passionflower *(Passiflora incarnata)* and the bark of Devil's Club *(Oplopanax horridus)* (Kavasch and Baar 1999: 179).

Nonbotanical folk treatments for depression in North America include iodine solution mixed with sugar water (UCLA Folklore Archives 15_5597). The flesh of screech owls was eaten by both Native Americans and black Americans and was thought to be good for melancholy (Hudson 1960: 13). More poetically, the music played on pipes made from cinnamon bark *(Cinnamomum aromaticum)* is recommended for melancholy (Leland 1892: 188). In the Native American culture music is widely used for healing. This usage, it has been claimed, is largely based on the "actual power of rhythm" (Densmore 1954: 109). The color red has been associated with cheerfulness, and in the Mexican culture wearing something red is held to combat depression. A red dress may be worn (Hatch 1969: 164) or a gold ring threaded on a red ribbon (Kay 1972: 178).

There has been a folk belief that burned bread can cause depression (Puckett 1981: 290).

*See also* **Blacksmith, Cabbage, Chamomile, Color, Ivy, Mexican tradition, St. John's wort, Sassafras, Yarrow.**

### References

Beith, Mary. *Healing Threads: Traditional Medicines of the Highlands and Islands.* Edinburgh: Polygon, 1995.

Brown, Frank C. *Collection of North Carolina Folklore.* 7 vols. Durham, NC: Duke University Press, 1952–1964.

Densmore, Frances. "Importance of Rhythm in Songs for the Treatment of the Sick by American Indians." *Scientific Monthly* 79(2) (August 1954): 109–112.

*The Diary of a Farmer's Wife 1796–1797.* Harmondsworth: Penguin, 1981.

Gruber, John. Hagerstown, MD: Hagerstown Town and Country Almanac, 1852–1914.

Hatch, E. Le Roy. "Home Remedies Mexican Style." *Western Folklore* 28 (1969): 163–168.

Herrick, James William. *Iroquois Medical Botany.* Ph.D. thesis, State University of New York, Albany, 1977.

Hudson, Arthur Palmer. "Animal Lore in Lawson's and Brickell's Histories of North Carolina." *North Carolina Folklore* 8(2) (1960): 1–15.

Kavasch, E. Barrie, and Karen Baar. *American Indian Healing Arts: Herbs, Rituals and Remedies for every Season of Life.* New York: Bantam Books, 1999.

Kay, Margarita Artschwager. *Healing with Plants in the American and Mexican West.* Tucson: University of Arizona Press, 1996.

———. *Health and Illness in the Barrio: Women's Point of View.* Ph.D. dissertation, University of Arizona, 1972.

Leland, Charles Godfrey. "The Folklore of Straw." *Journal of American Folklore* 5 (1892): 186–188.

Martin, M. *A Description of the Western Islands of Scotland.* 2nd. ed. London, 1716 (facsimile James Thin, 1976).

McWhorter, Bruce. "Superstitions from Russell County, Kentucky." *Kentucky Folklore Record* 12 (1966): 11–14.

Meyer, Clarence. *American Folk Medicine.* Glenwood, IL: Meyerbooks, 1985.

Moerman, Daniel E. *Native American Ethnobotany.* Portland, OR: Timber Press, 1998.

Moore, A.W. *Folk-Medicine in the Isle of Man.*" *Yn Lioar Manninagh* 3 (1898): 303–314.

Prince, Dennis. *Grandmother's Cures: An A–Z of Herbal Remedies.* London: Fontana, 1991.

Puckett, Newbell Niles. *Popular Beliefs and Superstitions: A Compendium of American Folklore from the Ohio Collection of Newbell Niles Puckett.* Edited by Wayland D. Hand, Anna Casetta, and Sondra B. Thiederman. 3 vols. Boston: G. K. Hall, 1981.

Rafinesque, C. S. *Medical Flora; or Manual of the Medical Botany of the United States of North America.* 2 vols. Philadelphia: Atkinson and Alexander, 1828–1830.

Souter, Keith. *Cure Craft: Traditional Folk Remedies and Treatment from Antiquity to the Present Day.* Saffron Walden: C. W. Daniel, 1995.

Swank, George R. *The Ethnobotany of the Acoma and Laguna Indians.* M.A. thesis, University of New Mexico, Albuquerque, 1932.

Willard, Terry. *Edible and Medicinal Plants of the Rocky Mountains and Neighbouring Territories.* Calgary: Wild Rose College of Natural Healing, 1992.

Wilson, Charles Bundy. "Notes on Folk-Medicine." *Journal of American Folklore* 21 (1908): 68–73.

# Dew

Bathing in early-morning dew on the first day of May was recommended in British folk medicine for improving the complexion and removing freckles. In folk medicine dew was used especially for eye troubles (Tongue 1965: 39). The custom of bathing in May dew for eye ailments was observed by Samuel Pepys's wife in 1667 and was still being followed in Edinburgh until recently (Radford and Radford 1974: 134). In Ireland dew was also recommended for preserving the eyesight (Logan 1972: 60). May dew was collected and used to bathe weak children (Addy 1895: 92). The dew from particular flowers was used in official medicine and also in folk medicine. Since the time of Pliny, the water collecting in the leaf-bases of teasel *(Dipsacus fullonum)* has been regarded as magical. This water has been used in England for sore eyes and also for removing warts (Vickery 1995: 368). The dew shaken from the flowers of chamomile was believed to cure tuberculosis (Trevelyan 1909: 315). Running barefoot in the dew is recommended for chilblains (Souter 1995: 143).

In North American folk medicine, as in Britain, dew has been widely recommended for removing freckles (Brown 1952–1964: 196–198). Again as in Britain, it has been used to treat warts (Brown 1952–1964, 6: 333) and sore eyes (Boudreaux 1971: 140). A number of other conditions too have been treated with dew: rashes (Brown 1952–1964, 6: 253), sweaty feet, ringworm (Hyatt 1965: 221, 328), bed-wetting, rheumatism, fever, and hay fever (Puckett 1981: 98, 108, 388, 431).

*See also* **Bed-wetting, Chamomile, Chilblains, Eye problems, Fevers, Freckles, Hay fever, Rheumatism, Ringworm, Tuberculosis, Warts.**

## References

Addy, Sidney Oldall. *Household Tales with Other Traditional Remains Collected in the Counties of York, Lincoln, Derby and Nottingham.* London, 1895.

Boudreaux, Anna M. "Les Remèdes du Vieux Temps: Remedies and Cures of the Kaplan Area in Southwestern Louisiana." *Southern Folklore Quarterly* 35 (1971): 121–140.

Brown, Frank C. *Collection of North Carolina Folklore.* 7 vols. Durham, NC: Duke University Press, 1952–1964.

Hyatt, Harry Middleton. *Folklore from Adams County Illinois.* 2nd rev. ed. New York: Memoirs of the Alma Egan Hyatt Foundation, 1965.

Logan, Patrick. *Making the Cure: A Look at Irish Folk Medicine.* Dublin: Talbot Press, 1972.

Puckett, Newbell Niles. *Popular Beliefs and Superstitions: A Compendium of American Folklore from the Ohio Collection of Newbell Niles Puckett.* Edited by Wayland D. Hand, Anna Casetta, and Sondra B. Thiederman. 3 vols. Boston: G. K. Hall, 1981.

Radford, E., and M. A. Radford. *Encyclopaedia of Superstitions.* Edited and revised by Christina Hole. London: Book Club Associates 1974.

Souter, Keith. *Cure Craft: Traditional Folk Remedies and Treatment from Antiquity to the Present Day.* Saffron Walden: C. W. Daniel, 1995.

Tongue, Ruth L. *Somerset Folklore.* County Folklore 8. Edited by Katharine Briggs. London: Folklore Society, 1965.

Trevelyan, Marie. *Folk-Lore and Folk-Stories of Wales.* London: Elliot Stock, 1909.

Vickery, Roy. *A Dictionary of Plant Lore.* Oxford: Oxford University Press, 1995.

# Diabetes

This illness was recognized and named more than two millennia ago by the pre-Christian Greek physicians. It is not clear to what extent diabetes was recognized in folk medicine; there are relatively few records of folk treatments for the condition. In Sussex, powdered mice were recommended (Allen 1995: 115). In Herefordshire, eating peanuts *(Arachis hypogea)* was said to be good for diabetes (Vickery 1995: 278). Other plant remedies used for diabetes include a mixture of chickweed and comfrey (Hatfield MS), and a wormwood *(Artemisia absinthium)* preparation was used in the Isle of Man (Fargher n.d.). In Ireland, an infusion of herb Robert *(Geranium robertianum)* was recommended (Moloney 1919), or one of dandelion (Allen and Hatfield, in press). Boiled nettles were also used to treat diabetes (EFS 112). The "hungry grass" well known in Irish folklore, probably *Agrostis stolonifera,* was held by some to cause not only hunger when trodden on, but also diabetes (Allen and Hatfield, in press).

In North American folk medicine there are some dietary recommendations for diabetes. Drinking goat's milk (UCLA Folklore Archives 11_6283) or buttermilk (Puckett 1981: 360) is recommended. Taking a small amount of vinegar before every meal is also advised (UCLA Folklore Archives 13_5586), as is eating honey (UCLA Folklore Archives 10_6283). Drinking sauerkraut juice has been found helpful (Puckett 1981: 360). "Winter" diabetes has been treated with a mixture of sulphur and molasses (Cannon 1984: 138). Salt and soda is another suggestion (Rogers 1941: 15–16). Drinking one's own urine has been held to be beneficial in diabetes (Brown 1952–1964, 6: 169). A strange-sounding suggestion to cure diabetes is to allow a poisonous snake to bite the sufferer (Browne 1958: 57). It is suggested that eating brown sugar rather than white is helpful in avoiding diabetes (Cannon 1984: 138).

Among plant remedies recommended in North American folk medicine, one of the most widespread is the roots of huckleberry (*Vaccinium* sp.) (Puckett 1981: 360). A tea made from the "heart" of mullein has been used (Wintemberg 1925: 621), or one made from alfalfa *(Medicago sativa)* (Cannon 1984: 104). Other suggestions are an infusion of queen of the meadow *(Eupatorium purpureum),* devil's shoestrings (*Yucca filamentosa*) (Browne 1958: 57), sage brush (*Artemisia* sp.) (Smithers 1961: 37), yarrow blossoms (Musick 1964: 51), or horsetail grass (*Equisetum* sp.) (Carey 1970: 27). Infusions of Spanish moss *(? Tillandsia usneoides)* (Michael and Barrow 1967: 781–782) or of bugle weed (*Lycopus* sp.) (Lathrop 1961: 16) are alternatives.

Among Native American plant remedies are sumac leaves (*Rhus* sp.) (Vogel 1970: 199) and devil's club root *(Oplopanax horridus)* (MacDermot 1949: 181), as well as devil's shoestring (Hamel and Chiltoskey 1975: 25).

*See also* **Chickweed, Comfrey, Dandelion, Mullein, Nettle, Soda, Urine, Yarrow.**

**References**
Allen, Andrew. *A Dictionary of Sussex Folk Medicine.* Newbury: Countryside Books, 1995.
Allen, David E., and Gabrielle Hatfield. *Medicinal Plants in Folk Tradition.* Portland, OR: Timber Press, in press.
Brown, Frank C. *Collection of North Carolina Folklore.* 7 vols. Durham, NC: Duke University Press, 1952–1964.
Browne, Ray B. *Popular Beliefs and Practices from Alabama.* Folklore Studies 9. Berkeley and Los Angeles: University of California Publications, 1958.
Cannon, Anthon S. *Popular Beliefs and Superstitions from Utah.* Edited by Wayland D. Hand and Jeannine E. Talley. Salt Lake City: University of Utah Press, 1984.
Carey, George G. "An Introductory Guide to Maryland Folklore and Folklife." In *Final Report of the Study Commission on Maryland Folklife.* Bethesda, MD, 1970, 25–27.
EFS. Manuscript notes from English Folklore Survey, 1960s. Held in University College London.
Fargher, D. C. *The Manx Have a Word for It: 5. Manx Gaelic Names of Flora.* Port Erin: privately published (mimeo), n.d.
Hamel, Paul B., and Mary U. Chiltoskey. *Cherokee Plants and Their Uses: A 400 Year History.* Sylva, NC: Herald, 1975.
Lathrop, Amy. "Pioneer Remedies from Western Kansas." *Western Folklore* 20 (1961): 1–22.
MacDermot, J. H. "Food and Medicinal Plants Used by the Indians of British Columbia." *Canadian Medical Association Journal* 61(2) (August 1949): 177–183.
Michael, Max, Jr., and Mark V. Barrow. "Old Timey Remedies of Yesterday and Today." *Journal of the Florida Medical Association* 54(8) (August 1967): 778–784.
Moloney, Michael F. *Irish Ethno-Botany and the Evolution of Medicine in Ireland.* Dublin: M. H. Gill and Son, 1919.
Musick, Ruth M. (ed.). "Superstitions." *West Virginia Folklore* 14 (1964): 38–52.
Puckett, Newbell Niles. *Popular Beliefs and Superstitions: A Compendium of American Folklore from the Ohio Collection of Newbell Niles Puckett.* Edited by Wayland D. Hand, Anna Casetta, and Sondra B. Thiederman. 3 vols. Boston: G. K. Hall, 1981.
Rogers, E. G. *Early Folk Medical Practices in Tennessee.* Murfreesboro, TN: Mid-South, 1941.
Smithers, W. D. "Nature's Pharmacy and the Curanderos." *Sul Ross State College Bulletin* 41(3) (1961).

Vickery, Roy. *A Dictionary of Plant Lore.* Oxford: Oxford University Press, 1995.

Vogel, Virgil J. *American Indian Medicine.* Norman: University of Oklahoma Press, 1970.

Wintemberg, W. J. "Some Items of Negro-Canadian Folklore." *Journal of American Folklore* 38 (1925): 621.

# Diarrhea

Diarrhea resulting from contaminated water and food must have been a serious hazard for both children and adults before adequate sanitation and food preservation. A very large number of plant remedies, many of them "astringents" rich in tannins, were used in the domestic treatment of diarrhea. Among them are the bark and acorns of oak, and ribwort plantain (*Plantago lanceolata*) (Hatfield 1994: 36). Meadow sweet *(Filipendula ulmaria)* has been used in both England and Ireland (Allen and Hatfield, in press). Other plant remedies for diarrhea include leaves of mulberry tree *(Morus nigra)* (Taylor MSS), raspberry leaves *(Rubus idaeus)* (Vickery 1995: 306), bilberry (Vaccinium myrtillus) (Beith 1995: 205), shepherd's purse *(Capsella bursa-pastoris),* tormentil *(Potentilla erecta)* (Beith 1995: 208), and wood avens (*Geum urbanum*) (Vesey-Fitzgerald 1944: 22). Mullein has been used particularly in Ireland to treat diarrhea (Allen and Hatfield, in press). The berries and the inner bark of blackthorn *(Prunus spinosa)* have been used throughout Britain (Allen and Hatfield, in press). An intriguing remedy from the Scottish Highlands is the use of the so-called bonduc bean (*Caesalpinia bonduc*), boiled in milk for dysentery and diarrhea (Beith 1995: 208). This and other exotic species of nuts are washed ashore on the Hebrides by the Gulf Stream; they were valued both as amulets and for their use in folk medicine. Though it is surprising to find that they are used in Hawaii as a laxative (Akana 1922: 47), these two uses are

not mutually exclusive. Apples, for example, are claimed to "regulate" the bowels, aiding both diarrhea and constipation. Red lavender, as much as could be absorbed on a lump of sugar, was a cure used in Wiltshire (Prince 1991: 94) but originating elsewhere.

Nonplant remedies in use in British folk medicine include eating a hard-boiled egg (still in use today). In the Highlands of Scotland, where whisky is regarded as a panacea, setting fire to a glassful and letting it burn for a couple of minutes, then drinking it, was said to cure stubborn diarrhea (Beith 1995: 116).

North American folk medicine includes a wide array of remedies for diarrhea. Boiled milk, cream, the oil from mutton suet, scorched corn or flour, burned cork, charcoal, eggs in various forms, vinegar and salt, and lemonade are all dietary recommendations that occur widely (Meyer 1985: 90–96). Among the large number of plant remedies recorded, burdock, mullein, blackberry, raspberry, cranesbill, shepherd's purse, bistort, elder, and tormentil are all used in North American as well as British folk medicine. Mullein, with its large, velvety leaves, has been named "Adam's Flannel" or "Beggar's Flannel," and the leaves have been used in lieu of toilet paper; the central leaves, steeped in milk, were given to children with diarrhea or dysentery (Meyer 1985: 91, 194). Many other plants native to North America and not to Britain have been used in North American folk medicine to treat diarrhea. Among them are sassafras, white pine bark (*Pinus* sp.), Canada fleabane *(Conyza canadensis),* spotted spurge (*Euphorbia* sp.), boneset (*Eupatorium* spp.), sweetfern *(Comptonia peregrina),* black birch *(Betula nigra),* dewberry (*Rubus* spp.), slippery elm *(Ulmus rubra),* alum root (*Heuchera* spp.), black cohosh, and sumac (*Rhus* spp.) (Meyer 1985: 90–99). *Spiraea tomentosa* leaves and flowers were commonly used in colonial New England (Meyer 1985: 93). Josselyn recorded the use of water lily roots, and of powdered aloes (*Aloe* sp.) in apple pulp (Josselyn 1833: 264, 333). A broth prepared from dethorned prickly pear has been recommended (UCLA Folklore Archives 20_5359), or an infusion of rose leaves (Hendricks 1980: 82), or eating the inside of an acorn (as recorded in Britain too, see above) (UCLA Folklore Archives 9_5358). Smartweed tea (*Polygonum* spp.) has been drunk for diarrhea (Wilson 1968: 72).

Many of these plant remedies have been used in the Native American tradition. Thus sassafras (*Sassafras albidum*) was used by the Cherokee to treat diarrhea (Hamel and Chiltoskey 1975: 54); Canadian fleabane (*Conyza canadensis*) was used by the Blackfoot in the Dakotas (Johnston 1987: 56) and the Cree, who lived along Hudson Bay (Holmes 1884: 303). Smartweed (*Polygonum hydropiper*) is given by the Cherokee (Hamel and Chiltoskey 1975: 55) to children with diarrhea. Mullein was used by the Iroquois for diarrhea (Herrick 1977: 431). The list could be continued. (For other plants used by the Native Americans in treatment of diarrhea, see Moerman 1998: 770–771).

Finally, if all this plethora of remedies fail, the Yuma suggest that singing may stop diarrhea! (Harrington 1908: 335).

*See also* **Amulet, Apple, Beans, Birch, Black cohosh, Boneset, Elm, Mullein, Plantain, Sassafras.**

### References

Akana, Akaiko. *Hawaiian Herbs of Medicinal Value.* Honolulu: Pacific Book House. 1922.

Allen, David E., and Gabrielle Hatfield. *Medicinal Plants in Folk Tradition.* Portland, OR: Timber Press (in press).

Beith, Mary. *Healing Threads: Traditional Medicines of the Highlands and Islands.* Edinburgh: Polygon, 1995.

Collyns, W. "On the Economical and Medical Uses to Which Various Common Wild Plants Are Applied by the Cottagers in Devonshire." *Gardener's Magazine* 2 (1827): 160–162.

Hamel, Paul B., and Mary U. Chiltoskey. *Cherokee Plants and Their Uses: A 400 Year History.* Sylva, NC: Herald, 1975.

Harrington, John Peabody. "A Yuma Account of Origins." *Journal of American Folklore* 21 (1908): 324–348.

Hatfield, Gabrielle. *Country Remedies: Traditional East Anglian Plant Remedies in the Twentieth Century.* Woodbridge: Boydell, 1994.

Hendricks, George D. *Roosters, Rhymes and Railroad Tracks: A Second Sampling of Superstitions and Popular Beliefs in Texas.* Dallas: Southern Methodist University Press, 1980.

Herrick, James William. *Iroquois Medical Botany.* Ph.D. thesis, State University of New York, Albany, 1977.

Holmes, E. M. "Medicinal Plants used by Cree Indians, Hudson's Bay Territory." *Pharmaceutical Journal and Transactions* 15 (1884).

Johnston, Alex. *Plants and the Blackfoot.* Lethbridge, ALTA: Lethbridge Historical Society, 1987.

Josselyn, John. *An Account of Two Voyages to New England Made during the Years 1638, 1662, 1674.* Reprint 1833.

Meyer, Clarence. *American Folk Medicine.* Glenwood, IL: Meyerbooks, 1985.

Moerman, Daniel E. *Native American Ethnobotany.* Portland, OR: Timber Press, 1998.

Prince, Dennis. *Grandmother's Cures: An A-Z of Herbal Remedies.* London: Fontana, 1991.

Taylor, Mark R. Manuscript notes in Norfolk Record Office, Norwich. MS4322.

Vesey-Fitzgerald, B. "Gypsy Medicine." *Journal of the Gypsy Lore Society* 23 (1944).

Vickery, Roy. *A Dictionary of Plant Lore.* Oxford: Oxford University Press, 1995.

Wilson, Gordon, Sr. *Folklore of the Mammoth Cave Region.* Bowling Green, KY: Kentucky Folklore Series 4. 1968.

# Dizziness

In British folk medicine there is a small number of remedies for dizziness. One is to drink the blood of a black cat mixed with wine (Souter 1995: 153). "Cupping" with a cow or sheep's horn was practiced in the Scottish Highlands for dizziness (Beith 1995: 163–164). Also in Scotland, kelp soup (made from seaweed) was thought to help (Souter 1995: 153). In some parts of Ireland, hemlock was used as a cure for giddiness (Barbour 1897). A more harmless-sounding remedy was to snuff up dew through the nostrils (Radford and Radford 1974: 133).

In North American folk medicine, carrying salt in the pocket was recommended for dizziness (Brown 1952–1964, 6: 171). Feverfew *(Tanacetum parthenium)* was recommended by the Shakers, as it was also by official herbalists and doctors on both sides of the Atlantic from the sixteenth century onward (Crellin and Philpott 1990: 209–210). A tea made from mistletoe has been used (Wilson 1968: 323), as has an infusion of goldenrod (*Solidago* sp.) (UCLA Folklore Archives 10_5361). Taking the waters at Schooley's Mountain was recommended for dizziness, among other ailments. A louse hidden in the sufferer's bread was a suggested cure in Indiana (Knortz 1913: 127). The brain of a mountain goat was another possibility (Saul 1949: 75). Among the Native Americans, tansy *(Tanacetum vulgare)*, a plant related to the feverfew mentioned above, was used by the Cheyenne (Grinnell 1972: 190). A mixture of charcoal and bear gall worked into the skin was another Native American remedy (Mahr 1951: 348). A cure among the Papago was to sing the Owl Song (Wilson 1950: 339).

*See also* **Dew, Hemlock, Mistletoe, Shakers, Water.**

### References

Barbour, John H. "Some Country Remedies and Their Uses." *Folk-Lore* 8 (1897): 386–390.

Beith, Mary. *Healing Threads: Traditional Medicines of the Highlands and Islands.* Edinburgh: Polygon, 1995.

Brown, Frank C. *Collection of North Carolina Folklore.* 7 vols. Durham, NC: Duke University Press, 1952–1964.

Crellin, John K., and Jane Philpott. *A Reference Guide to Medicinal Plants.* Durham, NC: Duke University Press, 1990.

Grinnell, George Bird. *The Cheyenne Indians: Their History and Ways of Life.* Vol. 2. Lincoln: University of Nebraska Press, 1972.

Knortz, Karl. *Amerikanischer Aberglaube der Gegenwart: Ein Beitrag zur Volkskunde.* Leipzig: T. Gerstenberg, 1913.

Mahr, August C. "Materia Medica and Therapy among the North American Forest Indians." *Ohio State Archaeological and Historical Quarterly* 60 (October 1951): 331–354.

Radford, E., and M. A. Radford. *Encyclopaedia of Superstitions.* Edited and revised by Christina Hole. London: Book Club Associates, 1974.

Saul, F. William. *Pink Pills for Pale People.* Philadelphia: Dorrance, 1949.

Souter, Keith. *Cure Craft: Traditional Folk Remedies and Treatment from Antiquity to the Present Day.* Saffron Walden: C. W. Daniel, 1995.

Wilson, Eddie W. "The Owl and the American Indian." *Journal of American Folklore* 63 (1950): 336–344.

Wilson, Gordon. "Local Plants in Folk Remedies in the Mammoth Cave Region." *Southern Folklore Quarterly* 32 (1968): 320–327.

# Dock (*Rumex* spp.)

Rubbing dock leaves on to nettle stings is probably the most commonly known country remedy in Britain today, but even this is the vestige of very much wider uses of the plant. Until the recent past, dock leaves were eaten as a vegetable in both Scotland and England; they were tied onto cuts and grazes to stop the bleeding (Hatfield 1994: 32; Vickery 1995: 108), and they were used to treat sunburn (Vickery 1994: 108), chapped skin (Hatfield 1994: 48), and rheumatism (Vickery 1994: 108). The roots of various species of dock were boiled and the decoction drunk to clear boils (Hatfield 1994: 22) and to treat skin rashes (Hatfield 1994: 50). Dock has even been used in folk medicine in the treatment of cancer (Taylor MSS). The root of Yellow Dock *(Rumex crispus)* was used to treat indigestion (Souter 1995: 169). In Scotland, dock has been used for treating scurvy and for cleaning teeth; the roots were made into poultices for treating nettle and bee stings and other inflammations (Beith 1995: 214). In County Donegal, Ireland, it was said that a bag of dock seeds worn under the left oxter prevents barrenness in women (St. Clair 1971: 58). Other species of Rumex, such as garden sorrel *(Rumex acetosa)* and sheep's sorrel *(Rumex acetosella),* were used both in folk medicine and official herbalism in Britain as salad herbs, for treating skin complaints, and as a cooling drink for fevers.

Docks have not been as important in North American folk medicine. Yellow dock is not native to North America but has been introduced. In eighteenth-century New Jersey it was eaten as a vegetable, while in twentieth-century Maine it was a constituent of a spring tonic (Coffey 1993: 60). Meyer reports the use of mashed leaves of yellow dock in treating burns (Meyer 1985: 54). Sorrel is native to North America and, as in Britain, was used to treat fevers (Meyer 1985: 138). In the Mexican tradition, the roots of various species of dock were used to treat coughs, colds, and sore throat (Kay 1996: 239).

Native Americans used various species of docks for a very wide range of conditions (Moerman 1998: 495–499). The root of the yellow dock *(Rumex crispus)* was used to treat liver disorders, as well as diarrhea (Willard 1992: 77). The Iroquois regarded it as a panacea (Herrick 1977: 311). Swellings were treated by the Blackfoot with willow-leaved dock *(Rumex salicifolius)* (McClintock 1909: 274). *Rumex obtusifolius* was used for many skin conditions (Densmore 1928: 350) and as a tonic (Her-

rick 1977: 313), uses similar to those in general folk medical use in North America. Several species of dock were used for treating rheumatism. Water dock *(Rumex orbiculatus)* treated foul ulcers, while the winged dock *(Rumex venosus)* was known by the Shoshone in Nevada as "burn medicine." The roots were used, mashed as a poultice, or dried and powdered. (Coffey 1993: 62, 63).

*See also* **Boils, Burns, Cancer, Chapped skin, Colds, Coughs, Cuts, Indigestion, Insect bites and stings, Poultice, Rheumatism, Scurvy, Sore throat, Sunburn, Tonic.**

## References

Beith, Mary. *Healing Threads: Traditional Medicines of the Highlands and Islands.* Edinburgh: Polygon, 1995.

Coffey, Timothy. *The History and Folklore of North American Wildflowers.* New York: Facts On File, 1993.

Densmore, Frances. "Uses of Plants by the Chippewa Indians." Smithsonian Institution—*Bureau of American Ethnology Annual Report* 44 (1928): 273–379.

Hatfield, Gabrielle. *Country Remedies: Traditional East Anglian Plant Remedies in the Twentieth Century.* Woodbridge: Boydell, 1994.

Herrick, James William. *Iroquois Medical Botany.* Ph.D. thesis, State University of New York, Albany, 1977.

Kay, Margarita Artschwager. *Healing with Plants in the American and Mexican West.* Tucson: University of Arizona Press, 1996.

McClintock, Walter. "Materia Medica of the Blackfeet." *Zeitschrift für Ethnologie* 11 (1909): 273–276.

Meyer, Clarence. *American Folk Medicine.* Glenwood, IL: Meyerbooks, 1985.

Moerman, Daniel E. *Native American Ethnobotany.* Portland, OR: Timber Press, 1998.

Souter, Keith. *Cure Craft: Traditional Folk Remedies and Treatment from Antiquity to the Present Day.* Saffron Walden: C. W. Daniel, 1995.

St. Clair, Sheila. *Folklore of the Ulster People*. Cork: Mercier Press, 1971.

Taylor MSS. Manuscript notes of Mark R. Taylor in the Norfolk Records Office, Norwich. MS 4322.

Vickery, Roy. *A Dictionary of Plant Lore*. Oxford: Oxford University Press, 1995.

Willard, Terry. *Edible and Medicinal Plants of the Rocky Mountains and Neighbouring Territories*. Calgary: Wild Rose College of Natural Healing, 1992.

# Doctrine of signatures

The "doctrine of signatures" states that the healing properties of a plant are indicated by features of its appearance resembling the ailment to be treated. Yellow-flowered plants will be good for curing jaundice, simply because their flowers are yellow. Although frequently cited as a dogma of folk medicine, the doctrine was in fact formulated by the fifteenth-century physician Philippus Theophrastus Bombastus von Hohenheim (1493–1541), who came to be known as Paracelsus (Griggs 1981: 43–53). Subsequent herbalists elaborated on the theme, and many, such as Culpeper, made it a central tenet of their materia medica. Robert Turner, writing in the seventeenth century, stated, "God hath imprinted upon the Plants, Herbs, and Flowers, as it were in Hieroglyphicks, the very signature of their Vertues" (Arber 1953: 254).

It is plausible to suggest that the doctrine was in fact a misinterpretation of what was originally a practical system of mnemonics. Folk medicine depends on oral transmission almost entirely. It is easier to remember which plant was used for which ailment if a salient feature of the plant can be used as a reminder. Thus the pile-like swellings on the tuber of the lesser celandine (*Ranunculus ficaria*) could remind the collector that this was a treatment for hemorrhoids. The "doctrine," however, was developed to an extreme extent by some writers, such as the seventeenth-century Richard Sanders (Hatfield 1999: 141). It blended into imitative magic and the principle of like curing like. Imitative magic was and is widespread, in both folk and official medicine, and can be found in cultures as widely separated as the fenmen of East Anglia (Porter 1974: 47–48) and the Seminole Indians of Florida (Snow and Stans 2001). Examples are the use of bloodstone or of red thread to cure nosebleed, and of bryony root resembling the human form as an aphrodisiac; among the Seminole Indians, a forked tree branch of the relevant plant is favored for treating women's problems (Snow and Stans 2001: 39).

*See also* **Bryony, Nosebleed.**

## References

Arber, Agnes. *Herbals: Their Origin and Evolution*. 2nd ed. Cambridge: Cambridge University Press, 1953.

Griggs, Barbara. *Green Pharmacy: A History of Herbal Medicine*. London: Jill Norman and Hobhouse, 1981.

Hatfield, Gabrielle. *Memory, Wisdom and Healing: The History of Domestic Plant Medicine*. Phoenix Mill: Sutton, 1999.

Porter, Enid. *The Folklore of East Anglia*. London: Batsford, 1974.

Snow, Alice Micco, and Susan Enns Stans. *Healing Plants. Medicine of the Florida Seminole Indians*. Gainesville: University Press of Florida, 2001.

# Dog

Dog saliva has widely been regarded as curative, a belief that to modern ears sounds unhygienic. There is a famous sixteenth-century story of a great Italian mathematician whose life was saved by having a fearful facial wound licked by his pet dog (Root-Bernstein and Root-Bernstein 2000: 110). In the Scottish Highlands, dog lick was recommended for healing running sores (Gregor 1881: 127). A more recent instance is cited in the British medical journal *Lancet* in 1970 (Verrier 1970: 615). Recent chemical analysis has shown saliva to contain a wide range of antimicrobial substances, which may account for the apparent success of dog lick as a treatment for wounds (Root-Bernstein and Root-Bernstein 2000: 110–118). Dog saliva has been shown to be much richer than human in so-called transforming growth factors, which could speed healing (Allen 1995: 58). Obviously pathogens too can be introduced into wounds in this way, and it is not a method that can be recommended today. In folk medicine, dogs were sometimes used as victims of transference. An eighteenth-century cure for gout recommends laying a dog on the patient's feet, so that the pain will pass from human to dog (Clerk of Penicuik papers 1740–1751). In both Scotland and England, whooping cough was "transferred" to a dog by feeding it some of the child's hair in bread and butter; in Ireland, ague was cured by making a barley cake with the sufferer's urine, which was then fed to a dog (Black 1883: 35). In other instances, a dog has been a sacrificial victim, as in a cure for convulsions that involved eating the heart of a white hound baked with meal (Black 1883: 117), and in a fever remedy of carrying the right foot of a black dog (Black 1883: 148). In the seventeenth century, dog bones were hung around the neck as amulets for moles (Wright 1912: 231). A piece of a dog's tongue hung around the neck was used in Yorkshire as an amulet to cure scrofula, and the fat of dogs was used in a rheumatism cure in Ireland (Barbour 1897: 387).

In North American folk medicine many similar beliefs and practices concerning dogs have been recorded. Dog lick has been credited with healing wounds (Musick 1964: 51), sores (Thomas and Thomas 1920: 115), and snake bites (Brown 1952–1964, 6: 279). Sleeping with a dog has been widely recommended for rheumatism

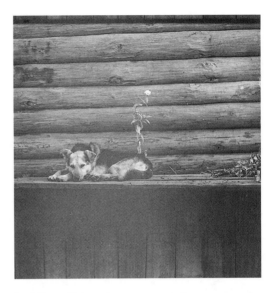

In folk medicine, dogs were sometimes used as victims of transference, and in North America, sleeping with a dog has been widely recommended for rheumatism. Dog saliva (dog lick) has been credited with healing wounds, sores, and snake bites. (Library of Congress)

(Brown 1952–1964, 6: 255). Other diseases have been "transferred" to dogs too. Asthma has been "cured" by sleeping with a Chihuahua (Anderson 1968: 194). For warts, applying butter and allowing a dog to lick it off (Hyatt 1965: 306) has been suggested. Fevers have been "transferred" to dogs by feeding them beef cooked in the patient's urine (Brendle and Unger 1935: 93). Thrush has been treated by rubbing a child's mouth with a piece of meat and feeding the meat to a dog (Browne 1958: 27). Various medicines have been prepared from dogs. As in Ireland, dog grease has been valued for rheumatism (Brown 1952–1964, 6: 256). Sometimes a black dog is specified. Alternatively, the disemboweled carcass of a dog has been used to poultice a sore limb (Grumbine 1905–1906: 278). For tuberculosis, soup made from a black dog (UCLA Folklore Archives 5_5517) or eating the hind leg of a dog (Thomas and Thomas 1920: 100) are suggested. Dog lard has been used to treat bruises (Puckett 1981: 332). The blood of a black dog has been considered a cure for smallpox (Randolph 1933: 4). Dog excrement has been used in a number of folk treatments: for diphtheria (UCLA Folklore Archives 10_6261), sore throat (Saxon 1945: 532), hives, colic, and bedwetting (Hyatt 1965: 246, 267, 289).

Dogs were used in the Native American tradition too. Burns and scalds were treated with dog excrement by the Opata (Vogel 1970: 214). Native Americans of British Columbia fed a child's shed tooth to a dog, presumably to ensure the child would have strong teeth like a dog (Radbill 1964: 138).

*See also* **Amulet; Asthma; Bed-wetting; Bruises; Colic; Color; Epilepsy; Excreta; Fevers; Hives; Mad dog, bite of; Rheumatism; Smallpox; Sore throat; Transference; Tuberculosis; Warts; Whooping cough.**

## References

Allen, Andrew. *A Dictionary of Sussex Folk Medicine.* Newbury: Countryside Books, 1995.

Anderson, John Q. "Magical Transference of Disease in Texas Folk Medicine." *Western Folklore* 27 (1968): 191–199.

Barbour, John H. "Some Country Remedies and Their Uses." *Folk-Lore* 8 (1897): 386–390.

Black, William George. *Folk-Medicine: A Chapter in the History of Culture.* London: Folklore Society, 1883.

Brendle, Thomas R., and Claude W. Unger. "Folk Medicine of the Pennsylvania Germans: The Non-Occult Cures." *Proceedings of the Pennsylvania German Society* 45 (1935).

Brown, Frank C. *Collection of North Carolina Folklore.* 7 vols. Durham, NC: Duke University Press, 1952–1964.

Browne, Ray B. *Popular Beliefs and Practices from Alabama.* Folklore Studies 9. Berkeley and Los Angeles: University of California Publications, 1958.

Clerk of Penicuik, Sir John. Manuscript papers in the Scottish Record Office, Edinburgh. SRO 18/2142.

Gregor, Walter. *Notes on the Folk-lore of the North-East of Scotland.* London: Folk-lore Society, 1881.

Grumbine, E. "Folklore and Superstitious Beliefs of Lebanon County." *Papers and Addresses of the Lebanon County Historical Society* 3 (1905–1906): 252–294.

Hyatt, Harry Middleton. *Folklore from Adams County Illinois.* 2nd rev. ed. New York: Memoirs of the Alma Egan Hyatt Foundation, 1965.

Musick, Ruth Ann (ed.). Superstitions. *West Virginia Folklore* 14 (1964): 38–52.

Puckett, Newbell Niles. *Popular Beliefs and Superstitions: A Compendium of American Folklore from the Ohio Collection of Newbell Niles Puckett.* Edited by Wayland D. Hand, Anna Casetta, and Sondra B. Thiederman. 3 vols. Boston: G. K. Hall, 1981.

Radbill, Samuel X. "The Folklore of Teething." *Keystone Folklore Quarterly* 9 (1964): 123–143.

Randolph, Vance. "Ozark Superstitions." *Journal of American Folklore* 46 (1933): 1–21.

Root-Bernstein, Robert, and Michèle Root-Bernstein. *Honey, Mud, Maggots and other Medical Marvels: The Science behind Folk Remedies and Old Wives' Tales.* London: Pan Books, 2000.

Saxon, Lyle. *Gumbo Ya-Ya.* Boston: Houghton Mifflin, 1945.

Thomas, Daniel Lindsay, and Lucy Blayney Thomas. *Kentucky Superstitions.* Princeton, NJ: Princeton University Press, 1920.

Verrier, L. "Dog Licks Man." *Lancet* (1970): Part I: 615.

Vogel, Virgil J. *American Indian Medicine.* Norman: University of Oklahoma Press, 1970.

Wright, A. R. "Seventeenth Century Cures and Charms." *Folk-Lore* 23 (1912): 230–236, 490–497.

# Dropsy

Among the plants used in British folk medicine to treat dropsy, foxglove is probably the most famous, since observations of its use by Withering in the eighteenth century led to his development of foxglove for treating heart conditions, and eventually to the development of the drug digoxin. Other plants use include broom (*Cytisus scoparius),* used, for example, in the Scottish Highlands (Beith 1995: 209), and butcher's broom *(Ruscus aculeatus),* used in Ireland (Vickery 1995: 54). Dandelion made into tea or wine was used in Norfolk to treat dropsy (Taylor MSS), and bogbean was widely used throughout Britain, as was juniper *(Juniperus communis)* (Allen and Hatfield, in press). Elder, among its many uses, was recommended for dropsy (Porter 1969: 80). Wild carrot *(Daucus carota)* has also been used (Allen and Hatfield, in press). In Ireland an infusion of nettles, especially those growing in a churchyard, was recommended for dropsy (Wilde 1919: 201). Wearing an iron ring was supposed to prevent dropsy (Black 1883: 174). In Scotland, the same cure recorded for jaundice of drinking urine passed during fasting was used to treat dropsy (Souter 1995: 75).

Some of these same remedies are to be found in North American folk medicine. Drinking one's fasting urine was recommended among the Pennsylvania Germans (Brendle and Unger 1935: 191). Wearing a brass ring was thought to prevent dropsy, and whipping the body was thought to help (Brown 1952–1964, 6: 172, 173). A preparation of dandelion root has been used to treat dropsy (Harris 1968: 99), as has one of elder root or bark (Brown 1952–1964, 6: 173). Juniper berries have been used in a mixture to treat dropsy (Brown 1952–1964, 6: 172). A large number of other plants have also been used, most of them not native to Britain. They include sourwood *(Oxydendrum arboreum),* ragweed (*Ambrosia* sp.), and mullein (Brown 1952–1964, 6: 173). A bath of hemlock infusion was another recommendation (Lick and Brendle 1922: 281). An infusion of bulrush (*Scirpus* sp.) or of watermelon seed *(Citrullus lanatus)* has also been used (Parler 1962, 3: 602, 603), or a preparation of skunk cabbage *(Symplocarpus foetidus)* (Lick and

Brendle 1922: 54) or of black snakeroot (*Sanicula* sp.) (Pickard and Buley 1945: 44).

Interestingly, most of the plants listed above were used by Native Americans in treating heart disease, which is, of course, the main cause of dropsy (Moerman 1998: 801–802).

*See also* **Bogbean, Dandelion, Elder, Heart trouble, Hemlock, Jaundice, Mullein, Stinging nettle, Urine.**

## References

Allen, David E., and Gabrielle Hatfield. *Medicinal Plants in Folk Tradition.* Portland, OR: Timber Press, in press.

Beith, Mary. *Healing Threads: Traditional Medicines of the Highlands and Islands.* Edinburgh: Polygon, 1995.

Black, William George. *Folk-Medicine: A Chapter in the History of Culture.* Folklore Society, London, 1883.

Brendle, Thomas R., and Claude W. Unger. "Folk Medicine of the Pennsylvania Germans: The Non-Occult Cures." *Proceedings of the Pennsylvania German Society* 45 (1935).

Brown, Frank C. *Collection of North Carolina Folklore.* 7 vols. Durham, NC: Duke University Press, 1952–1964.

Harris, Bernice Kelly (ed.). *Southern Home Remedies.* Murfreesboro, NC: Johnson, 1968.

Lick, David E., and Thomas R. Brendle. "Plant Names and Plant Lore among the Pennsylvania Germans." *Proceedings and Addresses of the Pennsylvania German Society* 33 (1922).

Moerman, Daniel E. *Native American Ethnobotany.* Portland, OR: Timber Press, 1998.

Parler, Mary Celestia, and University Student Contributors. *Folk Beliefs from Arkansas.* 15 volumes. Fayetteville: University of Arkansas, 1962.

Pickard, Madge E., and R. Carlyle Buley. *The Midwest Pioneer, His Ills, Cures and Doctors.* Crawfordsville, IN: R. E. Banta, 1945.

Porter, Enid. *Cambridgeshire Customs and Folklore.* London: Routledge, 1969.

Souter, Keith. *Cure Craft: Traditional Folk Remedies and Treatment from Antiquity to the*

*Present Day.* Saffron Walden: C. W. Daniel, 1995.

Taylor MSS. Manuscript notes of Mark R. Taylor, Norfolk Record Office, Norwich. MS4322.

Vickery, Roy. *A Dictionary of Plant Lore.* Oxford: Oxford University Press, 1995.

Wilde, Lady (Jane). *Ancient Legends, Mystic Charms and Superstitions of Ireland.* London: Chatto and Windus, 1919.

# Drunkenness

According to Pliny, the ancient Celts used betony *(Betonica officinalis)* to prevent drunkenness and to cure hangover (Beith 1995: 205). In the seventeenth century, in the Western Isles of Scotland, the dried root tubers of bitter-vetch *(Lathyrus linifolius)* were chewed to prevent drunkenness (Henderson and Dickson 1994: 80). In the sixteenth and seventeenth centuries a popular cure for drunkenness was prepared in Sussex from glow-worms (Allen 1995: 80). Also in the seventeenth century, a liquid distilled from acorns was used to control drunkenness and hangover (Radford and Radford 1974: 254). Until the twentieth century, willow bark was chewed for the headache of a hangover in Lincolnshire. Alternatives were celery or the seeds of the wild poppy (Hatfield 1994: 40). Raw cabbage was chewed for a hangover (Vickery 1995: 58). An infusion of hops has been suggested too (Souter 1995: 83). A decoction for curing drunkenness was prepared from iron sulphate, magnesia, peppermint water, and nutmeg, administered on a lump of sugar (Prince 1991: 23). A drastic-sounding remedy for drunkenness was to drink beer or wine in which a frog had been drowned (Souter 1995: 131). Hangovers could be transferred to slugs or snails by rubbing them on the forehead and throwing them away (Souter 1995: 164). Placing a live eel in someone's drink was reputedly a cure for alcoholism (Radford and Radford 1974: 148). Dietary advice for a hangover includes drinking more alcohol the morning after, eating fried food, and, probably more sensibly, drinking plenty of water. Epsom salts and all kinds of proprietary preparations have also been suggested.

In North American folk medicine there are some similar suggestions for drunkenness and hangover, including, as in Britain, drinking more of the same drink the following morning—advice known as the "hair of the dog that bit you" (Hand 1970: 119). Whisky in which a toad has been soaked (Wheeler 1892–1893) or with water added in which ten tiny fish have soaked (Moya 1940: 74) has been recommended as a cure for alcoholism. Among the Ozarks it has been suggested that owl eggs cure drunkenness (Rayburn 1941: 322). Dietary advice for a hangover is abundant, ranging from greasy food to elaborate cocktails (see, for example, Paulsen 1961: 152–168). Cabbage in various forms, both raw and as juice, has been recommended for a hangover (Micheletti 1998: 183). In New England in colonial times an infusion of Indian St. John's wort was used for drunkenness (Spicer 1937: 153). Chamomile tea has been recommended for a hangover (UCLA Folklore Archives 22_6331). In Mexico, an infusion of an herb called huevo de torro (? *Ruellia* sp.) was used to treat a hangover (Hendricks 1966: 46). Willow and rattle box *(Crotalaria pallida)* are among the plants that feature in the "on the wagon" medicine used by the Seminole Indians (Snow and Stans 2001: 87). A Native American recommendation for a hangover is to wear the leaves of species of alder under one's hat (Willard 1992: 69).

*See also* **Alder, Chamomile, Hops, Poppy, St. John's wort, Snail, Transference, Willow.**

## References

Allen, Andrew. *A Dictionary of Sussex Folk Medicine.* Newbury: Countryside Books, 1995.

Beith, Mary. *Healing Threads: Traditional Medi-*

*cines of the Highlands and Islands.* Edinburgh: Polygon, 1995.

Hand, Wayland D. "North Carolina Folk Beliefs and Superstitions Collected in California." *North Carolina Folklore* 18 (1970): 117–123.

Hatfield, Gabrielle. *Country Remedies: Traditional East Anglian Plant Remedies in the Twentieth Century.* Woodbridge: Boydell, 1994.

Henderson, D. M., and J. H. Dickson. *A Naturalist in the Highlands: James Robertson, His Life and Travels in Scotland 1767–1771.* Edinburgh: Scottish Academic Press, 1994.

Hendricks, George D. *Mirrors, Mice and Mustaches: A Sampling of Superstitions and Popular Beliefs in Texas.* Austin: Texas Folklore Society, 1966.

Micheletti, Enza (ed.). *North American Folk Healing: An A-Z Guide to Traditional Remedies.* New York and Montreal: Reader's Digest Association, 1998.

Moya, Benjamin S. *Superstitions and Beliefs among the Spanish-Speaking People of New Mexico.* Master's thesis, University of New Mexico, 1940.

Paulsen, Frank M. "A Hair of the Dog and Some Other Hangover Cures from Popular Tradition." *Journal of American Folklore* 74 (1961): 152–168.

Prince, Dennis. *Grandmother's Cures: An A-Z of Herbal Remedies.* London: Fontana, 1991.

Radford, E., and M. A. Radford. *Encyclopaedia of Superstitions.* Edited and revised by Christina Hole. London: Book Club Associates, 1974.

Rayburn, Otto Ernest. *Ozark Country.* New York: Duell, Sloan and Pearce, 1941.

Snow, Alice Micco, and Susan Enns Stans. *Healing Plants. Medicine of the Florida Seminole Indians.* Gainesville: University Press of Florida, 2001.

Souter, Keith. *Cure Craft: Traditional Folk Remedies and Treatment from Antiquity to the Present Day.* Saffron Walden: C. W. Daniel, 1995.

Spicer, Dorothy Gladys. "Medicine and Magic in the New England Colonies." *Trained Nurse* 99 (1937): 153–156.

Vickery, Roy. *A Dictionary of Plant Lore.* Oxford: Oxford University Press, 1995.

Wheeler, Helen M. "Illinois Folk-Lore." *Folk-Lorist* 1 (1892–1893): 55–68.

Willard, Terry. *Edible and Medicinal Plants of the Rocky Mountains and Neighbouring Territories.* Calgary, ALTA: Wild Rose College of Natural Healing, 1992.

# Dysentery

Amoebic dysentery, now confined to the tropics, was once prevalent in Britain too. In the seventeenth century the botanist John Ray reported the use in Wales of a dysentery treatment made from moonwort *(Botrychium lunaria)* (Ray 1670: 199). In the same century one of the St. John's wort species *(Hypericum elodes)* was used in Ireland for treating dysentery; its Gaelic name translates as "dysentery herb" (Lankester 1848: 319). In the eighteenth century in Ireland, purple loosestrife *(Lythrum salicaria)* was used to treat diarrhea and dysentery (Threlkeld 1726). In more recent times in the Isle of Man, sanicle *(Sanicula europaea)* (Quayle 1973: 70), wood sage *(Teucrium scorodonia)* (Moore 1898), and mallow (Quayle 1973), have been used. Mallow was similarly used in Devon (Collyns 1827).

Dysentery was one of the diseases introduced in the sixteenth century to North and South America. It is an irony of history that one of the most valuable plant remedies for treating it, ipecacuanha *(Cephaelis ipecacuanha),* was actually imported to Europe from South American usage and became an established drug of Western practitioners.

In North American folk medicine the inner leaves of mullein were given to children with dysentery (Meyer 1985: 91). Navy beans ground into powder were also used (UCLA Folklore Archives 19_5362). A tea of broom straw *(Andropogon* sp.) and pine needles was another recommendation (UCLA Folklore Archives 7_5362). Other plants used include red oak bark, low myrtle (? *Myrica* sp.) and dewberry *(Rubus* sp.)

(Brown 1952–1964, 6: 174). Spruce bark (*Picea* sp.), elderberries, and blackberries have all been used too (Meyer 1985: 95, 96). Remedies not involving plants include eggs, chalk, vinegar mixed with salt, charcoal (Meyer 1985: 94–95), and a mixture of flour and milk (Brown 1952–1964, 6: 174).

In the Native American tradition, dysentery was treated with sassafras root (Meyer 1985: 96). The inner bark of pine was used by the Alabama for treating dysentery (Taylor 1940: 5). Steeple bush *(Spiraea tomentosa)* was used by the Mohegan (Tantaquidgeon 1928: 266).

*See also* **Blackberry, Diarrhea, Elder, Mallow, Mullein, Pine, St. John's wort, Sassafras.**

## References

Brown, Frank C. *Collection of North Carolina Folklore.* 7 vols. Durham, NC: Duke University Press, 1952–1964.

Collyns, W. "On the Economical and Medical Uses to Which Various Common Wild Plants Are Applied by the Cottagers in Devonshire." *Gardener's Magazine* 2 (1827): 160–62.

Lankester, Edwin (ed.). *The Correspondence of John Ray.* London: Ray Society, 1848.

Meyer, Clarence. *American Folk Medicine.* Glenwood, IL: Meyerbooks, 1985.

Moore, A. W. "Folk-Medicine in the Isle of Man." *Yn Lioar Manninagh* 3 (1898): 303–314.

Quayle, George E. *Legends of a Lifetime: Manx Folklore.* Douglas: Courier Herald, 1973.

Ray, John. *Catalogus Plantarum Angliae, et Insularum Adjacentium.* London: John Martyn, 1670.

Tantaquidgeon, Gladys. "Mohegan Medicinal Practices, Weather-Lore and Superstitions." *Smithsonian Institution-Bureau of American Ethnology Annual Report* 42 (1928): 264–270.

Taylor, Linda Averill. *Plants Used as Curatives by Certain Southeastern Tribes.* Cambridge, MA: Botanical Museum of Harvard University, 1940.

Threlkeld, Caleb. *Synopsis Stirpium Hibernicarum.* Dublin: F. Davys et al., 1726.

# E

## Earache

Earache is typical of an ailment where, until the recent past, domestic medicine would be used initially. A vast number of folk medical treatments have been used on both sides of the Atlantic. In Britain, onion has probably been the most frequently used remedy. In the commonest form of the remedy, a small roast onion is inserted into the ear. Sometimes a poultice of cooked onions is applied (see, for example, Vickery 1995: 265, 266). Other plant remedies include the juice of houseleek *(Sempervivum tectorum)*, or of stinging nettle *(Urtica dioica)* dripped into the ear (Hatfield MSS). A Norfolk country remedy was to take an infusion of the wild poppy *(Papaver rhoeas)*; the urban equivalent of this remedy, recorded from Essex, was to buy a poppy seed head (presumably an opium poppy, *Papaver somniferum*) from the chemist and bind it round the ear (Hatfield 1994: 37). In both England (Black 1883: 158) and Ireland (Logan 1972: 34), froth from a pricked snail dropped into the ear was used for earache. Ash sap was also used to treat earache (Vickery 1995: 20). In the Highlands of Scotland, a drop of cave water from a particular cave on the Black Isle had the reputation of curing earache (Beith 1995: 132). Less exotic measures, such as applying a hot water bottle, still help today. Variants on this were to apply a poultice of hot salt or a mustard leaf behind the ear (Prince 1991: 22). An interesting example of transference is given by Souter. Here the sufferer removed wax from the aching ear, rubbed it on some bread, and threw the bread for the birds. The birds would take the pain away with them (Souter 1995: 154).

In North America, folk remedies for earache have been even more diverse. In the Mexican West, a variety of plants have been used to treat earache, of which the juice of Rue *(Ruta graveolens)* is the most commonly used (Kay 1996: 61). In the Appalachians a great variety of plants have been used traditionally to treat earache. They include chinaberry juice *(Melia azedarach)*, oil warmed with peach pits *(Prunus persica)*, persimmon *(Diospyros virginiana)*, prickly ash *(Xanthoxylum americanum)*, and yucca *(Yucca filamentosa)*. A drop of molasses or the smoke from tobacco have also been reported (Crellin and Philpott 1990: 159, 324, 336, 354, 406, 430, 467). Intriguingly, Meyer reports the juice from a green ash stick *(Fraxinus* sp.), dripped into the ear for earache (Meyer 1985: 101), just as in Britain. Persimmon juice has been used similarly, and the method of obtaining the juice is the same as for ash: one end of a persimmon stick is heated in a fire, and the juice that drips from the other end is collected (Parler 1962, 6: 610). As in Britain, roast onion and roast garlic appear frequently among folk treatments for earache

(Meyer 1985: 100, 101). Alternative treatments include lemon juice *(Citrus limon),* or even of the juice of roast mutton (Meyer 1973: 101). Tobacco smoke was blown into the ears for earache (UCLA Folklore Archives 22_5368). Wild honey, warmed and put in the ear was an alternative (Browne 1958: 58). To clear wax from the ear, a wide variety of plant juices were employed, such as sowthistle *(Sonchus oleraceus),* houseleek, and, rather surprisingly, foxglove *(Digitalis purpurea)* (Meyer 1985: 103). Animal oils were used too for this purpose, including hedgehog oil, skunk oil, and eel's oil (Meyer 1985: 103). Ear wax from a healthy person has been another recommendation (Cannon 1984: 105). Human milk has been used (UCLA Folklore Archives 2_5364), as has urine from either a cow (Koch 1980: 61) or a human (Brown 1952–1964, 6: 175). A drop of blood from a Betsy bug (UCLA Folklore Archives 7_5365) or the juice of a cockroach (Brown 1952–1964, 6: 175) has been dripped into a sore ear. A preparation of worms has also been used (Bergen 1899: 73).

Numerous plants were used by Native Americans in the treatment of earache, including members of more than seventy genera (Moerman 1998: 791). Some of the remedies are similar to those already mentioned in general North American folk medicine. Ash sap, from *Fraxinus americana,* was used for treating earache by the Iroquois (Rousseau 1945: 60) and by the Algonquin (Black 1980: 218). Tobacco smoke (in this case from native species of *Nicotiana*) was blown into aching ears by the Cahuilla (Bean and Saubel 1972: 90), among others. Among the Diegueño a sprig of rue was placed in the sore ear (Hinton 1975: 218). The warmed juice of houseleek was used by the Cherokee (Hamel and Chiltoskey 1975: 42). In addition, there were a large number of other plants used. The Native Americans of Appalachia used oil of mullein flowers to treat earache, while those of Nevada used the root pulp of false Solomon's seal (*Smilacina* spp.) (Willard 1992: 54, 186).

*See also* **Ash, Houseleek, Mullein, Poultice, Snail, Transference.**

### References

Bean, Lowell John, and Katherine Siva Saubel. *Temalpakh (From the Earth): Cahilla Indian Knowledge and Usage of Plants.* Banning, CA: Malki Museum Press, 1972.

Beith, Mary. *Healing Threads: Traditional Medicines of the Highlands and Islands.* Edinburgh: Polygon, 1995.

Bergen, Fanny D. "Animal and Plant Lore Collected from the Oral Tradition of English Speaking Folk." *Memoirs of the American Folk-Lore Society* 7 (1899).

Black, Meredith Jean. *Algonquin Ethnobotany: An Interpretation of Aboriginal Adaptation in South Western Quebec.* Mercury Series 65. Ottawa: National Museums of Canada, 1980.

Black, William George. *Folk-Medicine: A Chapter in the History of Culture.* London: Folklore Society, 1883.

Brown, Frank C. *Collection of North Carolina Folklore.* 7 vols. Durham, NC: Duke University Press, 1952–1964.

Browne, Ray B. *Popular Beliefs and Practices from Alabama.* Folklore Studies 9. Berkeley and Los Angeles: University of California Publications, 1958.

Cannon, Anthon S. *Popular Beliefs and Superstitions from Utah.* Edited by Wayland D. Hand and Jeannine E. Talley. Salt Lake City: University of Utah Press, 1984.

Crellin, John K., and Jane Philpott. *A Reference Guide to Medicinal Plants.* Durham, NC: Duke University Press, 1990.

Hamel, Paul B., and Mary U. Chiltoskey. *Cherokee Plants and Their Uses: A 400 Year History.* Sylva, NC: Herald, 1975.

Hatfield, Gabrielle. *Country Remedies: Traditional East Anglian Plant Remedies in the Twentieth Century.* Woodbridge: Boydell, 1994.

Hinton, Leanne. "Notes on La Huerta Diegueño Ethnobotany." *Journal of California Anthropology* 2 (1975): 214–222.

Kay, Margarita Artschwager. *Healing with Plants*

in the American and Mexican West. Tucson: University of Arizona Press, 1996.

Koch, William E. Folklore from Kansas: Beliefs and Customs. Lawrence, KS: Regent Press, 1980.

Logan, Patrick. Making the Cure: A Look at Irish Folk Medicine. Dublin: Talbot Press, 1972.

Meyer, Clarence. American Folk Medicine. Glenwood, IL: Meyerbooks, 1985.

Moerman, Daniel E. Native American Ethnobotany. Portland, OR: Timber Press, 1998.

Parler, Mary Celestia, and University Student Contributors. Folk Beliefs from Arkansas. 15 vol. Fayetteville: University of Arkansas, 1962.

Prince, Dennis. Grandmother's Cures: An A-Z of Herbal Remedies. London: Fontana, 1991.

Rousseau, Jacques. "Le Folklore Botanique de Caughnawaga." Contributions de l'Institut Botanique de l'Université de Montréal 55 (1945): 7–72.

Souter, Keith. Cure Craft: Traditional Folk Remedies and Treatment from Antiquity to the Present Day. Saffron Walden: C. W. Daniel, 1995.

Vickery, Roy. A Dictionary of Plant Lore. Oxford: Oxford University Press, 1995.

Willard, Terry. Edible and Medicinal Plants of the Rocky Mountains and Neighbouring Territories. Calgary, ALTA: Wild Rose College of Natural Healing, 1992.

# Earth

A number of folk remedies in British folk medicine involve partial or complete burial of the patient in the earth. In the eighteenth century a treatment for rheumatism was reported that involved burial up to the neck for several hours at a time. Similar treatment was advised for the victim of a lightning strike. For colic, a turf laid on the stomach was recommended (Radford and Radford 1974: 147–148). Earth from a grave was used in Shetland to treat a stitch (Radford and Radford 1974: 147), and in Sandbach to treat fits (Black 1883: 95). Some remedies involved removing a turf and laying it face downward; in Cornwall this was used to cure warts; as the grass withered, so the wart would disappear (Radford and Radford 1974: 148). Wesley suggested as a remedy for consumption that the sufferer breathe into a hole made by removing the turf (Trimmer 1965: 166). In Fifeshire a miner partially asphyxiated was laid over a shallow hole in the earth and when recovered was put to bed with the piece of turf from the hole laid on his pillow (Buchan 1994: 40). In the mid-twentieth century a practice known as "turning the sod" was still in use for treating the disease known as "foul" in cattle (Doherty 2002: 49–51). Whooping cough was sometimes treated by holding the child over a hole in the earth.

A remedy from Virginia for a bruised foot involves cutting out the turf around the foot and reversing it, grass downward. Other foot ailments such as bunions, sores, and felons (infected sores, usually under the finger nail), were treated similarly by the Pennsylvania Germans (Brendle and Unger 1935: 75). John Wesley's treatment for consumption was evidently used in North American folk medicine too (Pickard and Buley 1945: 42). For removing a foreign body from the head, the patient was placed with his head in a circular hole and the turf removed was placed on his head. Someone then sat upon the turf (Parler 1962, 6: 684).

See also **Bruises, Colic, Epilepsy, Felons, Rheumatism, Tuberculosis, Whooping cough.**

### References

Black, William George. Folk-Medicine: A Chapter in the History of Culture. London: Folklore Society, 1883.

Brendle, Thomas R., and Claude W. Unger. "Folk Medicine of the Pennsylvania Germans: The Non-Occult Cures." Proceedings of the Pennsylvania German Society 45 (1935).

Buchan, David, ed. Folk Tradition and Folk Medicine in Scotland: The Writings of David Rorie. Edinburgh: Canongate Academic, 1994.

Doherty, Michael L. "The Folklore of Cattle Diseases: A Veterinary Perspective." *Béaloideas* 70 (2002): 41–75.

Parler, Mary Celestia, and University Student Contributors. *Folk Beliefs from Arkansas.* 15 volumes. Fayetteville: University of Arkansas, 1962.

Pickard, Madge E., and R. Carlyle Buley. *The Midwest Pioneer, His Ills, Cures and Doctors.* Crawfordsville, IN: R. E. Banta, 1945.

Radford, E., and M. A. Radford. *Encyclopaedia of Superstitions.* Edited and revised by Christina Hole. London: Book Club Associates 1974.

Trimmer, Eric J. "Medical Folklore and Quackery." *Folklore* 76 (1965): 161–175.

# Echinacea

This genus, also known as coneflower, is not native to Britain and does not appear in its folk medicine, but many of the folk medicinal uses in North America have been incorporated into British medical herbalism since the eighteenth century. Currently the plant is the subject of pharmacological research worldwide, and its ability to boost the immune system is exploited in a large number of herbal preparations for coughs, colds, and other infections. It is also the subject of anti-AIDS research. Herbalists recommend it for postviral fatigue syndrome (myalgic encephalomyelitis [ME]) (Chevallier 1996: 90).

The species most widely used in herbal medicine are *Echinacea angustifolia* and *E. purpurea;* they occur throughout central North America but are now cultivated, both in North America and in Europe, for medicinal use. Today, *Echinacea* is the most widely sold herbal in both North America and Germany (Micheletti 1998: 135). In North American folk medicine, the coneflower was seen as a "blood purifier" and was recommended as a tonic, often in combination with other herbs such as burdock and yellow dock (Meyer 1985: 41). It was also recommended as both treatment for

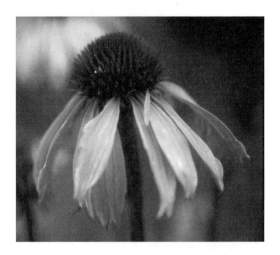

In North American folk medicine, echinacea has been used as a tonic. Native Americans used it in addition for treating pain and infections. The plant is now known to boost the immune system. (Sarah Boait)

and preventative against boils (Meyer 1985: 44).

The Native Americans used the plant in a large number of ailments. The rhizome produces a numbing sensation when chewed. As a painkiller, it has been used, for example, by the Cheyenne to treat sore throat (Grinnell 1905:188); by the Dakota to treat toothache, headache, burns and snakebite (Gilmore 1919: 131); and by the Sioux for bowel pain (Densmore 1913: 270). The related species *E. pallida* has been used by the Cheyenne as an antirheumatic and as a treatment for boils (Hart 1981: 20). Coneflower's antibacterial and antiviral properties were evidently recognized too by the Native Americans, who used the plant for tonsillitis (Kraft 1990: 47), venereal disease (Tantaquidgeon 1972: 33), smallpox, mumps, and measles (Hart 1992: 38), as well as coughs (Campbell 1951: 288) and colds (Hart 1981: 20).

*See also* **Boils, Burdock, Burns, Dock, Headache, Snake bite, Sore throat, Toothache.**

## References

Campbell, T. N. "Medicinal Plants Used by Choctaw, Chickasaw and Creek Indians in the Early Nineteenth Century." *Journal of the Washington Academy of Sciences* 41(9) (1951): 285–290.

Chevallier, Andrew. *The Encyclopedia of Medicinal Plants.* London: Dorling Kindersley, 1996.

Densmore, Frances. *Teton Sioux Music.* Smithsonian Institution-Bureau of American Ethnology Bulletin, no. 53, 1913.

Gilmore, Melvin R. *Uses of Plants by the Indians of the Missouri River Region.* Bureau of American Ethnology Annual Report 33. Washington, DC: Smithsonian Institution, 1919.

Grinnell, George Bird. "Some Cheyenne Plant Medicines." *American Anthropologist* 7 (1905): 37–43.

Hart, Jeffrey A. "The Ethnobotany of the Northern Cheyenne Indians of Montana." *Journal of Ethnopharmacology* 4 (1981): 1–55.

Hart, Jeffrey A. *Montana Native Plants and Early Peoples.* Helena: Montana Historical Society Press, 1992.

Kraft, Shelly Katherine. *Recent Changes in the Ethnobotany of Standing Rock Indian Reservation.* M.A. thesis, University of North Dakota, Grand Forks, 1990.

Meyer, Clarence. *American Folk Medicine.* Glenwood, IL: Meyerbooks, 1985.

Micheletti, Enza (ed.). *North American Folk Healing: An A-Z Guide to Traditional Remedies.* New York and Montreal: Reader's Digest Association, 1998.

Tantaquidgeon, Gladys. "Folk Medicine of the Delaware and Related Algonkian Indians." *Pennsylvania Historical Commission Anthropological Papers,* no. 3, 1972.

# Eczema

Since the term "eczema" is not always used in folk medicine, there are probably many folk records concealed under such headings as "skin complaints," "dry, itchy skin," or "tetter," a term that seems to have been used to cover a number of skin conditions, sometimes including eczema.

In British folk medicine a number of common native plants have been used over the centuries in the treatment of eczema. Different parts of the elder have been used all over Britain to treat this as well as a number of other skin conditions. In the Highlands of Scotland an ointment was made from the flowers (including particularly the pollen) of the tree, mixed with lard (Beith 1995: 215). In England also, elder has been used for treating eczema in both humans and animals (Hatfield 1995: 51). Chickweed, a widespread and common weed of cultivated land, has been used, crushed, in the form of a poultice (Prince 1991: 123). Under the local name of "markery," another weed of cultivated land, good King Henry *(Chenopodium bonus-henricus),* was used in Cambridgeshire (Porter 1974: 47). In Ireland, white dead-nettle *(Lamium album),* was made into an ointment with mutton suet and used for eczema (Logan 1972: 73). In the Scottish Highlands moistened foxglove *(Digitalis purpurea)* leaves were used (Beith 1995: 218). Another plant, not native to Britain but widely naturalized, has been used right up to the present time in eczema treatment. The juicy leaves of the houseleek have been split and bound on the affected area, or, for larger areas, a poultice has been made of the crushed leaves, mixed with single cream (Hatfield 1994: 51; Taylor MSS). Boiled ivy shoots have been recommended in Derbyshire (Vickery 1995: 203), while in Scotland a cap of ivy leaves was placed on a child's head to treat eczema (Simpkins 1914: 411). In Essex the root of the dock was boiled and mixed with lard to form an eczema ointment (Taylor MSS). In Suffolk in the twentieth century, rue—not a native plant of Britain, so presumably grown in the garden—was used. The instructions were to boil a few sprigs of rue and when cool to "bathe the inflammation of the skin and poultice with a few of the leaves on parts that burn and tingle and itch" (Taylor

MSS). Elm wood *(Ulmus procera)* tea was drunk in Hampshire to treat eczema. In Ireland, the bark of the birch was used similarly (Allen and Hatfield, in press).

Miscellaneous remedies reported from Suffolk include application of milk and the touch of a dead man's hand (Rolleston 1940: 79).

In North American folk medicine, a wide diversity of plant remedies have been used in the treatment of eczema, most of them native to North America and not to Britain. Poke root was recommended, as well as prince's pine *(Chimaphila sp.)*, sassafras and sarsaparilla, mountain grape *(Mahonia aquifolium),* Indian turnip (probably *Arisaema triphyllum*), bloodroot, tag alder *(Alnus serrulata),* and checkerberry *(Gaultheria probumbens)* (Meyer 1985: 104–107). In addition, there were some plants used that although native in Britain have not been traced there in the folk records for eczema. These include strawberry *(Fragaria vesca)* leaves, burdock, and watercress *(Rorippa nasturtium-aquaticum).* Elm, dock, and elder were used in both British and North American folk medicine for this ailment.

Corn oil was used by the settlers both internally and externally in the treatment of eczema (Micheletti 1998: 111); it is recorded as a part of Vermont folk medicine by Jarvis (Jarvis 1961: 149). An ointment made from unsalted butter or lard and the buds of the balm of Gilead is recorded from Georgia (UCLA Folklore Archives 17_5368).

Some of these folk uses can be correlated with Native American usage of the plants. A salve made from balm of Gilead *(Populus balsamifera)* was used by the Cherokee and the Potawatomi (Micheletti 1998: 44; Smith 1933: 80, 81). Prince's pine *(Chimaphila maculata)* was used by the Cherokee for "tetter and ringworm," the former perhaps a reference to eczema (Hamel and Chiltoskey 1975: 62). More definitely, the root of poke *(Phytolacca americana)* was used by the Cherokee for treating eczema (Hamel and Chiltoskey 1975: 50). In addition, the powdered root of black cohosh was used (Micheletti 1998: 97). Pine *(Pinus virginiana)* was used by the Cherokee on "scald head, tetterworm" (Hamel and Chiltoskey 1975: 49).

Apart from all these plant remedies used in the treatment of eczema, a number of common household substances have been used as well. Glycerine (UCLA Folklore Archives 11_5367) has been recommended in North American folk medicine, and castile soap, alum, vinegar, and sulphur have all been applied (Meyer 1985: 104). More poetically, May dew has been applied, a remedy of Pennsylvanian German origin (White 1897: 79). As in the treatment of both acne and freckles, the use of urine has also been suggested (UCLA Folklore Archives 6_6244).

*See also* **Acne, Alder, Balm of Gilead, Birch, Black cohosh, Bloodroot, Burdock, Chickweed, Corn, Dead man's hand, Dew, Dock, Elder, Elm, Freckles, Houseleek, Ivy, Pine, Poke, Poultice, Sarsaparilla, Sassafras, Urine.**

### References

Allen, David E., and Gabrielle Hatfield. *Medicinal Plants in Folk Tradition.* Portland, OR: Timber Press, in press.

Beith, Mary. *Healing Threads: Traditional Medicines of the Highlands and Islands.* Edinburgh: Polygon, 1995.

Hamel, Paul B., and Mary U. Chiltoskey. *Cherokee Plants and Their Uses: A 400 Year History.* Sylva, NC: Herald, 1975.

Hatfield, Gabrielle. *Country Remedies: Traditional East Anglian Plant Remedies in the Twentieth Century.* Woodbridge: Boydell, 1994.

Jarvis, D. C. *A Doctor's Guide to Good Health.* London: Pan Books, 1961.

Logan, Patrick. *Making the Cure: A Look at Irish Folk Medicine.* Dublin: Talbot Press, 1972.

Meyer, Clarence. *American Folk Medicine.* Glenwood, IL: Meyerbooks, 1985.

Micheletti, Enza (ed.). *North American Folk Healing: An A-Z Guide to Traditional Remedies.* New York and Montreal: Reader's Digest Association, 1998.

Porter, E. M. *The Folklore of East Anglia.* London: Batsford, 1974.

Prince, Dennis. *Grandmother's Cures: An A-Z of Herbal Remedies.* London: Fontana, 1991.

Rolleston, J. D. "Dermatology and Folk-Lore, Part II." *The British Journal of Dermatology and Syphilis* 52 (March 1940): 74–86.

Simpkins, John Ewart. *Examples of Printed Folklore concerning Fife, with Some Notes on Clackmannan and Kinross-shire.* London: Sidgwick and Jackson, 1914.

Smith, Huron H. "Ethnobotany of the Forest Potawatomi Indians." *Bulletin of the Public Museum of the City of Milwaukee* 7 (1933): 1–230.

Taylor MSS. Manuscript notes of Mark R. Taylor in Norfolk Records Office, Norwich. MS4322.

Vickery, Roy. *A Dictionary of Plant Lore.* Oxford: Oxford University Press, 1995.

White, Emma Gertrude. "Folk-Medicine among Pennsylvania Germans." *Journal of American Folklore* 10 (1897): 78–80.

# Eggs

Hen's eggs have been used in a number of ways in British folk medicine. In the past doubtless eggs from other birds were used too. The eggs of gannets were eaten raw for a chest infection on the island of St. Kilda (Beith 1995: 172). A whole hen's egg steeped in vinegar with honey added has been a widespread cure for a cough (Prince 1991: 115). Hard-boiled eggs have been recommended as a treatment for diarrhea, a remedy still in use (Jones 1980: 62). Egg white has been used as a dressing for fractures. In Ireland, it was believed to improve the complexion (Sharkey 1985: 88). Egg shells ground up in milk or water were given in Lincolnshire to children to cure them of bedwetting (Radford and Radford 1974: 151). The membrane of an egg has been used as a natural plaster for a cut or

wound; this is another remedy still in use within living memory (Hatfield MSS). The water in which eggs have been cooked has been credited both with causing and curing warts.

In North American folk medicine a similar array of remedies have been used involving eggs. Egg white beaten with lemon and sugar has been used as a cough cure (Brown 1952–1964, 6: 219). A sore mouth has been treated with a mixture of egg, honey, and alum (Brown 1952–1964, 6: 234–235). Egg white has been applied to a sty on the eye (Brown 1952–1964, 6: 294). Eating eggs has been recommended for "phthisic" (tuberculosis) (Brown 1952–1964, 6: 248). The egg membrane, or the egg white raw with honey, or an egg hard-boiled, has been used to "draw" a boil (Brown 1952–1964, 6: 130). An egg laid on Good Friday was believed to be a cure for colic (Brown 1952–1964, 6: 156). As in Britain, eggs have been used to treat warts and have also been claimed to cause them (Brown 1952–1964, 6: 309).

*See also* **Bed-wetting, Boils, Colic, Coughs, Diarrhea, Fractures, Tuberculosis, Warts.**

**References**
Beith, Mary. *Healing Threads: Traditional Medicines of the Highlands and Islands.* Edinburgh: Polygon, 1995.

Brown, Frank C. *Collection of North Carolina Folklore.* 7 vols. Durham, NC: Duke University Press, 1952–1964.

Jones, Anne E. "Folk Medicine in Living Memory in Wales." *Folk Life* 18 (1980): 58–68.

Prince, Dennis. *Grandmother's Cures: An A-Z of Herbal Remedies.* London: Fontana, 1991.

Radford, E., and M. A. Radford. *Encyclopaedia of Superstitions.* Edited and revised by Christina Hole. London: Book Club Associates, 1974.

Sharkey, Olive. *Old Days, Old Ways: An Illustrated Folk History of Ireland.* Dublin: O'Brien Press, 1985.

# Elder

Every part of the elder tree has been used in British folk medicine. The tree's semimagical status in folklore, including the superstition that one must never cut down an elder tree (without first asking the druids)—or that burning green elder branches can cause rheumatism (Hatfield 1999: 76)—may reflect simply the great usefulness of this tree in medicine in the past, which would lead to its protection. In Ireland the tree was so highly valued medicinally that even the clay from around the roots was said to cure toothache (Sharkey 1985: 145). The root has been boiled and used to treat rheumatism in Ireland (Vickery 1995: 124). The bark has been used to treat rheumatism, and in powdered form as a laxative in Scotland (Beith 1995: 215) and in Devon (Lafont 1984: 35). The crushed leaves have been used to treat insect bites and stings, or warmed and laid on the forehead for a headache (Quelch 1941: 80).

In Devon they have been chewed for toothache, and bandaged on leg sores (Lafont 1984: 35). They have been made into an all-purpose ointment, used especially for treating eczema, and for healing stubborn cuts (Hatfield MS). Even the buds were used in domestic medicine; they were candied and given to children as a gentle laxative (Quelch 1941: 80). The flowers in infusion have treated fevers, and been used as a cosmetic, as well as to remove sunburn (Hatfield MS). In Northumberland, the skin was rubbed with an elder flower preparation to keep midges away (Vickery 1995: 122), a use reminiscent of the well-known practice of tying elder branches to the horse's harness to keep flies away (Vickery 1995: 122). In Scotland the flowers were boiled with birch bark to make a tonic (Beith 1995: 214). In Ireland, an ointment was made from the flowers, with particular care to gather the pollen too. This ointment was used for eczema, chapped skin, and nettle stings (Beith 1995: 214). Particularly in Ireland, burns and scalds were treated with elder ointment (Allen and Hatfield, in press). In Gloucestershire a similar ointment was made and used for aches, sprains, and whitlows (Vickery 1995: 124). In Worcestershire, hot elderflower tea was used to treat fevers and even pneumonia (Vickery 1995: 125). The berries, made into wine, produce a drink for pleasure and for the treatment of sore throat, colds, and flu, as well as for bronchitis and asthma. An amulet for epilepsy was to wear nine pieces of elder cut from between two knots (Black 1883: 120). The pith of elder wood has been used in Gloucestershire to treat ringworm (Hartland 1895: 54).

Even the plants that grow in the shade of an elder tree are believed to take on something of its powers. The Gaelic name for figwort (*Scrophularia nodosa),* a plant revered in folk medicine, translates as "under elder" (Allen and Hatfield, in press). The fungi that grow on elder have been used in folk medicine too—for example, the fungus from elder bark was used in the Scottish Highlands for treating sore throat (Beith 1995: 215). Warts have been treated by cutting notches into an elder tree equal in number to the warts; or by rubbing the warts with a green elder stick and burying the stick. The latter remedy was recorded in the seventeenth century by Francis Bacon (Bacon 1631: 258), and recorded again in the mid-twentieth century, in use by a schoolchild (Opie 1959: 315). A spring rising from the ground under an elder tree yielded water believed to cure sore eyes (Quelch 1941: 79).

In North America, the native elder species is *Sambucus canadensis,* but the European species has been naturalized in North America since the seventeenth century and has been used by North American Indians, by Shakers, and by Appalachian healers. Many of the same uses have been recorded for Britain and North America. Folk medical records do not always distinguish between the native *S. canadensis* and the introduced *S. nigra* (Crellin and Philpott 1998: 200). Meyer records the use of elder leaves for asthma and boils, and of the bark for liver complaints and eczema (Meyer 1985: 31, 37, 43, 106). The flowers simmered in lard made a salve for sore breasts, and with the inner bark were used to treat burns. The flowers were also used for colds and flu and for constipation in children (Meyer 1985: 55, 66, 75). The berries were simmered in brandy for dysentery, the leaves laid over the eyes to clear the eyes and brow (Meyer 1985: 96, 106, 110). The inner bark was simmered in hen's oil for frostbite and mixed with cream and chamomile for treating piles (Meyer 1985: 133, 196). Both the flowers and the leaves were used as a tonic (Meyer 1985: 258). Elder leaves were held to attract maggots out of a wound (Shelby 1959:10). A necklace made from elder stems has been used as a teething aid (Fowler and Fowler 1950: 175). Leaves of elder placed in the hat were claimed to protect from sunstroke (Fogel 1915: 138). Simply carrying elder leaves in the pocket was thought to help galled arms (Musick 1964: 48). For croup a child was touched with an elderberry wand which was kept where neither sun nor moon could shine upon it (Brendle and Unger 1935: 136).

In Native American practice, the American elder *(Sambucus canadensis)* was very widely used, by at least seventeen different tribes (Moerman 1998 : 511), and many of the same uses recorded by Meyer are recognizable in Native American practice, suggesting that this was probably the species most widely employed in folk medicine generally. By contrast, the European elder *(Sambucus nigra)* seems only to have been specifically selected by the Cherokee, for rheumatism, burns, skin eruptions and fevers, as a diuretic, and as an emetic (Hamel and Chiltoskey 1975: 33). Among the Mohegan, the bark of *S. canadensis* was scraped

upward to obtain an emetic, downward to obtain a laxative (Tantaquidgeon 1928: 265). Other species too, such as the blue elder *(Sambucus cerulea)* and scarlet elder *(Sambucus racemosa),* were used medicinally, though not quite as widely as American elder. *S. racemosa* seems to be the only species used in childbirth (see, for instance, Reagan 1936: 69).

*See also* **Amulet, Asthma, Birch, Burns, Childbirth, Colds, Constipation, Croup, Cuts, Dysentery, Eczema, Epilepsy, Eye problems, Fevers, Frostbite, Headache, Insect bites and stings, Piles, Rheumatism, Ringworm, Shakers, Sore throat, Sunburn, Teething, Tonic, Toothache, Warts.**

## References

Allen, David E., and Gabrielle Hatfield. *Medicinal Plants in Folk Tradition.* Portland, OR: Timber Press, in press.

Bacon, F. *Sylva Sylvarum.* 3rd ed. London, 1631.

Beith, Mary. *Healing Threads: Traditional Medicines of the Highlands and Islands.* Edinburgh: Polygon, 1995.

Black, William George. *Folk-Medicine: A Chapter in the History of Culture.* London: Folklore Society, 1883.

Brendle, Thomas R., and Claude W. Unger. "Folk Medicine of the Pennsylvania Germans: The Non-Occult Cures." *Proceedings of the Pennsylvania German Society* 45 (1935).

Crellin, John K., and Jane Philpott. *A Reference Guide to Medicinal Plants.* Durham, NC: Duke University Press, 1998.

Fogel, Edwin Miller. "Beliefs and Superstitions of the Pennsylvania Germans." *Americana Germanica* 18 (1915).

Fowler, David C., and Mary Gene Fowler. "More Kentucky Superstitions." *Southern Folklore Quarterly* 14 (1950): 170–176.

Hamel, Paul B., and Mary U. Chiltoskey. *Cherokee Plants and Their Uses: A 400 Year History.* Sylva, NC: Herald, 1975.

Hartland, Edwin Sidney. *County Folklore: Gloucestershire.* Printed Extracts 1, Vol. 37. London: Folk-Lore Society, 1895.

Hatfield, Gabrielle. *Memory, Wisdom and Heal-*

*ing: The History of Domestic Plant Medicine.* Phoenix Mill: Sutton, 1999.

Lafont, Anne-Marie. *Herbal Folklore.* Bideford: Badger Books, 1984.

Meyer, Clarence. *American Folk Medicine.* Glenwood, IL: Meyerbooks, 1985.

Moerman, Daniel E. *Native American Ethnobotany.* Portland, OR: Timber Press, 1998.

Musick, Ruth Anne (ed.). "Superstitions." *West Virginia Folklore* 14 (1964): 38–52.

Opie, Iona, and Peter Opie. *The Lore and Language of Schoolchildren.* Oxford: Oxford University Press, 1959.

Quelch, Mary Thorne. *Herbs for Daily Use.* London: Faber and Faber, 1941.

Reagan, Albert B. "Plants Used by the Hoh and Quileute Indians." *Kansas Academy of Sciences* 37 (1936): 55–70.

Sharkey, Olive. *Old Days, Old Ways.* Dublin: O'Brien Press, 1985.

Shelby, Carolyn. "Folklore of Jordan Springs, Tennessee." *Tennessee Folklore Society Bulletin* 25 (1959): 6–17.

Tantaquidgeon, Gladys. "Mohegan Medicinal Practices, Weather-Lore and Superstitions." *Smithsonian Institution-Bureau of American Ethnology Annual Report* 43 (1928): 264–270.

Vickery, Roy. *A Dictionary of Plant Lore.* Oxford: Oxford University Press, 1995.

# Elm (*Ulmus spp.*)

Considering how widespread the elm tree was in Britain, at least until the outbreak of Dutch elm disease in the 1970s, the number of ways in which it has been used in folk medicine is relatively small. There is a record of one particular tree in Bedfordshire that grew at the spot where a murderer had been executed being used to cure ague (fever). The patient nailed some of his hair or nail clippings to the tree, and the fever was transferred to the tree (Vickery 1995: 127). The inner bark of the elm has been chewed or boiled and made into a jelly-like liquid, to treat colds and sore throats (Vickery 1995: 127). In Ireland, the liquid obtained from boiling the bark has been used at least since the eighteenth century for treating burns (Threlkeld 1726). It has also been used in Ireland for treating sprains, swellings, and jaundice (Allen and Hatfield, in press), as well as for staunching bleeding (Maloney 1972).

In North America, the slippery elm *(Ulmus rubra)* is widespread and has been extensively used in folk medicine as well as in official medicine and herbalism. Many of the uses of this species of elm are similar to the British ones for their native elms *(Ulmus procera, U. glabra and U. minor)*, but the use of slippery elm in North American folk medicine seems to have been much more extensive. The bark has been chewed for sore throats and coughs (just as the native species of elm have been used in England), and it was also made into proprietary lozenges (Micheletti 1998: 114). Meyer recorded the use of slippery elm, or simply "elm," for a large range of ailments in addition to sore throat. The list includes skin ailments (Meyer 1985: 106, 108), eye ailments (Meyer 1985: 109–114), kidney complaints (Meyer 1985: 157–161), piles (Meyer 1985: 194–196), heartburn, and upset stomach (Meyer 1985: 235, 242).

Native Americans had many uses for elm. The bark was chewed for sore throats (Densmore 1928: 342) and made into an infusion for coughs (Tantaquidgeon 1972: 31). A poultice of the bark was used to treat burns and wounds (Hamel and Chiltoskey 1975: 33) and also swellings, including tubercular glands (Herrick 1977: 304). The plant was in addition used to treat bleeding cuts (Reagan 1928: 231), as well as bleeding lungs (Chandler, Freeman, and Hooper 1979: 63). (For further Native American uses of this and other species of elm, see Moerman 1998: 576–578.)

Though slippery elm is not native to Britain, its use has been imported by herbalists into Britain, and it now forms a staple of many herbal preparations there also.

*See also* **Bleeding, Burns, Colds, Coughs, Eye problems, Indigestion, Jaundice, Sore throat, Sprains, Transference, Wounds.**

## References
Allen, David E., and Gabrielle Hatfield. *Medicinal Plants in Folk Tradition.* Portland, OR: Timber Press, in press.

Chandler, R. Frank, Lois Freeman, and Shirley N. Hooper. "Herbal Remedies of the Maritime Indians." *Journal of Ethnopharmacology* 1 (1979): 49–68.

Densmore, Frances. "Uses of Plants by the Chippewa Indians." *Smithsonian Institution-Bureau of American Ethnology Annual Report* 44 (1928): 273–379.

Hamel, Paul B., and Mary U. Chiltoskey. *Cherokee Plants and Their Uses: A 400 Year History.* Sylva, NC: Herald, 1975.

Herrick, James William. *Iroquois Medical Botany.* Ph.D. thesis, State University of New York, Albany, 1977.

Maloney, Beatrice. "Traditional Herbal Cures in County Cavan: Part 1." *Ulster Folklife* 18 (1972): 66–79.

Meyer, Clarence. *American Folk Medicine.* Glenwood, IL: Meyerbooks, 1985.

Micheletti, Enza (ed.). *North American Folk Healing: An A-Z Guide to Traditional Remedies.* New York and Montreal: Reader's Digest Association, 1998.

Moerman, Daniel E. *Native American Ethnobotany.* Portland, OR: Timber Press, 1998.

Reagan, Albert B. "Plants Used by the Bois Fort Chippewa (Ojibwa) Indians of Minnesota." *Wisconsin Archaeologist* 7(4) (1928): 230–248.

Tantaquidgeon, Gladys. "Folk Medicine of the Delaware and Related Algonkian Indians." *Pennsylvania Historical Commission Anthropological Papers,* no. 3 (1972).

Threlkeld, Caleb. *Synopsis Stirpium Hibernicarum.* Dublin: F. Davys et al., 1726.

Vickery, Roy. *A Dictionary of Plant Lore.* Oxford: Oxford University Press, 1995.

# Epilepsy

This disease has always been regarded with fear and superstition, and it still is today. This unease is reflected in the wide range of magical and semi-magical "cures" in British folk medicine. In Aberdeenshire, Scotland, there was a belief that burning the clothes of a person who had had a fit would produce a cure (Black 1883: 72). Some of the remedies for epilepsy have a strong association with death. In Ireland, grated human skull has been ingested to cure epilepsy, and in Scotland too the bones of a man were regarded as a cure for a woman, and those of a woman for a man. Again, the skull was particularly valued (Black 1883: 96, 97). A medal made from coffin handles was worn as an amulet against epilepsy in the Scottish Highlands (Souter 1995: 37). Other amulets include the skin of a wolf, which was valued in England as well as on the continent of Europe (Black 1883: 153). An alternative was to wear nine pieces of elder, cut from between two knots (Black 1883: 120). Mistletoe was thought to prevent harm from witches. It was reputedly used by the Druids against epilepsy (Souter 1995: 41), and even the eminent eighteenth-century physician Sir Thomas Browne recommended that it be worn as a precaution against epilepsy (Black 1883: 196).

Rings that had been hallowed by the king were another popular charm against epilepsy, particularly during the sixteenth century; they were distributed by reigning monarchs until the death of Mary Tudor (Thomas 1978: 235). Originally they had been made from "Maundy Money," the royal offering to the church on Maundy Thursday, but later they were purpose-made. A strange survival of the idea of coins curing epilepsy is recorded from Sussex in the twentieth century. The mother of a young child suffering from fits was told to collect seven threepenny bits from seven strange men, without telling them what they were for. These were then placed secretly in a bag around the child's neck. The child had no further fits until the bag was

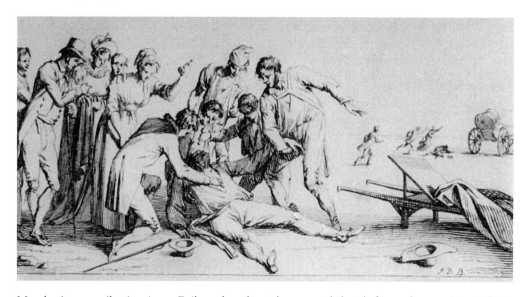

Man having an epileptic seizure. Epilepsy has always been regarded with fear and superstition. This is reflected in the wide range of magical and semi-magical 'cures' in British folk medicine. Some of the remedies for epilepsy have a strong association with death. (National Library of Medicine)

seen by another child (Esdaile 1942). There was a belief that a piece of coal found under a mugwort plant *(Artemisia vulgaris)* was a cure for epilepsy (Radford and Radford 1961).

In a symbol of rebirth, large standing stones with a hole in them were employed as a gateway to health. For example, in Cornwall a person suffering from epilepsy would be passed naked through the hole of the "Men-an-Tol" (Souter 1995: 37). In Sussex and elsewhere in England there was belief that sleeping under a walnut tree could lead to fits or madness (Souter 1995: 172). Another Sussex belief was that eating ashes of a roast cuckoo was a cure for fits (Allen 1995: 42). Interestingly, the plant known as cuckoo-flower *(Cardamine pratense)* had a reputation in the Scottish Highlands for soothing epileptic fits (Beith 1995: 213), while "cuckoo sorrel" *(Rumex acetosa)* was similarly used in Cumbria (Newman and Wilson 1951: 252–266). There is on record from the early twentieth century the story of a cure for epilepsy practiced in the Isle of Lewis by a healer, a cure that com-bines many of these different epilepsy treatments in one. The patient had to drink blood taken from his left foot. He had toe and finger nail clippings and hair clippings from moustache and eyebrows wrapped in parcels. A cross of ropes was laid on his body, the ends of the ropes being knotted. The knots were then cut off and wrapped and, together with the clippings were buried in a place where neither sun, wind, nor rain could reach them. A black cock was buried at the place where the patient had had his first fit. The patient was then in-structed to drink water out of a human skull (Henderson 1910: 319–320). Near the head of Loch Torridon in Wester Ross there is a well that within living memory was used to treat a man suffering from epilepsy. He was instructed to drink its water from the skull of a suicide and thereafter to abstain from excessive alcohol and not to act as a coffin bearer (Beith 1995: 131).

Herbal treatments for epilepsy in British folk medicine are comparatively few in number. Mistletoe was used especially in southern England, also in southern Ireland

(Allen and Hatfield, in press). Juniper berries *(Juniperus communis)* were used in the Scottish Highlands (Carmichael 1900–1971, 4: 268), and in Cavan the fern known as spleenwort *(Asplenium rutamuraria)* was infused in milk to treat epilepsy (Maloney 1972: 66–79).

All the elements of folk healing discussed above are also to be found in North American remedies for epilepsy. In Alabama there was a belief that if a baby has convulsions, burning its clothes will stop them (Browne 1958: 23). If an epileptic's shirt is burned (Kanner 1930: 208) or pulled over his head and pulled up through the chimney of the house and buried (UCLA Folklore Archives 2_6805), the fits will cease. Many of the remedies show an association with blood or death. A woman who had epilepsy witnessed an execution at Karis, collected some of the dead man's blood, and drank it to cure herself (Hand 1970: 325). A piece of rope with which someone had hanged himself was believed to be a cure for epilepsy (Fogel 1915: 292). The fresh blood of a turtle dove, drunk, was a suggested cure for epilepsy in Pennsylvania (Smith 1950: 4). Hair cuttings from the patient, buried either under the bed (Wilson 1908: 70) or in a hole in an oak tree (Simons 1954: 3), were believed to stop epilepsy. Cuckoo ashes were recommended for epilepsy, as in Britain (McAtee 1955: 172). Less drastically, holding a child in the smoke from burned black chicken feathers was a cure suggested in Alabama (Browne 1958: 23). Rubbing a naked baby with a newly born pig is an example of transference in epilepsy treatment (Bourke 1894: 119). An idea remarkably similar to one found in Britain is to dig under the roots of red wormwood, take two pieces of coal from there, then eat one and wear the other as a cure for epilepsy (Brendle and Unger 1935: 105). Miscellaneous "cures" for epilepsy include getting the patient to drink out of a dish from which a crossbill has drunk (Brendle and Unger 1935: 108); eating beaver fat (Hendricks 1953: 126); and, from Arizona, passing a worm dipped in alcohol down the sufferer's throat on a thread during a fit and pulling it up gradually (UCLA Folklore Archives 4_6245).

To avoid "catching" epilepsy, wearing an amulet made from the backbone of a rattlesnake is a suggested precaution in California (UCLA Folklore Archives record number 3_6245). Another precaution against getting epilepsy is to crush the shells of eggs after eating them (Kanner 1930: 192).

Herbal treatments for epilepsy, as in Britain, are not very numerous in North America. They include nibbling the end of a hop *(Humulus lupulus)* vine every morning for seven mornings in the spring before sunrise (Hyatt 1965: 248). Other herbal remedies involve fresh parsley *(Petroselinum crispum)* (Randolph 1947: 110); cow parsnip seeds *(Heracleum maximum)* (Partridge 1838: 286–288), pansies *(Viola* sp.) (UCLA Folklore Archives record number 2_6245), and dog fennel *(Anthemis cotula)* (Pickard and Buley 1945: 44). Of these herbal treatments, dog fennel is used by the Cherokee to treat epilepsy (Hamel and Chiltoskey 1975: 32), and cowparsnip is used similarly by the Winnebago (Gilmore 1919: 107), suggesting a Native American origin for these remedies. A large number of other plant genera were employed by the Native Americans in treating epilepsy (Moerman 1998: 769–770).

*See also* **Amulet, Elder, Mistletoe, Mugwort, Skull, Witch.**

### References

Allen, Andrew. *A Dictionary of Sussex Folk Medicine.* Newbury: Countryside Books, 1995.

Allen, David E., and Gabrielle Hatfield. *Medicinal Plants in Folk Tradition.* Portland, OR: Timber Press, in press.

Beith, Mary. *Healing Threads: Traditional Medicines of the Highlands and Islands.* Edinburgh: Polygon, 1995.

Black, William George. *Folk-Medicine: A Chapter in the History of Culture.* London: Folklore Society, 1883.

Bourke, John G. "Popular Medicine, Customs and Superstitions of the Rio Grande." *Journal of American Folklore* 7 (1894): 119–146.

Brendle, Thomas R., and Claude W. Unger. "Folk Medicine of the Pennsylvania Germans: The Non-Occult Cures." *Proceedings of the Pennsylvania German Society* 45 (1935).

Browne, Ray B. *Popular Beliefs and Practices from Alabama.* Folklore Studies 9. Berkeley and Los Angeles: University of California Publications, 1958.

Carmichael, Alexander. *Carmina Gadelica: Hymns and Incantations.* 6 vols. (3 and 4 ed. J. Carmichael Watson, 5 and 6 ed. Angus Matheson). Edinburgh: Constable (1900); Oliver and Boyd (1940–54); Scottish Academic Press (1971).

Esdaile, K. A. *Sussex Notes and Queries.* Lewes: Sussex Archaeological Society, Vol. 9 (1942).

Fogel, Edwin Miller. "Beliefs and Superstitions of the Pennsylvania Germans." *Americana Germanica* 18 (1915).

Gilmore, Melvin R. "Uses of Plants by the Indians of the Missouri River Region." *Smithsonian Institution-Bureau of American Ethnology Annual Report,* no. 33 (1919).

Hamel, Paul B., and Mary U. Chiltoskey. *Cherokee Plants and Their Uses: A 400 Year History.* Sylva, NC: Herald, 1975.

Hand, Wayland D. "Hangmen, the Gallows and the Dead Man's Hand in American Folk Medicine." In *Medieval Literature and Folklore Studies: Essays in Honour of Francis Lee Utley,* edited by Jerome Mandell and Bruce A. Rosenberg, 323–329, 381–387. New Brunswick, NJ: Rutgers University Press, 1970.

Henderson, George. *The Norse Influence on Celtic Scotland.* Glasgow: James Maclehose, 1910.

Hendricks, George D. "Misconceptions Concerning Western Wild Animals." *Western Folklore* 12 (1953): 119–127.

Hyatt, Harry Middleton. *Folklore from Adams County Illinois.* 2nd rev. ed. New York: Memoirs of the Alma Egan Hyatt Foundation, 1965.

Kanner, Leo. "The Folklore and Cultural History of Epilepsy." *Medical Life* 37 (1930): 167–214.

Maloney, Beatrice. "Traditional Herbal Cures in County Cavan: Part 1." *Ulster Folklife* 18 (1972): 66–79.

McAtee, W. L. "Odds and Ends of North American Folklore on Birds." *Midwest Folklore* 5 (1955): 169–183.

Moerman, Daniel E. *Native American Ethnobotany.* Portland, OR: Timber Press, 1998.

Newman, L. F., and E. M. Wilson. "Folk-Lore Survivals in the Southern 'Lake Counties' and in Essex: A Comparison and Contrast. Part I." *Folk-Lore* 62 (1951): 252–266.

Partridge, Oliver. "Of the Cow-Parsnip." *Boston Medical and Surgical Journal* 18 (1838): 18.

Pickard, Madge E., and R. Carlyle Buley. *The Midwest Pioneer, His Ills, Cures and Doctors.* Crawfordsville, IN: R. E. Banta, 1945.

Radford, E., and M. A. Radford. *Encyclopaedia of Superstitions.* Edited and revised by Christina Hole. London: Hutchinson, 1961.

Randolph, Vance. *Ozark Superstitions.* New York: Columbia University Press, 1947.

Simons, Isaak Shirk. "Dutch Folk-Beliefs." *Pennsylvania Dutchman* 5(14) (March 15, 1954): 2–3, 15.

Smith, Richard. "Collecting Folk Cures in Lebanon County." *Pennsylvania Dutchman* 2(8) (September 15, 1950).

Souter, Keith. *Cure Craft: Traditional Folk Remedies and Treatment from Antiquity to the Present Day.* Saffron Walden: C. W. Daniel, 1995.

Thomas, Keith. *Religion and the Decline of Magic.* London: Peregrine, 1978.

Wilson, Charles Bundy. "Notes on Folk Medicine." *Journal of American Folklore* 21 (1908): 68–73.

# Eryngo

The roots of sea-holly (*Eryngium maritimum* and other species) were highly prized in the past in both official and folk medicine as a tonic and worm-treatment (Ó Síocháin 1962), a cure for coughs and colds (*Shenstone* 1887), and as an aphrodisiac. In the latter role they are mentioned by Shakespeare in *The Merry Wives of Windsor* (5.5).

Colchester in Essex was famous for many centuries as the center of the eryngo trade. Though *Eryngium maritimum* is not native to North America, other members of the genus are, and these have been used in a variety of ways in North American folk medicine.

*See also* **Button snakeroot.**

### References

Ó Síocháin, P. A. *Aran, Islands of Legend.* Dublin: Foilsiúcháin Éireann, 1962.

Shenstone, J. C. "A Report on the Flowering Plants Growing in the Neighbourhood of Colchester." *Essex Naturalist* 1 (1887): 30–33.

# Erysipelas

In Christian times, this disease, also known as St. Anthony's fire, became associated with Saint Anthony, and by the sixteenth century he was credited with the power not only of relieving it but also of inflicting it (Thomas 1973: 29). Apart from numerous charms (preferably including a line of Latin [Beith 1995: 197]), the ailment attracted a number of folk remedies involving either fire, water, or blood. In Wales, it was believed that the sparks struck from stone and steel against the face would cure erysipelas (Radford and Radford: n.d., 115). In the seventeenth century in Perthshire, Scotland, washing in running water and applying hog's lard was considered effective (Perth Kirk Session Record, May 1623). Individuals were sometimes credited with the power of healing erysipelas. In Ireland, the blood of a member of the Keogh, Walch, or Cahill family was considered to be an erysipelas cure (Black 1883: 140). In East Anglia, up to the nineteenth century, in rural areas leeches were applied to remove the "bad blood" of erysipelas (Rider Haggard 1974: 17). In Ireland, the disease was sometimes called "wild fire," and cures for it include the blood of a black cat (Wilde 1898: 30). The left shoe of a person of the opposite sex from the patient, reduced to ashes and ingested, was once considered a cure for erysipelas (Black 1883: 190). An amulet made from elder on which the sun had never shone was a seventeenth-century remedy for erysipelas (Blochwich 1665: 54). More prosaically, in Ulster, salted butter was a cure for erysipelas (Hickey 1938: 268). Frogspawn was used in the Scottish Highlands (Beith 1995: 176).

Herbs used to treat the condition in Scotland were stonecrop *(Sedum acre),* blackberry leaves (Beith 1995: 244, 209), and herb Robert *(Geranium robertianum)* (Gregor 1881: 47). In East Anglia, agrimony was used *(Agrimonia eupatoria)* (Taylor MSS).

In North American folk medicine, a similar medley of magical and practical remedies for erysipelas has been reported. Amulets worn for erysipelas include elder (as in Britain) (Puckett 1981: 368) and green glass beads (Whitney and Bullock 1925: 93). There are a number of cures involving fire—for instance, passing a shovel of burning coal in front of a patient, practiced in Maryland (Whitney and Bullock 1925: 90), or striking sparks from an Indian arrowhead (Hyatt 1965: 264). In Pennsylvania there was a blacksmith credited with the power to heal erysipelas (Shoemaker 1951: 2). There, as in Ireland, the disease was also known as "wildfire." Blood from either a black cat (as in Ireland) or black hen was used in Pennsylvania (Weiser 1954: 6, 14). Rubbing with a dead toad was suggested in Indiana (Brown 1952–1964, 6: 179). Also from Indiana comes the suggestion of collecting nine catkins from a birch branch on a Friday morning, without speaking to anyone, and rubbing them on the affected area (Pickard and Buley 1945: 79). In Pennsylvania, an ointment for treating erysipelas was made from sheep tallow, elder scrapings, and goose dung (Fogel 1915: 270).

Simple household remedies for erysipelas include boric acid solution, sprinkling with starch or wheat flour, and bathing with a solution of sodium bicarbonate or with a mixture of salt and brandy, with buttermilk, with glycerine, or with egg wine. Poultices prepared from beans, or from onions and bran, have also been used (Meyer 1985: 107–108). Herbal treatments for the condition include a poultice of cranberries *(Vaccinium vitis-idaea)* (Meyer 1985: 108), a preparation made from sumac roots *(Rhus* sp.) (Michael and Burrow 1967: 782) or the oil from infusing blossoms of dog fennel *(?Anthemis cotula)* in the sunshine (UCLA Folklore Archives 5_6245). In Georgia, a poultice was made from cornmeal and peach leaves *(Prunus persica)* (Brown and Ledford 1967: 28). In Nebraska, a poultice was prepared from red beets and fresh-cut chewing tobacco (Black 1935: 18). Other herbal poultices include aralia roots *(Aralia* sp.) (Pickard and Buley 1945: 45) and houseleek (Browne 1958: 61). Sweet fern *(Comptonia peregrina)* and berries or roots of poke have also been used (Meyer 1985: 108). At least some of these remedies are probably borrowed from Native American usage; *Anthemis cotula* was given by the Iroquois to children with "red spots" (Herrick 1977: 471), and peach leaves were used by the Cherokee for a number of skin conditions (Hamel and Chiltoskey 1975: 47), while the roots of *Rhus copallinum* were used by the Delaware to treat skin eruptions (Tantaquidgeon 1972: 32). In addition, a very large number of other plants were used in treating skin complaints in Native American practice (Moerman 1998: 783–788).

*See also* **Amulet, Blackberry, Blacksmith, Houseleek, Poke, Poultice, Toads and frogs.**

## References
Beith, Mary. *Healing Threads: Traditional Medicines of the Highlands and Islands.* Edinburgh: Polygon, 1995.

Black, Pauline Monette. *Nebraska Folk Cures.* Studies in Language, Literature, and Criticism 15. Lincoln: University of Nebraska, 1935.

Black, William George. *Folk-Medicine: A Chapter in the History of Culture.* London: Folklore Society, 1883.

Blochwich, Martin. *Anatomia Sambuci: or, the Anatomie of the Elder.* 1665.

Brown, Frank C. *Collection of North Carolina Folklore.* 7 vols. Durham, NC: Duke University Press, 1952–1964.

Brown, Judy, and Lizzie Ledford. Superstitions. *Foxfire* 1(2), (1967): 25–28.

Browne, Ray B. *Popular Beliefs and Practices from Alabama.* Folklore Studies 9. Berkeley and Los Angeles: University of California Publications, 1958.

Fogel, Edwin Miller. "Beliefs and Superstitions of the Pennsylvania Germans." *Americana Germanica* 18 (1915).

Gregor, Walter. *Notes on the Folk-Lore of the North-East of Scotland.* London: Publications of the Folklore Society, vol. 7, 1881.

Hamel, Paul B., and Mary U. Chiltoskey. *Cherokee Plants and Their Uses: A 400 Year History.* Sylva, NC: Herald, 1975.

Herrick, James William. *Iroquois Medical Botany.* Ph.D. thesis, State University of New York, Albany, 1977.

Hickey, E. M. "Medical Superstitions in Ireland." *Ulster Medical Journal* 2 (1938).

Hyatt, Harry Middleton. *Folklore from Adams County Illinois.* 2nd rev. ed. New York: Memoirs of the Alma Egan Hyatt Foundation, 1965.

Meyer, Clarence. *American Folk Medicine.* Glenwood, IL: Meyerbooks, 1985.

Michael, Max, Jr., and Mark V. Burrow. "'Old Timey' Remedies of Yesterday and Today." *Journal of the Florida Medical Association* 54(8) (August 1967): 778–784.

Moerman, Daniel E. *Native American Ethnobotany.* Portland, OR: Timber Press, 1998.

Perth Kirk Session Record, May 1623.

Pickard, Madge E., and R. Carlyle Buley. *The Midwest Pioneer, His Ills, Cures and Doctors.* Crawfordsville, Indiana: R. E. Banta, 1945.

Puckett, Newbell Niles. *Popular Beliefs and Super-*

*stitions: A Compendium of American Folklore from the Ohio Collection of Newbell Niles Puckett.* Edited by Wayland D. Hand, Anna Casetta, and Sondra B. Thiederman. 3 vols. Boston: G. K. Hall, 1981.

Radford, E., and M. A. Radford. *Encyclopaedia of Superstitions.* London, n.d.

Rider Haggard, Lilias (ed.). *I Walked by Night.* Woodbridge: Boydell Press, 1974.

Shoemaker, Alfred L. "Blacksmith Lore." *Pennsylvania Dutchman* 3(6) (August 1, 1951).

Tantaquidgeon, Gladys. "Folk Medicine of the Delaware and Related Algonkian Indians." *Pennsylvania Historical Commission Anthropological Papers,* no. 3 (1972).

Taylor MSS. Manuscript notes of Mark R. Taylor in the Norfolk Record Office, Norwich. MS4322.

Thomas, Keith. *Religion and the Decline of Magic.* Harmondsworth: Penguin Books, 1973.

Weiser, Rev. Daniel. "Braucherei." *Pennsylvania Dutchman* 5(14) (March 15, 1954).

Whitney, Annie Weston, and Caroline Canfield Bullock. "Folklore from Maryland." *Memoirs of the American Folklore Society* 18 (1925).

Wilde, Lady (Jane). *Ancient Charms, Cures and Usages of Ireland.* London: Ward and Downey, 1898.

# Evil eye

The idea that disease can be caused by being "overlooked" (i.e., looked at) by someone with evil powers is a very ancient one, recorded in ancient Babylon five thousand years ago (Souter 1995: 29). It still lingers today in folk medicine across the world. Protection against the evil eye has often been provided by wearing amulets. The ancient Egyptians used as an amulet the eye of Horus, while in Rome horseshoes were nailed to the doors of houses to provide protection against the evil eye (Souter 1995: 31), a practice still current in Britain and elsewhere. In the nineteenth century in both England and Scotland there was still a firm belief that certain individuals possessed the evil eye, and its effects were countered with elaborate ceremonies (Black 1883: 22–23). As recently as the early years of the twentieth century, Tongue recalls as a child being hidden when a certain woman passed by. The woman was thought to have the evil eye since she praised a young child who subsequently died (Tongue 1965: 68). Porter describes several twentieth-century individuals in East Anglia who were thought to possess the evil eye (Porter 1974: 154–155). Protection against it could be obtained by using certain plants, such as mugwort (Black 1883: 201). A witch in a Norfolk village in the twentieth century was reported to have obtained services free from her neighbors, for fear of her powers of "overlooking." She was never allowed to look at a newborn baby, "for fear of the Evil Eye" (Taylor 1929: 129–130).

Similar beliefs are to be found in North American folk medicine. As in Britain, certain people regarded as having the evil eye were not allowed to look at a baby (UCLA Folklore Archives 11_5413). Headaches in babies were thought to be caused by the evil eye (Jones 1951: 17). Amulets worn to avert the evil eye include a locket in the shape of a heart and a red spot on the forehead. When meeting a cross-eyed person it has been suggested that one must cross one's fingers to avert the evil eye (Brown 1952–1964, 7: 136). A red ribbon helped to protect a baby against the evil eye; alternatively, written prayers could be used as an amulet, or crossing oneself could provide protection (Puckett 1981: 131, 1078, 1079). Snake skin or snake heads have also been used as amulets (Cannon 1984: 319). In the Mexican tradition there was a belief that when admiring a child, it was necessary to touch the child at the same time, to ward off the evil eye (Dodson 1932: 84). Protection could be had by embroidering spiders on the child's clothing or giving it coral to wear (Baca 1969: 2174). In the Native American tradition garlic, among its many powers, was thought to ward off the evil eye (UCLA Folklore Archives 9_6794).

See also **Amulet, Mexican tradition, Mugwort, Native American tradition, Witch.**

## References

Baca, Josephine Elizabeth. "Some Health Beliefs of the Spanish Speaking." *American Journal of Nursing* 69 (October 1969): 2172–2176.

Black, William George. *Folk-Medicine: A Chapter in the History of Culture.* London: Folklore Society, 1883.

Brown, Frank C. *Collection of North Carolina Folklore.* 7 vols. Durham, NC: Duke University Press, 1952–1964.

Cannon, Anthon S. *Popular Beliefs and Superstitions from Utah.* Edited by Wayland D. Hand and Jeannine E. Talley. Salt Lake City: University of Utah Press, 1984.

Dodson, Ruth. "Folk Curing among the Mexicans." *Publications of the Texas Folklore Society* 10 (1932): 82–98.

Jones, Louis C. "The Evil Eye among European-Americans." *Western Folklore* 10 (1951): 11–25.

Porter, Enid. *The Folklore of East Anglia.* London: Batsford, 1974.

Puckett, Newbell Niles. *Popular Beliefs and Superstitions: A Compendium of American Folklore from the Ohio Collection of Newbell Niles Puckett.* Edited by Wayland D. Hand, Anna Casetta, and Sondra B. Thiederman. 3 vols. Boston: G. K. Hall, 1981.

Souter, Keith. *Cure Craft: Traditional Folk Remedies and Treatment from Antiquity to the Present Day.* Saffron Walden: C. W. Daniel, 1995.

Taylor, Mark R. "Norfolk Folklore." *Folk-Lore* 40 (1929): 113–133.

Tongue, Ruth L. *Somerset Folklore.* Edited Katharine Briggs. County Folklore 8. London: Folklore Society, 1965.

# Excreta

The dung of a wide range of animals has been used in British folk medicine from early times to the present day. It is not al-ways appreciated that official medicine employed animal products, including their feces, and that at least some of the folk uses may in fact have been derived from book knowledge. William Salmon's *English Physician* of 1693 gives the official uses of the dung of no fewer than thirty-four different birds and beasts (Salmon 1693). In folk medicine the excreta of various animals has been used. Sheep droppings have been used in the Scottish Highlands as an infusion in milk for smallpox, and fresh pig dung has served to staunch a nosebleed (Marwick 1975: 130). Sheep's dung and water have been used to treat jaundice and whooping cough in Scotland (Gregor 1881: 46). Mixed with porter and sulphur, it was used to treat children in Ireland with measles in the nineteenth century (Black 1883: 157). Cowpats were used to poultice wounds in Hampshire in the nineteenth century (Black 1883: 161) and to help in the removal of splinters (Hatfield 1994: 11). As a hot poultice, cow dung has been used to treat a badly swollen knee (Prince 1991: 111) and to bring an abscess to a head (Allen 1995: 42). A Yorkshire remedy for arthritis was a poultice of cow dung and vinegar (Souter 1995: 135). In Scotland cow dung has also been used to treat blotches on the face, as well as "quinsy," or tonsillitis (Beith 1995: 172). Bird dung has been used as a remedy for baldness. The white part of hen's dirt has been used to draw pus (Beith 1995: 173). Human feces, dried and powdered, have been blown into the eyes for blindness (Beith 1995: 173). In the eighteenth century, in his *Flora Scotica*, Lightfoot (Lightfoot 1777) recorded the use of human feces as a poultice for snake bite (Beith 1995: 173). Logan records the use of human excrement in Ireland in the treatment of quinsy, inflammation, scalds and burns, gout, and erysipelas (Logan 1972: 154).

In North American folk medicine there is a similar usage of dung. Human excrement has been used to treat "felons" (infected sores usually under the finger nail) (see, for example, Welsch 1966: 368). In Spanish American folk medicine, it has been used to treat scorpion bites (UCLA Folklore Archives 12_6180) and cramps (Espinosa 1910: 411). It has been claimed to be commonly used to treat toothache in the New World and Spain (Foster 1953: 213–214.) Dried and powdered, it has been recommended for epilepsy and for intermittent fevers (Saul 1949: 65). Burying in a hole in a tree the excrement of a person suffering from asthma is said to be a cure of African American origin (Hyatt 1970, 1: 386). Chicken excrement has been used to treat hives in children (Hendricks 1966: 48), as well as warts (Puckett 1981: 474), diphtheria (UCLA Folklore Archives 9_6261), whooping cough (Anderson 1970: 91), and as a deterrent to thumb-sucking (Frankel 1977: 128). Sheep dung has been used particularly in the treatment of measles (see, for instance, Wheeler 1892–1893: 66), as in Ireland. This practice has also been recorded among the Mohegan (Tantaquidgeon 1928: 268). It has also been used to treat scarlet fever (Brendle and Unger 1935: 90) and hives (Anderson 1970: 42). The water collecting on cowpats has been used to treat warts (Waugh 1918: 23). Cow excrement has been used, like that of sheep, as an infusion to treat measles (Anderson 1970: 51). As a poultice it has been applied to boils (Wintemberg 1950: 11) and for rheumatism (Wintemberg 1918: 127). The dung specifically of a black cow has been suggested as a treatment for a whitlow (inflammation of finger or toe, especially at the nail) (Riddell 1934: 43), and again the cowpat and urine of a black cow are recommended for scabs (Bourke 1894: 139–140). Dog excrement has been applied to the stomach for indigestion (Brown 1952–1964, 6: 220). White dog feces are specified as a treatment for sore throat (Saucier 1956: 23) and

pneumonia (Parler 1962: 819). There are records of the use of dog feces among Native Americans in Mexico in the treatment of burns and scalds (Vogel 1970: 214). Hog dung has been used to treat diphtheria (Hoffman 1889: 29), nosebleed (Riddell 1934: 43), and mumps (Brendle and Unger 1935: 137). Goose dung has been used to treat burns and erysipelas (Brendle and Unger 1935: 82, 153). Finally, wolf dung was recorded by Josselyn in the seventeenth century as a treatment for colic (Josselyn 1833: 238).

*See also* **Abscesses, Asthma, Baldness, Boils, Burns, Colic, Cramp, Erysipelas, Eye problems, Felons, Gout, Hives, Indigestion, Jaundice, Nosebleed, Poultice, Quinsy, Rheumatism, Smallpox, Snake bite, Sore throat, Toothache, Warts, Whooping cough, Wounds.**

## References

Allen, Andrew. *A Dictionary of Sussex Folk Medicine.* Newbury: Countryside Books, 1995.

Anderson, John Q. *Texas Folk Medicine.* Austin: Encino Press, 1970.

Beith, Mary. *Healing Threads: Traditional Medicines of the Highlands and Islands.* Edinburgh: Polygon, 1995.

Black, W. G. *Folk-Medicine: A Chapter in the History of Culture.* London: Folklore Society, 1883. Reprinted New York: Burt Franklin, 1970.

Bourke, John G. "Popular Medicine, Customs and Superstitions of the Rio Grande." *Journal of American Folklore* 7 (1894): 119–146.

Brendle, Thomas R., and Claude W. Unger. "Folk Medicine of the Pennsylvania Germans: The Non-Occult Cures." *Proceedings of the Pennsylvania German Society* 45 (1935).

Brown, Frank C. *Collection of North Carolina Folklore.* 7 vols. Durham, NC: Duke University Press, 1952–1964.

Espinosa, Aurelio M. "New Mexican Spanish Folk-Lore." *Journal of American Folklore* 23 (1910): 395–418.

Foster, George M. "Relationships between Spanish and Spanish-American Folk Medicine."

*Journal of American Folklore* 66 (1953): 201–217.

Frankel, Barbara. *Childbirth in the Ghetto: Folk Beliefs of Negro Women in a North Philadelphia Hospital Ward.* San Francisco: R and E Research Associates, 1977.

Gregor, Walter. *Notes on the Folk-Lore of the North-East of Scotland.* London: Publications of the Folk-Lore Society, vol. 7, 1881.

Hatfield, Gabrielle. *Country Remedies: Traditional East Anglian Plant Remedies in the Twentieth Century.* Woodbridge: Boydell, 1994.

Hendricks, George D. *Mirrors, Mice and Mustaches: A Sampling of Superstitions and Popular Beliefs in Texas.* Austin: Texas Folklore Society, 1966.

Hoffman, W. J. "Folk-Lore of the Pennsylvania Germans." *Journal of American Folklore* 2 (1889): 23–35.

Hyatt, Harry Middleton. *Hoodoo, Conjuration, Witchcraft, Rootwork.* 5 vols. New York: Memoirs of the Alma Egan Hyatt Foundation, 1970.

Josselyn, John. *Two Voyages to New England.* Cambridge, MA: Historical Society Collection III, 1833.

Lightfoot, J. *Flora Scotica.* London, 1777.

Logan, Patrick. *Making the Cure: A Look at Irish Folk Medicine.* Dublin: Talbot Press, 1972.

Marwick, Ernest. *The Folklore of Orkney and Shetland.* London: Batsford, 1975.

Parler, Mary Celestia, and University Student Contributors. *Folk Beliefs from Arkansas.* 15 volumes. Fayetteville: University of Arkansas, 1962.

Prince, Dennis. *Grandmother's Cures: An A-Z of Herbal Remedies.* London: Fontana, 1991.

Puckett, Newbell Niles. *Popular Beliefs and Superstitions: A Compendium of American Folklore from the Ohio Collection of Newbell Niles Puckett.* Edited by Wayland D. Hand, Anna Casetta, and Sondra B. Thiederman. 3 vols. Boston: G. K. Hall, 1981.

Riddell, William Renwick. "Some Old Canadian Folk Medicine." *Canada Lancet and Practitioner* 83 (August 1934): 41–44.

Salmon, William. *The Compleat English Physician.* London: 1693.

Saucier, Corinne L. *Traditions de la Paroisse des Avoyelles en Louisiande.* Philadelphia: American Folklore Society, 1956.

Saul, F. William, MD. *Pink Pills for Pale People.* Philadelphia: Dorrance, 1949.

Souter, Keith. *Cure Craft: Traditional Folk Remedies and Treatment from Antiquity to the Present Day.* Saffron Walden: C. W. Daniel, 1995.

Tantaquidgeon, Gladys. "Mohegan Medicinal Practices, Weather Lore and Superstitions." In *Forty-third Annual Report of the Bureau of American Ethnology*, 1925–1926. Washington, DC: 1928.

Vogel, Virgil J. *American Indian Medicine.* Norman: University of Oklahoma Press, 1970.

Waugh, F. W. "Canadian Folk-Lore from Ontario." *Journal of American Folklore* 31 (1918): 4–82.

Welsch, Roger L. *A Treasure of Nebraska Pioneer Folklore.* Lincoln: University of Nebraska Press, 1966.

Wheeler, Helen M. "Illinois Folk-Lore." *The Folk-Lorist* 1 (1892–1893): 55–68.

Wintemberg, W. J. "Folk-Lore Collected in Toronto and Vicinity." *Journal of American Folklore* 31 (1918): 125–134.

Wintemberg, W. J. *Folk-Lore of Waterloo County, Ontario.* Bulletin 116. Anthropological Series 28. Ontario: National Museum of Canada, 1950.

# Eye problems

British folk medicine has recommendations for most eye problems. For foreign bodies in the eye, the seeds of clary (*Salvia verbenaca*) were used (Allen and Hatfield, in press). In contact with the film of water on the surface of the eye, the mucilaginous seeds swell up, and particles in the eye can be easily removed along with the swollen seed. For stys, infections of the rim of the eye, rubbing with hair from the tail of a black cat or with a gold wedding ring was recommended (Black 1883: 116, 173). In Ireland, a cure was to pick ten thorns of the gooseberry *(Ribes uva-crispa).* One was thrown away, nine were pointed to the eye and then buried (Vickery 1995: 155). Zinc sulphate solution was used to bathe sore eyes (Prince 1991: 107).

In the Scottish Highlands, individuals were credited with the power to soothe eye inflammations by rubbing the eye with a stone on which they had placed soot and spittle (Beith 1995: 94). Foreign particles were often removed from a child's eyes by the mother licking them out (Beith 1995: 103); this was thought to be more effective if a frog's eye were licked first (Beith 1995: 176). For a sty one recommendation in the Scottish Highlands was to stand on one's head in the sea until nine waves had passed over, or to count to one hundred without drawing breath (Beith 1995: 135). Asking a man on a white horse to remove a sty was a method practiced in Aberdeenshire (Beith 1995: 178). Among the Celts, the gall of the hare was used to treat eye problems (Beith 1995: 177). In the west Highlands, a cure for blindness was to dry and powder human excrement and blow it into the eyes (Beith 1995: 173). For inflammation of the eyelid, a poultice of watercress (Rorippa nasturtium-aquaticum) was used in East Anglia (Hatfield 1994: 37). If just one eye was sore, a remedy from Suffolk suggested an ointment of egg white, red ochre, bay salt, and finely chopped leaves of hemlock (Conium maculatum), to be applied to the healthy eye (Porter 1974: 43). Water collected among the basal leaves of teasel (Dipsacus fullonum) was widely suggested to sooth sore eyes (Latham 1878: 45). The liquid from boiled mallow leaves was used to bathe sore eyes in Cornwall (Vickery 1995: 230). In parts of Norfolk, the common speedwell (Veronica chamaedrys) was known as "sore eyes" because an infusion of the little blue flowers was used for this purpose (Hatfield 1994: 37). The juice of houseleek was dripped into children's eyes to treat conjunctivitis (Hatfield 1994: 37). For infections of the eye the herb eyebright (Euphrasia officinalis), as its country name suggests, was widely used. In the Scottish Highlands eyebright was infused in milk and applied to the eye with a feather (Beith

1995: 215). Daisy flowers (Bellis perennis) were also used in Scotland for eye troubles, as were the flowers of plantains (Plantago lanceolata and Plantago media) (Beith 1995: 213, 234). For eyestrain and tired eyes, a slice of cucumber laid on the closed eyes, or a moistened teabag were recommended. Compresses made from the flowers of chamomile and infusions made from the shoots of ground ivy (Glechoma hederacea) were other applications used for sore eyes (Hatfield 1994: 37). For a black eye, witch hazel (Hamamelis virginiana) was recommended, or a piece of raw steak laid on the eye. In the Scottish Highlands, a slice of raw potato was used (Beith 1995: 235). Eating raw seaweed was thought to improve eyesight (Beith 1995: 241). For failing eyesight, the flowers of the cornflower (Centaurea cyanus) have been used as an infusion at least since the eighteenth century. This flower, once a common field weed, is now comparatively scarce. In the eighteenth century it was known as "break spectacles water," so high was its reputation (Gunton Household Book). Ulcers of the eye used to be termed "kennings"; a country remedy for these was an ointment made from the creeping buttercup (Ranunculus repens), which in some parts of England was known as "kenning herb." Another herb used for this purpose was the greater celandine (Chelidonium majus) (Davey, 1909: 10, 23). In Devon scarlet pimpernell (Anagallis arvensis) was used to treat sore eyes (Vickery 1995: 336). In Cornwall leaves of the tree mallow (Lavatera arborea) were used to treat kennings or stys (Vickery 1995: 375).

In North American folk medicine many of the same remedies as in Britain have been recorded, as well as many more besides. For sore eyes, zinc sulphate was again recommended as an eyewash, or boracic powder, or simply warm water or milk, ordinary tea, diluted witch hazel extract (Hamamelis virginiana), cheeseplant (Malva neglecta) leaves, or roots in infusion, or water in which seeds of quince *(Cydonia oblonga)* have been soaked. Sassafras twigs boiled and with mare's milk added, an infusion of blue violet *(Viola cucullata)* tops and roots, the bark of green ozier *(Cornus circinata),* roots of basswood *(Tilia americana),* chamomile *(Chamaemelum nobile)* simmered in milk, the old leaves of a beech tree *(Fagus grandifolia)* steeped in water, rosewater and witch hazel, eyebright *(Euphrasia officinalis),* and purple loosestrife *(Lythrum salicaria)*—all formed eyewashes. Poultices for soothing sore eyes were made from grated raw potato, beetroot, slippery elm *(Ulmus fulva),* or cold tea. Fumes from cajuput oil *(Melaleuca cajuputi)* were found beneficial. Golden seal *(Hydrastis canadensis),* sometimes combined with other herbs, was widely used (Meyer 1985: 109–114). Flaxseed *(Linum* spp.) was widely used to treat eye problems. The seeds were used, like those of clary in Britain, to aid removal of foreign particles in the eye. The plant was also used to treat eye problems in general and was still found to be widely used in the 1960s (Humphrey 1970: 287–290). For a black eye, raw steak was used, as in Britain. Other recommendations include a poultice of slippery elm or of the fresh mashed roots of Solomon's Seal *(Polygonatum* spp.), or bathing with hot water, an infusion of hyssop *(Hyssopus officinalis)* leaves, or a decoction of the roots of soapwort *(Saponaria officinalis)* (Meyer 1985: 112).

The amount of folklore surrounding the subject of stys is enormous. As in Britain, the tail of a black cat or rubbing with a gold ring are suggested cures (Kimmerle and Gelber 1976 [unpublished]: 31). Conversely, there is an idea that cats cause stys (Cannon 1984: 126). Another frequently cited "cause" is urinating on the sidewalk (Puckett 1981: 456). Even looking at another person's stys can cause them in the viewer (Parler 1962, 3: 939). Carrying a nutmeg as an amulet is claimed to prevent stys (Bergen 1899: 100), while carrying a

sweet potato is said to cure them (Parler 1962, 3: 938). Other cures include salt pork (Simon 1953: 93) or fresh urine (UCLA Folklore Archives 1_6515). Passing over the sty a pebble or a doorknob that has gathered dew is a suggested cure from the western South (Perez 1951: 110). There are about a thousand cures for stys recorded in the UCLA Folklore Archive.

Many of the plants mentioned in these cures have been reported in use by Native Americans for eye problems. Witch hazel, for instance, has been used by the Chippewa to treat sore eyes (Gilmore 1933: 31). Sassafras has been used by five different tribes as an eye medicine (Moerman 1998: 519–520). Slippery elm bark has been used by the Iroquois, the Catawba, and the Potawatomi for sore eyes (Moerman 1998: 577). Flaxseed *(Linum* spp.) has been used by the Great Basin Indian, the Paiute, the Shoshoni, the White Mountain Apache, and the Ramah Navajo to prepare eye medicine (Moerman 1998: 309). Eyedrops have been prepared from Golden Seal by the Iroquois (Moerman 1998: 270). In addition, a great number of other plants have been used in the treatment of eyes by Native Americans; about two hundred different genera are recorded by Moerman (Moerman 1998: 793–794).

*See also* **Amulet, Dew, Elm, Excreta, Golden seal, Houseleek, Mallow, Poultice, Sassafras, Toads and frogs.**

### References

Allen, David E., and Gabrielle Hatfield. *British and Irish Plants in Folk Medicine.* Portland, OR: Timber Press, in press.

Beith, Mary. *Healing Threads: Traditional Medicines of the Highlands and Islands.* Edinburgh: Polygon, 1995.

Bergen, Fanny D. "Animal and Plant Lore Collected from the Oral Tradition of English Speaking Folk." *Memoirs of the American Folklore Society* 7 (1899).

Black, William George. *Folk-Medicine: A Chapter*

*in the History of Culture.* London: Folklore Society, 1883.

Cannon, Anthon S. *Popular Beliefs and Superstitions from Utah.* Edited by Wayland D. Hand and Jeannine E. Talley. Salt Lake City: University of Utah Press, 1984.

Davey, F. Hamilton. *Flora of Cornwall.* Penryn: F. Clegwidden,1909.

Gilmore, Melvin R. *Some Chippewa Uses of Plants.* Ann Arbor: University of Michigan Press, 1933.

Gunton Household Book. Collection of seventeenth and eighteenth-century remedies, Church of St. Peter Mancroft, Norwich.

Hatfield, Gabrielle. *Country Remedies: Traditional East Anglian Plant Remedies in the Twentieth Century.* Woodbridge: Boydell, 1994.

Humphrey, William T. "Flaxseeds in Ophthalmic Folk Medicine." *American Journal of Ophthalmology* 70(2) (August 1970): 287–290.

Kimmerle, Marjorie, and Mark Gelber. *Popular Beliefs and Superstitions from Colorado.* Boulder: University of Colorado, 1976 (unpublished).

Latham, C. "Some West Sussex Superstitions Still Lingering in 1868." *Folk-Lore Record* 1 (1878): 1–67.

Meyer, Clarence. *American Folk Medicine.* Glenwood, IL: Meyerbooks, 1985.

Moerman, Daniel E. *Native American Ethnobotany.* Portland, OR: Timber Press, 1998.

Parler, Mary Celestia, and University Student Contributors. *Folk Beliefs from Arkansas.* 15 volumes. Fayetteville: University of Arkansas, 1962.

Perez, Soledad. "Mexican Folklore from Austin, Texas." *Publications of the Texas Folklore Society* 24 (1951): 71–127.

Porter, Enid. *The Folklore of East Anglia.* London: Batsford, 1974.

Prince, Dennis. *Grandmother's Cures: An A-Z of Herbal Remedies.* London: Fontana, 1991.

Puckett, Newbell Niles. *Popular Beliefs and Superstitions: A Compendium of American Folklore from the Ohio Collection of Newbell Niles Puckett.* Edited by Wayland D. Hand, Anna Casetta, Sondra B. Thiederman. 3 vols. Boston: G. K. Hall, 1981.

Simon, Gladys Hughes. "Beliefs and Customs Reported by Students at Tokyo American School." *Western Folklore* 12 (1953): 85–93.

Vickery, Roy. *A Dictionary of Plant Lore.* Oxford: Oxford University Press, 1995.

# F

## Fat

Animal fats have been used as remedies for a wide variety of ailments, as well as the basis of ointments. In the Scottish Highlands, bruises were treated with butter or fat bacon, and butter with oatmeal was used to bring boils to a head and to soothe chapped skin. The fat of deer was especially valued as a basis for ointments and was also used to treat chapped hands and feet. Snake bites were treated with butter from a cow of one color (preferably white) (Beith 1995: 173–174). In England, goose grease was applied to burns (a practice not recommended today) and, spread on brown paper, was used as a wrap for the chest during the winter, to help ward off colds and infection. It was also used to treat chapped hands (Souter 1995: 142). In Wales, pork fat has been used to treat ringworm, and smeared on muslin it has formed a wrap for sore throat. Butter was rubbed onto sore lips or noses, and into the hair to treat head lice. Goose grease was rubbed into swollen joints (Jones 1980: 62). Clarified lard (usually pork lard) was used as the basis for many ointments (Prince 1991: 107).

In North American folk medicine, fats have been used similarly. Pork fat has treated boils; lard and brown sugar have been applied to bruises; butter or lard has been applied to burns (Brown 1952–1964, 6: 130, 135–137). Goose grease has been rubbed into muscles to make them supple and with molasses has been used to treat croup (Brown 1952–1964, 6: 167, 236). Lard has been used as the basis for ointments—for example, for treating piles (Brown 1952–1964, 6: 249). Grease from a buzzard, goat, or black dog has been used as a rheumatism treatment (Brown 1952–1964, 6: 255–256). Pork fat and snake fat have both been used to treat snake bites (Brown 1952–1964, 6: 278–279). Bear fat was highly regarded in nineteenth-century domestic medicine and was used to treat quinsy and stiff joints (Meyer 1985: 19). Hedgehog fat, eel oil, and skunk oil have all been used to clear the wax from ears (Meyer 1985: 103), and whale oil has been applied to athlete's foot (Meyer 1985: 116).

*See also* **Boils, Bruises, Burns, Chapped skin, Colds, Croup, Piles, Quinsy, Rheumatism, Ringworm, Snake bite, Sore throat.**

### References

Beith, Mary. *Healing Threads: Traditional Medicines of the Highlands and Islands.* Edinburgh: Polygon, 1995.

Brown, Frank C. *Collection of North Carolina Folklore.* 7 vols. Durham, NC: Duke University Press, 1952–1964.

Jones, Anne E. "Folk Medicine in Living Memory in Wales." *Folk Life* 18 (1980): 58–68.

Meyer, Clarence. *American Folk Medicine.* Glenwood, IL: Meyerbooks, 1985.

Prince, Dennis. *Grandmother's Cures: An A-Z of Herbal Remedies.* London: Fontana, 1991.

Souter, Keith. *Cure Craft: Traditional Folk Remedies and Treatment from Antiquity to the Present Day.* Saffron Walden: C. W. Daniel, 1995.

# Felons

In folk medicine this term has been applied mainly to the inflamed sores on fingers known today as "whitlows." However, it has also sometimes referred to other skin conditions. Various native plants have been used in British folk medicine to treat felons. Navelwort *(Umbilicus rupestris)* has been used in the Isle of Man (Roeder 1897). In the seventeenth century, Parkinson recorded that country people used crushed berries of bittersweet *(Solanum dulcamara)* to treat felons (Parkinson 1640: 350), and in some English counties this plant is known as felon-wood or felon-wort. Parkinson also recorded the use of butterwort *(Pinguicula vulgaris)* for hands chapped by wind, known as felons (Parkinson 1640: 534). In the eighteenth century a poultice of the very poisonous hemlock waterdropwort *(Oenanthe crocata)* was used for felons (Watson 1746: 228). In Ireland, hounds tongue *(Cynoglossum officinale)* was used to treat arm rashes, known as felons (Colgan 1904: 309). There are a number of folk medical records from Ireland for treating whitlows, named as such, in the twentieth century. They include gorse *(Ulex europaeus)*, bugle *(Ajuga reptans)*, mouse-ear hawkweed *(Hieracium pilosella)*, daisy *(Bellis perennis)*, chamomile *(Chamaemelum nobile)*, and bluebell *(Hyacinthoides nonscripta)* (Allen and Hatfield, in press). So-called whitlow-grass *(Draba verna)* was recommended in the herbals, but there are no convincing records of its use in folk as opposed to official medicine.

In North American folk medicine there are various miscellaneous cures for felons, such as tying on a toad bone or applying a salve of soap and turpentine (Brown 1952–1964, 6: 186). A hand that has squeezed a mole to death is believed to be capable of curing a felon (Porter 1894: 111). Placing the sore finger into the ear of a cat (Fogel 1915: 272) is a felon cure that depends on transference. An alternative was to place the palm of the hand on the grass and cut out the turf in the shape of the hand. The sod was then turned, and in the time the grass took to rot away the felon would heal (Puckett 1981: 375). In the African tradition, felons, also known as "ring-arounds," were treated with the patient's urine, with cow dung or by pressing the affected finger into the mud (Hyatt 1965: 327). Plant remedies include lemon, sweet potato leaves, and red pepper pods (Brown 1952–1964, 6: 186). Poultices of raw onion or of sassafras root bark, smartweed *(Polygonum* sp.), yellow dock root, blue flag root *(Iris versicolor)*, white birch bark *(Betula papyrifera)*, poke root, Jack-in-the-pulpit *(Arisaema* sp.), or true love leaves *(Trillium erectum)* are other recommendations (Meyer 1985: 120–123). Poultices of red oak bark *(Quercus* sp.) (Browne 1958: 64) or jimson weed *(Datura* sp.) (Puckett 1981: 375) have been recommended. In the Mexican tradition, warmed prickly pear with the thorns removed was used as a poultice (Dodson 1932: 85–86). A remedy from the Native American tradition is a salve prepared from the bark of wild red cherry *(Prunus serotina)* (Meyer 1985: 122).

*See also* **African tradition, Birch, Dock, Earth, Excreta, Mexican tradition, Poke, Poultice, Sassafras, Transference, Urine.**

### References

Brown, Frank C. *Collection of North Carolina Folklore.* 7 vols. Durham, NC: Duke University Press, 1952–1964.

Browne, Ray B. *Popular Beliefs and Practices from Alabama.* Folklore Studies 9. Berkeley and

Los Angeles: University of California Publications, 1958.

Colgan, Nathaniel. *Flora of the County Dublin.* Dublin: Hodges, Figgis, 1904.

Dodson, Ruth. "Folk Curing among the Mexicans." *Publications of the Texas Folklore Society* 10 (1932): 82–98.

Fogel, Edwin Miller. "Beliefs and Superstitions of the Pennsylvania Germans." *Americana Germanica* 18 (1915).

Hyatt, Harry Middleton. *Folklore from Adams County Illinois.* 2nd rev. ed. New York: Memoirs of the Alma Egan Hyatt Foundation, 1965.

Meyer, Clarence. *American Folk Medicine.* Glenwood, IL: Meyerbooks, 1985.

Parkinson, John. *Theatrum Botanicum.* London: Thomas Cotes, 1640.

Porter, J. Hampden. "Notes on the Folk-Lore of the Mountain Whites of the Alleghenies." *Journal of American Folklore* 7 (1894): 105–111.

Puckett, Newbell Niles. *Popular Beliefs and Superstitions: A Compendium of American Folklore from the Ohio Collection of Newbell Niles Puckett.* Edited by Wayland D. Hand, Anna Casetta, and Sondra B. Thiederman. 3 vols. Boston: G. K. Hall, 1981.

Roeder, C. "Contribution to the Folk Lore of the South of the Isle of Man." *Yn Lioar Manninagh* 3 (1897): 129–191.

Watson, W. "Critical observations concerning the *Oenanthe aquatica, succo viroso crocante* of Lobel..," *Philosophical Transactions of the Royal Society* 44 (1746): 227–242.

# Fevers

Until late in the nineteenth century, malaria was endemic in large areas of Britain. This was one of the illnesses often referred to as "ague." Folk medical treatment for it included willow bark. It was observation of this practice by the Rev. Edward Stone in the eighteenth century that eventually led to identification of the salicylates and later to the development of aspirin. Other tree barks too were employed in fever treatment, notably poplar (Tongue 1965: 40). In the fenland districts of England, where the abundant marshes made malaria a particular problem, opium poppies were frequently grown for the relief they could bring. As commercial "laudanum" became available and cheap, it rapidly became a household item for most fenland families.

In the seventeenth century, according to the botanist John Ray, many people wore leaves of toadflax *(Linaria vulgaris)* under the soles of their feet to ward off certain types of fever (Ewen and Prime 1975: 80). Fuller's teasel *(Dipsacus fullonum)* was used as a fever cure in some parts of England (Black 1883: 202). Tansy *(Tanacetum parthenium)* leaves were worn in the shoes to prevent ague (Borlase 1758: 126). Blackthorn berries *(Prunus spinosa)* were used in the Scottish Highlands for treating fevers (Beith 1995: 205). In the Inner Hebrides, poultices of chickweed were applied to the neck and shoulders of a person recovering from fever. Ladies smock *(Cardamine pratense)* and butterbur *(Petasites albus)* are other plants used to treat fevers in the Scottish Highlands (Beith 1995: 209, 213). In the eighteenth century, tea was made from dried mistletoe for treating fevers, a remedy still in use at the end of the nineteenth century (Beith 1995: 227–228). Onions hung in the house were thought to attract fevers, and the survival of one family in an epidemic that wiped out most of the village in the eighteenth century in Angus, Scotland, was attributed to the fact that the house had been "hung about" with onions (Hatfield 1999: 108). The great Celtic hero CuChulainn was said to have been cured of a fever by bathing in a meadowsweet infusion *(Filipendula ulmaria)* (Beith 1995: 236). In Bedfordshire one woman was renowned for her cures of fevers using meadowsweet and green wheat (Aubrey 1881: 255). An infusion of sorrel *(Rumex acetosa)* was given as a cooling drink during fevers (Beith 1995: 243). Wood-sorrel *(Oxalis acetosella)* was used similarly (Beith 1995: 251). Pine bark was used in the Scottish Highlands in the treatment of agues (Beith 1995: 233).

Some fever treatments depended on transference; for example, ague was sometimes treated by making a cake with barley meal and the urine of the sufferer, and giving the cake to a dog to eat (Black 1883: 35). In parts of Scotland, blue woollen threads worn around the neck were thought to avert fever (Black 1883: 113). In Northamptonshire a lace given freely by a woman must be worn by a fever sufferer for nine days (Notes and Queries: 36). In East Anglia in the nineteenth century, notches in a stick were cut equal in number to the attacks of fever. A stone was then tied to the stick, which was secretly thrown into a pond, taking the fever with it (Black 1883: 58). A spider worn in a nutshell around the neck was held to cure fever. This remedy, still practiced in Leicestershire in the nineteenth century, can be traced back to Dioscorides (Black 1883: 59). In the west of Scotland, pills made from cobwebs were used to treat fevers (Black 1883: 60). The right foot of a dead black dog hung on the arm was said in Scotland to be a fever cure (Black 1883: 148). Pieces of rose quartz known as "fever stones" were also used in Scotland. They were dipped into water, and the water was drunk to cure the fever (Beith 1995: 154). Also in the Highlands of Scotland, otter skin was used to make a potion for curing fevers (Beith 1995: 180). Apples, combined with charms, were also used to treat a fever (Beith 1995: 203). In Hampshire, ague patients were given the snuff of a tallow candle on sugared bread and butter to eat (Black 1883: 183).

In Ireland, a son born after his father's death was held to have the power to cure fevers, as was the seventh son of a seventh son (Wilde 1919: 205). Inhaling the smell of a burning leather shoe was claimed to prevent fevers in Nottinghamshire (Addy 1895: 92).

Some folk medical treatments were thought to "draw out" the fever. Warmed salt placed inside socks is a gypsy cure reported from Hampshire (Prince 1991: 124). In South Wales, a woollen sock was filled with earthworms and placed around a feverish child's neck (Prince 1991: 119). "Melts" from the butcher's shop tied to a child's feet were another fever remedy from Hampshire (Prince 1991: 109).

In North American folk medicine, various poultices were similarly applied to the soles of the feet to "draw" fevers. Onions were used in this way, as were heated bags of hops, slices of potato, and horseradish leaves (Meyer 1985: 128). Salt has been used similarly, as in Britain (Brown 1952–1964: 149). A freshly killed chicken split open and applied to the chest was a remedy from Indiana (Brown 1952–1964: 187). Examples of transference of fevers from North American folk medicine include boring a hole in the south side of a tree; the patient blows into the hole, which is then plugged (UCLA Folklore Archives 1_5684). A method reported from New England involved cutting a number of willow rods corresponding to the hour of the day, then burning the rods one at a time, pronouncing at the same time that as the rod burns, the ague will depart (Black 1883: 58).

Amulets used to cure fevers include a spider worn around the neck, as in Britain (Simons 1954: 2). A bag of asafoetida *(Ferula assafoetida)* hung around the neck was claimed to ward off fevers (Lary 1953: 11). An undyed woollen cord worn by a mother was thought to protect a child from fevers until it was weaned (Editor 1893: 66) (compare this with the blue woollen thread mentioned above as used in Scotland). A suggestion from Pennsylvania is that three kinds of food set out on the window sill on Christmas Eve and eaten the following morning will prevent fevers, as will eating hailstones on Ascension Day (Brendle 1951: 1, 7). In North Carolina it has been

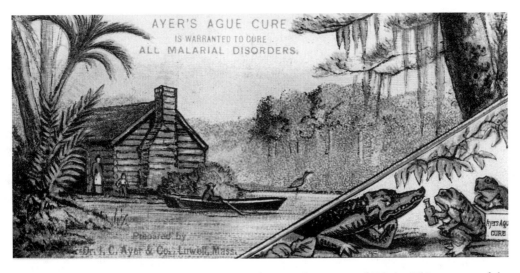

Until the late nineteenth century, malaria was endemic in large areas of Britain. This was one of the illnesses often referred to as "ague." Pictured here is Ayer's Ague Cure "Warranted To Cure All Malarial Disorders." (National Library of Medicine)

suggested that keeping an ear of purple corn in the house will keep away fevers (Clark 1961: 11) From Mississippi there is a report of a custom of hanging empty blue quinine bottles on tree limbs beside a house to ward off fevers (Orr 1969: 109).

Of cures ingested for fever, one of the nastiest-sounding is pills made from dried and powdered human excrement (Saul 1949: 65). Rattlesnake gall mixed with clay was made into pills for fever (Masterson 1946: 185).

Dietary recommendations in fevers were very numerous in North American folk medicine. Eating water melons or bilberries (two kinds, black and sky colored) (Cobb 1917: 103) was recommended, and drinking sarsaparilla mead was very popular in the eighteenth century (Pickard and Buley 1945: 267). Peppermint tea was also recommended (Puckett 1981: 377). Strawberry leaf tea was another cooling drink recommended during fevers (Hoffman 1889: 29).

Herbal preparations used in North American folk medicine for fever treatment are very numerous and include willow (as

in Britain, although probably different species) and snakeroot (*Aristolochia* sp.), combined with white-walnut bark peeled upward *(Juglans cinerea)* (Pickard and Buley 1945: 40). In Tennessee pennyroyal tea *(Hedeoma pulegioides)* and lobelia tea were given for a "slow fever" to clear out the poison, while feverweed tea *(?Triosteum perfoliatum)* was given to counteract the high temperature of the patient (Rogers 1941: 15, 17). Another simple remedy for fevers from Tennessee was to swallow peppercorns as pills (Wilson 1965: 36). Other plants used in fever treatment include boneset, also known as "ague weed," borage (*Borago* sp. or ?*Cryptantha* sp.), and slippery elm (Lick and Brendle 1922: 70, 86). Dogwood *(Cornus sanguinea)* has been used particularly in the treatment of malaria (Cadwallader and Wilson 1965: 221). In Kansas, a tea made from black oak *(Quercus velutina)* was used to treat malaria (Parler 1962: 516).

Among numerous other plant remedies for fevers, a tea made from the black jack vine *(Berchemia scandens)* or a poultice made from castor bean leaves *(Ricinus com-*

*munis)* was used in Georgia (Campbell 1953: 3). A tea made from cherry and apple bark mixed was used in North Carolina (Brown 1952–1964: 187). In the eastern states a tea was made from evening primrose *(Oenothera biennis)* for fevers (Bergen 1893: 142). A tea made from five finger grass *(Potentilla* sp.) has been used in Alabama (Browne 1958: 65); broom weed *(?Gutierrezia* sp.) in Texas (UCLA Folklore Archives record number 11_5379); and the root of wolfsbane *(Aconitum* sp.) in the Great Smokies (Peattie 1943: 118). Other suggestions for fever treatment include the inner membrane of the pomegranate (Bourke 1894: 127) and a poultice of cinnamon and saliva, used in California (UCLA Folklore Archives record number 3_6249). Many of these plant remedies clearly originate from Native American practice—for example, the use of slippery elm and of boneset in fevers (Vogel 1970: 303). Others, such as asafoetida, may have their origins in official herbalism. Yet others, such as elder, could have come from either tradition. (For the numerous other plants used by the Native Americans to treat fevers, see Moerman 1998: 794–796.)

*See also* **Amulet, Apple, Boneset, Chickweed, Dog, Elder, Elm, Excreta, Lobelia, Mistletoe, Onion, Otter, Poppy, Poultice, Seventh son, Spider, Transference, Willow.**

## References

Addy, Sidney Oldall. *Household Tales with Other Traditional Remains Collected in the Counties of York, Lincoln, Derby and Nottingham.* London, 1895.

Aubrey, John. *Remaines of Gentilisme and Judaisme.* Edited and annotated by James Britten. London, 1881.

Beith, Mary. *Healing Threads: Traditional Medicines of the Highlands and Islands.* Edinburgh: Polygon, 1995.

Bergen, Fanny D. "Popular American Plant Names II." *Journal of American Folklore* 6 (1893): 135–142.

Black, W. G. *Folk Medicine. A Chapter in the History of Culture.* London: Folklore Society, 1883.

Borlase, William. *The Natural History of Cornwall.* Oxford: privately published, 1758.

Bourke, John G. "Popular Medicine, Customs, and Superstitions of the Rio Grande." *Journal of American Folklore* 7 (1894): 119–146.

Brendle, Rev. Thomas R. "Customs of the Year in the Dutch Country." *Pennsylvania Dutchman* 3 (November 15, 1951): 12.

Brown, Frank C. *Collection of North Carolina Folklore.* 7 vols. Durham, NC: Duke University Press, 1952–1964.

Browne, Ray B. *Popular Beliefs and Practices from Alabama.* Folklore Studies 9. Berkeley and Los Angeles: University of California Publications, 1958.

Cadwallader, D. E., and F. J. Wilson. "Folklore Medicine among Georgia's Piedmont Negroes after the Civil War." *Collections of the Georgia Historical Society* 49 (1965): 217–221.

Campbell, Marie. "Folk Remedies from South Georgia." *Tennessee Folklore Society Bulletin* 19 (1953): 1–4.

Clark, Joseph D. "Superstitions from North Carolina." *North Carolina Folklore* 9(2) (1961): 4–22.

Cobb, Carolus M. "Some Medical Practices among the New England Indians and Early Settlers." *Boston Medical and Surgical Journal* 177(4) (1917): 97–105.

Editor. "Folk-Lore Scrap Book." *Journal of American Folklore* 6 (1893): 63–67.

Ewen A. H., and C. T. Prime. *Ray's Flora of Cambridgeshire.* Hitchin: Wheldon and Wesley, 1975.

Hatfield, Gabrielle. *Memory, Wisdom and Healing: The History of Domestic Plant Medicine.* Phoenix Mill: Sutton, 1999.

Hoffman, W. J., MD. "Folk-Lore of the Pennsylvania Germans." *Journal of American Folklore* 2 (1889): 23–35.

Lary, Preston A. "William's Township Lore." *Pennsylvania Dutchman* 5(2) (June 1953).

Lick, David E., and Thomas R. Brendle. "Plant

Names and Plant Lore among the Pennsylvania Germans." *Proceedings and Addresses of the Pennsylvania German Society* 33 (1922).

Masterson, James R. "Travellers' Tales of Colonial Natural History." *Journal of American Folklore* 59 (1946): 51–67, 174–188.

Meyer, Clarence. *American Folk Medicine.* Glenwood, IL: Meyerbooks, 1985.

Moerman, Daniel E. *Native American Ethnobotany.* Portland, OR: Timber Press, 1998.

Notes and Queries. London. 1st series, 2: 36.

Orr, Ellen. "The Bottle Tree." *Mississippi Folklore Register* 3(2) (1969): 109–111.

Parler, Mary Celestia, and University Student Contributors. *Folk Beliefs from Arkansas.* 15 vols. Fayetteville: University of Arkansas, 1962.

Peattie, Roderick (ed.). *The Great Smokies and the Blue Ridge.* New York: Vanguard Press, 1943.

Pickard, Madge E., and R. Carlyle Buley. *The Midwest Pioneer, His Ills, Cures and Doctors.* Crawfordsville, IN: R. E. Banta, 1945.

Prince, Dennis. *Grandmother's Cures: An A-Z of Herbal Remedies.* London: Fontana, 1991.

Puckett, Newbell Niles. *Popular Beliefs and Superstitions: A Compendium of American Folklore from the Ohio Collection of Newbell Niles Puckett.* Edited by Wayland D. Hand, Anna Casetta, and Sondra B. Thiederman. 3 vols. Boston: G. K. Hall, 1981.

Rogers, E. G. *Early Folk Medical Practice in Tennessee.* Murfreesboro, TN, 1941.

Saul, F. William, MD. *Pink Pills for Pale People.* Philadelphia: Dorrance, 1949.

Simons, Isaac Shirk. "Dutch Folk Beliefs." *Pennsylvania Dutchman* 5(14) (March 15, 1954).

Tongue, R. L. *Somerset Folklore.* County Folklore 8. Edited by K. M. Briggs. London: Folklore Society, 1965.

Vogel, Virgil J. *American Indian Medicine.* Norman: University of Oklahoma Press, 1970.

Wilde, Lady. *Ancient Legends, Mystic Charms and Superstitions of Ireland.* London: Chatto and Windus, 1919.

Wilson, Gordon. "Studying Folklore in a Small Region. VI: Folk Remedies." *Tennessee Folklore Society Bulletin* 31 (1965): 33–41.

# Figwort (*Scrophularia spp.*)

This plant has been highly valued in British and especially in Irish folk medicine. In Ireland it was known as "queen of herbs" and was used as a tonic and was made into salves for treating piles and skin conditions. One of its Irish names translates as "under elder," indicating that it shared the magical powers of that tree. Like mistletoe, it was thought to lose its effectiveness if it touched the ground (Allen and Hatfield, in press). It was used in England similarly for skin conditions, but less widely (Lafont 1984: 36).

Different species of figwort are native to North America. Their use in folk medicine is relatively slight. They have been used as a blood tonic and for treating erysipelas (Meyer 1985: 40, 108). In Native American medicine they have been used for skin conditions and as a blood tonic after childbirth, as well as for poor vision (Moerman 1998: 524).

*See also* **Elder, Erysipelas, Mistletoe, Piles, Tonic.**

### References
Allen, David, and Gabrielle Hatfield. *Medicinal Plants in Folk Tradition.* Portland, OR: Timber Press, in press.

Lafont, Anne-Marie. *Herbal Folklore.* Bideford: Badger Books, 1984.

Meyer, Clarence. *American Folk Medicine.* Glenwood, IL: Meyerbooks, 1985.

Moerman, Daniel E. *Native American Ethnobotany.* Portland, OR: Timber Press, 1998.

# Fish

In British folk medicine there are a number of remedies involving fish. For whooping cough, placing a live fish in the mouth has been widely recommended (Black 1883: 36); when it is released in the water, it swims away taking the illness with it, a very clear example of transference. The tench, known as the doctor fish, was used to treat jaundice (Radford and Radford 1974: 339). In East Anglia in the days of steam trawlers, an ointment prepared from the liver of a fish was taken on board to heal burns, a frequent occurrence on these vessels (Hatfield MSS). In the Scottish Highlands, the juice of the cuddy fish was used to treat indigestion, and boiled herring was similarly used. Dogfish oil was given to asthma sufferers (Beith 1995: 174). Oil from the liver of a sting-ray was used to treat rheumatism.

In North American folk medicine, the fish has also been used as a whooping-cough treatment (Brown 1952–1964, 6: 351). Rubbing a teething child's gums with a minnow and returning the fish to the water is another example of transference (Barker 1941: 250). Fish oil has been rubbed into sore joints (UCLA Folklore Archive 12_5423), and rubbed over the throat for mumps (UCLA Folklore Archives 5_5435). Fish have been bound onto sore feet (Hyatt 1965: 222), and also applied to the feet for treating typhoid fever (Stout 1936: 190). Slime from the skin of a fish has been used to soothe nettle stings (Welsch 1966: 359). Cod-liver oil, for most people nowadays a "shop medicine" and only marginally a part of folk medicine, has been widely used to treat rickets (Brown 1952–1964, 6), as well as arthritis, boils, burns and piles (Micheletti 1998: 61, 69, 153, 194).

Some Native Americans used fish-liver oil to treat rickets.

*See also* **Asthma, Boils, Burns, Indigestion, Jaundice, Piles, Rheumatism, Rickets, Sore feet, Transference, Whooping cough.**

## References

Barker, Catherine S. *Yesterday Today.* Caldwell, ID: Caxton, 1941.

Beith, Mary. *Healing Threads: Traditional Medicines of the Highlands and Islands.* Edinburgh: Polygon, 1995.

Black, William George. *Folk-Medicine: A Chapter in the History of Culture.* London: Folklore Society, 1883.

Brown, Frank C. *Collection of North Carolina Folklore.* 7 vols. Durham, NC: Duke University Press, 1952–1964.

Hyatt, Harry Middleton. *Folklore from Adams County Illinois.* 2nd rev. ed. New York: Memoirs of the Alma Egan Hyatt Foundation, 1965.

Micheletti, Enza (ed.). *North American Folk Healing: An A-Z Guide to Traditional Remedies.* New York and Montreal: Reader's Digest Association, 1998.

Radford, E., and M. A. Radford. *Encyclopaedia of Superstitions.* Edited and revised by Christina Hole. London: Book Club Associates, 1974.

Stout, Earl J. "Folklore from Iowa." *Memoirs of the American Folklore Society* 29 (1936).

Welsch, Roger L. *A Treasury of Nebraska Pioneer Folklore.* Lincoln: University of Nebraska Press, 1966.

# Flax (*Linum* spp.)

So-called fairy flax, *Linum catharticum,* is native to Britain and has been used in folk medicine for centuries as a purge and, especially in the Highlands of Scotland, for "suppressed menses" (Robertson 1768, quoted in Beith 1995: 96). It has also been used to treat rheumatism (Pratt 1855). Cultivated flax, *Linum usitatissimum,* has been grown as a source of fiber and of linseed, which has been used in cattle feed but also as a basis for poultices for man and beast alike. In present-day herbalism such poultices are still used. The seeds of flax swell in water to form a thick mucilaginous mass, the basis for a poultice for treating boils and respiratory complaints (Chevallier 1996: 227).

In North America, *Linum catharticum* has been introduced. The cultivated flax *(Linum usitatissimum)*, being the most readily available, is probably the species most widely used in folk medicine. The major use of flax in folk medicine has been to poultice swellings (Meyer 1985: 243), boils (UCLA Folklore Archives 1_5296), and stys (Puckett 1981: 456). Its use has extended to the treatment of sore teeth and gums (Meyer 1985: 247) or of a sore and swollen throat (Meyer 1985: 253). As in Britain, the plant has also been used to treat respiratory complaints: pneumonia has been treated with a poultice of mustard and flaxseed (Brown 1952–1964, 6: 250); whooping cough has been treated with a mixture of honey and flaxseed (Clark 1970: 34); and tuberculosis with lemon, honey, and flaxseed (Brown 1952–1964, 6: 308). A flaxseed poultice has treated chicken pox (Lathrop 1961: 5) and smallpox (Lathrop 1961: 14), as well as infected wounds (UCLA Folklore Archives 6_5292) and even (during the eighteenth century) bullet wounds (Vogel 1970: 129). In addition, flaxseed has been used to treat a miscellany of other conditions. Flax seeds, which swell in water, have been used to remove foreign particles from the eye (Puckett 1981: 360) and splinters from the flesh (Lewis 1938: 267). Flaxseed has also been used as the basis of a soothing drink during fevers (Meyer 1985: 132), as a mild diuretic (Meyer 1985: 154), and for kidney trouble (Koch 1980: 63). The plant has been used to treat piles; linseed oil has been rubbed on piles, or an emulsion of the seeds used as an enema (Meyer 1985: 192). Constipation has been relieved by eating flaxseed (Randolph 1947: 97), while diarrhea has been treated using the scraped root of flax (Browne 1958: 41). The water in which flaxseed has been boiled has been applied for headache (UCLA Folklore Archives 3_1913) and drunk as an aid to digestion (UCLA Folklore Archives

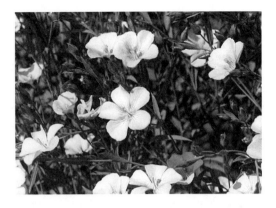

The major use of flax in folk medicine has been to poultice swellings, boils, and styes. Its use has extended to the treatment of sore teeth and gums or a sore and swollen throat. (Library of Congress)

3_5360), to ease labor (Puckett 1981: 20), and to treat diabetes (Puckett 1981: 360). It has even been drunk for heart ailments (Marie-Ursule 1951: 174). Both hand lotion and hair-setting lotions have been prepared from flaxseed (Cannon 1984: 85; UCLA Folklore Archives 1_5910). Flaxseed meal and vinegar have been used to relieve pain (Puckett 1981: 422).

It is not surprising that a plant with so many uses has in addition been credited with the power to prevent or avert disease. Flax fiber has been braided around the neck to prevent mumps (Levine 1941: 490). String or cloth made from flax has been worn to prevent croup (UCLA Folklore Archives 4_7593), while a child failing to grow has been passed through a loop of flax thread: as the thread wears out, so will the child grow (Fogel 1915: 136).

In Native American medicine, many of these same uses are found. The species of flax most widely used is the prairie flax, *Linum lewisii*. This has been used for swellings, as an eyewash, and to aid digestion (Moerman 1998: 309). Another species, *Linum australe,* has been used to treat headache and to ease labor (Moerman 1998: 308).

*See also* **Boils, Childbirth, Constipation, Croup, Diabetes, Diarrhea, Eye problems, Fevers, Headache, Heart trouble, Piles, Poultice, Rheumatism, Smallpox, Sore throat, Tuberculosis, Whooping cough, Wounds.**

## References

Beith, Mary. *Healing Threads: Traditional Medicines of the Highlands and Islands.* Edinburgh: Polygon, 1995.

Brown, Frank C. *Collection of North Carolina Folklore.* 7 vols. Durham, NC: Duke University Press, 1952–1964.

Browne, Ray B. *Popular Beliefs and Practices from Alabama.* Folklore Studies 9. Berkeley and Los Angeles: University of California Publications, 1958.

Cannon, Anthon S. *Popular Beliefs and Superstitions from Utah.* Edited by Wayland D. Hand and Jeannine E. Talley. Salt Lake City: University of Utah Press, 1984.

Chevallier, Andrew. *The Encyclopedia of Medicinal Plants.* London: Dorling Kindersley, 1996.

Clark, Joseph D. "North Carolina Popular Beliefs and Superstitions." *North Carolina Folklore* 18 (1970): 1–66.

Fogel, Edwin Miller. "Beliefs and Superstitions of the Pennsylvania Germans." *Americana Germanica* 18 (1915).

Koch, William E. *Folklore from Kansas: Beliefs and Customs.* Lawrence, KS: Regent Press, 1980.

Lathrop, Amy. "Pioneer Remedies from Western Kansas." *Western Folklore* 20 (1961): 1–22.

Levine, Harold D. "Folk Medicine in New Hampshire." *New England Journal of Medicine* 224 (1941): 487–492.

Lewis, Gabe. "Old-Time Remedies from Madison County." *Publications of the Texas Folklore Society* 14 (1938): 267–268.

Marie-Ursule, Soeur. "Civilisation Traditionelle des Lavalois." *Les Archives de Folklore* 5–6 (1951): 1–403.

Meyer, Clarence. *American Folk Medicine.* Glenwood, IL: Meyerbooks, 1985.

Moerman, Daniel E. *Native American Ethnobotany.* Portland, OR: Timber Press, 1998.

Pratt, Anne. *The Flowering Plants and Ferns of Great Britain.* 5 vols. London: Society for Promoting Christian Knowledge, 1855.

Puckett, Newbell Niles. *Popular Beliefs and Superstitions: A Compendium of American Folklore from the Ohio Collection of Newbell Niles Puckett.* Edited by Wayland D. Hand, Anna Casetta, and Sondra B. Thiederman. 3 vols. Boston: G. K. Hall, 1981.

Randolph, Vance. *Ozark Superstitions.* New York: Columbia University Press, 1947.

Vogel, Virgil J. *American Indian Medicine.* Norman: University of Oklahoma Press, 1970.

# Forge water

The water in which a blacksmith had quenched iron was regarded as therapeutic in British folk medicine. In the East Anglian fens it was recommended for whooping cough (J.C., pers. com. 1994). More generally, it was considered a good tonic for anemia and weakness (Souter 1995: 122). In Suffolk it was recommended for "delicate boys" and for toughening fighters' fists (EFS MSS). It was recommended in Ireland for tiredness as well as for chilblains and for warts (Logan 1972: 68, 120, 140).

In North American folk medicine, forge water was used to treat a number of skin conditions including warts (Parler 1962, 3: 1078), pimples (Wilson 1967: 300), eczema (Hyatt 1965: 263), and freckles (Brown 1952–1964, 6: 198). It was used as a mouthwash for a sore mouth (Wintemberg 1950: 13) and as a soak for sore hands and feet (UCLA Folklore Archives 7_7592).

*See also* **Anemia, Blacksmith, Chilblains, Eczema, Freckles, Sore feet, Warts, Whooping cough.**

## References

Brown, Frank C. *Collection of North Carolina Folklore.* 7 vols. Durham, NC: Duke University Press, 1952–1964.

EFS. English Folklore Survey, Manuscript notes at University College London, 1960s.

Hyatt, Harry Middleton. *Folklore from Adams*

*County Illinois.* 2nd rev. ed. New York: Memoirs of the Alma Egan Hyatt Foundation, 1965.

Logan, Patrick. *Making the Cure: A Look at Irish Folk Medicine.* Dublin: Talbot Press, 1972.

Parler, Mary Celestia, and University Student Contributors. *Folk Beliefs from Arkansas.* 15 vols. Fayetteville: University of Arkansas, 1962.

Souter, Keith. *Cure Craft: Traditional Folk Remedies and Treatment from Antiquity to the Present Day.* Saffron Walden: C. W. Daniel, 1995.

Wilson, Gordon W. "Swallow It or Rub It On: More Mammoth Cave Remedies." *Southern Folklore Quarterly* 31 (1967): 296–303.

Wintemberg, W. J. *Folk-Lore of Waterloo County, Ontario.* Bulletin 116, Anthropological Series 28. Ontario: National Museum of Canada, 1950.

# Foxglove (*Digitalis purpurea*)

Thanks to Withering's careful research in the eighteenth century into a Shropshire folk remedy for dropsy, the development of digoxin in treatment of heart disease has made foxglove one of the best known plants of herbal medicine. In British folk medicine, before the days of Withering, the plant was widely known to be poisonous but was nevertheless used in a number of ailments. It formed an all-purpose salve, used for treating boils and other skin conditions, for example in the Isle of Man (Fargher 1969) and in the Highlands (Beith 1995: 219). In the Forest of Dean up to the twentieth century, the large leaves of the foxglove were wrapped around the breasts to stop lactation at weaning (Hatfield MS).

In Orkney, after it was noticed that geese died after eating the plant, it was not used at all in human folk medicine. In Shropshire, children suffering from scarlet fever were given leaves of the foxglove to wear in their shoes for a year (Vickery 1995: 141); presumably this custom arose out of knowl-

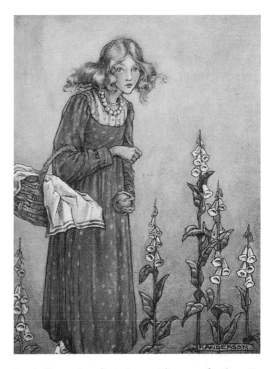

Book illustration depicting a girl among foxglove. In British folk medicine, the foxglove plant was widely known to be poisonous, but was nevertheless used in a number of ailments. The foxglove was introduced to North America in colonial times. (Blue Lantern Studio/CORBIS)

edge of the plant's dangers when taken internally. There are numerous records of fatalities among children in Scotland through drinking foxglove tea (Dalyell 1834: 113), although, according to Withering's son, some people in Derbyshire used the brew as a cheap form of intoxication (Withering 1830). Foxglove tea was used in the treatment of coughs, colds and fevers—for example, in Fife in Scotland (Simpkins 1914: 133). This was a widely used remedy in Ireland (Allen and Hatfield, in press).

The folk records for the treatment of heart disease, of which there are a number, particularly from Ireland, may represent a secondary use, infiltrating from learned medicine and from the publicity surrounding Withering's work.

The foxglove is not native to North America but was introduced in colonial times. Meyer records a nineteenth-century folk remedy for deafness caused by accumulation of wax in the ears. It uses the fresh juice of flowers, leaves, and stalks of foxglove, mixed with brandy and used as ear drops (Meyer 1985: 103). Foxglove was mixed with white rose petals, elder flowers, St. John's wort, and lard to make an ointment for hard swellings (Meyer 1985: 244). It was also used for sores (the fresh juice) and for healing wounds (the fresh leaves bound on) (Meyer 1985: 273). No Native American records of medicinal usage have been traced.

*See also* **Boils, Colds, Coughs, Deafness, Dropsy, Fevers, St. John's wort.**

### References

Allen, David E., and Gabrielle Hatfield. *Medicinal Plants in Folk Traditions.* Portland, OR: Timber Press (in press).

Beith, Mary. *Healing Threads: Traditional Medicines of the Highlands and Islands.* Edinburgh: Polygon, 1995.

Dalyell, J. G. *The Darker Superstitions of Scotland.* Edinburgh: Waugh and Innes, 1834.

Fargher, D. C. *The Manx Have a Word for It. 5. Manx Gaelic Names of Flora.* Port Erin: privately published, 1969.

Meyer, Clarence. *American Folk Medicine.* Glenwood, IL: Meyerbooks, 1985.

Simpkins, John Ewart. *Examples of Printed Folklore Concerning Fife, with Some Notes on Clackmannan and Kinross-shire.* London: Sidgwick and Jackson, 1914.

Vickery, Roy. *A Dictionary of Plant Lore.* Oxford: Oxford University Press, 1995.

Withering, William, Jr. (ed.). *An Arrangement of British Plants.* 7th ed. London: Longman, 1830.

# Fractures

By far the commonest plant remedy in British folk medicine used for helping bones to heal is comfrey. Extract of the root produces a sludgelike putty that can be moulded around a broken limb. With expert splinting, it can produce remarkable results (Hatfield 1994: 6). Sometimes, as in Somerset, a charm accompanied the application (Tongue 1965: 37). In the Scottish Isle of Skye in the seventeenth century, barley and white of egg was applied to a broken limb, which was then splinted (Beith 1995: 204). Goldenrod *(Solidago virgaurea)* was also used in Scotland for healing broken bones (Beith 1995: 221; Martin 1934 [1703]: 230). Mallow was occasionally used in Ireland for treating fractures (Allen and Hatfield, in press). St. John's wort was used throughout Britain to help heal broken bones (Carmichael 1900–1971, 4: 208). In the Isle of Man, a preparation of sanicle *(Sanicula europaea)* was used (Quayle 1973: 70). An alternative in the rural past was a visit to a "bonesetter," who was often the local blacksmith (Buchan 1994: 27–30).

The Mexican equivalent of Scotland's bonesetter was the *sobador* (or *sobradora*), skilled in massage and manipulation (Micheletti 1998: 236). In northern Mexico, chewed peyote root *(Lophophora williamsii)* was applied to fractures (Vogel 1970: 166). A poultice of Yerba Pasma was used to relieve the swelling of fractures (UCLA Folklore Archives 7_6259). In general North American folk medicine, a dressing of egg white beaten with salt was used for simple fractures (cf. the remedy from Skye, above) (Puckett 1981: 330). Carrying a raw potato in the pocket was supposed to prevent fractures or to avoid complications (Puckett 1981: 330, 402). Dressings of cow dung were sometimes applied to fractures (Randolph 1947: 99). There were some strange folk beliefs concerning fractures; stepping over someone's leg could cause it to break; killing a wren could lead to a broken arm shortly afterward (Brown 1952–1964, 6: 193). Even acting as though an arm was broken could cause a later breakage of the arm (Browne 1958: 42).

In the Native American tradition, a poultice of mallow was used to help the healing of fractures (Herrick 1977: 385). Various species of *Artemisia* were used as bone setters, as were species of biscuitroot *(Lomatium* spp.) (Turner et al. 1990: 154, 170). Birch bark and rawhide were used to form splints (Wells 1954: 282), as were cottonwood (*Populus* sp.) and cedar branches (Micheletti 1998: 315). The root of jimson weed was used as an anaesthetic during setting of fractures (Vogel 1970: 84), and spruce gum *(Pinus rigida)* was used to immobilize fractures (MacDermot 1949: 182).

*See also* **Birch, Blacksmith, Comfrey, Excreta, Mallow, Poultice, St. John's wort, Sprains, Thornapple.**

### References

Allen, David E., and Gabrielle Hatfield. *Medicinal Plants in Folk Tradition.* Portland, OR: Timber Press (in press).

Beith, Mary. *Healing Threads: Traditional Medicines of the Highlands and Islands.* Edinburgh: Polygon, 1995.

Brown, Frank C. *Collection of North Carolina Folklore.* 7 vols. Durham, NC: Duke University Press, 1952–1964.

Browne, Ray B. *Popular Beliefs and Practices from Alabama.* Folklore Studies 9. Berkeley and Los Angeles: University of California Publications, 1958.

Buchan, David, ed. *Folk Tradition and Folk Medicine in Scotland: The Writings of David Rorie.* Edinburgh: Canongate Academic, 1994.

Carmichael, Alexander. *Carmina Gadelica: Hymns and Incantations.* 6 vols. (3 & 4, ed. J. Carmichael Watson; 5 & 6, ed. Angus Matheson). Edinburgh: Constable, 1900; Oliver and Boyd, 1940–54; Scottish Academic Press, 1971.

Hatfield, Gabrielle. *Country Remedies: Traditional East Anglian Plant Remedies in the Twentieth Century.* Woodbridge: Boydell, 1994.

Herrick, James William. *Iroquois Medical Botany.* Ph.D. thesis, State University of New York, Albany, 1977.

MacDermot, J. H. "Food and Medicinal Plants Used by the Indians of British Columbia." *Canadian Medical Association Journal* 61(2) (August 1949): 177–183.

Martin, Martin. *A Description of the Western Isles of Scotland.* London: A. Bell, 1703. (Page references cited are from the 4th edition of 1934 [Stirling: Eneas Mackay]: ed. Donald J. Macleod.)

Micheletti, Enza (ed.). *North American Folk Healing: An A-Z Guide to Traditional Remedies.* New York and Montreal: Reader's Digest Association, 1998.

Puckett, Newbell Niles. *Popular Beliefs and Superstitions: A Compendium of American Folklore from the Ohio Collection of Newbell Niles Puckett.* Edited by Wayland D. Hand, Anna Casetta, and Sondra B. Thiederman. 3 vols. Boston: G. K. Hall, 1981.

Quayle, George E. *Legends of a Lifetime: Manx Folklore.* Douglas: Courier Herald, 1973.

Randolph, Vance. *Ozark Superstitions.* New York: Columbia University Press, 1947.

Tongue, Ruth L. *Somerset Folklore.* Edited by Katharine Briggs. County Folklore 8. London: Folklore Society, 1965.

Turner, Nancy J., Laurence C. Thompson, M. Terry Thompson, and Annie Z. York. *Thompson Ethnobotany: Knowledge and Usage of Plants by the Thompson Indians of British Columbia.* Victoria: Royal British Columbia Museum, 1990.

Vogel, Virgil J. *American Indian Medicine.* Norman: University of Oklahoma Press, 1970.

Wells, Warner. "Surgical Practice in North Carolina: A Historical Commentary." *North Carolina Medical Journal* 15 (1954): 281–287.

# Freckles

Freckles are in no way a serious medical condition, which makes the frequency of folk remedies for them surprising. One of the most poetic British remedies is to bathe in early morning dew, preferably on the first day of May (Hatfield MSS). Another widely used remedy was to wash them in an infusion of elderflowers. This country remedy was also used to remove the blackish discoloration of skin from sunburn. Lemon juice was also recommended. In Scotland, buttermilk in which the leaves of silverweed *(Potentilla anserina)* had been steeped for nine days formed a face wash for removing freckles (Black 1883: 119). The juice of sundew *(Drosera* spp.) mixed with milk was used on Colonsay in Scotland; evidently the addition of milk made this "an innocent and safe application to remove freckles and sunburn" (McNeill 1910: 123). Honeysuckle flowers *(Lonicera periclymenum)* crushed in boiling water were used to remove freckles and sunburn in the Highlands of Scotland (Beith 1995: 223). An infusion of fumitory *(Fumaria* spp.) was used in Wiltshire (Vickery 1995: 143).

In North American folk medicine, numerous plants were used to remove freckles. An infusion of elderflowers was recommended, or the juice from chickweed, or an infusion of meadowsweet *(Filipendula ulmaria),* or the seeds of marshmallow *(Malva* sp.) bruised in vinegar (Meyer 1985: 225). An infusion of cleavers *(Galium aparine)* has been recommended, both applied externally and drunk (Willard 1992: 189). Freshly cut potato has been used (Anderson 1970: 36). Grated horseradish *(Armoracia rusticana)* is another suggestion (Bishop 1979: 130). Dandelion juice was claimed to prevent freckles (Cannon 1984: 109). Nonplant remedies include buttermilk applied (UCLA Folklore Archives 1_5385), or carbonic sulphur, salt, and alcohol (UCLA Folklore Archives 12_5385). Morning dew appears in freckle remedies in North America, as in Britain. In one, washing the face in red clover in the morning dew is claimed to prevent freckles (UCLA Folklore Archives 14_5387). Applying vinegar (UCLA Folklore Archives 10_5988), or egg-white and alum (Wilson 1908: 71), or ammonia, lavender water, and rainwater (UCLA Folk-

lore Archives 11_5385) have also been suggested. As in Scotland, urine was claimed to be effective (Brown 1952–1964, 6: 194). Other suggestions are to lie face down in cow manure (Brown 1952–1964, 6: 194) or to plaster the freckles with red mud (Brown 1952–1964, 6: 195). In the Native American tradition, Yucca roots and cornmeal make a face mask recommended for all kinds of skin blemishes (Kavasch and Baar 1999).

*See also* **Chickweed, Dandelion, Dew, Elder, Excreta, Native American tradition, Sunburn, Urine.**

## References

Anderson, John. *Texas Folk Medicine.* Austin: Encino Press, 1970.

Beith, Mary. *Healing Threads: Traditional Medicines of the Highlands and Islands.* Edinburgh: Polygon, 1995.

Bishop, Carol. *The Book of Home Remedies and Herbal Cures.* Toronto: Octopus, 1979.

Black, William George. *Folk-Medicine: A Chapter in the History of Culture.* London: Folklore Society, 1883.

Brown, Frank C. *Collection of North Carolina Folklore.* 7 vols. Durham, NC: Duke University Press, 1952–1964.

Cannon, Anthon S. *Popular Beliefs and Superstitions from Utah.* Edited by Wayland D. Hand and Jeannine E. Talley. Salt Lake City: University of Utah Press, 1984.

Kavasch, E. Barrie, and Karen Baar. *American Indian Healing Arts. Herbs, Rituals and Remedies for Every Season of Life.* New York and Toronto: Bantam Books, 1999.

McNeill, Murdoch. *Colonsay: One of the Hebrides.* Edinburgh: David Douglas, 1910.

Meyer, Clarence. *American Folk Medicine.* Glenwood, IL: Meyerbooks, 1985.

Vickery, Roy. *A Dictionary of Plant Lore.* Oxford: Oxford University Press, 1995.

Willard, Terry. *Edible and Medicinal Plants of the Rocky Mountains and Neighbouring Territories.* Calgary, ALTA: Wild Rose College of Natural Healing, 1992.

Wilson, Charles Bundy. "Notes on Folk-Medicine." *Journal of American Folklore* 21 (1908): 68–73.

# Frogs

See **Toads and frogs.**

# Frostbite

This is not a common enough problem in Britain to have attracted a repertoire of folk remedies. In North America, however, there are a host of suggestions for preventing and treating frostbite.

A newborn baby should have his or her feet and hands bathed in spring water to prevent suffering from frostbite later (UCLA Folklore Archives 12_5389). Wearing snuff (UCLA Folklore Archives 2_6305) or salt (Hyatt 1965: 221) in the shoes has been suggested as a means of warding off frostbite. Walking barefoot three times round the outside of the house in the first snow is a poetic alternative (Farr 1935: 318–336).

Suggestions for treating frostbite include bathing the feet in a westward-running stream (Thomas and Thomas 1920: 104) or soaking in rum (UCLA Folklore Archives 5_6305), or wiping with an old dishrag (Hyatt 1965: 221) or with a mixture of soda and molasses (Frazier 1936: 35). A mixture of water and wood ashes has been recommended (O'Dell 1944: 3). Rubbing with various oils has been tried—for example, olive oil (Browne 1958: 68) or skunk oil (Koch 1980: 1931) or rabbit grease (Puckett 1981: 383). Wrapping frostbitten feet in the skins of rabbits has also been suggested (Thomas and Thomas 1920: 103). Raw beefsteak (UCLA Folklore Archives 7_6834) or cow's gall (UCLA Folklore Archives 6_6834) has been applied, or chicken dung in hot water (Hyatt 1965: 221), or a poultice of cow manure and milk (Beck 1957: 45). Bread and milk has also been used as a poultice (Puckett 1981: 383).

Among numerous plant-based remedies are warm roast potato (Browne 1958: 67),

rotten apple (Cannon 1984: 109), and roast turnip (Meyer 1985: 133) as poultices. Elder bark boiled in hen's oil has been recommended (Meyer 1985: 133). The boiled inner bark of pine has been used (Beck 1957: 45), as has the inner bark of birch combined with cod oil (Bergen 1899: 110). The smoke from burning cedar boughs (*Juniperus* sp.) has been used (Frazier 1936: 35), as has a beech leaf poultice *(Fagus grandifolia)* (Maxwell 1918: 100). These last two remedies are probably of Native American origin. The Potawatomi use beech leaves to "restore" frost-bitten extremities (Smith 1933: 58). Cedar branches are burned to treat a large number of dermatological conditions (Moerman 1998: 282–292).

See also **Birch, Elder, Pine, Poultice, Soda.**

**References**

Beck, Horace P. *The Folklore of Maine.* Philadelphia and New York: J. B. Lippincott, 1957.

Bergen, Fanny D. *Animal and Plant Lore Collected from the Oral Tradition of English Speaking Folk.* Boston and New York: Memoirs of the American Folk-Lore Society 7, 1899.

Browne, Ray B. *Popular Beliefs and Practices from Alabama.* Folklore Studies 9. Berkeley and Los Angeles: University of California Publications, 1958.

Cannon, Anthon S. *Popular Beliefs and Superstitions from Utah.* Edited by Wayland D. Hand and Jeannine A. Talley. Salt Lake City: University of Utah Press, 1984.

Farr, T. J. "Riddles and Superstitions of Middle Tennessee." *Journal of American Folklore* 48 (1935): 318–336.

Frazier, Neal. "A Collection of Middle Tennessee Superstitions." *Tennessee Folklore Society Bulletin* 2 (1936): 33–48.

Hyatt, Harry Middleton. *Folklore from Adams County Illinois.* 2nd rev. ed. New York: Memoirs of the Alma Egan Hyatt Foundation, 1965.

Koch, William E. *Folklore from Kansas. Beliefs and Customs.* Lawrence, KS: Regent Press, 1980.

Maxwell, Hu. "Indian Medicines: Numerous Popular Remedies Obtained from Forest

Trees." *Scientific American Supplement* 86(2224) (August 1918): 100–103.

Meyer, Clarence. *American Folk Medicine.* Glenwood, IL: Meyerbooks, 1985.

Moerman, Daniel E. *Native American Ethnobotany.* Portland, OR: Timber Press, 1998.

O'Dell, Ruth W. "Signs and Superstitions." *Tennessee Folklore Society Bulletin* 10(2) (1944): 1–6.

Puckett, Newbell Niles. *Popular Beliefs and Superstitions: A Compendium of American Folklore from the Ohio Collection of Newbell Niles Puckett.* Edited by Wayland D. Hand, Anna Casetta, and Sondra B. Thiederman. 3 vols. Boston: G. K. Hall, 1981.

Smith, Huron H. "Ethnobotany of the Forest Potawatomi Indians." *Bulletin of the Public Museum of the City of Milwaukee* 7 (1933): 1–230.

Thomas, Daniel Lindsay, and Lucy Blayney Thomas. *Kentucky Superstitions.* Princeton, NJ: Princeton University Press, 1920.

# ❧ G ❧

## Garlic (*Allium sativum*)

Like the onion, garlic was cultivated in ancient Egypt, and it has been grown in European gardens since at least the sixteenth century (Grieve 1931: 343). Both the cultivated garlic and wild garlic or ramsons *(Allium ursinum)* have been used in folk medicine. There are records of garlic used for treating worms in children in eighteenth century Scotland (Lochead 1948: 338), and in twentieth century Suffolk (Hatfield 1999: 134), as well as in treatment of whooping cough in East Anglia, where it has variously been rubbed into the hands and feet, worn in the socks, or made into an ointment (Taylor MSS). A mixture of garlic and May butter was regarded as a cure-all in the Scottish Highlands (Beith 1995: 176). In the same area, garlic was used in poultices to treat diphtheria and bad knees (Beith 1995: 231). In Somerset, an ointment of garlic and lard was rubbed on the soles of the feet to treat bronchitis (Tongue 1965: 37). Wild garlic has been used especially in Ireland, where it has been carried as a prophylactic against fever, used to treat toothache, boils, colds, coughs, worms, and indigestion (Allen and Hatfield in press), and in the Aran Islands, it was even held to prevent blood clots (Ó h-Eithir). Its country name of "ramsons" is reflected in the name of "ramp" applied in North America (where this species does not occur) to *Allium tricoccum*. Both these species are eaten as a spring vegetable.

In recent North American folk medicine, as in Britain, records do not usually specify what type of garlic was involved. The number and diversity of ailments to which garlic has been applied in North American folk medicine are impressive. There seems to have been a widespread belief that many illnesses could be prevented by surrounding oneself with garlic. Garlic hung over the front door was thought to prevent disease entering the house (UCLA Folklore Archives 6_6352). During epidemics in Pennsylvania, some children were sent to school with garlic bags around their necks (Hand 1958: 65). Placing garlic under the pillow was another way of avoiding illness (UCLA Folklore Archives 5_6352). Worn on the person, garlic was thought to protect against smallpox (Brendle and Unger 1935: 97). In Utah, a bag of garlic has been claimed to keep away all infections (Cannon 1984: 113). The ultimate accolade also comes from Utah, where it has been suggested that all sickness can be combated or prevented by wearing a bag containing garlic, sulphur, and cheese, tied with a red ribbon (Cannon 1984: 80).

Wearing garlic has been used to treat as well as prevent disease. Worn around the neck, it has been credited with curing influenza (UCLA Folklore Archives 7_5423), mumps (UCLA Folklore Archives 7_5435),

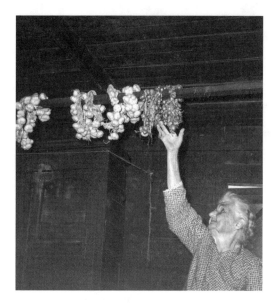

In North American folk medicine, there was a widespread belief that many illnesses could be prevented by surrounding oneself with garlic. Garlic hung over the front door was thought to prevent disease from entering the house. (Library of Congress)

goiter (Puckett 1981: 385), spasms in infants (Saucier 1956: 139), tuberculosis (Webb 1971: 297), colic (Louisiana State Guide 1941: 97), croup (Anderson 1970: 24), and, as in Britain, worms (Puckett 1981: 503). Garlic placed in the shoes is a remedy suggested for insomnia (Hyatt 1965: 270).

The fumes from garlic have been used to treat eye disease (Puckett 1981: 369), fainting (Puckett 1981: 373), and hiccups (Funk 1950: 66). Eating garlic has been recommended for sore throat (UCLA Folklore Archives 2_6499), and arthritis (Puckett 1981: 309), and to prevent snoring (Parler 1962: 891) or bedwetting (Browne 1958: 29). Garlic has been eaten to treat gout (Koch 1980: 128), tuberculosis (Puckett 1981: 468), malaria (UCLA Folklore Archives 15_64046), diabetes (UCLA Folklore Archives 6_5358), colds and whooping cough (Puckett 1981: 346, 501),

sinus problems (UCLA Folklore Archives 1_5467), croup (Davis 1945: 48) and asthma (Pickard and Buley 1945: 41). Garlic has been given to children to rid them of worms, as in Britain (UCLA Folklore Archives 10_587). It has been eaten to lower blood pressure (Clark 1970: 13) and to treat hardening of the arteries (Koch 1980: 127). It has been claimed that eating garlic will prevent mosquitoes from biting (UCLA Folklore Archives 6_6820).

As a topical application, the folk uses of garlic have been equally diverse. It has been applied to ringworm (Parler 1962: 864), to the stings of wasps (Parler 1962: 918), bees (Cannon 1984:114), and scorpions (Brown 1952–1964: 292) and to snake bites (Pickard and Buley 1945: 42). It has been rubbed onto the rash of poison oak (UCLA Folklore Archives 22_6429) and of shingles (UCLA Folklore Archives 13_7616). Worked into and around finger nails, it has been claimed to strengthen them (UCLA Folklore Archives 6_6003). It has been used to treat sores (UCLA Folklore Archives 9_2584), bunions (UCLA Folklore Archives 9_6200), stone bruises (Fentress 1934: 88), and stys (UCLA Folklore Archives 4_6485). The juice of garlic has been dripped into the ear for a migraine headache (UCLA Folklore Archive 19_2185) and rubbed into muscles to cure cramps (UCLA Folklore Archives 13_5592), or rubbed into the scalp for baldness (UCLA Folklore Archives 5_6830). An ointment for wrinkles has been made from garlic and honey (UCLA Folklore Archives 12_5964). Garlic has been widely used to treat toothache (see, for example, Anderson 1970: 76), and a clove of garlic has been placed in the ear for earache in much the same way as onions have been used in Britain (Doering 1945: 153). As a poultice, mashed garlic has treated headaches (Lick and Brendell 1922: 115), moles (Herrera 1972: 43), stomachache

(Puckett 1981: 453), pneumonia (Creighton 1968: 225), and yellow fever (Hendricks 1980: 109).

As an enema, garlic has been used to treat "locked intestines" (Kay 1972: 183), constipation (UCLA Folklore Archives 18_6276), hemorrhoids (Parler 1962: 811), and worms (Street 1959: 84).

In Native American practice, numerous species of Allium have been widely used as food and medicine. Cultivated garlic has been used by the Cherokee for scurvy, deafness, worms, croup, asthma and colic (Hamel and Chiltoskey 1975: 35). Vogel records how soldiers at Camp Missouri in 1819–1820 were cured of scurvy using green herbs and the bulbs of wild garlic (Vogel 1970: 109). For all the other numerous uses of garlic recorded in North American folk medicine, it is difficult to tell whether they arrived with immigrants or were borrowed from the Native American tradition.

Cultivated garlic is one of a number of plants in which there is currently a middle-class resurgence of interest, as part of the trend toward "natural" medicines. Where our forebears, on both sides of the Atlantic, depended largely on native plants for their folk medicine, we now buy packaged extracts of their cultivated relatives. Current research on the chemistry of garlic and other *Allium* species is vindicating a large number of earlier folk uses (Crellin and Philpott 1990: 319).

*See also* **Asthma, Bed-wetting, Boils, Colds, Colic, Constipation, Coughs, Cramp, Croup, Deafness, Diabetes, Earache, Fevers, Gout, Headache, Hiccups, Indigestion, Insect bites and stings, Piles, Poison oak, Poultice, Ringworm, Scurvy, Shingles, Sleeplessness, Smallpox, Snake bite, Sore throat, Toothache, Tuberculosis, Whooping cough, Worms.**

## References

Allen, David E., and Gabrielle Hatfield. *Medicinal Plants in Folk Tradition.* Portland, OR: Timber Press, in press.

Anderson, John Q. *Texas Folk Medicine.* Austin: Encino Press, 1970.

Beith, Mary. *Healing Threads: Traditional Medicines of the Highlands and Islands.* Edinburgh: Polygon, 1995.

Brendle, Thomas R., and Claude W. Unger. "Folk Medicine of the Pennsylvania Germans: The Non-Occult Cures." *Proceedings of the Pennsylvania German Society* 45 (1935).

Brown, Frank C. *Collection of North Carolina Folklore.* 7 vols. Durham, NC: Duke University Press, 1952–1964.

Browne, Ray B. *Popular Beliefs and Practices from Alabama.* Folklore Studies 9. Berkeley and Los Angeles: University of California Publications, 1958.

Cannon, Anthon S. *Popular Beliefs and Superstitions from Utah.* Edited by Wayland D. Hand and Jeannine E. Talley. Salt Lake City: University of Utah Press, 1984.

Clark, Joseph D. "North Carolina Popular Beliefs and Superstitions." *North Carolina Folklore* 18 (1970): 1-66.

Creighton, Helen. *Bluenose Magic, Popular Beliefs and Superstitions in Nova Scotia.* Toronto: Ryerson Press, 1968.

Crellin, John K., and Jane Philpott. *A Reference Guide to Medicinal Plants.* Durham, NC: Duke University Press, 1990.

Davis, Julia. *The Shenandoah: Rivers of America.* New York: Rinehart and Company, 1945.

Doering, J. Frederick. "More Folk Customs from Western Ontario." *Journal of American Folklore* 58 (1945): 150-155.

Fentress, Elza E. *Superstitions of Grayson County (Kentucky).* MA thesis, Western State Teachers College, 1934.

Funk, William D. "Hiccup Cure." *Western Folklore* 9 (1950): 66-67.

Grieve, Mrs. M. *A Modern Herbal.* Edited by Mrs. C. F. Leyel. London: Jonathan Cape, 1931.

Hamel, Paul B., and Mary U. Chiltoskey. *Cherokee Plants and Their Uses: A 400 Year History.* Sylva, NC: Herald, 1975.

Hand, Wayland D. "Popular Beliefs and Superstitions from Pennsylvania." *Keystone Folklore Quarterly* 3 (1958): 61–74.

Hatfield, Gabrielle. *Memory, Wisdom and Healing: The History of Domestic Plant Medicine.* Phoenix Mill: Sutton, 1999.

Hendricks, George D. *Roosters, Rhymes and Railroad Tracks: A Second Sampling of Superstitions and Popular Beliefs in Texas.* Dallas: Southern Methodist University Press, 1980.

Herrera, Mary Armstrong. "The Miseries and Folk Medicine." *North Carolina Folklore* 20 (1972): 42–46.

Hyatt, Harry Middleton. *Folklore from Adams County Illinois.* 2nd rev. ed. New York: Memoirs of the Alma Egan Hyatt Foundation, 1965.

Kay, Margarita Artschwager. *Health and Illness in the Barrio: Women's Point of View.* Ph.D. dissertation, University of Arizona, 1972.

Koch, William E. *Folklore from Kansas: Beliefs and Customs.* Lawrence, KS: Regent Press, 1980.

Lick, David E., and Thomas R. Brendle. "Plant Names and Plant Lore among the Pennsylvania Germans." *Proceedings and Addresses of the Pennsylvania German Society* 33 (1922).

Lochead, Marion. *The Scots Household in the Eighteenth Century.* Edinburgh: Moray Press, 1948.

*Louisiana State Guide.* New York, Federal Writers Project, 1941.

Ó hEithir, Ruarí. *Folk Medical Beliefs and Practices in the Aran Islands, Co. Galway.* Master's thesis, National University of Ireland, 1983.

Parler, Mary Celestia, and University Student Contributors. *Folk Beliefs from Arkansas.* 15 vols. Fayetteville: University of Arkansas, 1962.

Pickard, Madge E., and R. Carlyle Buley. *The Midwest Pioneer, His Ills, Cures and Doctors.* Crawfordsville, IN: R. E. Banta, 1945.

Puckett, Newbell Niles. *Popular Beliefs and Superstitions: A Compendium of American Folklore from the Ohio Collection of Newbell Niles Puckett.* Edited by Wayland D. Hand, Anna Casetta, and Sondra B. Thiederman. 3 vols. Boston: G. K. Hall, 1981.

Saucier, Corinne L. *Traditions de la Paroisse des Avoyelles en Louisiane.* Philadelphia: American Folklore Society, 1956.

Street, Anne C. "Medicine Populaire des Iles Saint-Pierre et Miquelon." *Arts et Traditions Populaires* 7 (January–June 1959): 75–85.

Taylor MSS. Mark R. Taylor Manuscript notes in the Norfolk Record Office, Norwich. MS4322.

Tongue, Ruth L. *Somerset Folklore.* Edited by K. M. Briggs. County Folklore 8. London: Folklore Society, 1965.

Vogel, Virgil J. *American Indian Medicine.* Norman: University of Oklahoma Press, 1970.

Webb, Julie Yvonne. *Louisiana Voodoo and Superstitions Related to Health.* HSMHA Health Reports, 86 (April 1971): 291–301.

# Ginger (*Zingiber officinale*)

The name of this Asian spice has passed into colloquial English as a verb meaning to stimulate, indicating one of its medicinal roles. The plant is not native to Britain, nor can it be readily cultivated there. It is therefore unsurprising to find that its uses in British folk medicine are very limited. It formed a constituent of the official Materia Medica, in both Scotland (Beith 1995: 60) and England (Pechey 1694: 262) and is used in official herbalism today (Chevallier 1996: 153). Its only apparent role in British folk medicine is a recent one: it is used as a home remedy to check nausea and indigestion (Souter 1995: 169, 179).

The plant has a quite different history in North American folk medicine. Introduced into North America by the Spaniards, it became naturalized there, was cultivated, and became a valuable export during the sixteenth century (Grieve 1931: 353). Not only has it been used in official medicine and herbalism, but it has a well-established place in North American folk medicine as well. It has been used to treat nausea and vomiting, as a digestive tonic, and to treat an upset stomach (Meyer 1985: 239, 256, 261). Ginger and honey tea has been taken as a cure for stomach ulcers (Clark 1966:

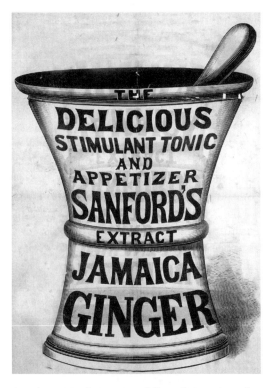

Popular in North American folk medicine, ginger has been widely used as a digestive tonic. It also has been used to treat nausea, vomiting, upset stomach, and a number of respiratory conditions. (Library of Congress)

10). Ginger ale is recommended for hiccups (Barrick 1964: 106). For diarrhea and dysentery, an infusion of ground ginger has been used (Browne 1958: 41). Ginger has treated a number of respiratory conditions. Sprinkled on brown paper, it has formed a poultice for a chest cold (Neal 1955: 286). With molasses it has formed a cough syrup (UCLA Folklore Archives 4_7597). It has been an ingredient of a syrup taken for asthma (Miller 1958: 64), and another for sore throat (Puckett 1981: 446). Ginger has helped bring out a rash (Puckett 1981: 430), treat a fever (Wilson 1968: 78), and relieve a hangover (Paulsen 1961: 157). It has treated fainting (a remedy from the Chinese tradition) (UCLA Folklore Archives 22_6303), headaches (Browne 1958:

70), high blood pressure (Puckett 1981: 402), and insomnia (Roy 1955: 76). It has had varied gynecological uses: for leucorrhoea, for obstructed menstruation, for painful or profuse periods (Meyer 1985: 165, 171, 174, 175). It has relieved neuralgia (Meyer 1985: 186) and formed the basis of a "drawing" poultice, in addition to being used in the treatment of rheumatism and as a constituent of a tooth-cleaning powder (Meyer 1985: 201, 217, 246).

In Native American practice, ginger seems to have played only a minor role (Moerman 1998: 613). The so-called wild ginger (*Asarum canadense* and other species of *Asarum*) is botanically unrelated, belonging to the birthwort family. Wild ginger has been widely and variously used in Native American practice.

*See also* **Asthma, Colds, Coughs, Diarrhea, Dysentery, Fevers, Headache, Hiccups, Indigestion, Nausea, Poultice, Rheumatism, Sleeplessness, Sore throat.**

## References

Barrick, Mac E. "Folk Medicine in Cumberland County." *Keystone Folklore Quarterly* 9 (1964): 100–110.

Beith, Mary. *Healing Threads: Traditional Medicines in the Highlands and Islands.* Edinburgh: Polygon, 1995.

Browne, Ray B. *Popular Beliefs and Practices from Alabama.* Folklore Studies 9. Berkeley and Los Angeles: University of California Publications, 1958.

Chevallier, Andrew. *The Encyclopedia of Medicinal Plants.* London: Dorling Kindersley, 1996.

Clark, J. D. "North Carolina Superstitions." *North Carolina Folklore* 14: 1 (1966): 3–40.

Grieve, Mrs. M. *A Modern Herbal.* Edited by Mrs. C. E. Leyel. London: Jonathan Cape, 1931.

Meyer, Clarence. *American Folk Medicine.* Glenwood, IL: Meyerbooks, 1985.

Miller, Mary E. "A Folklore Survey of Dickson County, Tennessee." *Tennessee Folklore Society Bulletin* 24 (1958): 57–71.

Moerman, Daniel E. *Native American Ethnobotany.* Portland, OR: Timber Press, 1998.

Neal, Janice C. "Grandad-Pioneer Medicine

Man." *New York Folklore Quarterly* 11 (1955): 277–291.

Paulsen, Frank M. "A Hair of the Dog and Some Other Hangover Cures from Popular Tradition." *Journal of American Folklore* 74 (1961): 152–168.

Pechey, John. *The Compleat Herbal of Physical Plants.* London: 1694.

Puckett, Newbell Niles. *Popular Beliefs and Superstitions: A Compendium of American Folklore from the Ohio Collection of Newbell Niles Puckett.* Edited by Wayland D. Hand, Anna Casetta, and Sondra B. Thiederman. 3 vols. Boston: G. K. Hall, 1981.

Roy, Carmen. *La Littérature Orale en Gaspésie.* Bulletin 134, 36 de la Serie Anthropologique. Ottawa: Ministre de Nord Canadien et des Ressources Nationales, 1955.

Souter, Keith. *Cure Craft: Traditional Folk Remedies and Treatment from Antiquity to the Present Day.* Saffron Walden: C. W. Daniel, 1995.

Wilson, Gordon, Sr. *Folklore of the Mammoth Cave Region.* Bowling Green, KY: Kentucky Folklore Society, Folklore Series 4. 1968.

# Ginseng (*Panax* spp.)

In China ginseng has been used as a medicinal plant for several thousand years. In Britain, where no ginseng species is native, the plant did not reach official medicine and herbalism until the eighteenth century (Chevallier 1996: 116), and the plant has played no part in British folk medicine.

In North America, various species of *Panax* are native. The one most commonly used medicinally is the American ginseng, *Panax quinquefolius.* This has been prized in both official and folk medicine, and since it is the root that has been mainly used, its use has endangered the plant in the wild and driven up its price (Micheletti 1998: 174–175). In folk medicine the plant has been used as a tonic, a treatment for hives, to soothe nervousness (Meyer 1985: 141, 185), and to "comfort the bowels" (Brown, 1952–1964: 134). It has been chewed to ward off heart attack (Clark 1970: 23), and the smoke from burning dried ginseng has been inhaled for asthma (Redfield 1937: 14). The root chewed can soothe a tickling throat (Meyer 1985: 255).

Usage among the Native Americans has been similar. *Panax quinquefolius* has been widely valued as a tonic, even as a panacea (Smith 1928: 204). It has also been recommended for its aphrodisiac properties—for example, by the Pawnee (Gilmore 1919: 106). Numerous other ailments, ranging from intestinal worms to tuberculosis, have also been treated with ginseng by Native Americans (Moerman 1998: 373–377). Among the Seminole, ginseng has been so highly valued that long after being displaced from their original territories, they have continued to import it from other tribes (Snow and Stans 2001: 43).

*See also* **Asthma, Hives, Tonic, Tuberculosis, Worms.**

### References

Brown, Frank C. *Collection of North Carolina Folklore.* 7 vols. Durham, NC: Duke University Press, 1952–1964.

Chevallier, Andrew *The Encyclopedia of Medicinal Plants.* London: Dorling Kindersley, 1996.

Clark, Joseph D. "North Carolina Popular Beliefs and Superstitions." *North Carolina Folklore* 18 (1970): 1–66.

Gilmore, Melvin R. "Uses of Plants by the Indians of the Missouri River Region." *Smithsonian Institution-Bureau of American Ethnology Annual Report* 33 (1919).

Meyer, Clarence. *American Folk Medicine.* Glenwood, IL: Meyerbooks, 1985.

Micheletti, Enza (ed.). *North American Folk Healing: An A–Z Guide to Traditional Remedies.* New York and Montreal: Reader's Digest Association, 1998.

Moerman, Daniel E. *Native American Ethnobotany.* Portland, OR: Timber Press, 1998.

Redfield, W. Adelbert. "Superstitions and Folk Beliefs." *Texas Folklore Society Bulletin* 3 (1937): 11–40.

Smith, Huron. "Ethnobotany of the Meskwaki

Indians." *Bulletin of the Public Museum of the City of Milwaukee* 4 (1928): 175–326.

Snow, Alice Micco, and Susan Enns Stans. *Healing Plants: Medicine of the Florida Seminole Indians.* Gainesville: University Press of Florida, 2001.

# Gold

Especially in the form of a wedding ring, gold has been used quite extensively in British folk medicine. Rubbing a sty with a gold ring is a commonly known remedy in British folk medicine (Porter 1974: 43). Gold rings have also been used to treat warts and cuts "throughout Christendom" (Black 1883: 173). In Fife, Scotland, a gold ring has also been used to treat ringworm (Buchan, ed., 1994: 242). Wearing one or more gold rings was held to prevent epilepsy (Tongue 1965: 39). Earrings, often of gold, were worn to improve eyesight or treat inflammation of the eyes (Buchan, ed., 1994: 242). A golden goblet, obviously a remedy only for the wealthy, was considered to protect the person who drank from it from leprosy, jaundice, and heart disease (Souter 1995: 43).

In North America a similar range of conditions has been treated with gold in folk medicine. A gold ring has been rubbed on a sty and on ringworm (Brown 1952–1964, 6: 270, 295), as well as cold sores (UCLA Folklore Archives 4_6275). Wearing a gold ring has been thought to guard against leprosy (Cannon 1984: 116). Earrings of gold have been worn to strengthen the eyes and to prevent sore eyes (Brown 1952–1964, 6: 183, 274). A string of gold beads has been worn around the neck to prevent or treat goiter and quinsy (Brown 1952–1964, 6: 201, 253). A suggested cause of heart trouble is to wear a gold watch near the heart.

*See also* **Cuts, Epilepsy, Eye problems, Heart trouble, Jaundice, Ringworm, Warts.**

## References

Black, William George. *Folk-Medicine: A Chapter in the History of Culture.* London: Folklore Society, 1883.

Brown, Frank C. *Collection of North Carolina Folklore.* 7 vols. Durham, NC: Duke University Press, 1952–1964.

Buchan, David, ed. *Folk Tradition and Folk Medicine in Scotland: The Writings of David Rorie.* Edinburgh: Canongate Academic, 1994.

Cannon, Anthon S. *Popular Beliefs and Superstitions from Utah.* Edited by Wayland D. Hand and Jeannine E. Talley. Salt Lake City: University of Utah Press, 1984.

Porter, Enid. *The Folklore of East Anglia.* London: Batsford, 1974.

Souter, Keith. *Cure Craft: Traditional Folk Remedies and Treatment from Antiquity to the Present Day.* Saffron Walden: C. W. Daniel, 1995.

Tongue, Ruth L. *Somerset Folklore.* Edited by Katharine Briggs. County Folklore 8. London: Folklore Society, 1965.

# Golden seal (*Hydrastis canadensis*)

This plant, native to Canada and the eastern United States, has been extensively used in folk medicine both by Native Americans and by settlers. Native Americans used the plant as a tonic and soother of the digestive tract, as well as for sore eyes (Grieve 1931: 363). The Iroquois used it in addition for liver trouble, fever, pneumonia, and scrofula (Herrick 1977). The Cherokee used it as a tonic and to treat local inflammations (Hamel and Chiltoskey 1975: 36). (For other uses by Native Americans, see Moerman 1998: 270.)

Settlers in North America adopted the plant and found numerous uses for it, ranging from abortion (Micheletti 1998: 180) to prevention of pitting from smallpox (Grieve 1931: 364). Among the uses for it described by Meyer in folk medicine are treatment of weak eyes, impetigo, and indigestion (Meyer 1985: 113, 239, 336). In combination with other herbs, he reports its use for bronchitis, chicken pox, diarrhea, sore eyes, female "weakness," as a tonic after flu, to help alcoholism, for jaundice, liver complaints, heavy periods, sore mouth, gastric ulcer, sore throat, and as a general tonic (Meyer 1985: 51, 60, 93, 112, 124, 133, 135, 147, 151, 168, 175, 179, 243, 250, 256). Clearly the plant was very widely used. It was used for kidney troubles (Clark 1970: 24) and lack of appetite (Roy 1955: 66), and the dry root was powdered and applied to wounds (Randolph 1947: 101). Long records its use for treating night sweats and constipation and adds that it was regarded as a cure-all (Long 1962: 3). During the nineteenth century its reputation spread, and the plant was adopted by the Thomsonian herbalists and by European herbalists, who still use it and prize it. Over-collection in the wild brought the plant near to extinction, but it is now cultivated for medicinal use. Golden seal is not native to Britain and is not easily grown there.

*See also* **Abortion; Constipation; Diarrhea; Eye problems; Fevers; Indigestion; Jaundice; Smallpox; Sore throat; Thomson, Samuel; Tonic; Tuberculosis; Wounds.**

**References**

Clark, Joseph D. "North Carolina Popular Beliefs and Superstitions." *North Carolina Folklore* 18 (1970): 1–66.

Grieve, Mrs. M. *A Modern Herbal.* Edited by Mrs. C. F. Leyel. London: Jonathan Cape, 1931.

Hamel, Paul B., and Mary U. Chiltoskey. *Cherokee Plants and Their Uses: A 400 Year History.* Sylva, NC: Herald, 1975.

Herrick, James William. *Iroquois Medical Botany.* Ph.D. thesis, State University of New York, Albany, 1977.

Long, Grady M. "Folk Medicine in McMinn, Polk, Bradley and Meigs Counties, Tennessee, 1910–1927." *Tennessee Folklore Society Bulletin* 28 (1962): 1–8.

Meyer, Clarence. *American Folk Medicine.* Glenwood, IL: Meyerbooks, 1985.

Micheletti, Enza (ed.). *North American Folk Healing: An A–Z Guide to Traditional Remedies.* New York and Montreal: Reader's Digest Association, 1998.

Moerman, Daniel E. *Native American Ethnobotany.* Portland, OR: Timber Press, 1998.

Randolph, Vance. *Ozark Superstitions.* New York: Columbia University Press, 1947.

Roy, Carmen. *La Littérature Orale en Gaspésie.* Bulletin 134, 36 de la Serie Anthropologique. Ottawa: Ministre de Nord Canadien et des Ressources Nationales, 1955.

# Gout

There were a number of herbal and dietary recommendations for gout in British folk medicine. Among the plants used, ground elder *(Aegopodium podagraria)* is also known as goutweed and was used in both official medicine and in folk medicine (Vickery 1995: 162). A poultice of horse-radish root *(Armoracia rusticana)* was also used (Taylor MSS) or a preparation of tansy *(Tanacetum vulgare)* (Vickery 1995: 367). Roasted hemlock roots were used to treat gout (Radford and Radford 1974: 189). Other plant remedies include bryony, a seventeenth-century remedy (Lankester 1848: 238), and vervain *(Verbena officinalis)* used as a plaster in the eighteenth century (Quincy 1718: 133). In more recent times, herb Robert *(Geranium robertianum)* was used in Devon (Lafont 1984: 46). In Ireland elder has been used (Maloney 1972), as well as comfrey (Logan 1972: 125) and ash leaves (Allen and Hatfield, in press). In the seventeenth and eighteenth century, saffron (from the stigmas of *Crocus sativus*) was used in both official medicine and, where it was grown commercially, in folk medicine (Newman 1945: 355). From this plant colchicine was derived, still sometimes used today in the official treatment of gout.

In the Scottish island of St. Kilda, the ashes of a crow were used to treat gout (Beith 1995: 165). Walking through dew

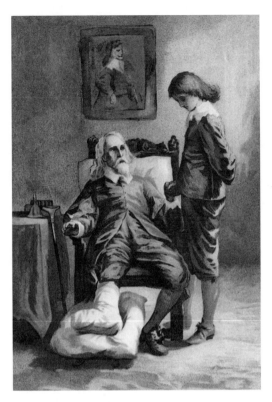

Man with gout. In British folk medicine, there were a number of herbal and dietary recommendations for gout. Ground elder was also known as goutweed and was used in both official medicine and in folk medicine. (National Library of Medicine)

was a seventeenth-century recommendation for gout (Radford and Radford 1974: 133). The foot of a frog wrapped in deerskin and worn as an amulet was thought to prevent gout (Black 1883: 63). Bathing the afflicted joint with urine was suggested in Ireland (Logan 1972: 77). Alternatively, gout could be transferred to a dog by laying on it the painful foot.

North American folk medicine offers dietary advice for gout: abstention from alcohol; eating fruit, such as apples (Browne 1958: 69), strawberries (Pickard and Buley 1945: 45), or cherries (UCLA Folklore Archives 6_5392); and eating bread and water (Puckett 1981: 386) or garlic morning and evening (Koch 1980: 128). Plants used in treating gout include thornapple (Aguirre

Beltran 1950: 494, 502), aralia (Pickard and Buley 1945: 45), and burdock (Clark 1970: 22). Other remedies included snake oil (Knortz 1913: 66) and placing the feet in manure (Carranco 1967: 171) or in hot water (UCLA Folklore Archives 19_5393). Spring waters were recommended too, such as Chippewa natural spring water (Saul 1949: 58). Miscellaneous treatments include tying a string dipped in meat grease around the toes, placing a bowl of water and turpentine under the bed (Parler 1962, 3: 662), burning a string equal in length to the patient's girth (Brown 1952–1964, 6: 201), or transferring the illness to a tree or to a cat or dog (Cantero 1929: 306).

Plant remedies used in the Native American tradition include boneset and a hallucinogenic mushroom called Teonanacatl (Vogel 1970: 164, 284).

There was considerable overlap between folk remedies for gout and for rheumatism.

*See also* **Amulet, Ash, Boneset, Bryony, Burdock, Comfrey, Dew, Elder, Excreta, Garlic, Hemlock, Rheumatism, Thornapple, Transference, Urine.**

### References

Aguirre Beltran, Gonzalo. "Las Daturas en la Colonia." *Anuario de la Sociedad Folkloria de Mexico* 6 (1950): 493–502.

Allen, David E., and Gabrielle Hatfield. *Medicinal Plants in Folk Tradition.* Portland, OR: Timber Press, in press.

Beith, Mary. *Healing Threads: Traditional Medicines of the Highlands and Islands.* Edinburgh: Polygon, 1995.

Black, William George. *Folk-Medicine: A Chapter in the History of Culture.* Folklore Society, London, 1883.

Brown, Frank C. *Collection of North Carolina Folklore.* 7 vols. Durham, NC: Duke University Press, 1952–1964.

Browne, Ray B. *Popular Beliefs and Practices from Alabama.* Folklore Studies 9. Berkeley and Los Angeles: University of California Publications, 1958.

Cantero, Antonio. "Occult Healing Practices in

French Canada." *Canadian Medical Association Journal* (New Series) 29 (1929) 303–306.

Carranco, Lynwood. "A Miscellany of Folk Beliefs from the Redwood Country." *Western Folklore* 26 (1967): 169–176.

Clark, Joseph D. "North Carolina Popular Beliefs and Superstitions." *North Carolina Folklore* 18 (1970): 1–66.

Knortz, Karl. *Amerikanischer Aberglaube der Gegenwart zur Volkskunde.* Leipzig: T. Gerstenberg, 1913.

Koch, William E. *Folklore from Kansas: Beliefs and Customs.* Lawrence, KS: Regent Press, 1980.

Lafont, Anne-Marie. *Herbal Folklore.* Bideford: Badger Books, 1984.

Lankester, Edwin, ed. *The Correspondence of John Ray.* London: Ray Society, 1848.

Logan, Patrick. *Making the Cure: A Look at Irish Folk Medicine.* Dublin: Talbot Press, 1972.

Maloney, Beatrice. "Traditional Herbal Cures in County Cavan. Part 1." *Ulster Folklife* 18 (1972): 66–79.

Newman, L. F. "Some Notes on Folk Medicine in the Eastern Counties." *Folk-Lore* 56 (1945): 349–360.

Parler, Mary Celestia, and University Student Contributors. *Folk Beliefs from Arkansas.* 15 vols. Fayetteville: University of Arkansas, 1962.

Pickard, Madge E., and R. Carlyle Buley. *The Midwest Pioneer, His Ills, Cures and Doctors.* Crawfordsville, IN: R. E. Banta, 1945.

Puckett, Newbell Niles. *Popular Beliefs and Superstitions: A Compendium of American Folklore from the Ohio Collection of Newbell Niles Puckett.* Edited by Wayland D. Hand, Anna Casetta, and Sondra B. Thiederman. 3 vols. Boston: G. K. Hall, 1981.

Quincy, John. *Pharmacopoeia Officinalis et Extemporanea.* London: A. Bell et al., 1718.

Radford, E., and M. A. Radford. *Encyclopaedia of Superstitions.* Edited and revised by Christina Hole. London: Book Club Associates 1974.

Saul, F. William. *Pink Pills for Pale People.* Philadelphia: Dorrance, 1949.

Taylor MSS. Manuscript Notes of Mark R. Taylor in the Norfolk Record Office MS 4322.

Vickery, Roy. *A Dictionary of Plant Lore.* Oxford: Oxford University Press, 1995.

Vogel, Virgil J. *American Indian Medicine.* Norman: University of Oklahoma Press, 1970.

# Gravel and stone

There are innumerable folk remedies for these painful conditions in British folk medicine. One gentleman in Scotland kept a diary of his own health matters during the seventeenth century and built up a collection of remedies for gravel and stone over the years. Though Clerk of Penicuik was a member of the landed gentry and therefore had access not only to medical books but also to the orthodox medicine of his day, some of the remedies he collected from individuals clearly fall into the category of folk medicine. From a wheelwright he had the suggestion of using grated carrot in white wine. Burdock was another suggestion. A remedy provided by the Laird of Innes consisted of the inner bark of the ash, dried and powdered (Clerk of Penicuik Papers).

In the Highlands of Scotland, the blood of wild goats was believed to dissolve both kidney and bladder stones (Beith 1995: 177). In Sutherland, the blaeberry *(Vaccinium myrtillus)* was valued as a remedy for kidney stones (Beith 1995: 206). Dietary advice included avoiding salt (Beith 1995: 160). Wild garlic was recommended for the stone, as was dulse *(Rhodymenia palmata)* boiled and eaten in its own juice (Beith 1995: 219, 241). In the West Midlands, parsley piert *(Aphanes arvensis)* was used to treat gravel (Vickery 1995: 276). An eighteenth-century Sussex remedy for the stone entails roasting a hedgehog skin and adding the powdered prickles to a drink (Allen 1995: 81). In Staffordshire, drinking one's own urine was recommended for gravel (Bergen 1899: 148). In Yorkshire, fasting spittle taken internally was recommended for gravel and stone (Gutch 1901: 177). More pleasantly, in Ireland, the water from a particular well at Larne was drunk to cure gravel (Foster 1951: 115). In Suffolk in the seventeenth century, beans were considered to promote formation of kidney stones (Packard, J. and F. Packard 1981: 9).

In North American folk medicine, a number of fruit and vegetables have been used in treating gravel and stone. Bean seeds, pods and leaves, have been used, as have parsnips and onions. A remedy for gravel consisting of red onion juice and horsemint tea was so successful that the patient gave his informant, a slave, his freedom in thanks for it (Meyer 1985: 161). The kernels of peach stones eaten first thing in the morning have brought great relief to some (Hohman 1930: 26–27). There are a large number of different herbal teas recommended for treating gravel and stone. They include watermelon seed tea (Harder 1956: 98), or an infusion made from corn silk, or pansy (*Viola* sp.), or sarsaparilla (Browne 1958: 69). As its alternative name of "gravel-root" implies, Joe-Pye weed *(Eupatorium purpureum)* was used to treat gravel, an infusion being made from the roots (Bergen 1899: 112). Infusions of flaxseed, buttonweed roots *(?Cephalanthus occidentalis)* (Puckett 1981: 409), or of the leaves and stems of huckleberry (*Vaccinium* sp.) (Yoder 1965–1966: 48) were also used. Other plants, used alone or in combination, include cleavers *(Galium aparine)*, nephritic plant *(Parthenium integrifolium)*, honeysuckle *(Diervilla lonicera)*, bearberry *(Arctostaphlos uva-ursi)*, mountain mint *(Pycnanthemum virginianum)*, spleenwort *(Asplenium trichomanes)*, broom tops *(Cytisus scoparius)*, smartweed *(Polygonum* spp.), milkweed *(Asclepias syriaca)*, shave grass *(Equisetum arvense)*, wild carrot (root and seeds) *(Daucus carota)*, and thimbleweed *(Anemone virginiana)* (Meyer 1985: 161–163). Tea made simply from "boiled grass" has been used (Brown, Frank C. 1952–1964, 6: 201). In North Carolina a tea made from sunflower seed (*Helianthus*

sp.), prickly pear (*Opuntia* sp.), and green coffee has been used (Parker 1907: 249). From the same area, there is a suggestion that applying to the abdomen a hot greasy plate used over cooking beans or meat can bring relief from pain.

To prevent formation of gravel and stones, eating strawberries is recommended (Meyer 1985: 161), or carrying a snail shell as an amulet (Brown 1952–1964, 6: 201).

Many of these plants have been used to treat urinary complaints by the Native Americans too. For instance, *Arctostaphylos uva-ursi* has been used as a tonic for the kidneys and bladder by the Okanagon (Perry 1952: 40); *Equisetum arvense* by the Potawatomi (Smith 1933: 55); and *Galium aparine* by the Ojibwa (Smith 1932: 386). Others, such as broom, may owe their place in North American folk medicine to the European tradition.

*See also* **Amulet, Ash, Burdock, Colic, Corn, Flax, Garlic, Peach, Sarsaparilla, Spit, Urine.**

### References
Allen, Andrew. *A Dictionary of Sussex Folk Medicine.* Newbury: Countryside Books, 1995.

Beith, Mary. *Healing Threads: Traditional Medicines of the Highlands and Islands.* Edinburgh: Polygon, 1995.

Bergen, Fanny D. "Animal and Plant Lore Collected from the Oral Tradition of English Speaking Folk." *Memoirs of the American Folk-Lore Society* 7 (1899).

Brown, Frank C. *Collection of North Carolina Folklore.* 7 vols. Durham, NC: Duke University Press, 1952–1964.

Browne, Ray B. *Popular Beliefs and Practices from Alabama.* Folklore Studies 9. Berkeley and Los Angeles: University of California Publications, 1958.

Clerk of Penicuik Papers, Scottish Record Office Edinburgh, GD18 2125.

Foster, Jeanne Cooper. *Ulster Folklore.* Belfast: H. R. Carter, 1951.

Gutch, Mrs. Eliza. *Examples of Printed Folk-Lore Concerning the North Riding of Yorkshire,*

*York and the Ainstie.* Vol. 2 of *County Folk-Lore.* London: Folk-Lore Society, 1901.

Harder, Kelsie B. "Home Remedies in Perry County, Tennessee." *Tennessee Folklore Society Bulletin* 22 (1956): 97–98.

Hohman, John George. *Long Lost Friend, or Book of Pow-Wows: A Collection of Mysterious and Invaluable Arts and Remedies for Man as Well as Animals.* Edited by A. Monroe Aurand, Jr., Harrisburg, PA: The Aurand Press 1930.

Meyer, Clarence. *American Folk Medicine.* Glenwood, IL: Meyerbooks, 1985.

Packard, J., and F. Packard. *Herbal Review.* Vol. 6 (1981). London: The Herb Society.

Parker, Haywood. "Folk-Lore of the North Carolina Mountaineers." *Journal of American Folklore* 20 (1907): 241–250.

Perry, F. "Ethno-Botany of the Indians in the Interior of British Columbia." *Museum and Art Notes* 2(2): 36–43 (1952).

Puckett, Newbell Niles. *Popular Beliefs and Superstitions: A Compendium of American Folklore from the Ohio Collection of Newbell Niles Puckett.* Edited by Wayland D. Hand, Anna Casetta, and Sondra B. Thiederman. 3 vols. Boston: G. K. Hall, 1981.

Smith, Huron H. "Ethnobotany of the Ojibwe Indians." *Bulletin of the Public Museum of Milwaukee* 4 (1932): 327–525.

———. "Ethnobotany of the Forest Potawatomi Indians." *Bulletin of the Public Museum of the City of Milwaukee* 7 (1933): 1–230.

Vickery, Roy. *A Dictionary of Plant Lore.* Oxford: Oxford University Press, 1995.

Yoder, Don. "Official Religion Versus Folk Religion." *Pennsylvania Folklife* 15(2) (Winter 1965/66): 36–52.

# H

## Hair Problems

Rosemary *(Rosmarinus officinalis)* is one of the most commonly recommended plants for hair problems. Native to southern Europe, it is cultivated worldwide. An infusion of the chopped leaves is added to the final rinse water (Vickery 1995: 319; Taylor MSS). Proprietary shampoos often contain rosemary extract, which thickens the hair and leaves it shiny. A gypsy cure for thinning hair was prepared from rosemary and hedgehog fat (Souter 1995: 164). Chamomile *(Chamaemelum nobile)* is widely used as a rinse, especially for blonde hair (Vickery 1995: 63). Sage *(Salvia officinalis)* has been used as a hair tonic and to darken hair going grey (Quelch 1941: 274). To prevent dandruff, a folk cure was to rub a raw egg into the scalp before washing (Prince 1991: 21). In the nineteenth century the juice of houseleek was used (Weston, Norfolk Record Office). To encourage regrowth of hair—for example, after ringworm—it was claimed that the powder of a burned cork rubbed into the scalp would help (Taylor MSS). Burdock has been claimed to aid regrowth of hair (Prince 1991: 95). Head lice have been treated with a preparation of spindle berries *(Euonymus europaeus)* (Freethy 1985: 100).

In North American folk medicine a remedy used by early settlers to thicken the hair was made from shavings of hartshorn mixed with oil (Robertson 1960: 6). Castor oil (from *Ricinus communis*) and corn oil (from *Zea mays*) have both been used in Vermont to improve the health of the hair and remove dandruff (Jarvis 1961: 146, 150). Olive oil to strengthen the hair and correct split ends is a remedy used in Mexico (UCLA Folklore Archives 3_5592). In Canada, Native Americans made a hair oil from the sunflower (*Helianthus* sp.) (Bourke 1895: 48). A hair oil was prepared by the Blackfoot from the balsam fir, *Abies lasiocarpa* (McClintock 1909: 273). Various species of *Yucca* (known as soapwort) have a reputation as a hair tonic and to prevent baldness (Willard 1992: 58). On the other hand, this plant apparently causes rashes in some people, and one Mexican remedy suggests instead the juice of the Cholla cactus (*Opuntia* sp.) (UCLA Folklore Archives 10_5590).

Specifically to treat falling hair, a number of folk remedies have been recorded from North America. Sagebrush tea (*Artemisia* spp.) was found to help hair grow and prevent greyness and hair loss (Fife 1957: 155). In Saskatchewan, a mixture of castor oil (from *Ricinus communis*) and iodine has been suggested (UCLA Folklore Archives 16_5393). Also in Saskatchewan, watercress *(Nasturtium officinale)* has been found useful to prevent falling hair (UCLA Folklore Archives 16_5391). In Texas, persimmon juice (*Diospyros* sp.) has been recommended

(Hendricks 1980: 85), and in Oregon, onions steeped in rum (UCLA Folklore Archives 12_5391). Cleaning the head with kerosene is an old-fashioned remedy for head lice used in both Britain (Hatfield MS) and North America (Cannon 1984: 116).

Among the Native Americans, various species of sage (*Salvia* spp.) have been used to strengthen the hair, dye it, and even, among the Cahuilla, straighten it (Bean and Saubel 1972: 136). The maidenhair fern (*Adiantum* spp.) has been used as a hair wash by the Lummi, Makah, and Skomish (Gunther 1973: 14). The Blackfoot used a wash of little blanket (*Apocynum cannabinum*) or of bear grass (*Yucca glauca*) to prevent hair falling out (McClintock 1909: 276, 274). Yucca root has been recommended for dandruff (UCLA Folklore Archives 20_6282). The berries of Devil's Club (*Oplopanax horridus*) were used as a hair tonic and to treat dandruff in young children (Willard 1992: 151). Among the Oweekeno, the berries were rubbed into the scalp to treat head lice (Compton 1993: 85). The Chinook used fermented urine for healthy, flea-free hair (LaBarre 1951: 175). In the nineteenth century, Josselyn reported the use of Hellebore root (probably *Veratrum viride*) in New England for the treatment of head lice (Josselyn 1833: 262). This plant is on record as used by the Kwakiutl for treating dandruff (Turner and Bell 1973: 273) and by the Shushwap to make hair grow on a bald head (Palmer 1975: 55).

Hair has always been regarded as a symbolic part of a person, hence many spells and curses employ hair from the would-be victim. Perhaps this explains in part the large number of superstitions surrounding hair. Of these, the commonest in North America seems to concern disposal of hair combings; if a bird acquires the combings, the owner will die, go mad, or lose all his

or her hair. Some suggest that March is an unlucky time to cut hair (Brown 1952–1964, 6: 121), others that cutting hair on the first day of March ensures its health (Puckett 1981: 163). A German-American belief is that to cut the hair when the moon is increasing will ensure a healthy luxuriant head of hair (Starr 1891: 322). In Britain it has been believed that hair should be cut when the moon is waxing to ensure it grows quickly, and when the moon is waning for slower growth (Radford and Radford 1974: 177). These beliefs are reported from North American too (Brown 1952–1964, 6: 202, 203).

Among Native Americans, the Micmac used an eel skin to tie the hair, which would ensure the hair grew long (Parsons 1926: 485). Oddly, there seems to have been a belief among African Americans that this same practice would cause lice to breed (Bergen 1899). Rattlesnake oil was used by the Nahuatl to make the hair grow "as long as a snake" (Madsen 1955: 132).

*See also* **Baldness, Burdock, Houseleek.**

**References**
Bean, Lowell John, and Katherine Siba Saubel. *Temalpakh (From the Earth): Cahuilla Indian Knowledge and Usage of Plants.* Banning, CA: Malki Museum Press, 1972.
Bergen, F. D. "Animal and Plant Lore." *Memoirs of the American Folklore Society* 7 (1899).
Bourke, John G. "Folk-Foods of the Rio Grande Valley and of Northern Mexico." *Journal of American Folklore* 8 (1895): 41–71.
Brown, Frank C. *Collection of North Carolina Folklore.* 7 vols. Durham, NC: Duke University Press, 1952–1964.
Cannon, Anthon S. *Popular Beliefs and Superstitions from Utah.* Edited by Wayland D. Hand and Jeannine E. Talley. Salt Lake City: University of Utah Press, 1984.
Compton, Brian Douglas. *Upper North Wakashan and Southern Tsimshian Ethnobotany: The Knowledge and Usage of Plants.* Ph.D. dis-

sertation, University of British Columbia, Vancouver, 1993.

Fife, Austin E. "Pioneer Mormon Remedies." *Western Folklore* 16 (1957): 153–162.

Freethy, Ron. *From Agar to Zenry.* Marlborough: Crowood Press, 1985.

Gunther, Erna. *Ethnobotany of Western Washington.* Rev. ed. Seattle: University of Washington Press, 1973.

Hendricks, George D. "Roosters, Rhymes and Railroad Tracks." In *A Second Sampling of Superstitions and Popular Beliefs in Texas.* Dallas, TX: Southern Methodist University Press, 1980.

Jarvis, D. C. *Folk Medicine.* London: Pan Books, 1961.

Josselyn, John. *An Account of Two Voyages to New England Made during the Years 1638, 1663.* Reprint 1833.

LaBarre, Weston. "Aymara Biologicals and Other Medicines." *Journal of American Folklore* 64 (1951): 171–178.

Madsen, William. "Hot and Cold in the Universe of San Francisco Tecospa, Valley of Mexico." *Journal of American Folklore* 68 (1955): 123–139.

McClintock, Walter. "Materia Medica of the Blackfeet." *Zeitschrift für Ethnologie* 11 (1909): 273–276.

Palmer, Gary. "Shuswap Indian Ethnobotany." *Syesis* 8 (1975): 29–51.

Parsons, Elsie Clews. "Micmac Notes." *Journal of American Folklore* 39 (1926): 460–485.

Prince, Dennis. *Grandmother's Cures: An A–Z of Herbal Remedies.* London: Fontana, 1991.

Puckett, Newbell Niles. *Popular Beliefs and Superstitions: A Compendium of American Folklore from the Ohio Collection of Newbell Niles Puckett.* Edited by Wayland D. Hand, Anna Casetta, and Sondra B. Thiederman. 3 vols. Boston: G. K. Hall, 1981.

Quelch, Mary Thorne. *Herbs for Daily Use.* London: Faber and Faber, 1941.

Radford, E., and M. A. Radford. *Encyclopaedia of Superstitions.* Edited and revised by Christina Hole. London: Book Club Associates 1974.

Robertson, Marion. *Old Settlers' Remedies.* Bar-rington, NS: Cape Sable Historical Society, 1960.

Souter, Keith. *Cure Craft: Traditional Folk Remedies and Treatment from Antiquity to the Present Day.* Saffron Walden: C. W. Daniel, 1995.

Starr, Frederick. "Some Pennsylvania German Lore." *Journal of American Folklore* 4 (1891): 321–326.

Taylor MSS. Manuscript notes of Mark R. Taylor in Norfolk Records Office, Norwich. MS4322.

Turner, Nancy Chapman, and Marcus A. M. Bell. "The Ethnobotany of the Southern Kwakiutl Indians of British Columbia." *Economic Botany* 27 (1973): 257–310.

Vickery, Roy. *A Dictionary of Plant Lore.* Oxford: Oxford University Press, 1995.

Weston, Maryanne. Diary notes in Norfolk Record Office, Norwich NRO MC 43/9.

Willard, Terry. *Edible and Medicinal Plants of the Rocky Mountains and Neighbouring Territories.* Calgary, ALTA: Wild Rose College of Natural Healing, 1992.

# Hand, Wayland D. (1907–1986)

Born in New Zealand and a student originally of German, Wayland Debs Hand taught at the University of Minnesota before joining the University of California at Los Angeles (UCLA). Here he developed his studies of folklore, a subject to which he devoted the rest of his life. He gave the first-ever undergraduate lectures in folklore at the university. His work in collecting and archiving folk medical remedies led directly to the formation of the Folklore Archive at UCLA, now a world-famous resource. Among his many publications, one of the most famous is *The Encyclopedia of American Popular Belief and Superstition,* published in 1976. He edited and annotated volumes 6 and 7 of the Frank C. Brown Collection of North Carolina Folklore. He was president and a fellow of the American

Folklore Society and was awarded a knighthood in Finland.

**Reference**

Cattermole-Tally, Frances. Obituary: Wayland Debs Hand (1907–1986). *Journal of American Folklore* 102(404) (1989): 183–185.

# Hawthorn (*Crataegus spp.*)

Also known as "may" in many country areas, this tree has attracted numerous superstitions, including the idea that it is unlucky to bring its flowers into the house (Vickery 1995: 166). In British folk medicine there are records from Devon and the Isle of Man of its use as a heart tonic (Lafont 1984: 44; Quayle 1973: 70) and from Scotland of its use in controlling blood pressure (Beith 1995: 221)—both uses familiar to modern-day herbalists.

In the Highlands of Scotland, the bark has also been used for sore throat (Beith 1995: 221). In East Anglia an infusion of the leaves has been used to ease labor pains (Newman and Wilson 1951), in much the same way raspberry leaves are widely used. The leaves were used as a poultice to bring boils to a head and to remove stubborn splinters (Souter 1995: 128). An infusion of the leaves was used to treat anxiety and to stimulate the appetite (Souter 1995: 134). The young leaves (known as "bread and cheese" in many country areas of England) are eaten by country children in the spring. Dew from the hawthorn tree, gathered on the first day of May, was thought to ensure a beautiful complexion (Souter 1995: 147). A twentieth-century toothache remedy from Ireland is to chew hawthorn bark (Westropp 1911: 57–58). Because the hawthorn was revered, some remedies gain power by being associated with it. Mistletoe growing specifically on hawthorn was regarded as a cure for epilepsy (Leather 1912: 79). A common wart cure involved rubbing

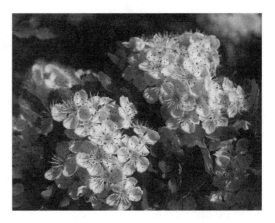

The hawthorn tree has attracted numerous superstitions, including the idea that it is unlucky to bring its flowers into the house. In Britain, rubbing the face with dew from a hawthorn bush on the first day of May was believed to remove freckles and ensure a good complexion. (Pat Jerrold)

the wart with a slug or snail, which was then impaled on a hawthorn twig. Hawthorn was often planted in the hedges around pastures, and traditionally the afterbirth of a cow was hung in the thorn to prevent milk fever and ensure fertility of the cattle for the following year (W.A., pers. com., Trunch, Norfolk 1980; Vickery 1995: 170).

English may (after which the *Mayflower* was named) was taken to North America by English settlers. Meanwhile, the numerous native species of hawthorn were already in use by Native Americans. Interestingly, some of these were used to improve blood circulation (e.g., *Crataegus spathulata* was used by the Cherokee [Hamel and Chiltoskey 1975: 37]). The "discovery" of hawthorn as a blood tonic is attributed to a nineteenth-century Irish physician (Chevallier 1996: 86), but evidently there was at least scattered knowledge of its use long before then. Other Native American uses for hawthorn include treatment of diarrhea, using berries and bark (e.g., Turner, Thompson et al. 1990: 258). (For further Native American uses of hawthorns see Moerman 1998: 182–183.)

In general North American folk medicine, hawthorn berries have been used in a mixture to treat rheumatism (Meyer 1985: 215). Simply wearing hawthorn around the neck as an amulet was an alternative recommended in Arkansas (Parler 1962, 3: 854). A French Canadian cure for stubborn ulcers was to hide the dressings under a hawthorn; anyone touching them would acquire the ulcers, an example of transference (Cantero 1929: 306). As in Britain, rubbing the face with dew from a hawthorn bush on the first day of May was believed to remove freckles and ensure a good complexion (Puckett 1981: 383).

*See also* **Amulet, Boils, Dew, Diarrhea, Freckles, Heart trouble, Mistletoe, Poultice, Rheumatism, Sore throat, Toothache, Transference, Warts.**

### References

Beith, Mary. *Healing Threads: Traditional Medicines of the Highlands and Islands.* Edinburgh: Polygon, 1995.

Cantero, Antonio. "Occult Healing Practices in French Canada." *Canadian Medical Association Journal.* Canadian Medical Association, New Series, 20 (1929): 303–306.

Chevallier, Andrew. *The Encyclopedia of Medicinal Plants.* London: Dorling Kindersley, 1996.

Hamel, Paul B., and Mary U. Chiltoskey. *Cherokee Plants and Their Uses: A 400 Year History.* Sylva, NC: Herald, 1975.

Lafont, Anne-Marie. *Herbal Folklore.* Bideford: Badger Books, 1984.

Leather, Ella Mary. *The Folk-Lore of Herefordshire Collected from Oral and Printed Sources.* Hereford and London: Jakeman and Carver, 1912.

Meyer, Clarence. *American Folk Medicine.* Glenwood, IL: Meyerbooks, 1985.

Moerman, Daniel E. *Native American Ethnobotany.* Portland, OR: Timber Press, 1998.

Newman, L. F. and E. M. Wilson. "Folk-Lore Survivals in the Southern 'Lake Counties' and in Essex: A Comparison and Contrast. Part I." *Folk-Lore* 62 (1951): 252–266.

Parler, Mary Celestia, and University Student Contributors. *Folk Beliefs from Arkansas.* 15 vols. Fayetteville: University of Arkansas, 1962.

Puckett, Newbell Niles. *Popular Beliefs and Superstitions: A Compendium of American Folklore from the Ohio Collection of Newbell Niles Puckett.* Edited by Wayland D. Hand, Anna Casetta, and Sondra B. Thiederman. 3 vols. Boston: G. K. Hall, 1981.

Quayle, George E. *Legends of a Lifetime: Manx-Folklore.* Douglas: Courier Herald, 1973.

Souter, Keith. *Cure Craft: Traditional Folk Remedies and Treatment from Antiquity to the Present Day.* Saffron Walden: C. W. Daniel, 1995.

Turner, Nancy J., Laurence C. Thompson, M. Terry Thompson, and Annie Z. York. *Thompson Ethnobotany: Knowledge and Usage of Plants by the Thompson Indians of British Columbia.* Victoria: Royal British Columbia Museum, 1990.

Vickery, Roy. *A Dictionary of Plant Lore.* Oxford: Oxford University Press, 1995.

Westropp, Thomas. "A Folklore Survey of County Clare." *Folk-Lore* 22 (1911): 49–60.

# Hay fever

One of the most interesting folk treatments for hay fever in Britain is the use of honey. Honey produced locally (and therefore containing the pollen from the local flora) and eaten throughout the winter has been found very helpful by some sufferers from hay fever (pers. com., 1977, 2002). Lime water and milk has been suggested as a hay fever medicine. Another remedy was to inhale the fumes from Friar's balsam and to drink sherry with hot milk and sugar (Prince 1991: 32). Inhaling the scent of mint, by placing it under the pillow and wearing a sprig during the day, is a remedy of gypsy origin (Vickery 1995: 240).

In North American folk medicine recommendations include rubbing the ears until they are red and hot, inhaling the fumes from coffee sprinkled on hot coals, or from vinegar and horseradish *(Armoracia rusti-*

*cana),* or from a pungent oil such as peppermint (cf. British remedy above) or rosemary. Inhaling salt and water has been suggested (UCLA Folklore Archives 1_6308), or bathing in vinegar and warm water (Doering 1944: 141). Lying on a pillow of hemlock boughs (*Tsuga* sp.), or inhaling the smell of freshly crushed milkweed (*Asclepias* sp.) are alternatives. It has been claimed that the leaves and flowers of ragweed (*Ambrosia* sp.) and golden rod (*Solidago* sp.) infused in boiling water can cure hay fever (Meyer 1985: 135–136). Other herbal treatments include inhalation of steamed camphor; smoking mullein leaves, use of snuff made from yellow dock root, and a pillow stuffed with "life everlasting" *(Gnaphalium obtusifolium)* (Micheletti 1998: 185). Smoking dried life everlasting, also known as rabbit tobacco, has been tried (Browne 1958: 70). Drinking sassafras tea in the spring was thought to help prevent hay fever (UCLA Folklore Archives 16_5394). Drinking an infusion of the weed thought to be the cause of the hay fever is another remedy (Parler 1962, 3: 708).

As in Britain, local honey is recommended to "immunize" against hay fever (Jarvis 1961: 115–119). Chewing honeycomb is also recommended (Hendricks 1966: 46). A poetic hay fever remedy is to eat the color out of violets in the spring (Cannon 1984: 110). Walking barefoot in the dew at the time of a new moon has also been suggested (Puckett 1981: 388). Alternatively, one can cut a willow branch the same length as the sufferer and put it in the loft. By the time it is dry, the hay fever will be better (Browne 1958: 70).

Biscuitroot *(Lomatium dissectum)* is one of the plants used by Native Americans to treat hay fever (Train, Henrichs, and Archer 1941: 97–100). Strawberry (*Fragaria* sp.) has also been used (Willard 1992: 112), as has mint (Hamel and Chiltoskey 1975: 427).

*See also* **Dew, Dock, Honey, Mullein, Sassafras.**

## References

Browne, Ray B. *Popular Beliefs and Practices from Alabama.* Folklore Studies 9. Berkeley and Los Angeles: University of California Publications, 1958.

Cannon, Anthon S. *Popular Beliefs and Superstitions from Utah.* Edited by Wayland D. Hand and Jeannine E. Talley. Salt Lake City: University of Utah Press, 1984.

Doering, J. Frederick. "Folk Remedies for Divers Allergies." *Journal of American Folklore* 57 (1944): 140–141.

Hamel, Paul B., and Mary U. Chiltoskey. *Cherokee Plants and Their Uses: A 400 Year History.* Sylva, NC: Herald, 1975.

Hendricks, George D. *Mirrors, Mice and Mustaches: A Sampling of Superstitions and Popular Beliefs in Texas.* Austin: Texas Folklore Society, 1966.

Jarvis, D. C. *Folk Medicine.* London: Pan Books, 1961.

Meyer, Clarence. *American Folk Medicine.* Glenwood, IL: Meyerbooks, 1985.

Micheletti, Enza (ed.). *North American Folk Healing: An A–Z Guide to Traditional Remedies.* New York and Montreal: Reader's Digest Association, 1998.

Parler, Mary Celestia, and University Student Contributors. *Folk Beliefs from Arkansas.* 15 vols. Fayetteville: University of Arkansas, 1962.

Prince, Dennis. *Grandmother's Cures: An A–Z of Herbal Remedies.* London: Fontana, 1991.

Puckett, Newbell Niles. *Popular Beliefs and Superstitions: A Compendium of American Folklore from the Ohio Collection of Newbell Niles Puckett.* Edited by Wayland D. Hand, Anna Casetta, and Sondra B. Thiederman. 3 vols. Boston: G. K. Hall, 1981.

Train, Percy, James R. Henrichs, and W. Andrew Archer. *Medicinal Uses of Plants by Indian Tribes of Nevada.* Washington, DC: U.S. Department of Agriculture, 1941.

Vickery, Roy. *A Dictionary of Plant Lore.* Oxford: Oxford University Press, 1995.

Willard, Terry. *Edible and Medicinal Plants of the Rocky Mountains and Neighbouring Territo-*

*ries.* Calgary, ALTA: Wild Rose College of Natural Healing, 1992.

# Head lice

*See* **Hair problems.**

# Headache

There are some very strange magico-medical folk cures for headache. In both Ireland and Scotland, a piece of the shroud of a man who had died prematurely was said to be good for headaches (Souter 1995: 165). The rope by which a man had been hanged was also thought to be a cure for headache (Black 1883: 100), a belief that can be traced back to the writings of Pliny (Peacock 1896: 272). A modification of this idea was to wrap round an aching head part of a sheet that had wrapped a corpse (Wilde 1919: 82). The sloughed skin of a snake, worn as a bandage, was said to help headaches; this remedy was in use in Sussex as recently as the nineteenth century (Allen 1995: 169). One man in Cambridge made an income from selling snakeskins for this purpose (Black 1883: 156).

Many more prosaic folk remedies for headache involve cold or hot compresses applied to the head, the simplest being a cloth wrung out in cold water and applied to the forehead. Water from a particular healing well was sometimes reckoned especially effective (Beith 1995: 142). Rhubarb and cabbage leaves were used in Britain as cooling applications (Hatfield 1994: 39). Jack and Jill's famous recipe of vinegar and brown paper has actually been in use in British folk medicine until very recent times. Interestingly, brown paper used to be made from pine wood, and the vinegar could have extracted some of the active ingredients of the pine (C.H., pers. com., 2001).

Other headache remedies relied on such actively painkilling remedies as willow

*(Salix* spp.*)* (from which aspirin was developed) and meadowsweet *(Filipendula ulmaria)* (Beith 1995: 123), also now known to contain salicylates. Various species of willow were used as poultices or infusions, or the bark was chewed (Hatfield 1994: 40). In Britain, the seeds of the wild poppy *(Papaver rhoeas)* were chewed for a hangover, a use that may have given the plant its country name of "headache flower" (Hatfield 1994: 40). Betony *(Stachys officinalis),* viper's bugloss *(Echium* spp.), and mint were all used in Somerset (Tongue 1965: 40). Yarrow leaves *(Achillea millefolium)* were used in Norfolk for soothing headache (Bardswell 1911: 132) and in Ireland for provoking a nosebleed and thus relieving headache (Allen and Hatfield, in press). In the Scottish Highlands, dried ground ivy *(Glechoma hederacea)* was ground into a snuff and sniffed up for headaches (Beith 1995: 221). Violet *(Viola* spp.) was also used as a headache cure in Scotland (Beith 1995: 250). In Suffolk, a garden plant, American cudweed *(Anaphilis margaritacea)* was smoked for headache (Jobson 1967: 59). Could this have been borrowed from the Native American tradition? (see below).

In the west of Scotland there was a belief that if hair cuttings were used by a bird to build its nest, the owner of the hair would suffer from headaches (Black 1883: 16).

In North American folk medicine there were many and miscellaneous folk cures for headache. Some of these are recognizably the same as British ones. The wearing of a snakeskin (Brown 1952–1964, 6: 208) or of the rattles from a rattlesnake (Wilson 1968: 63) have been widely reported from North America. Putting a tight band of some description around the head has been recommended, as has a towel wrapped tightly round (UCLA Folklore Archive 25_6290). Wearing a jet necklace (Brown 1952–1964: 210) or cornbeads (Roberts 1927: 166) has also been suggested.

Another cure was to wear around the neck a string with nine knots (Parler 1962, 3: 680), or alternatively a red ribbon (Hyatt 1965: 234). Other items carried as amulets to prevent headache include a nutmeg on a black thread (UCLA 4_6312) and a buckeye (Fentress 1934: 78). Cobwebs placed across the bridge of the nose were thought to be helpful for headache (as well as nosebleed) (UCLA Folklore Archive 7_6811). Salt placed on the head was recommended (Brown 1952–1964, 6: 210). Applying urine was also suggested (UCLA Folklore Archive 4_6312). Jack and Jill's vinegar and brown paper was widely recommended (Brown 1952–1964: 209). Having a seventh child blow into the ear of the sufferer was another folk cure for headache (Anderson 1970: 36). A remedy involving transference was to lean against a tree while someone hammered a nail into the opposite side of the tree (Anderson 1968: 198).

In North America, as in the west of Scotland, there seems to have been a widespread belief that if a bird used hair cuttings for its nest, the owner of the hair would suffer from headaches. It was therefore advisable to burn or bury hair cuttings. Perhaps as an extension of this idea, a headache cure was to bury secretly hair from the sufferer under a stone for seven days (UCLA Folklore Archives 22_6311). A simple remedy for a headache reported from Illinois was to watch a spider from the ceiling drop down to the floor (Hyatt 1965: 235). Allowing the head to get wet in the first rain of May was thought to ensure a headache-free year ahead (UCLA Folklore Archives 18_6811).

Meyer reports the smoking of dried sumach leaves (*Rhus* sp.) in a clay pipe to arrest a developing headache (Meyer 1985: 138). Coffee is found helpful in some headaches (UCLA Folklore Archive 3_5393) and is a component of many proprietary headache pills. Blowing smoke into the ear or inhaling the smoke from a burning hemp rope are other suggestions (UCLA Folklore Archive 1_5395; UCLA Folklore Archive 13_6289). A piece of raw potato bound to the head is another recommendation (Meyer 1985: 138). As in Britain, willow bark was chewed (Micheletti 1998: 190). Peppermint oil was a popular headache remedy in the early twentieth century (Micheletti 1998: 190). Among numerous plant remedies used in North American folk medicine are catnip (Campbell 1953: 3), cactus juice (Hendricks 1966: 47), an infusion of yarrow (UCLA Folklore Archive 11_6289) or elderflower (Roberts 1927: 166), cabbage leaves laid on the forehead (Puckett 1981: 390), or plantain leaves lightly salted and crushed (Curtin 1930: 190). The leaves of jimson weed or of mallow have been applied (Puckett 1981: 379; UCLA Folklore Archive 1_6287). A preparation of lady slipper (*Cypripedium* spp.) has been used (Clark 1970: 22). A pillow of pine needles has been used, particularly for a migraine headache (UCLA Folklore Archive 10_6288).

The Native Americans bound sliced raw potato to the head (Micheletti 1998: 191). The brown-paper remedy finds an echo in the use by the Ojibwa of steam from the crushed needles of white pine *(Pinus strobus)* or from the leaves and bark of red pine *(Pinus resinosa)* for treating headache (Hoffman 1891: 198). Another species of pine, Pinon *(Pinus edulis),* was used by the Navajo for treating headache (Vestal 1952: 12, 13). A relative of the poppy, Indian turnip *(Argemone triphyllum),* was used by the Pawnee as a dusting powder for headache (Micheletti 1998: 191). The California poppy *(Escholtzia californica)* was used in Mendocino County as a wash for headache (Chesnut 1902: 351). The leaves of the buttercup *(Ranunculus acris)* were crushed and sniffed for headache by the Montagnais Indians (Vogel 1970: 297). Yarrow was used by, for example, the Algonquin (Raymond 1945: 118) and the Iroquois (Herrick 1977: 469). Numerous other plants have also

been used by the Native Americans in headache treatment, including fleabane (*Erigeron* spp.) (Moerman 1998: 218, 219).
Pearly everlasting *(Anaphalis margaritacea)*
was used by the Cherokee for headache
(Hamel and Chiltoskey 1975: 48), as it was
in Suffolk, England.

Interestingly, feverfew *(Tanacetum parthenium),* which has received much attention recently as a treatment for migraine,
seems in the past to have been used in folk
medicine mainly for other ailments—especially, as its common name suggests, for
fever—although in official medicine it was
used for headaches and migraine too.

There is a reference to its use in "hemi-
crania" in John Pechey's herbal of 1694
(Pechey 1694: 81). On the whole its use in
folk medicine seems to have been as a general painkiller. In our own time it has become well known as a migraine treatment
(UCLA Folklore Archive 10_6288) and accepted by orthodox Western medicine after
successful clinical trials (Johnson et al.
1985: 569–573).

*See also* **Amulet, Cabbage, Catnip, Elder,
Hair problems, Mallow, Migraine,
Nosebleed, Pine, Plantain, Snake,
Thornapple, Transference, Urine, Yarrow.**

## References
Allen, Andrew. *A Dictionary of Sussex Folk Medi-
cine.* Newbury: Countryside Books, 1995.
Allen, David E., and Gabrielle Hatfield. *Medicinal
Plants in Folk Tradition.* Portland, OR:
Timber Press, in press.
Anderson, John. *Texas Folk Medicine.* Austin: En-
cino Press, 1970.
Anderson, John Q. "Magical Transference of Dis-
ease in Texas Folk Medicine." *Western Folk-
lore* 27 (1968): 191–199.
Bardswell, Frances Anne. *The Herb-Garden.* Lon-
don: A. and C. Black, 1911.
Beith, Mary. *Healing Threads: Traditional Medi-
cines of the Highlands and Islands.* Edin-
burgh: Polygon, 1995.
Black, William George. *Folk-Medicine: A Chapter
in the History of Culture.* London: Folklore
Society, 1883.
Brown, Frank C. *Collection of North Carolina
Folklore.* 7 vols. Durham, NC: Duke University Press, 1952–1964.
Campbell, Marie. "Folk Remedies from South
Georgia." *Tennessee Folklore Society Bulletin*
19 (1953): 1–4.
Chesnut, V. K. "Plants Used by the Indians of
Mendocino County, California." *Contri-
butions from the U.S. National Herbarium* 7
(1902): 295–408.
Clark, Joseph D. "North Carolina Popular Beliefs
and Superstitions." *North Carolina Folklore*
18 (1970): 1–66.
Curtin, L. S. M. "Pioneer Medicine in New Mex-
ico." *Folk-Say* (1930): 186–196.
Fentress, Eliza E. *Superstitions of Grayson County
(Kentucky).* M.A. thesis, Western State
Teachers College, 1934.
Hamel, Paul B., and Mary U. Chiltoskey. *Chero-
kee Plants and Their Uses: A 400 Year His-
tory.* Sylva, NC: Herald, 1975.
Hatfield, Gabrielle. *Country Remedies: Traditional
East Anglian Plant Remedies in the Twentieth
Century.* Woodbridge: Boydell, 1994.
Hendricks, George D. *Mirrors, Mice and Mus-
taches: A Sampling of Superstitions and Pop-
ular Beliefs in Texas.* Austin: Texas Folklore
Society, 1966.
Herrick, James William. *Iroquois Medical Botany.*
Ph.D. thesis, State University of New York,
Albany, 1977.
Hoffman, W. J. "The Midewiwin or 'Grand Med-
icine Society' of the Ojibwa." *Smithsonian
Institution-Bureau of American Ethnology
Annual Report No. 7.* Washington, DC:
1891.
Hyatt, Harry Middleton. *Folklore from Adams
County Illinois.* 2nd rev. ed. New York:
Memoirs of the Alma Egan Hyatt Foun-
dation, 1965.
Jobson, Allan. *In Suffolk Borders.* London: Robert
Hale, 1967.
Johnson, E. S., et al. *British Medical Journal* 291
(1985): 569–573.
Meyer, Clarence. *American Folk Medicine.* Glen-
wood, IL: Meyerbooks, 1985.
Micheletti, Enza (ed.). *North American Folk Heal-
ing: An A–Z Guide to Traditional Remedies.*

New York and Montreal: Reader's Digest Association, 1998.

Moerman, Daniel E. *Native American Ethnobotany.* Portland, OR: Timber Press, 1998.

Parler, Mary Celestia, and University Student Contributors. *Folk Beliefs from Arkansas.* 15 vols. Fayetteville: University of Arkansas, 1962.

Peacock, Mabel. "Executed Criminals and Folk Medicine." *Folk-Lore* 7 (1896): 268–283.

Pechey, John. *The Complete Herbal of Physical Plants.* London, 1694.

Puckett, Newbell Niles. *Popular Beliefs and Superstitions: A Compendium of American Folklore from the Ohio Collection of Newbell Niles Puckett.* Edited by Wayland D. Hand, Anna Casetta, and Sondra B. Thiederman. 3 vols. Boston: G. K. Hall, 1981.

Raymond, Marcel. "Notes Ethnobotaniques sur les Tête-de-Boule de Manouan." *Contributions de l'Institut Botanique de l'Université de Montréal* 55 (1945): 113–134.

Roberts, Hilda. "Louisiana Superstitions." *Journal of American Folklore* 40 (1927): 144–208.

Souter, Keith. *Cure Craft: Traditional Folk Remedies and Treatment from Antiquity to the Present Day.* Saffron Walden: C. W. Daniel, 1995.

Tongue, Ruth L. *Somerset Folklore.* Edited by Katharine Briggs. County Folklore 8. London: Folklore Society, 1965.

Vestal, Paul A. "The Ethnobotany of the Ramah Navaho." *Papers of the Peabody Museum of American Archaeology and Ethnology* 40(4) (1952): 1–94.

Vogel, Virgil J. *American Indian Medicine.* Norman: University of Oklahoma Press, 1970.

Wilde, Lady. *Ancient Legends, Mystic Charms and Superstitions of Ireland.* London: Chatto and Windus, 1919.

Wilson, Gordon, Sr. *Folklore of the Mammoth Cave Region.* Bowling Green, KY: Kentucky Folklore Society, Kentucky Folklore Series 4, 1968.

# Healer

British folk medicine has largely been community medicine, handed down by word of mouth. Those who administered it were often family members or friends, and very few documented records exist except in the recent past. Even then, we are often offered only tantalizing glimpses, such as a name only. Goody Shepherd was the wise woman of Upton, and widow Bernard was similarly regarded in Severn Stoke, both in Gloucestershire, but of their practices we have no details (Lawson 1884: 103). However, sometimes an individual became locally, or even nationally, famous for his or her "cures," and in such cases written records do sometimes exist. Examples of such local healers are Mrs. Eileen Pearsons in Ireland, who became famous and wealthy for her remedy for scrofula using brooklime *(Veronica becccabunga)* ("'Ó Clara'" 1978: 35), and, in East Anglia, Mrs. Wesby, who published pamphlets on her herbal cures in the mid-nineteenth century (Wesby 1855). In Aberdeenshire the life of Adam Donald of Bethelnie has been documented. He was born in 1703 into a poor family, was disabled and unfit for manual work, but prospered as a local healer (Anderson 1791). In Scotland, Ireland, and Wales the situation was somewhat different, in that local families became famous as physicians. The Beaton clan in the Scottish Highlands, and the thirteenth-century Physicians of Myddvai in Wales are examples. In these cases the boundaries between folk and official medicine break down almost entirely. In addition, certain trades were associated with healing; thus the blacksmith was often regarded as a healer. Local midwives, until the twentieth century, often doubled as herbal practitioners as well as layers-out of the dead.

In North American folk medicine the picture is more complex. So many different traditions have contributed to its folk medicine that generalizations are impossible. Doubtless within any given community there were individuals famous for their knowledge of herbs, such as Mrs. Benton, the woman who taught Samuel Thomson

(Fox 1924: 22). Another example is Mary Curby of Louisiana, after whom one species of Eryngium is named, "merry-curvye." She publicized its use for snake bite (Coffey 1993: 159). As in Britain, documentation of such people is largely lacking. Apart from individual experts, within each tradition there were recognized hierarchies of healers: the *curanderismo* in Mexico; the medicine men among many Native American tribes; and the so-called Indian root-doctors, who were herbalists, drawing on the Native American knowledge as well as their own. Tommy Bass in the Appalachians is an example of this type of healer; fortunately, his practice and life have been very well documented (Crellin and Philpott 1998).

*See also* **Blacksmith, Medicine man, Midwife, Snake bite, Specialist.**

### References

Anderson, Dr. James. "Life of Adam Donald." *Bee* 6 (December 21, 1791).

Coffey, Timothy. *The History and Folklore of North American Wildflowers.* New York: Facts On File, 1993.

Crellin, John K., and Jane Philpott. *Trying to Give Ease: Tommie Bass and the Story of Herbal Medicine.* Durham, NC: Duke University Press, 1998.

Fox, William. *Family Botanic Guide, or Every Man His Own Doctor.* Sheffield: William Fox and Sons, 1924.

Lawson, Emily M. *Nation in a Parish.* London, 1884.

"'Ó Clara, Padraig:' The Big Mrs. Pearson." *Cork Holly Bough* (Christmas 1978): 35.

Wesby, Mrs. E., Doctress. *A Few Words of Friendly Advice.* 1855. Uncatalogued pamphlet in Local Studies Library, Norwich.

# Heart trouble

Many of the symptoms of heart disease recognized in modern medicine were not related to the heart in folk medicine in the past. As a result, folk remedies specifically for heart conditions are probably underrepresented in the literature, some of them being "hidden" under the categories of breathlessness, dropsy, or chest pain, all of which are sometimes symptoms of heart disease. In Yorkshire, a traditional preventative of angina was to wear brown paper coated with fat and brown sugar (Souter 1995: 167). Fasting and drinking one's own urine were apparently recommended too (Souter 1995: 167). Wearing a cork as an amulet was reputed to prevent heart attacks (Notes and Queries, 1849: 449). In Oxfordshire, a heart patient was given the last nine drops of tea from the teapot after guests had departed (Kahn 1913: 93). In Ireland, a cup of oatmeal covered with a cloth was placed over the heart patient's chest and bandaged in place (Logan 1972: 29).

Especially in Irish folk medicine, a number of native plants have been used in treating heart disease. These include rock samphire *(Crithmum maritimum)* and watercress *(Rorippa nasturtium-aquaticum)* (Vickery 1995: 313, 384). In England an infusion of the flowers of wild pansy *(Viola tricolor),* also known as heart's-ease, was used (Wharton 1974: 185). Dandelion leaves were recommended in Irish folk medicine for every illness, including a weak heart (Vickery 1995: 104). Foxglove is probably one of the most famous plants of herbal medicine in the West. Although Withering developed the use of the plant in treating heart disease, in folk medicine it had, prior to that, been used mainly in the treatment of dropsy (in some cases a symptom of heart disease) and as a salve. Hawthorn was regarded as a heart tonic—for example, in Devon (Lafont 1984: 44)—and it is used in modern herbalism (Chevallier 1996: 86). In the Highlands of Scotland, bogbean was regarded as good for the heart (Beith 1995: 207). Mistletoe was also used for heart trouble in the Scottish Highlands (Beith 1995: 227–228) and in Gloucestershire, England (Kanner 1939: 922).

In North American folk medicine, there seems to have been a widespread association of metals with heart disease. Wearing a gold watch near the heart was said to cause heart disease, but wearing brass rings on the fingers could cure heart trouble (Brown 1952–1968, 6: 211). Wearing copper (Cannon 1984: 111) or a piece of silver (UCLA Folklore Archive 2_7608) has been recommended for heart trouble. Eating gold leaf and dried venison was claimed to help heart disease (UCLA Folklore Archives 7_5416). Wearing a nutmeg as an amulet above the heart was claimed to cure "fluttering" of the heart (Brown 1952–1964, 6: 211). Other amulets worn for heart disease include a wasp nest in the breast pocket (Campbell 1953: 2), a bag containing camphor (Puckett 1981: 395), a buckeye (Puckett 1981: 395), the rattles of a rattlesnake wrapped in silk (Hyatt 1965: 331), or a heart-shaped bag containing hair from a child born after the death of his or her father (Marie-Ursule 1951: 174). Tying a red tape around the chest was recommended in Canada for palpitations (Riddell 1934: 262), while in Illinois for strengthening a weak heart a black silk string was tied around the left arm (Hyatt 1965: 331).

Spitting three times on a stone and throwing it over the shoulder was reputed to cure palpitations (Fogel 1915: 286). Yellow clay poultices on the soles of the feet were a cure for palpitations from Illinois (Hyatt 1965: 331). White clay was eaten for heart trouble in Illinois (Hyatt 1965: 331). An infusion of porcupine quills has been recommended in Quebec for heart disease (Roy 1955: 28). In Louisiana, ants were considered good for heart trouble (Roberts 1927: 169). In Alabama, drinking buttermilk was recommended (Browne 1958: 72). From Alabama also comes the suggestion that smelling one's own farts will cure a heart attack (Puckett 1981: 395). General recommendations for avoiding or treating heart disease include always sleeping on the

right side (Lathrop 1961: 15) and sleeping in a north-south orientation (Hyatt 1965: 331). A glass of water recently brought from the river drunk on five consecutive nights was said to cure heart sickness (Dodson 1954: 265). Lukewarm tea rubbed into the chest was recommended for heart pains in Minnesota (Lathrop 1961: 10, note 12), a remedy reminiscent of the Oxfordshire cure above. In French Canada, eating plenty of honey was considered good for the heart (Roy 1955: 68).

There was a widespread belief in Europe and North America that roasted toads were good for heart trouble (UCLA Folklore Archives 1_5403). Perhaps surprisingly, this strange remedy is fully vindicated by modern science: toad skin has been shown to contain cardiac glycosides called bufadienolides, which have a direct action on the heart (Allen 1995: 159). A number of North American folk remedies for heart diseases involve ingesting the blood or the heart of an animal (UCLA Folklore Archives 6_5401). In Mexico, blood from a deer was mixed with powdered antler and given for heart trouble (Smithers 1961: 24). A recommendation from Texas was to kill a woodpecker and drink its blood (UCLA Folklore Archives 2_5404). Eating a boiled roadrunner was also suggested (Hendricks 1966: 47).

There are a very large number of plant remedies in North American folk medicine for treating the heart. For palpitations, clove water (from *Syzygium aromaticum*) was rubbed on (Vestal 1973: 168), or red clover tea *(Trifolium pratense)* was drunk (UCLA Folklore Archives 11_6437). Eating garlic every day was recommended for keeping the heart healthy (UCLA Folklore Archives 8_5416), a remedy imported from Austria. In Mexico, boiled sweet lemon (*Agastache* sp.) was recommended for pains in the heart (Woodhull 1930: 61), as was orange blossom tea (Kay 1972: 178). Dill seeds were used in New Mexico (Curtin

1930: 188). Chewing the root of butterfly root *(Asclepias tuberosa)* was recommended in Arkansas (Parler 1962: 687). A tea made from Lady's slipper *(Cypripedium* sp.) was drunk in Virginia (Musick 1948: 6). Among numerous other plants used to treat heart conditions are costmary *(Balsamita major)* (Puckett 1981: 395), cherry (Puckett 1981: 395), wintergreen *(Gaultheria* sp.) (Rayburn 1941: 250), bugleweed *(Lycopus* sp.) (Lathrop 1961: 16), heart's-ease or heal-all *(Prunella vulgaris)* (Bergen 1899: 110), and lily-of-the-valley (which could refer to the European lily-of-the-valley, *Convallaria majalis,* or to a species of *Maianthemum).*

Another plant also called heart's ease, or pipissewa *(Chimaphila umbellata),* was used for heart disease in New England (Levine 1941: 488). Chewing ginseng was recommended to ward off heart trouble (Clark 1970: 23). A broth of heart-shaped leaves has been claimed to cure heart trouble (UCLA Folklore Archives 3_6437). Other plant remedies that may be examples of sympathetic magic include the use of smartweed *(Polygonum persicaria)* (Bergen 1899: 115), which has heart-shaped spots on its leaves, and of the Yoloxochitl plant (Loomis 1944: 95), which has heart-shaped flowers. Simply wearing a bag of herbs around the neck has been suggested (Puckett 1981: 395). Cayenne pepper in a glass of cold water has been recommended for a heart attack (Cannon 1984: 111). A suggestion implying little faith in the medical profession is to take two-thirds of the prescribed medicine and bury it (Cannon 1984: 111).

In Native American practice, a large number of plants have been used to treat heart conditions. These include white cedar *(Thuja* sp.), known also as arbor-vitae (Tantaquidgeon 1972: 266), and skunk cabbage *(Symplocarpus foetidus)* (MacDonald 1959: 222), as well as the pisissewa and Prunella mentioned above in general folk medicine (Moerman 1998: 801–802). When in 1837 a party of Canadian Indians visited Dr. Deerfield, they offered him their medicine for the heart palpitations from which he was suffering and were offended when he declined. The preparation was composed of wild ginger root *(Asarum canadense)* (Vogel 1970: 391). Among the Cherokee, there was apparently a belief that heart trouble was caused by the lungs being wrapped around the heart, so a preparation of fern leaves, which in nature uncurl as they grow, was given (Brown 1952–1964, 6: 211). In Nahuatl lore, a person with heart disease should wear red clothes (Madsen, 1955: 130). (For other plants used by the Native Americans in heart disease, see Moerman 1998: 801–802.)

*See also* **Amulet, Bogbean, Cayenne, Cherry, Dandelion, Dropsy, Foxglove, Ginseng, Gold, Hawthorn, Mistletoe, Poultice, Sympathetic magic, Toads and frogs.**

## References
Allen, Andrew. *A Dictionary of Sussex Folk Medicine.* Newbury: Countryside Books, 1995.

Allen, David E., and Gabrielle Hatfield. *Medicinal Plants in Folk Tradition.* Portland, OR: Timber Press, in press.

Beith, Mary. *Healing Threads: Traditional Medicines of the Highlands and Islands.* Edinburgh: Polygon, 1995.

Bergen, Fanny D. "Animal and Plant Lore Collected from the Oral Tradition of English Speaking Folk." *Memoirs of the American Folk-Lore Society* 7 (1899).

Brown, Frank C. *Collection of North Carolina Folklore.* 7 vols. Durham, NC: Duke University Press, 1952–1964.

Browne, Ray B. *Popular Beliefs and Practices from Alabama.* Folklore Studies 9. Berkeley and Los Angeles: University of California Publications, 1958.

Campbell, Marie. Folk Remedies from South Georgia. *Tennessee Folklore Society Bulletin* 19 (1953): 1–4.

Cannon, Anthon S. *Popular Beliefs and Superstitions from Utah.* Edited by Wayland D.

Hand and Jeannine E. Talley. Salt Lake City: University of Utah Press, 1984.

Chevallier, Andrew. *The Encyclopedia of Medicinal Plants.* London: Dorling Kindersley, 1996.

Clark, Joseph D. "North Carolina Popular Beliefs and Superstitions." *North Carolina Folklore* 18 (1970): 1–66.

Curtin, L. S.M. "Pioneer Medicine in New Mexico." *Folk-Say* (1930): 186–196.

Dodson, Ruth. "The Curandero of Los Olmos." *Publications of the Texas Folklore Society* 26 (1954): 264–270.

Fogel, Edwin Miller. "Beliefs and Superstitions of the Pennsylvania Germans." *Americana Germanica* 18 (1915).

Hendricks, George D. *Mirrors, Mice and Mustaches: A Sampling of Superstitions and Popular Beliefs in Texas.* Austin: Texas Folklore Society, 1966.

Hyatt, Harry Middleton. *Folklore from Adams County Illinois.* 2nd rev. ed. New York: Memoirs of the Alma Egan Hyatt Foundation, 1965.

Kahn, Max. "Vulgar Specifics and Therapeutic Superstitions." *Popular Science Monthly* 83 (1913): 81–96.

Kanner, Leo. "Mistletoe, Magic and Medicine." *Bulletin of the History of Medicine* 7 (1939): 875–936.

Kay, Margarita Artschwager. *Health and Illness in the Barrio: Women's Point of View.* Ph.D. dissertation, University of Arizona, 1972.

Lafont, Anne-Marie. *Herbal Folklore.* Bideford: Badger Books, 1984.

Lathrop, Amy. "Pioneer Remedies from Western Kansas." *Western Folklore* 20 (1961): 1–22.

Levine, Harold D. "Folk Medicine in New Hampshire." *New England Journal of Medicine* 224 (1941): 487–492.

Logan, Patrick. *Making the Cure: A Look at Irish Folk Medicine.* Dublin: Talbot Press, 1972.

Loomis, C. Grant. "Some Mexican Lore Prior to 1670." *California Folklore Quarterly* 3 (1944): 91–101.

MacDonald, Elizabeth. "Indian Medicine in New Brunswick." *Canadian Medical Association Journal* 80(3) (1959): 220–224.

Madsen, William. "Hot and Cold in the Universe of San Francisco Tecospa, Valley of Mexico." *Journal of American Folklore* 68 (1955): 123–139.

Marie-Ursule, Soeur. "Civilisation traditionelle des Lavalois." *Les Archives de Folklore* 5–6 (1951): 1–403.

Moerman, Daniel E. *Native American Ethnobotany.* Portland, OR: Timber Press, 1998.

Musick, Ruth Ann. "Western Virginia Folklore." *Hoosier Folklore* 7 (1948): 1–14.

Notes and Queries. London: 1849. Vol. 123.

Parler, Mary Celestia, and University Student Contributors. *Folk Beliefs from Arkansas.* 15 vols. Fayetteville: University of Arkansas, 1962.

Puckett, Newbell Niles. *Popular Beliefs and Superstitions: A Compendium of American Folklore from the Ohio Collection of Newbell Niles Puckett.* Edited by Wayland D. Hand, Anna Casetta, and Sondra B. Thiederman. 3 vols. Boston: G. K. Hall, 1981.

Rayburn, Otto Ernest. *Ozark Country.* New York: Duell, Sloan and Pearce, 1941.

Riddell, William Renwick. "Some Old Canadian Folk Medicine." *Medical Record* 140 (1934): 262.

Roberts, Hilda. "Louisiana Superstitions." *Journal of American Folklore* 40 (1927): 144–208.

Roy, Carmen. *La Littérature Orale en Gaspésie.* Bulletin 134, 36 de la Serie Anthropologique. Ottawa: Ministre de Nord Canadien et des Ressources Nationales, (1955): 61–105; 107–136.

Smithers, W. D. "Nature's Pharmacy and the Curanderos." *Sul Ross State College Bulletin* 41(3) (1961): 24.

Souter, Keith. *Cure Craft: Traditional Folk Remedies and Treatment from Antiquity to the Present Day.* Saffron Walden: C. W. Daniel, 1995.

Tantaquidgeon, Gladys. "Folk Medicine of the Delaware and Related Algonkian Indians." *Pennsylvania Historical Commission Anthropological Papers,* no. 3 (1972).

Vestal, Paul K., Jr. "Herb Workers in Scotland and Robeson Counties." *North Carolina Folklore* 21 (1973): 166–170.

Vickery, Roy. *A Dictionary of Plant Lore.* Oxford: Oxford University Press, 1995.

Vogel, Virgil J. *American Indian Medicine.* Norman: University of Oklahoma Press, 1970.

Wharton, C. *The Folklore of South Warwickshire: A Field Collection with Comparative Annotations and Commentary.* Ph.D. thesis, University of Leeds, 1969.

Woodhull, Frost. "Ranch Remedios." *Publications of the Texas Folklore Society* 8 (1930): 9–73.

# Heartburn

*See* **Indigestion.**

# Hemlock (*Conium maculatum*)

Despite its very poisonous nature, this plant has been used in British folk medicine. The name "hemlock" has been applied to various other species of umbellifers too, particularly to "water-hemlock," *Oenanthe crocata,* so that it is not always possible to assign a record with certainty to the "true" hemlock. A Suffolk ointment for sore eyes was prepared from hemlock but was applied to the healthy eye, not the sore one! (Porter 1969: 43). A similar salve was used in Yorkshire by the Fairfax family, but in this instance it was applied to the arm on the opposite side from the sore eye (Radford and Radford 1974: 189). Hemlock was a constituent of pills given to procure abortion (Porter 1969: 11). The most widespread use of hemlock in British folk medicine has been as an external poultice applied to sores and ulcers (Hart 1898: 378), and even to cancers. This latter use may have been influenced by the eighteenth-century cancer "cure" promoted by the Viennese physician Storck, but evidently folk medicine in some instances adopted the plant for this use. In Cornwall a man claimed to have cured himself of cancer by drinking hemlock juice (Polwhele 1806: 76). In Ireland the plant was also used for treating rheumatism (Allen and Hatfield, in press).

Hemlock was introduced into North America. Its use there in folk medicine ap-

pears to have been only slight. Among the Klamma Native Americans it was rubbed on a woman's body to make her attractive to men (Gunther 1973: 42). The name hemlock in North America generally refers to the unrelated hemlock spruce.

*See also* **Abortion, Cancer, Eye problems, Hemlock spruce, Poultice, Rheumatism.**

### References

Allen, David E., and Gabrielle Hatfield. *Medicinal Plants in Folk Tradition.* Portland, OR: Timber Press, in press.

Gunther, Erna. *Ethnobotany of Western Washington.* Rev. ed. Seattle: University of Washington Press, 1973.

Hart, Henry Chichester. *Flora of the County Donegal.* Dublin: Sealy, Bryers, and Walker, 1898.

Polwhele, Richard. *The Civil and Military History of Cornwall.* Vol. 5. London: Cadell and Davies, 1806.

Porter, Enid. *Cambridgeshire Customs and Folklore.* London: Routledge, 1969.

Radford, E., and M. A. Radford. *Encyclopaedia of Superstitions.* Edited and revised by Christina Hole. London: Book Club Associates 1974.

# Hemlock spruce (*Tsuga spp.*)

This tree is not native in Britain and is unknown there in folk medicine. In North America, the twigs of hemlock pounded with lard have been used to treat chilblains. Essence of hemlock was an ingredient of cough medicines. The inner bark of the hemlock tree has been used to treat dysentery and as a constituent of a tonic (Meyer 1985: 62, 81, 96, 257). Lying on fresh hemlock boughs has been found to help hay fever. Hemlock bark has been used in urinary incontinence and in a mixture for rheumatism. The pulverized bark has been used for chafed skin (Meyer 1985: 135, 156, 215, 224). The water in which hemlock bark has been boiled has been used to treat dandruff (Beck 1957: 78). The same infusion has been used to treat itches and sore feet (UCLA Folklore Archives 5_5418), as well as dropsy (Lick and Brendle 1922: 281). Hemlock tea has been used to treat measles (Puckett 1981: 413).

In Native American medicine these uses and many others have been recorded (Moerman 1998: 570–573). Additional uses include burns (Smith 1929: 51), gynecological problems (Hamel and Chiltoskey 1975: 38), and tuberculosis (Herrick 1977: 268). The gum of the tree has been used to treat eye inflammation (Boas 1932: 190). Hemlock is believed by some to be the plant used in the sixteenth century by Native Americans to cure the explorer Jacques Cartier's men of scurvy (Vogel 1970: 316).

Confusingly, hemlock in Britain refers to the unrelated and highly poisonous plant *Conium maculatum.*

*See also* **Burns, Chapped skin, Chilblains, Coughs, Dropsy, Dysentery, Hay fever, Hemlock, Rheumatism, Scurvy, Sore feet, Tonic, Tuberculosis.**

### References

Beck, Horace P. *The Folklore of Maine.* Philadelphia and New York: J. B. Lippincott, 1957.
Boas, Franz. "Current Beliefs of the Kwakiutl Indians." *Journal of American Folklore* 45 (1932): 177–260.
Hamel, Paul B., and Mary U. Chiltoskey. *Cherokee Plants and Their Uses: A 400 Year History.* Sylva, NC: Herald, 1975.
Herrick, James William. *Iroquois Medical Botany.* Ph.D. thesis, State University of New York, Albany, 1977.
Lick, David E., and Thomas R. Brendle. "Plant Names and Plant Lore among the Pennsylvania Germans." *Proceedings and Addresses of the Pennsylvania German Society* 33 (1922).
Meyer, Clarence. *American Folk Medicine.* Glenwood, IL: Meyerbooks, 1985.
Moerman, Daniel E. *Native American Ethnobotany.* Portland, OR: Timber Press, 1998.
Puckett, Newbell Niles. *Popular Beliefs and Superstitions: A Compendium of American Folklore from the Ohio Collection of Newbell Niles Puckett.* Edited by Wayland D. Hand, Anna Casetta, and Sondra B. Thiederman. 3 vols. Boston: G. K. Hall, 1981.
Smith, Harlan I. "Materia Medica of the Bella Coola and Neighboring Tribes of British Columbia." *National Museum of Canada Bulletin* 56 (1929): 47–68.
Vogel, Virgil J. *American Indian Medicine.* Norman: University of Oklahoma Press, 1970.

## Hemorrhoids

*See* **Piles.**

## Hiccups

For a usually trivial ailment, this has gathered a surprising amount of folk-lore. Recommendations in British folklore include holding the breath, drinking from the far side of a glass of water, drinking water while standing on one's head, and persuading someone to give the sufferer a fright. A nineteenth-century "cure" is to spit on the forefinger of the right hand and make a cross on the front of the left shoe while saying the Lord's prayer backward (Hawke 1973: 28). Holding the nose, closing the mouth, and counting to twenty backward is a Somerset suggestion (Tongue 1965: 40). Various plants found to soothe digestive problems have been used, such as chamomile tea or peppermint *(Mentha x piperita).* In Ireland gorse *(Ulex europaeus)* has been used to treat hiccups (Lucas 1960: 185).

In North America, there is a wealth of hiccup cures. In addition to those mentioned for Britain, they include swallowing sugar or vinegar, breathing into a paper bag, snuffing up pepper to provoke sneezing, and pulling on the tongue (Micheletti

1998: 195). Placing a hand on the pit of the stomach and applying pressure is another suggestion (Meyer 1985: 139). Drinking sips of water of varying number and with deep breaths between was a common recommendation (Brown 1952–1964, 6: 213–215). Holding the breath has often been found to help, as has giving the sufferer a shock (Brown 1952–1964, 6: 215–217). Sipping sugared water, chewing crushed ice, and drinking cold soda water have all been tried; drinking sips of water while keeping the ears blocked is another suggestion, as is sucking a lump of sugar through a slice of lemon or tomato (Meyer 1985: 140). Herbal suggestions include cinnamon *(Cinnamomum verum),* dill *(Anethum graveolens),* fennel *(Foeniculum vulgare),* mint, and peppermint *(Mentha* x *piperita)* (Meyer 1985: 140). Chewing pine straws and eating damson jam have also been recorded (Brown 1952–1964, 6: 213).

Among Native Americans, an infusion of juniper *(Juniperus* spp.) or of valerian *(Valeriana* spp.) was recommended (Micheletti 1998: 195).

*See also* **Chamomile.**

**References**

Brown, Frank C. *Collection of North Carolina Folklore.* 7 vols. Durham, NC: Duke University Press, 1952–1964.

Hawke, Kathleen. *Cornish Sayings, Superstitions and Remedies.* Redruth: Dyllanson Truran, 1973.

Lucas, A. T. *Furze: A Survey and History of Its Uses in Ireland.* Dublin: Stationery Office, 1960.

Meyer, Clarence. *American Folk Medicine.* Glenwood, IL: Meyerbooks, 1985.

Micheletti, Enza (ed.). *North American Folk Healing: An A–Z Guide to Traditional Remedies.* New York and Montreal: Reader's Digest Association, 1998.

Tongue, Ruth L. *Somerset Folklore.* Edited by Katharine Briggs. County Folklore 8. London: Folklore Society, 1965.

# Hives

This is a disease commonly mentioned in folk medicine but difficult to define in terms of modern medicine. In Scotland, it refers to almost any condition in a child that involves skin eruptions thought to be caused by some internal disorder (Buchan 1994: 110). Use of the term extended further to different types of hives, such as "bowel-hives" (a form of diarrhea) and "bannock-hive," thought to be due to overeating. The word was even used as an adjective, "hivie," meaning that a child was ill from almost any cause. Treatment for hives included an infusion of herb Robert *(Geranium robertianum).* The Gaelic name for this plant means "plant for the hives" (Beith 1995: 223). In Ireland, ragwort *(Senecio* sp.) was used to treat bowel hives in children (Vickery MSS).

The term hives is used in North American medicine, where it seems to refer sometimes to an urticarial (nettle-like) rash (Buchan 1994: 111). Various teas were given to a baby to "bring out" the hives, as it was believed this was desirable. Bullnettle tea *(Cnidoscolus stimulosus)* was given for this purpose (Anderson 1970: 42), as was ground-ivy tea *(Glechoma hederacea)* (Mullins 1973: 38). Other infusions were used to treat the hives—for example, tea made from catnip (Brown 1952–1964, 6: 52–53), onions, mistletoe (Browne 1958: 20), mullein, or maple leaf *(Acer* sp.) (Parler 1962, 3: 250, 704). A more drastic treatment involved a form of cupping, where blood was sucked out from small slits made between the infant's shoulders (Brown 1952–1964, 6: 52–53). It was recommended to give a newborn baby a drop of its own blood to prevent it from dying of hives (Hatcher 1958: 152).

Other treatments for hives had a magical element. Water in which nine pieces of buckshot (Randolph 1947: 111) or a borrowed silver dollar (Frazier 1936: 34) had been soaked was suggested. A tea made from the hind legs of crickets (Parler 1962, 3: 702) or from the stings of nine honeybees (UCLA Folklore Archive 19_5890) was given to a child with hives. Wearing a nutmeg (Farr 1939: 113) or a bag containing nine silverfish (Browne 1958: 20) was claimed to cure hives. Passing a baby backward through a horse collar (UCLA Folklore Archive 5_5685) or allowing a stud horse to breathe on the child (Parler 1962, 3: 706) were other recommendations. The breath of various humans was considered curative. A seventh child could cure hives by blowing into a child's mouth (UCLA Folklore Archive 9_5415), as could a man who had never seen the baby's father (Hand 1971: 265) or a man born with a caul (Parler 1962, 3: 706).

To prevent hives occurring, it was suggested that a baby be exposed to the sunshine on three successive mornings (Brewster 1939: 36).

*See also* **Bee, Catnip, Caul, Cricket, Mistletoe, Mullein, Onion.**

### References

Anderson, John. *Texas Folk Medicine.* Austin: Encino Press, 1970.

Beith, Mary. *Healing Threads: Traditional Medicines of the Highlands and Islands.* Edinburgh: Polygon, 1995.

Brewster, Paul G. "Folk Cures and Preventives from Southern Indiana." *Southern Folklore Quarterly* 3 (1939): 33–43.

Brown, Frank C. *Collection of North Carolina Folklore.* 7 vols. Durham, NC: Duke University Press, 1952–1964.

Browne, Ray B. *Popular Beliefs and Practices from Alabama.* Folklore Studies 9. Berkeley and Los Angeles: University of California Publications, 1958.

Buchan, David, ed. *Folk Tradition and Folk Medicine in Scotland: The Writings of David Rorie.* Edinburgh: Canongate Academic, 1994.

Farr, T. J. "Tennessee Folk Beliefs Concerning Children." *Journal of American Folklore* 52 (1939): 112–116.

Frazier, Neal. "A Collection of Middle Tennessee Superstitions." *Tennessee Folklore Society Bulletin* 2 (1936): 33–48.

Hand, Wayland D. "The Folk Healer Calling and Endowment." *Journal of History of Medicine* 26 (1971): 263–275.

Hatcher, Mildred. "Superstitions in Middle Tennessee." *Southern Folklore Quarterly* 19 (1958): 150–155.

Mullins, Gladys. "Herbs of the Southern Highlands and Their Medicinal Uses." *Kentucky Folklore Record* 19 (1973): 26–41.

Parler, Mary Celestia, and University Student Contributors. *Folk Beliefs from Arkansas.* 15 vols. Fayetteville: University of Arkansas, 1962.

Randolph, Vance. *Ozark Superstitions.* New York: Columbia University Press, 1947.

Vickery MSS. Roy Vickery, manuscript material.

# Holly (*Ilex aquifolium*)

Christian symbolism now overlies what was probably a much older tradition of reverence for this tree. The holly not only symbolizes survival, with its tough evergreen leaves and its very slow rate of growth, but was used in the past to mark out boundaries—it was a crime to cut down such boundary hollies. This perhaps led to the idea still prevalent today that it is unlucky to cut down hollies (Vickery 1995: 181).

In British folk medicine, holly has been used for one purpose above all others—treating chilblains. By beating the affected toes and fingers until they bled, it was thought that the local circulation could be improved and the chilblains helped to heal. This practice has been recorded from Norfolk and Oxfordshire (Allen and Hatfield, in press). That the use of holly was not merely symbolic is shown by the fact that in some areas, including Wiltshire (Whitlock 1976: 167) and Essex (Hatfield 1994: 27), an ointment made up of holly berries and lard was used to treat chilblains.

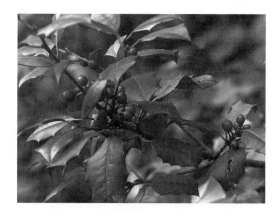

In British folk medicine, holly has been used to treat chilblains. In North America, influenza has been treated with a tea made from holly and holly leaf tea has been used to treat measles. (North Wind Picture Archive)

Rheumatism and arthritis were sometimes treated in a similar way, by beating with holly twigs—for example, in Somerset (Tongue 1965). In Waterford, Ireland, a stiff neck was treated similarly (Allen and Hatfield, in press). The belief is reported from Scotland that at Hogmanay (New Year's Eve) if a boy is beaten with holly he will live a year for every drop of blood spilt (Banks 1937–1941, 2: 42). An infusion of the leaves was used as a rheumatism treatment in Devon (Lafont 1984: 47), and there is a record from Hampshire of a treatment for whooping cough by drinking milk out of a cup made from wood from a variegated holly (Notes and Queries 1851: 227). There is also an isolated record from Limpsfield, Surrey, of the holly tree's being used in a cure for hernia in children, in much the same way that ash trees have been more generally used. In Meath, Ireland, holly leaves were used to treat burns (Allen and Hatfield, in press).

English holly was introduced in North America and arises occasionally in folk medicine. There is a record from New England of the use of powder of dried "French" holly (variegated garden holly) for treating worms in children (Fosbroke 1835: 165). Often there is no precise information about which species was used in folk medicine, and presumably one of the indigenous species was used by Swedish colonists for the treatment of stitches and pleuritic pains; the process involved drying and grinding the leaves, and boiling the powder in beer (Kalm 1747–1751: 185). Influenza has been treated with a tea made from holly (Wilson 1968: 323). Holly leaf tea has been used to treat measles (Brown 1952–1964, 6: 234). During the Civil War, a tea made of yaupon (holly) was used in the South to treat ulcers (Woodhull 1930: 66). A mixture of honey and holly ashes was used to treat thrush (Brown 1952–1964, 6: 65). Walking through a split trunk of holly as a cure for hernias, just as in England, has been reported from Ohio (Puckett 1981: 396). Evidently, holly leaf tea was regarded as a tonic (Clark 1970: 10), with one suggestion that "he-holly" is good for boys, "she-holly" for girls (Brown 1952–1964, 6: 114).

Some of these folk uses of holly are recognizable from Native American practice; for example, among the Micmac, the root of English holly *(Ilex aquifolium)* is used in treating coughs, consumption, and kidney complaints (Chandler, Freeman, and Hooper 1979: 57), and the plant is also used for treating fevers. *Ilex opaca* is used by the Catawaba to treat measles (Speck 1944: 41). The use of leaves of *Ilex opaca,* American holly, to scratch cramped muscles (Hamel and Chiltoskey 1975: 38) provides an interesting echo of the British folk uses for holly as a counter-irritant. *Ilex vomitoria,* as its specific name suggests, has provided an emetic, used by several Native American tribes to provoke vomiting and induce hallucinations (see, for example, Hamel and Chiltoskey 1975: 12, 62).

*See also* **Ash, Burns, Chilblains, Rheumatism, Tonic, Whooping cough.**

## References

Allen, David E., and Gabrielle Hatfield. *Medicinal Plants in Folk Tradition*. Portland, OR: Timber Press, in press.

Banks, Mrs. M. MacLeod. *British Calendar Customs: Scotland*. 3 vols. London: 1937–1941.

Brown, Frank C. *Collection of North Carolina Folklore*. 7 vols. Durham, NC: Duke University Press, 1952–1964.

Chandler, R. Frank, Lois Freeman, and Shirley N. Hooper. "Herbal Remedies of the Maritime Indians." *Journal of Ethnopharmacology* 1 (1979): 49–68.

Clark, Joseph D. "North Carolina Popular Beliefs and Superstitions." *North Carolina Folklore* 18 (1970): 1–66.

Fosbroke, John. "On the Effects of Male Fern Buds, in Cases of Worms." *Boston Medical and Surgical Journal* 13(11) (1835): 165–168.

Hamel, Paul B., and Mary U. Chiltoskey. *Cherokee Plants and Their Uses: A 400 Year History*. Sylva, NC: Herald, 1975.

Hatfield, Gabrielle. *Country Remedies: Traditional East Anglian Plant Remedies in the Twentieth Century*. Woodbridge: Boydell, 1994.

Kalm, P. *Travels in North America (1747–1751)*. Edited by A. P. Benson. New York: Wilson-Erickson, 1937. Reprint, Barre: Imprint Society, 1972.

Lafont, Anne-Marie. *Herbal Folklore*. Bideford: Badger Books, 1984.

*Notes and Queries,* series 1, 4 (1851): 227.

Puckett, Newbell Niles. *Popular Beliefs and Superstitions: A Compendium of American Folklore from the Ohio Collection of Newbell Niles Puckett*. Edited by Wayland D. Hand, Anna Casetta, and Sondra B. Thiederman. 3 vols. Boston: G. K. Hall, 1981.

Speck, Frank G. "Catawba Herbals and Curative Practices." *Journal of American Folklore* 57 (1944): 37–50.

Tongue, Ruth L. *Somerset Folklore*. Ed. K. M. Briggs. London: Folklore Society, 1965.

Vickery, Roy. *A Dictionary of Plant Lore*. Oxford: Oxford University Press, 1995.

Whitlock, Ralph. *The Folklore of Wiltshire*. London: Batsford, 1976.

Wilson, Gordon. "Local Plants in Folk Remedies in the Mammoth Cave Region." *Southern Folklore Quarterly* 32 (1968): 320–327.

Woodhull, Frost. "Ranch Remedios." *Publications of the Texas Folklore Society* 8 (1930): 9–73.

# Honey

As far back as records go and on both sides of the Atlantic, honey has been used in the treatment of wounds. It was used, for example, by the ancient Egyptians and by the Aztec. Recent scientific studies have largely vindicated its use, showing that, alone or mixed with sugar, honey can accelerate the healing of obstinate sores and help in the treatment of burns (Root-Bernstein 2000: 31–43). Modern clinical studies pioneered in Argentina and in Mississippi are demonstrating the use of honey and sugar in aiding the clean healing of surgical wounds (Root-Bernstein 2000: 36). Here is one folk remedy that will not go away; in time it may well be adopted and adapted into mainstream medicine.

Other folk uses include its use (often mixed with lemon juice or vinegar) to soothe a sore throat (EFS 155 Sf). Oatmeal gruel mixed with honey was used for treating coughs in the Highlands of Scotland (Beith 1995: 231). Pure honey, or honey mixed with meal, was used to treat infected wounds and bites in Suffolk (EFS 155 Sf). Honey made by local bees and eaten throughout the winter seems to confer protection against hay fever, at least for some sufferers. Honey is an important ingredient of many salves and cosmetic products. Hand cream was once made from honey and lard (EFS 241).

In North American folk medicine, honey was used in many of the same ways. Mixed with butter and sulphur it has been used to treat burns (Anderson 1970: 11). Red clover honey has been recommended for a sore throat (Smith 1930: 76). Local honey has been recommended for pollen allergies in Oklahoma (UCLA Folklore Archive

3_5256). Honey with sulphur has been taken for asthma (Welsch 1966: 360). Mixed with vinegar, it has been used for rheumatism (UCLA Folklore Archive 2_6466). Honey has even been used to treat bee stings (Rayburn 1941: 60). In addition, there have been many cosmetic uses of honey. Early settlers infused honey with vine tendrils and rosemary tops to form a wash to thicken hair, while with egg-yolk, hog's lard, rosewater, oatmeal and almond-paste it formed a remedy for chapped hands (Robertson 1960: 6, 10). Meyer gives numerous folk medical uses of honey, in preparations to treat ailments as diverse as bee-stings and bronchitis, burns, and rheumatism (Meyer 1985: 38, 50, 53, 217). Jarvis, the well-known exponent of cider vinegar, gives numerous folk uses of honey in his books (e.g., Jarvis 1961: 95–119).

In Native American medicine, both whole bees and honey are widely used in healing preparations. Other products of the bee are also used in folk medicine.

*See also* **Asthma, Bee, Burns, Chapped skin, Coughs, Hay fever, Insect bites and stings, Rheumatism, Sore throat, Wounds.**

### References

Anderson, John. *Texas Folk Medicine.* Austin: Encino Press, 1970.

Beith, Mary. *Healing Threads: Traditional Medicines of the Highlands and Islands.* Edinburgh: Polygon, 1995.

EFS. English Folklore Survey. Manuscript notes from the 1960s, in University College London.

Jarvis, D. C. *Folk Medicine.* London: Pan Books, 1961.

Meyer, Clarence. *American Folk Medicine.* Glenwood, IL: Meyerbooks, 1985.

Rayburn, Otto Ernest. *Ozark Country.* New York: Duell, Sloan, and Pearce, 1941.

Robertson, Marion. *Old Settlers' Remedies.* Barrington, NS: Cape Sable Historical Society, 1960.

Root-Bernstein, Robert, and Michèle Root-Bernstein. *Honey, Mud, Maggots, and Other Medical Marvels: The Science Behind Folk Remedies and Old Wives' Tales.* London: Pan Books, 2000.

Smith, Walter R. "Northwestern Oklahoma Folk Cures." *Publications of the Texas Folklore Society* 8 (1930): 74–85.

Welsch, Rogers L. *A Treasury of Nebraska Pioneer Folklore.* Lincoln: University of Nebraska Press, 1966.

# Hops (*Humulus lupulus*)

The pollen of this plant has been identified from prehistoric sites in Britain, making it likely that it is native. However, it has also been widely cultivated in Britain since the sixteenth century, when it replaced ground-ivy (*Glechoma hederacea*) as a flavoring for beer. Folk medical supplies of the plant may therefore have come mostly from the cultivated plant. It is thought to help insomnia, and hop pillows are sold commercially. There are records of its use in folk medicine as a sedative, especially in Ireland (Allen and Hatfield, in press). In England a poultice of bread and hops was used as a dressing for obstinate sores and ulcers (Quelch 1941: 99).

In North America the plant has a surprisingly high profile in folk medicine, given that the plant is not native there. Whether the so-called American hop (*Humulus lupulus* var. *lapuloides)* is in fact a native is a matter of disagreement (Crellin and Philpott 1990: 248). Either way, the plant has been widely used in general North American folk medicine as a sedative. In addition, it has been used as an external poultice for inflamed bowels, mixed with other herbs taken internally for bronchitis; as a chest poultice on the lungs and throat for chest colds (Meyer 1985: 46, 51, 67); as a hot fomentation applied externally for pleurisy; as a fomentation on its own or mixed with lobelia or thornapple for constipation; and as a component of cough mixtures

(Meyer 1985: 71, 80, 198). It has been used in the treatment of erysipelas, applied in heated bags to the feet and wrists for a fever, given as a tea for headache, and heated in a pillow for headache and neuralgia (Meyer 1985: 109, 128, 137, 139). As a syrup with sugar it has been given for jaundice; as an infusion for period pain, as a mouthwash for thrush; as a fomentation for the after pains of childbirth; as an infusion drunk for indigestion; in a mixture inhaled for sore throat or tonsillitis; and as a constituent of a general tonic (Meyer 1985: 152, 174, 180, 210, 238, 251, 252, 258). Flannels dipped in a hot infusion of hops have been used to poultice mumps (UCLA Folklore Archives 17_6410), and the hop shoots themselves have been used as a chest poultice for colds (Pope 1965: 43).

A recommendation for asthma has been to sleep on a pillow filled with hops (Puckett 1981: 312). Hop tea has been drunk for bladder inflammation (Browne 1958: 33). Hops fried in lard have been applied to caked breasts (Browne 1958: 42). Wild hops have been made into a brew to feed to babies (Lathrop 1961: 5). Folk faith in hops extends to the use of a hop-filled pillow under the bed to treat rheumatism (Cannon 1984: 121), or a bag of hops carried as an amulet to prevent motion sickness (Thomas 1920: 121). Hops have even figured in a treatment for epilepsy, a regimen involving visiting a hop vine for seven consecutive mornings and biting the end of a shoot (Hyatt 1965: 248).

Some of these uses can be traced in the records of Native American medicine, suggesting that they may have been learned from there rather than imported from European usage. As in general folk medicine, a warm application of the herb is a common method of preparation. In this way it was used to treat earache and toothache among the Delaware (Tantaquidgeon 1972: 31) and pneumonia among the Shinnecock (Carr and Westey 1945: 120). A decoction of the fruit has been used to treat intestinal pain and fever among the Dakota (Gilmore 1913: 32). An infusion of the blossom has been widely used as a sedative—for example, by the Mohegan (Tantaquidgeon 1972: 130) and the Cherokee (Hamel and Chiltoskey 1975: 39). (For other Native American uses of hops see Moerman 1998: 269–270.)

*See also* **Amulet, Asthma, Breast problems, Childbirth, Colds, Coughs, Earache, Epilepsy, Erysipelas, Fevers, Headache, Indigestion, Jaundice, Lobelia, Poultice, Rheumatism, Sleeplessness, Thornapple, Tonic, Toothache.**

## References

Allen, David E., and Gabrielle Hatfield. *Medicinal Plants in Folk Tradition.* Portland, OR: Timber Press, in press.

Browne, Ray B. *Popular Beliefs and Practices from Alabama.* Folklore Studies 9. Berkeley and Los Angeles: University of California Publications, 1958.

Cannon, Anthon S. *Popular Beliefs and Superstitions from Utah.* Edited by Wayland D. Hand and Jeannine E. Talley. Salt Lake City: University of Utah Press, 1984.

Carr, Lloyd G., and Carlos Westey. "Surviving Folktales and Herbal Lore among the Shinnecock Indians." *Journal of American Folklore* 58 (1945): 113–123.

Crellin, John C., and Jane Philpott. *A Reference Guide to Medicinal Plants: Herbal Medicine Past and Present.* Durham, NC: Duke University Press, 1990.

Gilmore, Melvin R. "Some Native Nebraska Plants with Their Uses by the Dakota." *Collections of the Nebraska State Historical Society* 17 (1913): 358–370.

Hamel, Paul B., and Mary U. Chiltoskey. *Cherokee Plants and Their Uses: A 400 Year History.* Sylva, NC: Herald, 1975.

Hyatt, Harry Middleton. *Folklore from Adams County Illinois.* 2nd rev. ed. New York: Memoirs of the Alma Egan Hyatt Foundation, 1965.

Lathrop, Amy. "Pioneer Remedies from Western Kansas." *Western Folklore* 20 (1961): 1–22.

Meyer, Clarence. *American Folk Medicine.* Glenwood, IL: Meyerbooks, 1985.

Moerman, Daniel E. *Native American Ethnobotany.* Portland, OR: Timber Press, 1998.

Pope, Genevieve. "Superstitions and Beliefs of Fleming Country." *Kentucky Folklore Record* 11 (1965): 41–51.

Puckett, Newbell Niles. *Popular Beliefs and Superstitions: A Compendium of American Folklore from the Ohio Collection of Newbell Niles Puckett.* Edited by Wayland D. Hand, Anna Casetta, and Sondra B. Thiederman. 3 vols. Boston: G. K. Hall, 1981.

Quelch, Mary Thorne. *Herbs for Daily Use.* London: Faber and Faber, 1941.

Tantaquidgeon, Gladys. "Folk Medicine of the Delaware and Related Algonkian Indians." *Pennsylvania Historical Commission Anthropological Papers,* no. 3 (1972).

Thomas, Daniel Lindsay, and Lucy Blayney Thomas. *Kentucky Superstitions.* Princeton, NJ: Princeton University Press, 1920.

# Horehound (*Marrubium vulgare*)

This common hedgerow plant has had a reputation in both official and folk medicine in Britain for treating coughs and colds. Horehound candy could still be bought in chemist shops in the late twentieth century. The plant was also made into beer, which was considered a good tonic. There were a few more minor uses for it in folk medicine: mixed with rue it was used in East Anglia as a contraceptive, and in Cumbria it was used to treat nosebleeds. Its uses in Ireland include headache, earache, as a heart tonic, and for treating rheumatism (Allen and Hatfield, in press).

It was introduced to North America, and although some of its uses there in folk medicine are similar, others seem to be unique to North America. As in Britain, its primary use has been for the treatment of respiratory complaints. It has been used to treat bronchitis (Meyer 1985: 51), asthma (Puckett 1981: 311), catarrh (Meyer 1985: 59),

croup (Rogers 1941: 18), colds (Cannon 1984: 99), and coughs (Meyer 1985: 80), including whooping cough (Brown 1952–1964: 353). In addition it has been used to treat sore throat (Smith 1929: 76), "female weakness" (Meyer 1985: 124), and, combined with raspberry, scanty or painful menstruation (Randolph 1947: 194). Both diarrhea (Black 1935: 19) and constipation (UCLA Folklore Archives 11_6391) have been treated using horehound, as have kidney and liver complaints (Meyer 1985: 157, 168). Horehound candy has been used for stomach ache and heartburn (Meyer 1985: 235). As a tea the plant has been used for colic (Wilson 1968: 71), as a diuretic (Browne 1958: 111), and to aid weight loss (Meyer 1985: 265). In either tea or candy form, the plant has been used to treat worms in children (Browne 1958: 30).

In the Mexican tradition, it has been used, as Marrubia, to treat jaundice (Campa 1950: 341). Horehound tea has been used as a tonic, as in Britain (Brown 1952–1964, 6: 114). Its use in Alabama to stop profuse bleeding and to soothe toothache has been reported (Browne 1958: 108). A slave in Carolina in the eighteenth century was awarded his freedom for revealing a cure for rattlesnake bite consisting of horehound and plantain (Schöpf 1788). Perhaps as an extension of this use, the juice has been recommended for poisons generally (Brown 1952–1964: 251).

In Native American practice the plant has had similar uses: for coughs, colds (Hamel and Chiltoskey 1975: 39), sore throat (Elmore 1944: 73), as a diuretic (Bean and Saubel 1972: 88), and for stomach ache (Vestal 1952: 41). In addition, it has been used to treat boils (Bocek 1984: 16) breast complaints (Hamel and Chiltoskey 1975: 39) and has been given before and after childbirth (Vestal 1952: 41).

*See also* **Asthma, Bleeding, Boils, Breast problems, Childbirth, Colds, Colic,**

Constipation, Contraception, Coughs, Croup, Diarrhea, Earache, Headache, Jaundice, Mexican tradition, Nosebleed, Rheumatism, Snake bite, Sore throat, Tonic, Toothache, Whooping cough, Worms.

## References

Bean, Lowell John, and Katharine Siva Saubel. *Temalpakh (From the Earth): Cahuilla Indian Knowledge and Usage of Plants.* Banning, CA: Malki Museum Press, 1972.

Black, Pauline Monette. *Nebraska Folk Cures.* University of Nebraska Studies in Language, Literature and Criticism 15. Lincoln: University of Nebraska, 1935.

Bocek, Barbara R. "Ethnobotany of Costanoan Indians, California: Based on Collections by John P. Harrington." *Economic Botany* 38(2) (1984): 240–255.

Brown, Frank C. *Collection of North Carolina Folklore.* 7 vols. Durham, NC: Duke University Press, 1952–1964.

Browne, Ray B. *Popular Beliefs and Practices from Alabama.* Folklore Studies 9. Berkeley and Los Angeles: University of California Publications, 1958.

Campa, Arthur L. "Some Herbs and Plants of Early California." *Western Folklore* 9 (1950): 338–347.

Cannon, Anthon S. *Popular Beliefs and Superstitions from Utah.* Edited by Wayland D. Hand and Jeannine E. Talley. Salt Lake City: University of Utah Press, 1984.

Elmore, Francis H. *Ethnobotany of the Navajo.* Santa Fe, NM: School of American Research, 1944.

Hamel, Paul B., and Mary U. Chiltoskey. *Cherokee Plants and Their Uses: A 400 Year History.* Sylva, NC: Herald, 1975.

Meyer, Clarence. *American Folk Medicine.* Glenwood, IL: Meyerbooks, 1985.

Puckett, Newbell Niles. *Popular Beliefs and Superstitions: A Compendium of American Folklore from the Ohio Collection of Newbell Niles Puckett.* Edited by Wayland D. Hand, Anna Casetta, and Sondra B. Thiederman. 3 vols. Boston: G. K. Hall, 1981.

Randolph, Vance. *Ozark Superstitions.* New York: Columbia University Press, 1947.

Rogers, E. G. *Early Folk Medical Practices in Tennessee.* Murfreesboro, TN: Rogers, 1941.

Schöpf, Johann David. *Travels in the Confederation (1783–1784).* Translated by A. J. Morrison. 1788. Reprint Philadelphia: Campbell, 1911.

Smith, Walter R. *Animals and Plants in Oklahoma Folk Cures: Folk-Say—A Regional Miscellany.* Edited by B. A. Botkin. Norman: Oklahoma Folk-Lore Society, 1929.

Vestal, Paul A. "The Ethnobotany of the Ramah Navaho." *Papers of the Peabody Museum of American Archaeology and Ethnology* 40(4) (1952): 1–94.

Wilson, Gordon., Sr. *Folklore of the Mammoth Cave Region.* Bowling Green, KY: Kentucky Folklore Society, Kentucky Folklore Series 4. 1968.

# Houseleek (*Sempervivum tectorum*)

This is a plant very widely used in British folk medicine and known by a variety of local names. One such name, sengreen, is of Anglo-Saxon origin and translates as "house plant." Though not a native of Britain, it must have been an early introduction from Central Europe. Botanically it is a sterile hybrid, which means that it is dependent for its spread on vegetative reproduction alone; the fact that it is now so common and widespread in Britain on walls and roofs probably is a direct result of its importance in folk medicine. The Romans claimed that it would protect a house from lightning and dedicated the plant to Jupiter (an association reflected in the name "thunder plant"). Country people had many more prosaic uses for it: it has been used for treating corns and warts, and the juice has been dropped into sore eyes and into ears for earache. It has been used within living memory in East Anglia, England, for treating eczema (Hatfield 1994: 50). In the Highlands of Scotland it was used for treating earache, deafness, shingles, and fevers (Beith 1995: 224). In Devon one of its uses

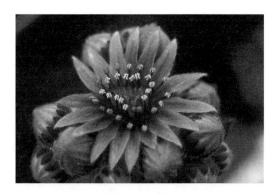

In Britain, houseleek is often grown on roofs and is claimed to protect the house from lightning. It has been widely used to treat skin, eye, and ear problems. (Sarah Boait)

was the treatment of chilblains (Lafont 1984: 48). In both England and Ireland, sore eyes were treated with its juice (Hatfield 1994: 37; Barbour 1897: 388). The plant has succulent rosettes of leaves and has been used as a poultice to treat abscesses (Hatfield 1994: 21), while there are also reports of its use in the treatment of asthma and epilepsy (Allen and Hatfield, in press). In Cambridgeshire, cancerous growths, after the application of a toad, had houseleek poultices applied to them (Porter 1974: 47).

In North American folk medicine, the plant has had similar, though not widespread, uses in folk medicine. There is a nineteenth-century report of its use for clearing blocked ears (Meyer 1985: 103), while it is claimed that the leaves of the houseleek "make the best salve known for wounds" (Meyer 1985: 273). The name "houseleek" has also been applied in North America to species of stonecrop, *Sedum* (Crellin and Philpott 1990: 256), which has also been used in treating skin complaints. In some of the folk records, it is not clear which plant is being used. Houseleek was used in an ointment to treat ringworm, and the fresh split leaf was applied to warts (Brown 1952–1964, 6: 269, 327). It was used for "risings" (Browne 1958: 92) and

for cuts, bruises, and swellings (UCLA Folklore Archive 9_6259). For improving the complexion, the juice was mixed with cream and applied (UCLA Folklore Archive 24_5615). It seems that the role of houseleek in treating burns in domestic medicine (Meyer 1985: 54) has largely been replaced in recent times by the use of aloe (Crellin and Philpott 1990: 46). In Native American practice, species of *Sempervivum* have been used in treatment of earache, corns, and salivary gland swelling (Moerman 1998: 526).

*See also* **Abscesses, Aloe vera, Asthma, Chilblains, Cuts, Deafness, Earache, Eczema, Epilepsy, Eye problems, Fevers, Poultice, Ringworm, Shingles, Toads and frogs, Warts.**

### References

Allen, David E., and Gabrielle Hatfield. *Medicinal Plants in Folk Tradition.* Portland, OR: Timber Press, in press.

Barbour, John H. "Some Country Remedies and Their Uses." *Folk-Lore* 8 (1897): 386–390.

Beith, Mary. *Healing Threads: Traditional Medicines of the Highlands and Islands.* Edinburgh: Polygon, 1995.

Brown, Frank C. *Collection of North Carolina Folklore.* 7 vols. Durham, NC: Duke University Press, 1952–1964.

Browne, Ray B. *Popular Beliefs and Practices from Alabama.* Folklore Studies 9. Berkeley and Los Angeles: University of California Publications, 1958.

Crellin, John K., and Jane Philpott. *A Reference Guide to Medicinal Plants.* Durham, NC: Duke University Press, 1990.

Hatfield, Gabrielle. *Country Remedies: Traditional East Anglian Plant Remedies in the Twentieth Century.* Woodbridge: Boydell, 1994.

Lafont, Anne-Marie. *Herbal Folklore.* Bideford: Badger Books, 1984.

Meyer, Clarence. *American Folk Medicine.* Glenwood, IL: Meyerbooks, 1985.

Moerman, Daniel E. *Native American Ethnobotany.* Portland, OR: Timber Press, 1998.

Porter, Enid. *The Folklore of East Anglia.* London: Batsford, 1974.

# Hunger

One of the ironies of modern civilization is the present quest for agents that will reduce appetite and so help in slimming, in communities where food is abundant. In the past, folk medicine has been more concerned with the suppression of appetite when food was scarce and work had to be done and journeys undertaken on an empty stomach. Some such agents are currently under investigation by pharmaceutical companies—for example, an African cactus is being developed as a slimming aid (Henderson 2001).

In British folk medicine, a number of plants were eaten to quell the sense of hunger, among them elm leaves (Hatfield MS). In Scotland, the root of a tuberous vetch (*Lathyrus linifolius*) was chewed to satisfy a sense of hunger (Pennant 1774: 310). The use of this plant in the Celtic tradition can be traced back at least to the first century A.D. When chewed, the roots taste like licorice (Beith 1995: 247–249). Among its other magico-medical properties, the butterwort plant (*Pinguicula* sp.) was thought to protect against hunger if simply carried as an amulet (Beith 1995: 207). While working on the seashore, Scottish highlanders chewed the seaweed known as dulse (*Rhodymenia palmata*) (Beith 1995: 240) to ward off hunger. As an actual slimming aid in the Highlands, water in which chickweed had been boiled was recommended (Beith 1995: 211). There is an anomalous tradition in parts of Ireland that walking on a certain type of grass makes one extremely tired. It is known as "hungry grass," and this tradition still survives (pers. com., County Meath, Ireland 2001; Vickery 1995: 199–200). In Gloucestershire, the buds of the ash tree were used as an aid to slimming (Allen and Hatfield, in press).

In Native American traditional herbal medicine, a large number of plants have been used to remove the sensation of hunger. The Devil's Club (*Oplopanax horridum*) has been used during fasts to relieve hunger and assist in visions (Willard 1992: 151). The inner bark of slippery elm was used much like chewing gum (Micheletti 1998: 307); like the tuberous vetch of Scotland, it tastes of licorice. Among the Cherokee, an infusion of the root of *Agrimonia gryposepala* was given to children to quell hunger (Hamel and Chiltoskey 1975: 22). The root of *Balsamorrhiza sagittata* was chewed and sucked for hunger among the Thompson tribe (Steedman 1928: 493). The powdered root of *Mirabilis multiflora* is mixed with flour and made into bread to decrease appetite among the Zuni (Camazine and Bye 1980: 377). An infusion of *Oenothera biennis* is taken by the Cherokee for reducing weight (Hamel and Chiltoskey 1975: 33), while among the Mahuna an infusion of witch grass, *Panicum capillare,* is used similarly (Romero 1954: 66). Canadian clearweed (*Pilea pumila*) was used by the Cherokee to curb excessive hunger in children (Hamel and Chiltoskey 1975: 52, 53). *Plantago patagonica,* woolly plantain, was used as a cold infusion by the Navajo and Ramah to reduce appetite (Vestal 1952: 45). *Saturejo douglasii* was used by the Pomo to help weight loss (Gifford 1967: 15). *Sassafras albidum* was used to help fight obesity both among the Native Americans (Perry 1975: 44) and in general folk medicine (Meyer 1985: 264). Other plants used in European-American folk medicine include chickweed, as used also in the Scottish Highlands, and sea-wrack (*Fucus vesiculosus*). The latter is a component of a number of modern proprietary slimming aids. A tea made from the leaves of the ash tree was drunk to reduce weight, a remedy echoing the English one above. An infusion of cleavers (*Galium aparine*) or of fennel seed (*Foeniculum vulgare*) was claimed to reduce the sense of hunger (Meyer 1985: 262, 264). Chewing tree leaves has been reported as a way of removing hunger (UCLA Folklore Archive 1_5725).

*See also* **Amulet, Ash, Celtic tradition, Chickweed, Elm, Sassafras.**

## References

Allen, David E., and Gabrielle Hatfield. *Medicinal Plants in Folk Tradition.* Portland, OR: Timber Press, in press.

Beith, Mary. *Healing Threads: Traditional Medicines of the Highlands and Islands.* Edinburgh: Polygon, 1995.

Camazine, Scott, and Robert A. Bye. "A Study of the Medical Ethnobotany of the Zuni Indians of New Mexico." *Journal of Ethnopharmacology* 2 (1980): 365–388.

Gifford, E. W. "Ethnographic Notes on the Southwestern Pomo." *Anthropological Records* 25 (1967): 10–15.

Hamel, Paul B., and Mary U. Chiltoskey. *Cherokee Plants and Their Uses: A 400 Year History.* Sylva, NC: Herald, 1975.

Henderson, Mark. "Cactus Pricks Obesity Problem." *(London) Times,* April 14, 2001.

Meyer, Clarence. *American Folk Medicine.* Glenwood, IL: Meyerbooks, 1985.

Micheletti, Enza (ed.). *North American Folk Healing: An A–Z Guide to Traditional Remedies.* New York and Montreal: Reader's Digest Association, 1998.

Pennant, Thomas. *A Tour in Scotland and Voyage to the Hebrides.* Chester: John Monk, 1774.

Perry, Myra Jean. *Food Uses of "Wild" Plants by Cherokee Indians.* M.S. thesis, University of Tennessee, Knoxville, 1975.

Romero, John Bruno. *The Botanical Lore of the California Indians.* New York: Vantage Press, 1954.

Steedman, E. V. "The Ethnobotany of the Thompson Indians of British Columbia." *Smithsonian Institution-Bureau of American Ethnology Annual Report* 45 (1928): 441–552.

Vestal, Paul A. "The Ethnobotany of the Ramah Navaho." *Papers of the Peabody Museum of American Archaeology and Ethnology* 40(4): (1952): 1–94.

Vickery, Roy. *A Dictionary of Plant Lore.* Oxford: Oxford University Press, 1995.

Willard, Terry *Edible and Medicinal Plants of the Rocky Mountains and Neighbouring Territories.* Calgary, ALTA: Wild Rose College of Natural Healing, 1992.

# Indigestion

There are numerous herbal infusions recommended in British folk medicine for treating indigestion. Among the most commonly used are infusions of various mints *(Mentha* spp.), and in particular peppermint *(Mentha piperita).* A mixture of sodium bicarbonate and peppermint has been recommended (Prince 1991: 33). Houseleek *(Sempervivum tectorum)* has been used similarly, and rue *(Ruta graveolens)* (Hatfield 1994: 54). In the Scottish Highlands, apples were regarded as a cure for indigestion (Beith 1995: 203), and the inner bark of barberry *(Berberis vulgaris)* was used there too (Beith 1995: 204). A preparation known as salep was also used in the Scottish Highlands for soothing indigestion. The main ingredient of this is the twayblade *(Listera ovata)* (Beith 1995: 232). Throughout Britain, chamomile was used to treat indigestion, a use made famous in Beatrix Potter's "Tale of the Flopsy Bunnies." Field gentian *(Gentiana campestris)* was a well known "bitter," considered to stimulate digestive juices and counter indigestion. The root of dandelion *(Taraxacum officinale)* has been similarly used (Taylor MSS).

In Northern Ireland in the nineteenth century there was a woman who specialized in curing indigestion. She eyed the patient from head to foot and measured him on three successive mornings before sunrise, using green thread; the patient then ate three dandelion leaves in the name of the Blessed Trinity on three successive mornings (M'Lintock 1899: 224). In the Scottish Highlands, dulse soup prepared from the seaweed *Rhodymenia palmata* was used as a treatment for indigestion (Beith 1995: 240). Dill *(Anethum graveolens)* has been used to treat indigestion especially in infants (Lafont 1984: 34). In Bedfordshire, sloe gin, prepared by pricking fresh sloes (berries of blackthorn, *Prunus spinosa)* with a silver pin and steeping them in gin (EFS 195Bd) was a pleasant remedy for indigestion. In Somerset, a tea prepared from the bark of white poplar *(Populus alba)* has been used (Tongue 1965: 40).

One of the simplest treatments in North American folk medicine for indigestion is to drink hot water (Meyer 1985: 237). Bathing in hot water was an alternative (Brown 1952–1964, 6: 223). Other simple household recommendations are sodium bicarbonate solution, salt and water, and lemon juice and water. Chicken gizzard, dried and powdered, has been used to treat indigestion (Meyer 1985: 238). In a variation on this remedy, the gizzard of the wild pigeon is used (McAtee 1955: 172). Coarse sand is another suggestion, recorded from both Canada and the United States (see, for example, Bradley 1964: 28). The Papago are reported to eat the red earth taken from under a fire with salt added as an indigestion cure (Vogel 1970: 202). Some other simple recommendations for indigestion are to bend over, turn over a rock, and walk straight forward without looking back (Musick 1964: 46). A remedy with an Irish origin reported from Nova Scotia is to pass a child with indigestion backward around a table leg seven times (Creighton 1968: 221). Performing a somersault is another suggestion (UCLA Folklore Archives record number 11_5414). Inhaling underarm smell is claimed to be good for indigestion (Brown 1952–1964, 6: 223). Cigar smoke inhaled is claimed to help indigestion (UCLA Folklore Archives record number 8_5494). To prevent indigestion, carrying a castor bean has been recommended as an amulet (Brown 1952–1964, 6: 221).

Among herbal recommendations are gentian (as in Britain), alder, golden seal, hops, samphire *(Salicornia maritima),* lovage *(Levisticum officinale),* chamomile (as in Britain), and bark of prickly ash root and mayapple root *(Podophyllum peltatum)* (Meyer 1985: 237–240). Dandelion roots have been used as in Britain, as has a tea made from the ashes of hickory wood *(Carya* sp.) or maplewood *(Acer* sp.), or an infusion of yarrow blossom in water (Browne 1958: 73, 74), or a tea made from white oak bark *(Quercus alba)* (Randolph 1947: 97), or poke root *(Phytolacca americana)* (Redfield 1937: 18). Eating raw parsley *(Petroselinum crispum)* (Lick and Brendle 1922: 182) or the root of Indian turnip *(Arisaema triphyllum)* (Wilson 1968: 323) are further suggestions for indigestion; others are chewing parched coffee, parched corn or pine rosin (Brown 1952–1964: 221, 222). The inner bark of the slippery elm, peeled and eaten, was found to help indigestion (Rogers 1941: 16). Calamus root *(Acorus calamus)* has been given for indigestion (Clark 1970: 23).

Some of the herbs mentioned above have been used in Native American practice for indigestion. Both slippery elm and calamus have been very widely used by Native American tribes (Moerman 1998: 46–48, 577). Alder *(Alnus rubra)* has been used by the Mendocino for stomachache (Chesnut 1902: 332). Golden seal *(Hydrastis canadensis)* has been used for dyspepsia by the Cherokee (Hamel and Chiltoskey 1975: 36). Hop has been used for intestinal pain by the Dakota (Gilmore 1919: 77) and chamomile by the Mahuna for unsettled stomachs (Romero 1954: 7). The Mendocino have used the leaves and flowers of yarrow for stomachache (Chesnut 1902: 391). White oak bark has been used for indigestion by the Cherokee (Hamel and Chiltoskey 1975: 46). Pine resin from *Pinus monophylla* has been used by the Paiute for indigestion (Train, Henrichs, and Archer 1941: 117). Several species of hickory have been used in Native American tribes to invigorate the stomach; *Carya alba* has been used in this way by the Cherokee (Hamel and Chiltoskey 1975: 38). The other herbs mentioned above do not appear to have been used for treating indigestion in Native American practice; presumably their use was developed by settlers.

*See also* **Alder, Amulet, Ash, Chamomile, Dandelion, Elm, Golden seal, Hops, Houseleek, Soda, Yarrow.**

### References

Beith, Mary. *Healing Threads: Traditional Medicines of the Highlands and Islands.* Edinburgh: Polygon, 1995.

Bradley, Francis W. "Sandlappers and Clay Eaters." *North Carolina Folklore* 12(2) (1964): 27–28.

Brown, Frank C. *Collection of North Carolina Folklore.* 7 vols. Durham, NC: Duke University Press, 1952–1964.

Browne, Ray B. *Popular Beliefs and Practice from Alabama.* Folklore Studies 9. Berkeley and Los Angeles: University of California Publications, 1958.

Chesnut, V. K. "Plants Used by the Indians of Mendocino County, California." *Contri-*

butions from the U.S. National Herbarium 7 (1902): 295–408.

Clark, Joseph D. "North Carolina Popular Beliefs and Superstitions." North Carolina Folklore 18 (1970): 1–66.

Creighton, Helen. Bluenose Magic, Popular Beliefs and Superstitions in Nova Scotia. Toronto: Ryerson Press, 1968.

EFS. English Folklore Survey, 1960s. Manuscript notes at University College London.

Gilmore, Melvin R. "Uses of Plants by the Indians of the Missouri River Region." Smithsonian Institution-Bureau of American Ethnology Annual Report, no. 33 (1919).

Hamel, Paul B., and Mary U. Chiltoskey. Cherokee Plants and Their Uses: A 400 Year History. Sylva, NC: Herald, 1975.

Hatfield, Gabrielle. Country Remedies: Traditional East Anglian Plant Remedies in the Twentieth Century. Woodbridge: Boydell, 1994.

Lafont, Anne-Marie. Herbal Folklore. Bideford: Badger Books, 1984.

Lick, David E., and Thomas R. Brendle. "Plant Names and Plant Lore among the Pennsylvania Germans." Proceedings and Addresses of the Pennsylvania German Society 33 (1922).

McAtee, W. L. "Odds and Ends of North American Folklore on Birds." Midwest Folklore 5 (1955): 169–183.

Meyer, Clarence. American Folk Medicine. Glenwood, IL: Meyerbooks, 1985.

M'Lintock, Letitia. "Some Superstitions of the Ulster Peasant." Gentleman's Magazine 286 (January–June 1899): 221–228.

Moerman, Daniel E. Native American Ethnobotany. Portland, OR: Timber Press, 1998.

Musick, Ruth Anne (ed.). "Superstitions." West Virginia Folklore 14 (1964): 38–52.

Prince, Dennis. Grandmother's Cures. An A-Z of Herbal Remedies. London: Fontana, 1991.

Randolph, Vance. Ozark Superstitions. New York: Columbia University Press, 1947.

Redfield, W. Adelbert. "Superstitions and Folk Beliefs." Tennessee Folklore Society Bulletin 3 (1937): 11–40.

Rogers, E. G. Early Folk Medical Practice in Tennessee. Murfreesboro, TN: Mid-South, 1941.

Romero, John Bruno. The Botanical Lore of the California Indians. New York: Vantage Press, 1954.

Taylor MSS. Manuscript notes of Mark R. Taylor in the Norfolk Records Office, Norwich MS4322.

Tongue, R. L. Somerset Folklore. Edited by K. M. Briggs. County Folklore 8. London: Folklore Society, 1965.

Train, Percy, James R. Henrichs, and W. Andrew Archer. Medicinal Uses of Plants by Indian Tribes of Nevada. Washington, DC: U.S. Department of Agriculture, 1941.

Vogel, Virgil J. American Indian Medicine. Norman: University of Oklahoma Press, 1970.

Wilson, Gordon. "Local Plants in Folk Remedies in the Mammoth Cave Region." Southern Folklore Quarterly 32 (1968): 320–327.

# Insect bites and stings

As a common minor emergency, insect bites and stings have attracted a whole host of household and botanical remedies in British folk medicine. Spit, urine, soda, the washday "blue bag," vinegar, and well-chewed tobacco have all been used within living memory. Plant remedies applied fresh, in the form of the crushed leaves, include plantain, dock, elder, chickweed, and dandelion (Vickery 1995: 105). In the Scottish Highlands, a poultice of dock root was applied to bee or nettle stings (Beith 1995: 214). Raw onion juice was widely used (Hatfield 1994: appendix). An onion was found to be particularly valuable for stings inside the mouth, which could otherwise cause swelling (Prince 1991: 117). The juice of houseleek, sometimes mixed with milk or cream, was another recommendation (Taylor MSS). Betony (Stachys officinalis) was made into an ointment with unsalted lard to treat bites and stings (Thompson 1925: 160). Scarlet pimpernel (Anagallis arvensis) was used in Devon (Vickery 1995: 336).

In North American folk medicine, remedies for bites and stings also include a number of domestic remedies, such as ammonia, vinegar, lemon juice, bicarbonate of soda, and rubbing alcohol. Olive oil, castor oil, sweet oil, and kerosene have all been used. Snuff has been suggested, especially for hornet or yellow jacket bites (Meyer 1985: 38), and damp tea leaves for wasp stings. There is a suggestion in Illinois that an insect bite will not swell if the body of the insect is rubbed on the wound (Hyatt 1965: 204). For a centipede bite, a suggestion is to rub it with brandy in which centipedes have been soaked (Brown 1952–1964, 6: 293). A remedy from Kansas for a spider bite is to split open a live chicken and put it on the wound (Koch 1980: 103). In Georgia, toad oil smeared on the body was claimed to immunize against insect bites. From the same area, a poultice made from ground peach seeds, dough, and honey was recommended for bee stings and mosquito and spider bites. (Killion and Waller 1972: 104). Plant remedies include preparations of lobelia or of chamomile flowers. As in Britain, both garlic and onion have been used, as well as sliced potato. Cabbage leaves have been recommended in Arkansas (Parler 1962: 912). Plantain leaves have been used, especially for spider stings, as has the juice of tobacco (Meyer 1985: 39). The powdered root of black cohosh was used to treat insect bites and stings (Micheletti 1998: 97). The crushed leaves of sassafras were used similarly.

Many plant remedies were used in Native American practice. A remedy from a Pawnee Indian was to use the juice of the wild locust shrub (? *Robinia* sp.) (Hewitt 1906: 184). Various species of plantain have been used in Native American practice to treat insect bites and stings. The Cherokee used *Plantago aristata* (Hamel and Chiltoskey 1975: 50), as well as *Plantago lanceolata* and *Plantago major*. The chewed leaves of *Rosa acicularis* were used for bee stings by the Okanagan-Colville (Turner, Bouchard, and Kennedy 1980: 131), and sassafras by the Koasati (Taylor 1940: 24).

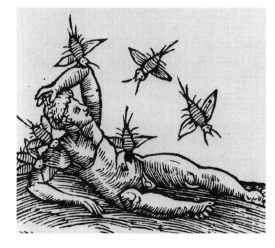

Insect bites and stings have attracted a whole host of household and botanical remedies in both British and North American folk medicine. Spit, urine, soda, ammonia, the washday "blue bag," vinegar, lemon juice, olive oil, and well-chewed tobacco have all been used. (National Library of Medicine)

Echinacea was used by the Dakota for bites and stings (Gilmore 1919: 131).

*See also* **Black cohosh, Cabbage, Chamomile, Chickweed, Dandelion, Dock, Echinacea, Elder, Garlic, Honey, Houseleek, Lobelia, Onion, Peach, Plantain, Poultice, Sassafras, Soda, Spit, Toads and frogs, Tobacco, Urine, Vinegar.**

## References

Beith, Mary. *Healing Threads: Traditional Medicines of the Highlands and Islands.* Edinburgh: Polygon, 1995.

Brown, Frank C. *Collection of North Carolina Folklore.* 7 vols. Durham, NC: Duke University Press, 1952–1964.

Gilmore, Melvin R. "Uses of Plants by the Indians of the Missouri River Region." *Smithsonian Institution-Bureau of American Ethnology Annual Report,* no. 33 (1919).

Hamel, Paul B., and Mary U. Chiltoskey. *Cherokee Plants and Their Uses: A 400 Year History.* Sylva, NC: Herald, 1975.

Hatfield, Gabrielle. *Country Remedies: Traditional East Anglian Plant Remedies in the Twentieth Century.* Woodbridge: Boydell, 1994.

Hewitt, Randall H. *Across the Plains and over the Divide.* New York: Broadway, 1906.

Hyatt, Harry Middleton. *Folklore from Adams County Illinois.* 2nd rev. ed. New York: Memoirs of the Alma Egan Hyatt Foundation, 1965.

Killion, Ronald G., and Charles Y. Waller. *A Treasury of Georgia Folklore.* Atlanta: Cherokee, 1972.

Koch, William E. *Folklore from Kansas: Beliefs and Customs.* Lawrence, KS: Regent Press, 1980.

Meyer, Clarence. *American Folk Medicine.* Glenwood, IL: Meyerbooks, 1985.

Micheletti, Enza (ed.). *North American Folk Healing: An A–Z Guide to Traditional Remedies.* New York and Montreal: Reader's Digest Association, 1998.

Parler, Mary Celestia, and University Student Contributors. *Folk Beliefs from Arkansas.* 15 vols. Fayetteville: University of Arkansas, 1962.

Prince, Dennis. *Grandmother's Cures: An A–Z of Herbal Remedies.* London: Fontana, 1991.

Taylor, Linda Averill. *Plants Used as Curatives by Certain Southeastern Tribes.* Cambridge, MA: Botanical Museum of Harvard University, 1940.

Taylor MSS. Manuscript notes of Mark R. Taylor in the Norfolk Record Office, Norwich. MS4322.

Thompson, T. W. "English Gypsy Folk-Medicine." *Journal of the Gypsy Lore Society* 3(4) (1925): 159–172.

Turner, Nancy J., R. Bouchard, and Dorothy I. D. Kennedy. *Ethnobotany of the Okanagan-Colville Indians of British Columbia and Washington.* Victoria: British Columbia Provincial Museum, 1980.

Vickery, Roy. *A Dictionary of Plant Lore.* Oxford: Oxford University Press, 1995.

## Insomnia

*See* **Sleeplessness.**

## Ivy (*Hedera helix*)

Common throughout Britain, this woody evergreen climber has been extensively used in British folk medicine. In the distant past it had religious and magical connotations. Bacchus's wreath was composed of ivy leaves, and ancient writers maintained that the plant could prevent intoxication. A bush of ivy was used as a sign outside British taverns, hence the saying, "A good wine needs no bush." In Scottish lore, a wreath of three plants twisted together—ivy, honeysuckle, and rowan—was placed over the lintel of a cow byre to protect the cattle from evil of all sorts (Darwin 1996: 72). In folk medicine, ivy has been used particularly extensively in the treatment of corns. Sometimes the leaves were soaked in vinegar (Hatfield 1994: 52). In other instances the leaves were simply worn inside socks. In one record, from Norfolk, UK, it is stipulated that an ivy leaf growing on an ash tree is a cure for corns (Hatfield 1994: 53), a remedy that perhaps reflects the reverence in which the ash tree is held in folk medicine worldwide. Crushed in oil, ivy leaves formed a treatment for burns , a remedy recorded from both Scotland and Ireland (Allen and Hatfield in press). It has been used for a variety of other skin complaints, including ringworm, boils, and eczema.

In Ireland it has been recorded that a cap made from ivy leaves was used as treatment for eczema, while in Shropshire drinking from a cup made from ivy wood was considered a cure for whooping cough (Notes and Queries, series 1, 7 [1853], 128). The juice of ivy leaves was used in Ireland to treat wounds (Logan 1972: 69). An infusion of ivy leaves has been used throughout Britain to treat sore eyes (Jobson 1967: 59). The juice of the leaves has been snuffed up the nose to cure a cold (Radford and Radford 1974). The berries have been used for aches and pains in Ireland (Barbour 1897: 386–390), for mumps in Devon (Lafont 1984: 49), and for "nerves" in Gloucestershire (Gibbs 1898: 57). From Devon there is a record of using a wash of ivy leaf infusion on the throat as a cure for stutters

(Prince 1991: 103). Warts have been treated with ivy leaves steeped in vinegar (Tongue 1965: 43).

No *Hedera* species is native to North America, although *Hedera helix* has become naturalized and ivies are grown horticulturally. Not surprisingly, ivy does not figure significantly in North American folk medicine. There are records of its use for kidney trouble (Peattie 1943: 113). Crushed leaves rubbed onto the forehead or the juice snuffed up the nose has been used for treating headache (UCLA Folklore Records 4_1904; 3_1904). A poultice of ivy leaves has been used to treat boils (Parr 1962: 9). An infusion of ivy leaves has been given to children suffering from hives (Rogers 1941: 38), and an infusion of the leaves has been given for croup (UCLA Folklore Archive 11_5355).

There is some confusion arising from the name "ivy," as it is also applied to the unrelated ground ivy *(Glechoma hederacea)* and to poison ivy *(Rhus radicans)*. It is possible that some of the records above may belong to one of these.

*See also* **Ash, Boils, Burns, Colds, Croup, Eczema, Eye problems, Headache, Hives, Poultice, Ringworm, Warts, Whooping cough, Wounds.**

**References**

Allen, David E., and Gabrielle Hatfield. *Medicinal Plants in Folk Tradition.* Portland, OR: Timber Press, in press.

Barbour, John H. "Some Country Remedies and Their Uses." *Folk-Lore* 8 (1897): 386–390.

Darwin, Tess. *The Scots Herbal: The Plant Lore of Scotland.* Edinburgh: Mercat Press, 1996.

Gibbs, J. Arthur. *A Cotswold Village.* London: John Murray, 1898.

Hatfield, Gabrielle. *Country Remedies: Traditional East Anglian Plant Remedies in the Twentieth Century.* Woodbridge: Boydell, 1994.

Jobson, Allan. *In Suffolk Borders.* London: Robert Hale, 1967.

Lafont, Anne-Marie. *Herbal Folklore.* Bideford: Badger Books, 1984.

Logan, Patrick. *Making the Cure: A Look at Irish Folk Medicine.* Dublin: Talbot Press, 1972.

*Notes and Queries,* series 1, vol. vii, p. 128. London, 1853.

Parr, Jerry S. "Folk Cures of Middle Tennessee." *Tennessee Folklore Society Bulletin* 28 (1962): 8–12.

Peattie, Roderick (ed.). *The Great Smokies and the Blue Ridge.* New York: Vanguard Press, 1943.

Prince, Dennis. *Grandmother's Cures: An A–Z of Herbal Remedies.* London: Fontana, 1991.

Radford, E., and M. A. Radford. *Encyclopaedia of Superstitions.* Edited by Christina Hole. London: Book Club Associates, 1974.

Rogers, E. G. *Early Folk Medical Practices in Tennessee.* Murfreesboro, TN: Mid-South, 1941.

Tongue, Ruth L. *Somerset Folklore.* Edited Katharine Briggs. County Folklore 8. London: Folklore Society, 1965.

# J

## Jaundice

In British folk medicine there are some unusual remedies for jaundice. A bizarre superstition from Staffordshire is that if a bladder is filled with the patient's urine and placed near the fire, as it dries out, the patient will recover (Black 1883: 56). In West Sussex, a live spider rolled up in its own web and swallowed as a pill is a cure for jaundice (Black 1883: 60). Live head lice ingested were a jaundice treatment in Westmoreland, and roasted and powdered earthworms have been used in Ireland (Radford and Radford 1961: 155, 218). In the seventeenth century, snails were recommended for jaundice (Antrobus 1929: 78). In Scotland, sheep's dung in water was reputedly used to treat jaundice (Black 1883: 157), as was cooked mouse (Black 1883: 159). Also in Scotland, there was a belief that jaundice could be cured by giving the patient a violent fright (Beith 1995: 103). A decoction of the common slater (woodlouse) in beer was also used in Scotland to treat jaundice (Beith 1995: 159). Sweetened urine was another remedy for jaundice used in the Highlands of Scotland (Beith 1995: 188). In Ireland, urine was mixed with milk and drunk for jaundice (Logan 1972: 47). A Yorkshire version of this remedy suggests baking a rye cake with the patient's urine and then burning it slowly; as it burns, the illness will abate (Gutch 1901: 191).

An issue of the *North British Mail* for 1883 records a jaundice remedy from the island of Tiree involving boiling nine stones in water taken from the crests of nine waves. The patient's shirt was then dipped in this water and put on while still wet. Alternatively, the water could come from nine springs where cresses grow (*North British Mail,* March 20, 1883).

There are a number of herbal remedies as well. Bogbean combined with raspberry and wild mint (*Mentha* spp.) was used for treating jaundice (Beith 1995: 207). Bogbean's name in Shetland, gulsa girse, means "yellow sickness plant" (Vickery 1995: 42). Barberry *(Berberis vulgaris)* is known in Cornwall as the "jaundice tree" and has been widely used in England and Ireland for treating jaundice. A decoction of the bark was used (Vickery 1995: 25). Broom *(Cytisus scoparius)* has also been used for treating jaundice (Vickery 1995: 51). Particularly in Ireland, dandelion *(Taraxacum officinale)* has been used, as were the flowers of gorse *(Ulex europaeus)* (Vickery 1995: 158). Ale made from nettle roots was used in Scotland for treating jaundice (Gregor 1884: 377). Infantile jaundice was treated in the Isle of Wight with a preparation of the greater celandine *(Chelidonium majus)* (Bromfield 1856: 26). Primrose *(Primula vulgaris)* has been used in Ireland, and cowslip in England, for treating jaundice. There is a record from Wales of the leaves of the "savage tree" (?*Juniperus* sp.) being used to treat jaundice (EFS record number 221). In East Anglia, chickweed and salsify (*Tragopogon porrifolius)* have been used in jaundice treatment (Newman 1945: 354). The inner bark of the elm (*Ulmus* spp.) boiled in milk was taken for jaundice in Herefordshire (Leather 1912: 80) and in Ireland (Vickery 1995: 127).

There is a similar, larger but equally miscellaneous, group of remedies for jaundice in North American folk medicine. Various forms of lice figure in a number of them. Sowbugs (the equivalent of the English woodlouse, Scottish slater) boiled in water have been taken to treat jaundice (Brown ca. 1930: 5). In Ohio parched wood lice have been given mixed with molasses (Puckett 1981: 407). Sheep lice in milk have been used in Illinois, as has goose-manure tea (Hyatt 1965: 329). Fishworms rolled in lard made an alternative (Randolph 1947: 107). Less unpleasant suggestions were pearls dissolved in vinegar (De Lys 1948: 285) and a mixture of horn scrapings and honey (Allen 1963: 86). Eating shellfish is a recommendation of Japanese origin (UCLA Folklore Archives, record number 23_5423). A remedy strikingly similar to the one reported from Yorkshire suggests baking a cornmeal cake with the patient's urine, burning it, and throwing it away (Hyatt 1965: 329).

There were numerous amulets used in North American folk medicine to protect against jaundice or to cure it. They include a copper necklace or penny worn around the neck (UCLA Folklore Archives record number 11_6404); red beets worn round the neck (Wine 1957: 151); amber (Curtin 1907: 465); a wedding ring worn round the neck, and a five dollar gold piece strapped to the chest (Puckett 1981: 407). From Pennsylvania the practice has been reported of dressing the patient in yellow clothes to cure jaundice, a custom apparently of Russian origin (Crosby 1927: 307). There are also examples of jaundice remedies involving transference. Hard-boiled eggs were placed under the armpits overnight (Hyatt 1965: 329) or strung on a necklace overnight. Next morning the egg-whites would be yellow, and the patient white (Rogers 1941: 31). Tying a fish against the stomach was a suggestion from California (UCLA Folklore Archives, record number 17_6404). Urinating through a bored-out carrot (Lick 1922: 107) or filling a scooped-out apple or turnip with urine (Hyatt 1965: 329) were other suggestions.

Miscellaneous remedies include having someone spit on the patient three times during the night without his or her knowing (Puckett 1981: 407) and, for a jaundiced baby, placing it between two pillows, to "bleach" out the jaundice (UCLA Folklore Archives record number 23_58900). "Taking the waters" at Schooley's Mountain in western Morris County was reckoned to be a cure for many ailments, including jaundice (Wildes 1943: 313).

There were a number of household remedies ingested for jaundice, including eggs, vinegar, new cider, and a tea made from oats (*Avena* sp.). Herbal remedies include dandelion, greater celandine, and barberry, as used in Britain. Sometimes the celandine (*Chelidonium majus*) was worn in the shoes (Lick and Brendle 1922: 215), sometimes ingested (Meyer 1985: 152). Other botanical remedies include the leaves or the bark of peach (*Prunus persica),* wild cherry bark, hops, boneset, walnut bark (*Juglans* sp.), black alder (*Ilex verticillata),* and cinquefoil (*Potentilla canadensis*) (Meyer 1985: 150–152). Strawberry leaves (*Fragaria* spp.) have been used (Lick and Brendle 1922: 35), as has a tea made from catnip (Puckett 1981: 407) or from mullein (Parler 1962: 735). Other herbal infusions used include St. John's wort (Wilson 1960: 317), yarrow (Hendricks et al. 1959: 112), mayapple root (*Podophyllum peltatum*) (Clark 1970: 24), mulberry roots *(Morus nigra)* (Mason

1957: 31), root of yellow dock *(Rumex crispus)* (Lick and Brendle 1922: 295), horehound (Campa 1950: 342), rosemary leaves *(Rosmarinus offficinalis)* (UCLA Folklore Archives record number 4_2092), calamus root *(Acorus calamus)* (Puckett 1981: 407), ironwood bark *(Carpinus caroliniana),* and crossvine *(Bignonia capreolata)* (Rogers 1941: 17). Several herbs were sometimes combined, as in a pleasant-sounding remedy from Carolina consisting of a tea brewed from wild oranges and basil (Brown 1952–1964, 6: 227). Bruised lobelia with red pepper pods in whisky was used by the pioneers in the Midwest (Pickard and Buley 1945: 43). A mixture of sarsaparilla root, red sumac *(Rhus* sp.), bitter root *(Lewisia* sp.), wild cherry bark *(Prunus* sp.), and wild poplar root *(Populus* sp.) was used in Indiana (Halpert 1950: 3–4). In New Mexico, logwood *(Haematoxylon* spp.) has been used to treat jaundice. The liquid extract is drunk, and a glassful is placed on a window sill for the patient to gaze at; the yellow color, it is hoped, transfers from the patient to the liquid (Curtin 1930: 195). A remedy unusual for combining plant and animal ingredients is a mixture of *Aralia racemosa,* molasses, and sowbugs (Mellinger 1968: 49).

Various vegetables were used in jaundice treatment, such as artichokes *(Helianthus tuberosus)* (UCLA Folklore Archive record number 6_7607) and collards *(Brassica oleracea)* (Browne 1958: 75). It was believed that tobacco *(Nicotiana* spp.) could destroy jaundice (Smith 1929: 74), while daisies *(Bellis perennis)* were credited with the ability to restore color after jaundice (Clark 1970: 11).

In Native American practice, a large number of plants have been used to treat liver disorders in general (Moerman 1998: 806). Specifically for treating jaundice, *Juglans cinerea* has been used by the Iroquois (Herrick 1977: 295). Various species of *Prunus* have been used; for instance, *Prunus cerasus* has been used by the Cherokee (Hamel and Chiltoskey 1975: 28). Collards were eaten for jaundice by the Catawba (Speck 1944: 46). Many other plants used to treat jaundice by Native Americans have not been traced in general folk usage in North America. Interestingly, swallowing a louse for jaundice was collected from Alberta as a Native American remedy (Adam 1945: 14).

*See also* **Amber, Amulet, Bogbean, Boneset, Cherry, Chickweed, Cowslip, Dock, Gold, Hops, Horehound, Lobelia, Mouse, Mullein, St. John's wort, Sarsaparilla, Snail, Spider, Stinging nettle, Transference, Urine, Yarrow.**

### References

Adam, Francois. "Duhamel." *Alberta Folklore Quarterly* 1 (1945), 12–17.
Allen, John W. *Legends and Lore of Southern Illinois.* Carbondale, IL: Southern Illinois University, 1963.
Antrobus, A. A. "Scraps of English Folklore, XVII." *Folk-Lore,* 40 (1929): 77–83.
Beith, Mary. *Healing Threads: Traditional Medicines of the Highlands and Islands.* Edinburgh: Polygon, 1995.
Black, William George. *Folk-Medicine: A Chapter in the History of Culture.* London: Folklore Society, 1883.
Bromfield, W. A. *Flora Vectensis.* London: 1856.
Brown, Charles E. *American Folklore: Insect Lore.* Madison, WI: State Historical Museum, ca. 1930.
Brown, Frank C. *Collection of North Carolina Folklore.* 7 vols. Durham, NC: Duke University Press, 1952–1964.
Browne, Ray B. *Popular Beliefs and Practices from Alabama.* Folklore Studies 9. Berkeley and Los Angeles: University of California Publications, 1958.
Campa, Arthur L. "Some Herbs and Plants of Early California." *Western Folklore* 9 (1950): 338–347.
Clark, Joseph D. "North Carolina Popular Beliefs and Superstitions." *North Carolina Folklore* 18 (1970): 1–66.
Crosby, Rev. John R. "Modern Witches of Penn-

sylvania." *Journal of American Folklore* 40 (1927): 304–309.

Curtin, L. S. M. "Pioneer Medicine in New Mexico." *Folk-Say* (1930): 186–196.

Curtin, Roland G. "The Medical Superstitions of Precious Stones, Including Notes on the Therapeutics of other Stones." *Bulletin of the American Academy of Medicine* 8 (December 1907): 444–494.

De Lys, Claudia. *A Treasury of American Superstitions.* New York: Philosophical Library, 1948.

EFS. English Folklore Survey, 1960s. Manuscript notes in University College London.

Gregor, W. "Unspoken Nettles." *Folk-Lore Journal* 2 (1884): 377–378.

Gutch, Mrs Eliza *Examples of Printed Folk-Lore Concerning the North Riding of Yorkshire, York and Ainsty.* County Folk-Lore 2, Printed extracts 4. London: Folklore Society, 1901.

Halpert, Violetta. "Folk Cures from Indiana." *Hoosier Folklore* 9 (1950): 1–12.

Hamel, Paul B., and Mary U. Chiltoskey. *Cherokee Plants and Their Uses: A 400 Year History.* Sylva, NC: Herald, 1975.

Hendricks, George D., et al. "Utah State University Folklore Collection." *Western Folklore* 18 (1959): 107–120.

Herrick, James William. *Iroquois Medical Botany.* Ph.D. thesis, State University of New York, Albany, 1977.

Hyatt, Harry Middleton. *Folklore from Adams County Illinois.* 2nd rev. ed. New York: Memoirs of the Alma Egan Hyatt Foundation, 1965.

Leather, Ella Mary. *The Folklore of Herefordshire Collected from Oral and Printed Sources.* Hereford: Jakeman and Carver; and London: Sidgwick and Jackson, 1912.

Lick, David E., and Thomas R. Brendle. "Plant Names and Plant Lore among the Pennsylvania Germans." *Proceedings and Addresses of the Pennsylvania German Society* 33 (1922).

Logan, Patrick. *Making the Cure: A Look at Irish Folk Medicine.* Dublin: Talbot Press, 1972.

Mason, James. "Home Remedies in West Virginia." *West Virginia Folklore* 7 (1957): 27–32.

Mellinger, Marie B. "Sang Sign." *Foxfire* 2(2) (1968): 15; 47–52.

Meyer, Clarence. *American Folk Medicine.* Glenwood, IL: Meyerbooks, 1985.

Moerman, Daniel E. *Native American Ethnobotany.* Portland, OR: Timber Press, 1998.

Newman, L. F. "Some Notes on Folk Medicine in the Eastern Counties." *Folk-Lore* 56 (1945): 349–360

Parler, Mary Celestia, and University Student Contributors. *Folk Beliefs from Arkansas.* 15 vols. Fayetteville: University of Arkansas, 1962.

Pickard, Madge E., and R. Carlyle Buley. *The Midwest Pioneer, His Ills, Cures and Doctors.* Crawfordsville, IN: R. E. Bantam, 1945.

Puckett, Newbell Niles. *Popular Beliefs and Superstitions: A Compendium of American Folklore from the Ohio Collection of Newbell Niles Puckett.* Edited by Wayland D. Hand, Anna Casetta, and Sondra D. Thiederman. 3 vols. Boston: G. K. Hall, 1981.

Radford, E., and M. A. Radford. *Encyclopedia of Superstitions.* Edited and revised by Christina Hole. London: Hutchinson, 1961.

Randolph, Vance. *Ozark Superstitions.* New York: Columbia University Press, 1947.

Rogers, E. G. *Early Folk Medical Practice in Tennessee.* Murfreesboro, Tenn.: Mid-South, 1941.

Smith, Walter R. *Animals and Plants in Oklahoma Folk Cures: Folk-Say—A Regional Miscellany.* Edited by B. A. Botkin. Norman: Oklahoma Folk-Lore Society, 1929.

Speck, Frank G. "Catawba Herbals and Curative Practices." *Journal of American Folklore* 57 (1944): 37–50.

Vickery, Roy. *A Dictionary of Plant Lore.* Oxford: Oxford University Press, 1995.

Wildes, Harry Emerson. *Twin Rivers (Rivers of America).* New York: Farrar and Rinehart 1943.

Wilson, Miki. "St. John's Wort." *Journal of the Indiana State Medical Association* 53(2) (February 1960): 316–317.

Wine, Martin L. "Superstitions Collected in Chicago." *Midwest Folklore* 7 (1957) 149–159.

# Jimson weed

*See* **Thornapple.**

# Josselyn, John

Born in the early years of the seventeenth century, Josselyn (1608–1675) made two visits to the colonies, where his brother was a wealthy landowner. He published two books as a result of his nine years spent in North America: *New England's Rarities Discovered in Birds, Beasts, Fishes, Serpents, and Plants of That Country* (London, 1672) and *An Account of Two Voyages to New-England, Made During the Years 1638, 1663* (London, 1674). The earlier of these books contained the first account of the local plants to be published in English. Much of the plant natural history that he recorded constituted a very valuable contribution to the knowledge of the plants of that region and their medicinal applications.

**Reference**

Felter, H. W. (ed.). "The Genesis of the American Materia Medica including a Biographical Sketch of Josselyn." *Bulletin Lloyd Library,* no. 25 (1927).

# K

---

## King's Evil

*See* **Tuberculosis.**

# L

## Lobelia (*Lobelia inflata*)

This herb has attracted a great deal of attention and even some notoriety among medical practitioners on both sides of the Atlantic. A native of North America, it was introduced to Britain by the Thomsonian school of herbalism in the nineteenth century. The plant is poisonous, and Samuel Thomson was actually tried for murder in 1809 after treating one of his patients unsuccessfully. It is still used in herbal practice in Britain but has no role there in folk medicine.

In North America it was one of the important herbal discoveries in early colonial days. Widely used by the Native Americans for a variety of respiratory problems, it was adopted into herbalism and then into folk medicine, especially as a treatment for coughs and asthma. It was one of the herbs grown commercially by the Shakers. It is often called Indian tobacco, and ironically it finds a use today in reducing nicotine addiction to the "true" tobacco, *Nicotiana* spp. (Chevallier 1996: 108). In Maine it is called asthma weed or pukeweed, reflecting its main uses in folk medicine. Described by a mid-nineteenth century writer as "a grand article to be relied upon for the alleviation or cure" of asthma, it was prepared in a number of ways. The dried seed pods were crushed and eaten, or the herb was boiled and sweetened to make a syrup (Meyer 1985: 32, 33). It has also been used, mixed with raspberry vinegar and honey, to soothe whooping cough. Other more minor uses in North American folk medicine include application of the herb as a fomentation to boils, felons, or the swellings of mumps, and as an eye wash for sore eyes (Meyer 1985: 44, 111, 123, 181). It was also used externally as a fomentation for treating neuralgia, colic, and sprains (Meyer 1985: 71, 187, 232). In cases of pneumonia the herb was used as a chest poultice (Brown 1952–1964, 6: 250). For croup in infants, it was given mixed with molasses (Jack 1964: 36). With red pepper and whisky, it formed a treatment for consumption (Richmond and Van Winkle 1958: 124). New Englanders called the plant "colic weed" and used it to treat gastritis (Jordan 1944: 146). Mixed with glycerine, a tincture of the plant was used to make ear drops for deafness (Stout 1936: 191).

In Native American usage, this species of lobelia has been used by the Cherokee in very similar ways; it has been applied externally for aches and pains, bites, and sores; it has been chewed for sore throat and given for croup as well as asthma; and, interestingly, it has been used to "break the tobacco habit" (Hamel and Chiltoskey 1975: 40). It seems likely that many of the American folk medical uses have been learned from Native American practice, as have many of the present-day uses in British herbalism.

Other species of lobelia have been used more extensively by Native Americans, especially *Lobelia cardinalis,* which had a wide variety of uses and was considered a panacea by the Iroquois (Herrick 1977: 453). A related species, *Lobelia siphilitica,* was, as its name implies, used to treat syphilis among both Native Americans and European settlers. Among the Meskwaki this plant was also used as a love medicine, eaten by a couple to avert divorce (Smith 1928: 231).

*See also* **Asthma; Boils; Colic; Coughs; Croup; Deafness; Felons; Poultice; Shakers; Sprains; Thomson, Samuel; Tuberculosis; Whooping cough.**

## References

Brown, Frank C. *Collection of North Carolina Folklore.* 7 vols. Durham, NC: Duke University Press, 1952–1964.

Chevallier, Andrew. *The Encyclopedia of Medicinal Plants.* London: Dorling Kindersley, 1996.

Hamel, Paul B., and Mary U. Chiltoskey. *Cherokee Plants and Their Uses: A 400 Year History.* Sylva, NC: Herald, 1975.

Herrick, James William. *Iroquois Medical Botany.* Ph.D. thesis, State University of New York, Albany. 1977.

Jack, Phil R. "Folk Medicine from Western Pennsylvania." *Pennsylvania Folklife* 14(2) (October 1964): 35–37.

Jordan, Philip D. "Botanic Medicine in the Western Country." *Ohio State Medical Journal* 40 (1944): 143–146.

Meyer, Clarence. *American Folk Medicine.* Glenwood, IL: Meyerbooks, 1985.

Richmond, W. Edson, and Elva Van Winkle. "Is There a Doctor in the House?" *Indiana History Bulletin* 35 (1958): 115–135.

Smith, Huron H. "Ethnobotany of the Meskwaki Indians." *Bulletin of the Public Museum of the City of Milwaukee* 4 (1928): 175–326.

Stout, Earl J. "Folklore from Iowa." *Memoirs of the American Folklore Society* 29 (1936).

# Lumbago

*See* **Backache.**

# M

## Mad dog, bite of

Fear of rabies, which even today is normally fatal to humans, has naturally led to a diversity of folk medical treatments for the bite of mad dogs. Black reports a practice in Scotland of drying the heart of a mad dog and giving it to the person bitten as a cure. Similarly, a case was reported in the 1860s of a child bitten by a rabid dog who died despite having been given a slice of its liver roasted (Black 1883: 51–52). These remedies are clearly sympathetic in nature. "Madstones" were used in treating hydrophobia and protecting against it. These were smooth, rounded stones, said to have been concretions formed inside one of a variety of animals. The distinction between bezoar and madstones is unclear. Such stones have been used therapeutically since the thirteenth century (Black 1883: 145). One such stone, found in Switzerland, was obtained by an Italian, who sold it to a farmer in Kentucky. The farmer is said to have used it to cure fifty-nine people of hydrophobia (Black 1883: 144). In South Wales, the grass in a particular churchyard was held to be a cure for hydrophobia (Black 1883: 96). In the sixteenth century, in order to tell whether a dog bite was that of a mad dog, it was held that a roasted walnut, laid over the bite, should be fed to a chicken: if it died, the dog causing the bite was a mad one (Allen 1995: 59–60). In Ireland, the touch of a seventh son was believed to cure hydrophobia (Wilde 1919: 201).

In British folk medicine, the ash-colored liverwort (*Peltigera canina*) was used, as it was also in official medicine, to treat hydrophobia. It was still in use in Caernarvonshire, Wales, in the early nineteenth century (Trevelyan 1909: 314). One of the Newmarket huntsmen of James II told the king of a cure for hydrophobia using a plant called "star-of-the-earth," which was subsequently shown to be buck's-horn plantain, *Plantago coronopus* (Cullum MS). A preparation of the leaves of scarlet pimpernel (*Anagallis arvensis*) was used in the past for treating the bites of mad dogs (Nuttall, n.d., 1: 181) and was still in use relatively recently in Glamorgan, Wales, for treating dog bites (Trevelyan 1909: 313). Salt was valued as a bandage for the bites of mad dogs (Black 1883: 131).

In North American folk medicine as in British, madstones were used in treatment of hydrophobia. One such was described in use in about 1806 in Frederick County. It was claimed to have cured eighty cases (Blanton 1935: 272). In Alabama, a madstone derived from a deer was recommended (Browne 1958: 78). The stone was sometimes applied warm to the bite, after being boiled in milk (Koch 1980: 90). As in Britain, various parts of the dog that had bitten were used in cures. The powdered jawbone was part of a mixture applied to bites (Pickard and Buley 1945: 80). The liver of the dog was claimed to cure the bite of the same dog (Bergen 1899: 77), much as in Scotland, above. A person bitten by a mad dog was advised to eat some of its hair in a bread and butter sandwich (Simon 1954: 2); remedies such as this are presumably the origin of the phrase "hair of the dog." Wearing a tooth taken from a mad dog as an amulet against hydrophobia was another suggestion (UCLA Folklore Archives 25_7597). A variety of substances were recommended as applications to the bite of a mad dog. They include deer gall (Browne 1958: 78), kerosene, or a mixture of soda, alcohol, and tobacco (McGlasson 1941: 18). Wrapping a chicken round the bite was suggested (Puckett 1981: 362). Cauterizing the wound with a hot metal bar made from a horseshoe was recommended (Brendle and Unger 1935: 215). As in Ireland, the touch of the hand of a seventh son was believed to cure the bite of a mad dog (Puckett 1981: 363).

Plant remedies used to treat hydrophobia in North American folk medicine include elecampane (*Inula helenium*) (UCLA Folklore Archives 8 6478), mugwort, and garlic and burdock (Brendle and Unger 1935: 214, 215); mint (*Mentha* sp.) mixed with salt (Clark 1970: 23); red chicken weed (*Anagallis arvensis*, known in Britain as scarlet pimpernel, see above) (Hetrick 1957: 249); and rattlesnake plantain (*Goodyera pubescens*) (Bergen 1899: 166).

*See also* **Amulet, Burdock, Garlic, Mugwort, Seventh son, Sympathetic magic.**

### References
Allen, Andrew. *A Dictionary of Sussex Folk Medicine.* Newbury: Countryside Books, 1995.
Bergen, Fanny D. "Animal and Plant Lore Collected from the Oral Tradition of English Speaking Folk." *Memoirs of the American Folk-Lore Society* 7 (1899).
Black, William George. *Folk-Medicine: A Chapter in the History of Culture.* London: Folklore Society, 1883.
Blanton, Wyndham B. "Madstones: With an Account of Several from Virginia." *Annals of Medical History* 7 (1935): 268–273.
Brendle, Thomas R., and Claude W. Unger. "Folk Medicine of the Pennsylvania Germans: The Non-Occult Cures." *Proceedings of the Pennsylvania German Society* 45 (1935).
Browne, Ray B. *Popular Beliefs and Practices from Alabama.* Folklore Studies 9. Berkeley and Los Angeles: University of California Publications, 1958.
Clark, Joseph D. "North Carolina Popular Beliefs and Superstitions." *North Carolina Folklore* 18 (1970): 1–66.
Cullum MS. Hand-written notes by Sir John Cullum in his copy of Hudson's *Flora Anglica.* 1762. Suffolk Record Office.
Hetrick, George. "Practice of Medicine in Berks from Time of Early Settlers to 1824." *Medical Record* 48(8) (October 1957): 247–250.
Koch, William E. *Folklore from Kansas: Beliefs and Customs.* Lawrence, KS: Regent Press, 1980.
McGlasson, Cleo. "Superstitions and Folk Beliefs of Overton County." *Tennessee Folklore Society Bulletin* 7 (1941): 13–27.
Nuttall, G. Clarke. *Wild Flowers as They Grow.* 5 vols. London: Waverley Book, n.d.
Pickard, Madge E., and R. Carlyle Buley. *The Midwest Pioneer, His Ills, Cures and Doctors.* Crawfordsville, IN: R. E. Banta, 1945.
Puckett, Newbell Niles. *Popular Beliefs and Superstitions: A Compendium of American Folklore from the Ohio Collection of Newbell Niles Puckett.* Edited by Wayland D. Hand, Anna Casetta, and Sondra B. Thiederman. 3 vols. Boston: G. K. Hall, 1981.
Simon, Isaak Shirk. "Dutch Folk-Beliefs." *Pennsylvania Dutchman* 5(14) (March 15, 1954): 2–3, 15.
Trevelyan, Marie. *Folk-Lore and Folk-stories of Wales.* London: Elliot Stock, 1909.
Wilde, Lady. *Ancient Legends, Mystic Charms and Superstitions of Ireland.* London: Chatto and Windus, 1919.

# Mallow (*Malva* spp.)

The common mallow (*Malva sylvestris*) has held an important place in British folk medicine. It is a common and widespread plant in Britain, and its flowering shoots have been crushed and used as a poultice for healing boils and abscesses, for treating cuts and sores, and for soothing sprains and rheumatic joints. In addition, the fruits have been eaten as a gentle laxative (Hatfield 1994: 28). These fruits were known as "cheeses" in East Anglia, and as "biscuities" in Scotland (Vickery 1995: 229). Other folk uses for the plant include treatment of burns, sore and strained eyes, ulcers, varicose veins, and sore feet (Tongue 1965: 37, 39, 42, 43). The crushed leaves have also been used for treating bruises (Hawke 1973: 28). The far less common marsh mallow *(Althaea officinalis),* famous for the sweets originally made from its root, was the mallow recommended by the herbals and used in official medicine in the past, and in present-day medical herbalism. Although this species is native in a few places in Britain, it has probably never been common enough to be exploited as a folk remedy on a large scale. However, there is inevitably some confusion here, since common mallow is also called "marshmallow" by many. In Devon, marsh mallow has been used to treat bruises and blisters, and the roots have been given to teething babies to soothe their gums (Lafont 1984: 53). Mallow has been widely used to treat coughs and colds and related complaints. Less common has been its use for kidney complaints (Allen and Hatfield, in press).

Like several other species of mallow, *Malva sylvestris* is naturalized in North America and has been used similarly for poulticing and reducing pain and inflammation. Sometimes known as the "cheese plant," mallow has also been made into an ointment for treating eczema and used to treat sore eyes, nettle rash, and gastric ulcers (Meyer 1985: 105, 110, 141, 243). Among a collection of "Old Settlers' Remedies" from Shelburne County, bruised mallows are recommended to soothe a wasp sting, while the root of marshmallow mixed with poppy heads and conserve of roses is suggested as a cough medicine (Robertson 1960: 12, 29). Meyer reports a similar use for an infusion of mallow flowers to loosen phlegm. The dried roots of marshmallow boiled in milk have been used for "chin-cough" (i.e., whooping cough); the seeds of marshmallow, mixed with vinegar, have been used to remove skin discoloration; while the mashed leaves can be used to remove splinters and made into an ointment for wounds and salves (Meyer 1985: 191, 225, 228, 267, 276). Mallow juice has been placed in the ear for earache (UCLA Folklore Archives 1_1545). An infusion has been used to treat falling hair (UCLA Folklore Archives 3_1890), colic (Valleta 1965: 37), skin rash, and sore feet (Lick and Brendle 1922: 77). The plant has also been used to treat kidney troubles (as a diuretic) (Lawton 1967: 12) and to treat bed-wetting (Fogel 1915: 281). Headache and fever have been treated with a poultice of mallow (Saucier 1956: 36). In these remedies, it is not clear which species of mallow is involved. In Ontario, the named species *Malva rotundifolia* has been used to treat wounds (Wintemberg 1950: 15). Cheeseweed *(Malva parviflora)* has been used to treat piles (Browne 1958: 84).

It is reported that a tea made of one mallow species *(Malva neglecta)* has been used in New Mexico to ease labor pains (Willard 1992: 139). *Malva rotundifolia,* known as "cheese plant," has been used similarly by Native Americans, and it still is today (Kavasch and Baar 1999: 143). In Mexico, this species has been used as an infusion to treat wounds, as a poultice for sore throat and mumps, and internally for stomach and kidney complaints. A modern use there is as a wash for treating hair loss after chemotherapy (Kay 1996: 188). Another mallow, *Malva parviflora,* has been used for headache, fever, sores, and digestive complaints (Kay 1996: 188). Among the Iroquois, *Malva neglecta* has been used to treat swellings and broken bones (Hamel and Chiltoskey 1975: 385). Several species of mallow have been used by Native Americans for treating headache and fevers (Moerman 1998: 334–335).

*See also* **Abscesses, Blisters, Boils, Bruises, Burns, Childbirth, Colds, Colic, Coughs, Cuts, Earache, Eczema, Eye problems, Fevers, Fractures, Headache, Insect bites and stings, Piles, Poultice, Rheumatism, Sore feet, Sprains, Whooping cough, Wounds.**

## References

Allen, David, and Gabrielle Hatfield. *Medicinal Plants in Folk Tradition*. Portland, OR: Timber Press, in press.

Browne, Ray B. *Popular Beliefs and Practices from Alabama*. Folklore Studies 9. Berkeley and Los Angeles: University of California Publications, 1958.

Fogel, Edwin Miller. "Beliefs and Superstitions of the Pennsylvania Germans." *Americana Germanica* 18 (1915).

Hamel, Paul B., and Mary U. Chiltoskey. *Cherokee Plants and Their Uses: A 400 Year History*. Sylva, NC: Herald, 1975.

Hatfield, Gabrielle. *Country Remedies: Traditional East Anglian Plant Remedies in the Twentieth Century*. Woodbridge: Boydell, 1994.

Hawke, Kathleen (comp.) *Cornish Sayings, Superstitions and Remedies*. Redruth: Dyllanson Truran, 1973.

Kavasch, E. Barrie, and Karen Baar. *American Indian Healing Arts: Herbs, Rituals and Remedies for Every Season of Life*. New York: Bantam Books, 1999.

Kay, Margarita Artschwager. *Healing with Plants in the American and Mexican West*. Tucson: University of Arizona Press, 1996.

Lafont, Anne-Marie. *Herbal Folklore*. Bideford: Badger Books, 1984.

Lawton, Arthur J. "Living History." *Pennsylvania Folklife* 16(4) (Summer 1967): 10–15.

Lick, David E., and Thomas R. Brendle. "Plant Names and Plant Lore among the Pennsylvania Germans." *Proceedings and Addresses of the Pennsylvania German Society* 33 (1922).

Meyer, Clarence. *American Folk Medicine*. Glenwood, IL: Meyerbooks, 1985.

Moerman, Daniel E. *Native American Ethnobotany*. Portland, OR: Timber Press, 1998.

Robertson, Marion. *Old Settlers' Remedies*. Barrington, NS: Cape Sable Historical Society, 1960.

Saucier, Corinne L. *Traditions de la Paroisse des Avoyelles en Louisiane*. Philadelphia: American Folklore Society, 1956.

Tongue, Ruth L. *Somerset Folklore*. Edited by Katharine Briggs. County Folklore 8. London: Folklore Society, 1965.

Valleta, Clement. "Italian Immigrant Life in Northampton County, Pennsylvania 1890–1915." *Pennsylvania Folklife* 14(3) (Spring 1965): 36–45.

Vickery, Roy. *A Dictionary of Plant Lore*. Oxford: Oxford University Press, 1995.

Willard, Terry. *Edible and Medicinal Plants of the Rocky Mountains and Neighbouring Territories*. Calgary, ALTA: Wild Rose College of Natural Healing, 1992.

Wintemberg, W. J. *Folklore of Waterloo County, Ontario*. Bulletin 116, Anthropological Series 28. Ontario: National Museum of Canada, 1950.

# Mandrake

In different cultures, this name has been applied to different plants. The botanically "true" mandrake *(Mandragora officinarum)* is a native of the Mediterranean and the Near East. It is especially revered in India and Persia (Simoons 1998: 101–133), where it is held sacred as well as used medicinally. The tap root of the plant is divided into two and bears some resemblance to the human form. It contains hallucinogenic, narcotic, and highly poisonous compounds and was used three thousand years ago in Persia as an anesthetic. The plant was brought to Britain by the Romans and cultivated for medicinal use through the medieval and Tudor periods. As a native of

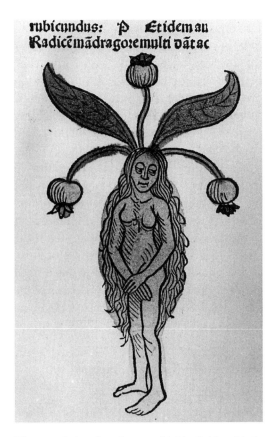

rubicundus: p Etidemau
Radicēmādragozemulti vātac

The mandrake plant became highly fashionable in official British medicine as a narcotic, hallucinogen, and aphrodisiac. In British medicine the mandrake has been "paired" with the unrelated black bryony *(Tamus communis)*; one was regarded as male, one female. (National Library of Medicine)

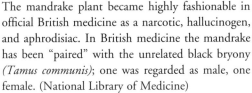

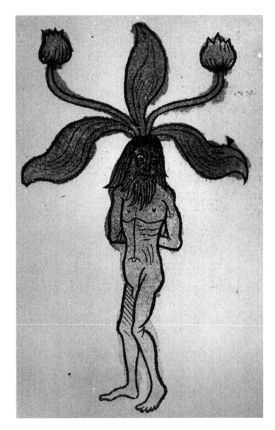

The idea of male and female mandrakes has persisted into recent times. (National Library of Medicine)

warmer climates, it was difficult to grow, and when the British climate became colder during the sixteenth century, its cultivation stopped, and the plant was imported instead.

The various legends that grew up around the plant included the suggestion that it shrieked when dug up and that the person who harvested it would die—so a dog should be used instead to uproot it. This legend was recorded by Gerard in his sixteenth-century herbal and has been repeated in Western writings ever since. The plant became highly fashionable in official medicine in Britain, as a narcotic, hallucin-

ogen, violent purgative, and aphrodisiac; it commanded a very high price. In time a thriving counterfeit industry grew up, in which fake mandrake roots were sold for high prices. On account of its cost, true mandrake probably never figured in British folk medicine, but other plants took its place, including white bryony, the tap root of which bears a resemblance to that of the true mandrake. This was one of the plants from which counterfeit mandrakes were produced from the seventeenth century onward. It became known as English mandrake, false mandrake, or, as in East Anglia, simply as mandrake. John Ray in 1691 came across an old woman who had cured her gout using this plant (Lankester 1848: 238). Particularly in horse medicine it was highly prized, though in light of the usual secrecy surrounding horsemen's remedies, it is difficult to find out how it was used, even in recent times. One man recalls that as a boy in the 1930s in Norfolk he went hunting for bryony roots because he could get a good price for them—half a crown (the equivalent of about ten pounds today). The horseman he supplied roasted and grated the root and fed it to his horses, ostensibly to improve the condition of their coats (Hatfield MS). In Sussex as recently as the twentieth century there was a mandrake seller who sold the roots of white bryony as mandrakes for healing rheumatism, malaria, indigestion, pains in the chest, and headaches (Allen 1995: 113). In recent folk medicine, white bryony figures occasionally—for example, as a chilblain remedy and carried as an amulet for rheumatism. Its reputation as an aphrodisiac has persisted into recent times, at least in Gloucestershire (Palmer 1994: 122).

Oddly, in British medicine this plant has been "paired" with the unrelated black bryony *(Tamus communis)*; one was regarded as male, one female. Probably this was due to early herbalists' identifying the white bryony and the black bryony respectively with the plants recorded by Dioscorides as "ampelos leuke" and "ampelos agria." The black bryony, which also has a large tap root, though much darker in color than that of white bryony, became known as he-mandrake, or just mandrake. White bryony was regarded as female, and some herbalists referred to it as womandrake (Allen 1995: 111). This concept spread into folk medicine, and, according to Rudkin, the "male" black bryony was used to treat women and mares, the "female" white bryony men and stallions (Rudkin 1933). The idea of male and female mandrakes has persisted in the fens into recent times (Randell 1966). In British folk medicine, black bryony was regarded as an aphrodisiac—for example, in

Lincolnshire (Woodruffe-Peacock 1894–1897)—and in addition was widely used for treating rheumatism, gout, and chilblains (see, for instance, Whitlock 1992: 104). Because of the confusion in names, it is very difficult to know to which plant any particular record refers. Any plant called "mandrake" would obviously share something of the "true" mandrake's aura of magic. North American medicine also has its "mandrake"; the mayapple *(Podophyllum peltatum)* is also known as the American mandrake, or as devil's apple. Like the "true" mandrake, it is a powerful purgative, and its medicinal use seems to have been adopted direct from Native American usage into official North American medicine (Crellin and Philpott 1990: 299).

*See also* **Amulet, Bryony, Chilblains, Gout, Headache, Indigestion, Rheumatism.**

### References

Allen, Andrew. *A Dictionary of Sussex Folk Medicine.* Newbury: Countryside Books, 1995.

Crellin, John K., and Jane Philpott. A *Reference Guide to Medicinal Plants.* Durham, NC: Duke University Press, 1990.

Lankester, Edwin (ed.). *The Correspondence of John Ray.* London: Ray Society, 1848.

Palmer, Roy. *The Folklore of Gloucestershire.* Tiverton: West Country Books, 1994.

Randell, Arthur R. *Sixty Years a Fenman.* Edited by Enid Porter. London: Routledge, 1966.

Rudkin, Ethel H. "Lincolnshire Folklore." *Folk-Lore* 44 (1933): 189–214.

Simoons, Frederick J. *Plants of Life, Plants of Death.* Madison: University of Wisconsin Press, 1998.

Whitlock, Ralph. *Wiltshire Folklore and Legends.* London: Robert Hale, 1992.

Woodruffe-Peacock, E. Adrian. *Lincolnshire Folk Names for Plants.* Lincolnshire Notes and Queries (1894–1897), 4.

# Medicine man

This name for a Native American healer is thought to have been invented by French

Jesuit missionaries in the seventeenth century. It is not quite synonymous with the term "shaman." Shamans depend for their powers on reaching an altered state of consciousness, whereas medicine men do not. Some individuals combine both roles (Lyon 1996: 168–169). The medicine man is responsible in many tribes for keeping the sacred medicine bundles used in ceremonies (Snow and Stans 2001: 27). It is the medicine man (or, more rarely, woman) who uses prayer and chants to render the medicine effective (Snow and Stans 2001: xi).

## References

Lyon, William S. *Encyclopedia of Native American Healing.* Santa Barbara, CA: ABC-CLIO, 1996.

Snow, Alice Micco, and Susan Enns Stans. *Healing Plants. Medicine of the Florida Seminole Indians.* Gainesville: University Press of Florida, 2001.

# Menopause

Because of the reticence surrounding so many "women's complaints," and the fact that many folklore authors are male, folk remedies for menopause as for other "women's complaints" are probably underrepresented in the literature. From Yorkshire comes the suggestion that eating a cock's liver after fasting will cure the hot flushes of menopause (EFS: 90Db). Drinking parsley tea *(Petroselinum crispum)* every day during the change of life was also recommended (EFS: 100Db). Teas made from sage *(Salvia officinalis)* (Hatfield 1994: 95) or from chamomile (Mrs I.P., Suffolk, pers. com., 1989) have also been used to treat the hot flushes of menopause.

In North America there is again a relative paucity of folk remedies. Meyer records the use of motherwort *(Leonurus cardiaca)* at change of life, and of nutmeg in Jamaica rum. A mixture called "mother's friend" was composed of white plantain *(Anten-*

*naria plantaginifolia),* sumac leaves *(Rhus glabra),* yellow dock *(Rumex crispus)* or burdock, and devil's bit *(Leatris spicata)* (Meyer 1985: 176). Chestnut leaf tea *(Castanea* sp.) was recommended in Alabama to be drunk during menopause (Browne 1958: 65), or a tea made from mayapple roots *(Podophyllum peltatum)* (UCLA Folklore Archives 12_5210). In Georgia, a tea prepared from parched eggshells or from green coffee was drunk during menopause (Killion and Waller 1972: 105). A remedy of French origin was to drink savory tea *(Satureja* sp.) (Roy 1955: 78). In California, Jamaica ginger *(Zingiber officinale)* tea was given (UCLA Folklore Archives 22_5431). In Arkansas chewing cinnamon bark *(Cinnamomum* sp.) was suggested (Parler 1962, 3: 1112). Chewing peach kernels was held to shorten menopause. Also from Arkansas comes the suggestion of curing hot flushes, or flashes, by placing under the bed an axe, a pan of water, and a sack of meal (Parler 1962, 3: 1112). Mexican American women use a tea made from the leaves of *Ambrosia* to treat menopausal symptoms (Kay 1996: 71). The Spanish-Americans of New Mexico use a tea made from the leaves of the wormwood *(Artemisia franserioides)* to treat the hot flushes of menopause (Kay 1996: 106). A remedy of Catawba origin was an infusion of sourwood *(Oxydendrum arboreum)* (Speck 1944: 47). The Iroquois used false Solomon's seal *(Maianthemum stellatum)* during menopause (Herrick 1977: 283). Many other plant remedies used in Native American practice are described as treating "female weakness" or "women's complaints." Doubtless some of these were used to ease menopause.

*See also* **Burdock, Chamomile, Peach.**

## References

Browne, Ray B. *Popular Beliefs and Practices from Alabama.* Folklore Studies 9. Berkeley and Los Angeles: University of California Publications, 1958.

EFS. English Folklore Survey. Manuscript notes, University College London.

Hatfield, Gabrielle. *Country Remedies: Traditional East Anglian Plant Remedies in the Twentieth Century.* Woodbridge: Boydell, 1994.

Herrick, James William. *Iroquois Medical Botany.* Ph.D. thesis, State University of New York, Albany, 1977.

Kay, Margarita Artschwager. *Healing with Plants in the American and Mexican West.* Tucson: University of Arizona Press, 1996.

Killion, Ronald G., and Charles T. Waller. *A Treasury of Georgia Folklore.* Atlanta: Cherokee, 1972.

Meyer, Clarence. *American Folk Medicine.* Glenwood, IL: Meyerbooks, 1985.

Parler, Mary Celestia, and University Student Contributors. *Folk Beliefs from Arkansas.* 15 vols. Fayetteville: University of Arkansas, 1962.

Roy, Carmen. *La Littérature Orale en Gaspésie.* Bulletin 134, 36 de la Serie Anthropologique. Ottawa: Ministre de Nord Canadien et des Ressources Nationales, 1955, 61–105, 107–136.

Speck, Frank G. "Catawba Herbals and Curative Practices." *Journal of American Folklore* 57 (1944): 37–50.

# Menstrual problems

Like other socially sensitive areas of enquiry, the folk treatment of menstrual problems is probably underreported in the literature. Perhaps women were forced to be more stoical in the past, but a lack of records seems to be a more likely explanation. Country people questioned about remedies used within living memory in East Anglia have mentioned only such simple measures as application of heat to ease period pain. Tansy *(Tanacetum vulgare)* is one of the few native British plants known to have been used to ease period pain (Hatfield 1994: appendix). Various tonics were recommended for the anemia that doubtless affected many. The waters of certain springs were thought to be rich in iron and therefore good for treating anemia. One such was the Hart Fell spa in Dumfriesshire, Scotland (Beith 1995: 132). Among plant remedies, one of the commonest was an infusion of nettles. With the benefit of modern knowledge, this is now known to be rich in iron and also to have hemostatic properties, so that it would have served the double function of correcting anemia and reducing menstrual flow.

A plant used in present-day herbalism to reduce heavy bleeding at menstruation is yarrow. Although there are many records of its use as a wound healer in the folk literature, the only record of a gynecological use comes from Devon, where it was used for heavy uterine bleeding (Collyns 1827). Chamomile, used generally in folk medicine as a painkiller, was used in Dorset for period pain (Dacombe 1935). Various plants have been used for "women's problems." In Scotland, fairy flax *(Linum catharticum)* was one of these (Allen and Hatfield in press). Mugwort was another "women's herb," used for period pain in England and in Scotland (Hatfield 1999: 79). Shepherd's purse *(Capsella bursapastoris)* has been used in Essex for heavy periods (Hatfield 1994: appendix). Irregular periods could be treated with one of a number of plant remedies, including raspberry tea. This subject is considered under abortion, since many so-called emmenagogues doubled as abortifacients.

In general, North American folk medicine information on this subject is less sparse. Warming spices such as ginger were recommended for period pain. Raspberry tea was used in much the same way as in Britain. Among the plants used in North American folk medicine generally, Meyer lists a number of plants used for period pain, including blue cohosh *(Caulophyllum thalictroides),* extract of Viburnum *(Viburnum* spp.), chamomile, hops, logwood *(Haematoxylon campechianum),* wormwood *(Artemisia* spp.), and pennyroyal *(Hedeoma pulegioides),* as well as the root of the cotton

**RISLEY'S**

**EXTRACT WITCH HAZEL**

Is the very best family medicine—composed entirely of simple vegetable substances—Bark of the Hamamelis Virginica, with sufficient pure spirit to preserve. Although the great secret of this popular remedy rests in the great care used in its preparation. The manufacturer feeling the need of a sure specific for the following ailments has given the profits usually retained by proprietors to the distressed by placing **RISLEY'S WITCH HAZEL** at their disposal at about half the price that other manufacturers of Extract of Witch Hazel are charging, and guarantee it as good, if not a better preparation for

**BURNS AND SCALDS.** It should be used liberally, as it will give prompt relief.

**CHILBLAINS OR FROST BITES.** It is highly recommended.

**BLISTERS AND CHAFINGS.** Allays all inflammation and soreness without pain.

**TOOTHACHE, EARACHE AND NEURALGIA.** Its effects are apparently magnetic.

**CATARRH OR COLD IN THE HEAD.** If used regularly will alleviate the disease, if not perform a radical cure.

**SWELLINGS OR INFLAMMATION.** It is unrivalled.

**FEMALE COMPLAINTS.** Ladies recommend it.

**SORE THROAT.** It is a prompt sure cure.

**NOSE BLEED OR HEMORRHAGES.** Is stopped promptly. And for

**ACHING PAINS,** It is undoubtedly the greatest healing preparation ever used, as physicians, nurses and mothers are forced to admit:

Six Oz. Bot. 25c.    Pint Bot. 50c.    Quart Bot. $1.00.

FOR PURIFYING, BLEACHING AND DISINFECTING

**ROSEGRANTS CHLORIDE OF LIME**
Stands preeminently the best.
Always put up in Diamond Blue Label Boxes.
¼ Lb. Boxes.    ½ Lb. Boxes.    1 Lb. Boxes.
ALL FIRST CLASS DRUGGISTS KEEP IT.

In North American folk medicine, witch hazel was used as a douche or taken in a mixture with bayberry and ginger to treat heavy menstrual flow. As shown in this advertisement, witch hazel was also used to treat nosebleeds, burns, inflammation, chilblains, and sore throat. (National Library of Medicine)

plant *(Gossypium herbaceum)*. For reducing the flow of heavy periods, Meyer mentions the use of a plain diet, avoidance of alcohol, and herbal preparations including yarrow and shepherd's purse *(Capsella bursa-pastoris)* (both used in Britain too, see above); black haw *(Viburnum prunifolium)* and wild alum root *(?Geranium maculatum* or *Heuchera americana);* and prince's feather or amaranth *(Amaranthus hypochon-driacus).* Another plant used was witch hazel *(Hamamelis virginiana),* as a douche or in a mixture with bayberry and ginger. To regulate periods, both mugwort and "Jill-grow-over-the ground" *(Glechoma hedera-cea)* have been used, both familiar in British folk medicine, as well as squaw weed *(?Senecio aureus)*. To provoke menstruation, tansy *(Tanacetum vulgaris)*, blue cohosh *(Caulophyllum thalictroides)*, juniper *(Juniperus* spp.), boneset *(Eupatorium perfoliatum)*, blood root *(Sanguinaria canadensis)*, motherwort *(Leonurus cardiaca)*, seneca snakeroot *(Polygala senega)*, fennel seed *(Foeniculum vulgare)*, and wintergreen *(Gaultheria procumbens)* have all been used (Meyer 1985: 171–176).

Trying to trace these remedies to their origins, it becomes evident that many of them are similar to, and presumably learned from, Native American practice. Blue cohosh was used, for instance by the Meskwaki, for profuse menstruation (Smith 1923: 205). Chamomile was used by the Cherokee as an abortifacient (Hamel and Chiltoskey 1975: 28, 30); tansy was used similarly by the Micmac (Chandler, Freeman, and Hooper 1979: 62), again illustrating the overlap between stimulating menstruation and achieving abortion. Kay records the use among Mexican Americans of various species of Artemisia to treat heavy periods. The roots of Ambrosia are used similarly. A douche of Ambrosia leaves, or one prepared from walnut or pecan, is used to clear out the uterus after menstruation (Kay 1996: 71). Moerman's extensive survey of Native American ethnobotany reveals that various species of Artemisia are widely used for menstrual and other gynecological problems (Moerman 1998: 799–800). These species include *Artemisia vulgaris,* the mugwort familiar in British folk medicine, and other species, such as *A. ludoviciana,* native to North America but not to Britain. Blue cohosh, *Caulophyllum thalictroides,* is used to treat profuse and painful menstruation by the Menominee (Smith 1923: 25), the Ojibwa (Smith 1932: 358), and the Potawatomi (Smith 1933: 43). *Erigeron* species are used for menstrual pain by the Thompson (Turner, Thompson, Thompson, and York 1990: 80) and the Navajo

(Vestal 1952: 50). Heavy menstrual flow is checked using red baneberry *(Actaea rubra)* among the Chippewa (Densmore 1928: 358) and the Woodlands Cree (Leighton 1985: 25); among the Iroquois *Viburnum acerifolium* is used similarly (Herrick 1977: 447). The list of other plants used in Native American practice to treat gynecological problems is enormous (Moerman 1998: 799–801), but these examples serve to demonstrate that some at least of this knowledge was evidently shared by them with the colonists. The use of cotton *(Gossypium* spp.) roots seems to come from the African American tradition, where the roots were used to procure an abortion.

*See also* **Abortion, African tradition, Chamomile, Hops, Mugwort, Stinging nettle, Yarrow.**

### References

Allen, David E., and Gabrielle Hatfield. *Medicinal Plants in Folk Tradition.* Portland, OR: Timber Press, in press.

Beith, Mary. *Healing Threads: Traditional Medicines of the Highlands and Islands.* Edinburgh: Polygon, 1995.

Chandler, R. Frank, Lois Freeman, and Shirley N. Hooper. "Herbal Remedies of the Maritime Indians." *Journal of Ethnopharmacology* 1 (1979): 49–68.

Collyns, W. "On the economical and medical uses to which various common wild plants are applied by the cottagers in Devonshire." *Gardener's Magazine* 2 (1827): 160–62.

Dacombe, Marianne R. (ed.). *Dorset up along and Down Along.* Dorchester: Dorset Federation of Women's Institutes, 1935.

Densmore, Frances. "Uses of Plants by the Chippewa Indians." *Smithsonian Institution-Bureau of American Ethnology Annual Report* 44 (1928): 273–379.

Hamel, Paul B., and Mary U. Chiltoskey. *Cherokee Plants and Their Uses: A 400 Year History.* Sylva, NC: Herald, 1975.

Hatfield, Gabrielle. *Country Remedies: Traditional East Anglian Plant Remedies in the Twentieth Century.* Woodbridge: Boydell, 1994.

Hatfield, Gabrielle. *Memory, Wisdom and Healing:*

*The History of Domestic Plant Medicine.* Phoenix Mill: Sutton, 1999.

Herrick, James William. *Iroquois Medical Botany.* Ph.D. thesis, State University of New York, Albany. 1977.

Kay, Margarita Artschwager. *Healing with Plants in the American and Mexican West.* Tucson: University of Arizona Press, 1996.

Leighton, Anna L. *Wild Plant Use by the Woodlands Cree (Nihithawak) of East-Central Saskatchewan.* Mercury Series 101. Ottawa: National Museums of Canada, 1985.

Meyer, Clarence. *American Folk Medicine.* Glenwood, IL: Meyerbooks, 1985.

Moerman, Daniel E. *Native American Ethnobotany.* Portland, OR: Timber Press, 1998.

Smith, Huron H. "Ethnobotany of the Menomini Indians." *Bulletin of the Public Museum of the City of Milwaukee* 4(1) (1923): 1–174.

Smith, Huron H. "Ethnobotany of the Ojibwe Indians." *Bulletin of the Public Museum of Milwaukee* 4(3) (1932): 327–525.

Smith, Huron H. "Ethnobotany of the Forest Potawatomi Indians." *Bulletin of the Public Museum of the City of Milwaukee* 7(1) (1933): 1–230.

Turner, Nancy J., Laurence C. Thompson, M. Terry Thompson, and Annie Z. York. *Thompson Ethnobotany: Knowledge and Usage of Plants by the Thompson Indians of British Columbia.* Victoria: Royal British Columbia Museum, 1990.

Vestal, Paul A. "The Ethnobotany of the Ramah Navaho." *Papers of the Peabody Museum of American Archaeology and Ethnology* 40(4): (1952): 1–94.

# Mexican tradition

The system of healing known as *curanderismo* embraces four categories of healers: midwives, herbalists, specialists in sprains and fractures, and the *curanderos* (or *curanderas*) themselves. In addition, as with other folk medical traditions, there is a broad spectrum of folk medical knowledge passed down orally from one generation to the next and held in common among the whole community. As far as healing with plants is concerned, Mexican ethnobotany uses a number of South American plants and in addition a large number of plant species endemic to the southwest of North America. The importance of these plant medicines in the past, including the recent past, would have been great for a people who historically have been impoverished and denied access to the health systems available to much of North America. There is in addition a significant number of Mediterranean herbs, such as rosemary, basil, and marjoram, whose use can be traced back to Spanish origins.

The Mexican tradition of folk medicine, though it uses physical agents such as herbs, has a strong spiritual side, as well—faith in the system, and particularly in the healer, forms a considerable part of the cure. Active participation of the patient is another important aspect of the treatment.

## References
Jones, Michael Owen, Patrick A. Polk, Ysamur Flores-Peña, and Roberta J. Evanchuk. "Invisible Hospitals: Botánicas in Ethnic Health Care." In *Healing Logics: Culture and Medicine in Modern Health Belief Systems,* edited by Erika Brady. Logan: Utah State University Press, 2001.

Kay, Margarita Artschwager. *Healing with Plants in the American and Mexican West.* Tucson: University of Arizona Press, 1996.

Maduro, R. "*Curanderismo* and Latino Views of Disease and Curing." *Western Journal of Medicine* 139(6): 868–874, 1983.

Micheletti, Enza (ed.). *North American Folk Healing: An A–Z Guide to Traditional Remedies.* New York and Montreal: Reader's Digest Association, 1998.

# Midwife

In rural Britain until well into the twentieth century communities were dependent on the local nurse/midwife, who often also attended the dying and laid out corpses. Often she was regarded as a "wise woman," and the few records that exist show that she often had a wide knowledge of herbs. One such person was Granny Davies from a village in Norfolk, who is fondly remembered by Mr. Wigby, brought into the world by her in the early years of the twentieth century (Wigby 1976). In Bedfordshire in the late years of the nineteenth century, Jane Cullip attended women in childbirth and administered raspberry tea (EFS 195). Among Highland communities the so-called henwife often served as midwife too (Beith 1995: 95), and it was she who made sure that traditional protective customs were observed. During labor the woman might have iron in her bed and a Bible under the pillow, appeasing both the pagan and the Christian deities (Beith 1995: 98). The midwife would ensure that all the locks in the house were open so that no ill could befall the mother and child. Straw from the woman's bed was formed into a rope and burned in the fire, again to protect from evil (Beith 1995: 98). A sea-bean was often used as an amulet during delivery, its use accompanied by prayers (Beith 1995: 208). As its first drink, the midwife would administer to the newly born child sap from an ash stick (Beith 1995: 208). In Ireland, midwives often invoked both God and the moon to protect the expectant mother (Black 1883: 128).

Since midwives were powerful figures in their own communities and were the first to make contact with newborn children, both church and state were anxious to limit their influence. Some midwives were accused of sorcery, and some even died as convicted witches in the sixteenth and seventeenth centuries (Donnison 1988: 17). By the eighteenth century the official role of the village midwife was becoming usurped, at least in urban settings and among the richer classes, by the medically trained obstetricians (Donnison 1988: 48); in rural Britain their role survived much longer.

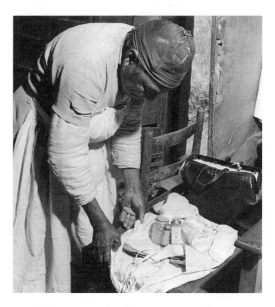

Midwife wrapping her kit to go on a call in Greene County, Georgia, 1941. (Library of Congress)

In colonial North America until the eighteenth century midwives were mostly untrained but experienced women. The first record of a non-Indian midwife in Canada is that of Catherine Guertin, elected as the community midwife by the citizens of Ville-Marie in 1713. It is a testimony to the skills of such midwives that fewer colonial women died in childbirth than among their English counterparts (Micheletti 1998: 147). This could have been partly due to healthier living conditions than in England's crowded cities; statistics are not available to show how the country midwives of the two nations compared. One such midwife, "Aunt Prudie," is said to have delivered nearly three thousand babies in her sixty-five years of practice in Mississippi (Meyer 1985: 4). After the eighteenth century, as in Europe generally, the role of the country midwife was largely taken over by "official" midwives, many of them men.

*See also* **Amulet, Ash, Beans, Childbirth, Pregnancy.**

## References

Beith, Mary. *Healing Threads: Traditional Medicines of the Highlands and Islands.* Edinburgh: Polygon, 1995.

Black, William George. *Folk-Medicine: A Chapter in the History of Culture.* London: Folklore Society, 1883.

Donnison, Jean. *Midwives and Medical Men: A History of the Struggle for the Control of Childbirth.* London: Historical Publications, 1988.

EFS. English Folklore Survey. Manuscript notes at University College London.

Meyer, Clarence. *American Folk Medicine.* Glenwood, IL: Meyerbooks, 1985.

Micheletti, Enza (ed.). *North American Folk Healing: An A–Z Guide to Traditional Remedies.* New York and Montreal: Reader's Digest Association, 1998.

Wigby, Frederick C. *Just a Country Boy.* Wymondham: Geo. R. Reeve, 1976.

# Migraine

A number of British folk remedies for migraine involve snuffing plant material into the nose. In Suffolk, primrose *(Primula vulgaris)* was used in this way (Jobson 1967: 60); in Wales, a mixture of betony leaves *(Stachys officinalis)* and primrose roots was used (Jones 1996: 89). Yarrow leaves were used similarly (Pratt 1855). Various seaweeds were used as poultices to relieve the pain of migraine. In the Isle of Skye, dulse *(Palmaria palmata)* and "linarich" *(?Ulva lactuca)* were both used (Martin 1703: 203). Feverfew, which has recently sprung to fame as a migraine treatment, was used in a number of folk remedies as a general pain reliever (Hatfield 1994: 90), but as a migraine treatment its use belonged until the twentieth century to official medicine. In Scotland, the brain of a hare was used to treat severe headache, including migraine (Beith 1995: 177).

In North American folk medicine there are a number of suggested applications to the head for easing migraine. They include rags dipped in vinegar (UCLA Folklore Archives 2_6290), horseradish leaves *(Armoracia rusticana)* wrapped around the head (UCLA Folklore Archives 14_5430), potato slices enclosed in a scarf similarly applied (UCL Folklore Archives 24_6288), resting the head on a pillow filled with pine needles (UCLA Folklore Archives 10_6288) or with dried hops (Puckett 1981: 414). Both corn (UCLA Folklore Archives 6_5394) and corn oil (Jarvis 1961: 149) have been recommended to mitigate migraine. To prevent it, wearing nutmeg around the neck has been suggested (UCLA Folklore Archives 8_6288), while placing the feet in plastic bags has been thought to ward off a migraine (Cannon 1984: 111).

In the Native American tradition, yarrow is used as a snuff for headaches much as in British folk medicine (Moerman 1998: 42).

Migraine has not always been distinguished in folk medicine from other headaches, and treatments overlap.

*See also* **Corn, Headache, Hops, Pine, Poultice, Yarrow.**

## References

Beith, Mary. *Healing Threads: Traditional Medicines of the Highlands and Islands.* Edinburgh: Polygon, 1995.

Cannon, Anthon S. *Popular Beliefs and Superstitions from Utah.* Edited by Wayland D. Hand and Jeannine E. Talley. Salt Lake City: University of Utah Press, 1984.

Hatfield, Gabrielle. *Country Remedies: Traditional East Anglian Plant Remedies in the Twentieth Century.* Woodbridge: Boydell, 1994.

Jarvis, D. C. *Folk Medicine.* London: Pan Books, 1961.

Jobson, Allan. *In Suffolk Borders.* London: Robert Hale, 1967.

Jones, Dewi. *The Botanists and Guides of Snowdonia.* Llanrwst: Gwasg Carreg Gwalch, 1996.

Martin, Martin. *A Description of the Western Isles of Scotland.* London: A. Bell, 1703. (Page references cited are from the fourth edition of 1934 [Stirling: Eneas Mackay], edited by Donald J. Macleod.)

Moerman, Daniel E. *Native American Ethnobotany.* Portland, OR: Timber Press, 1998.

Pratt, Anne. *The Flowering Plants and Ferns of Great Britain.* 5 vols. London: Society for Promoting Christian Knowledge, 1855.

Puckett, Newbell Niles. *Popular Beliefs and Superstitions: A Compendium of American Folklore from the Ohio Collection of Newbell Niles Puckett.* Edited by Wayland D. Hand, Anna Casetta, and Sondra B. Thiederman. 3 vols. Boston: G. K. Hall, 1981.

# Milk

Milk from a variety of animals has been used in folk medicine. In ancient healing rituals, milk was sometimes poured on the ground as a sacrificial offering (Beith 1995: 139). A bath of milk was said to have saved casualties of a Pictish battle (Beith 1995: 167). In the Scottish Highlands milk of a mare, a goat, or a donkey was particularly recommended as a drink for sufferers from tuberculosis (Beith 1995: 97). The milk from white cows was especially valued (Beith 1995: 168). Cow's milk, in the form of buttermilk, was recommended for tuberculosis too (Pennant 1776). Both butter and cream were valued for healing. Butter, especially from the milk of a white cow, was used for treating adder bites (Beith 1995: 174). In the Scottish borders butter made from the milk of cows grazed in churchyards reputedly cured a blacksmith's apprentice of tuberculosis (Black 1883: 96). Cream, boiled until oily, was applied to burns (Beith 1995: 168). Goat's milk was valued as a tonic, especially after influenza, and mare's milk was recommended for whooping cough (Beith 1995: 177, 178). The mold growing on milk was used in Mull, in western Scotland, for treating ulcerated legs (Beith 1995: 179). In Ireland, sow's milk was recommended for epilepsy (Notes and Queries 1849), and goat's milk was drunk for eczema (Logan 1972: 72).

Many of these uses for milk and more besides have been recorded in North American folk medicine. For tuberculosis, drinking the milk of a red cow was recommended (Hyatt 1965: 252). For the treatment of whooping cough both mare's milk (Cannon 1984: 38) and goat's milk (UCLA Folklore Archives 1_5570) have been recommended. Cream has been used to treat chapped skin (UCLA Folklore Archives 3_6835), sunburn, and burns (Anderson 1970: 12, 73). Human breast milk has been widely used for eye ailments, including stys (UCLA Folklore Archives 10_6515), sore eyes (Puckett 1981: 370), and even blindness at birth (Hyatt 1965: 241). Goat's milk has been used for treating menstrual pain (Hendricks 1980: 89), rashes (Puckett 1981: 430), diabetes (UCLA Folklore Archives 11_6283), typhoid (Hyatt 1965: 218), and ulcers (Puckett 1981: 468). It has also been drunk to prevent asthma (Anderson 1970: 5). Mare's milk has been rubbed on for croup (Campbell 1953: 2) and drunk for flu (Anderson 1970: 34), diphtheria, hives (Browne 1958: 57, 18), and measles (Creighton 1968: 223). Cow's milk has been used in innumerable ways, including warmed with honey as a drink for insomnia (UCLA Folklore Archives 11_6769); boiled for diarrhea (UCLA Folklore Archive 13_6284); drunk to aid healing of a fracture (Cannon 1984: 108); as a bath, mixed with wine, for a premature child (UCLA Folklore Archives 17_6095); and as an antidote to poisons (Puckett 1981: 450) and to germs in the atmosphere (Hyatt 1965: 195). To prevent one from getting old, drinking buttermilk is recommended! (UCLA Folklore Archives 3_6772).

*See also* **Asthma, Burns, Chapped skin, Color, Diabetes, Diarrhea, Eczema, Epilepsy, Eye problems, Fractures, Hives, Sleeplessness, Snake bite, Sunburn, Tonic, Tuberculosis, Whooping cough.**

## References

Anderson, John. *Texas Folk Medicine*. Austin, TX: Encino Press, 1970.

Beith, Mary. *Healing Threads: Traditional Medicines of the Highlands and Islands*. Edinburgh: Polygon, 1995.

Black, William George. *Folk-Medicine: A Chapter in the History of Culture*. London: Folklore Society, 1883.

Browne, Ray B. *Popular Beliefs and Practices from Alabama*. Folklore Studies 9. Berkeley and Los Angeles: University of California Publications, 1958.

Campbell, Marie. "Folk Remedies from South Georgia." *Tennessee Folklore Society Bulletin* 19 (1953): 1–4.

Cannon, Anthon S. *Popular Beliefs and Superstitions from Utah*. Edited by Wayland D. Hand and Jeannine E. Talley. Salt Lake City: University of Utah Press, 1984.

Creighton, Helen. *Bluenose Magic, Popular Beliefs and Superstitions in Nova Scotia*. Toronto: Ryerson Press, 1968.

Hendricks, George D. "Roosters, Rhymes and Railroad Tracks." *A Second Sampling of Superstitions and Popular Beliefs in Texas*. Dallas, TX: Southern Methodist University Press, 1980.

Hyatt, Harry Middleton. *Folklore from Adams County Illinois*. 2nd rev. ed. New York: Memoirs of the Alma Egan Hyatt Foundation, 1965.

Logan, Patrick. *Making the Cure: A Look at Irish Folk Medicine*. Dublin: Talbot Press, 1972.

Notes and Queries, London. 1849 ff. Vol. 11: 349.

Pennant, Thomas. 1776. *A Tour in Scotland and Voyage to the Hebrides, 1772*. Ed. 2. 2 vols. London: Benjamin White.

Puckett, Newbell Niles. *Popular Beliefs and Superstitions: A Compendium of American Folklore from the Ohio Collection of Newbell Niles Puckett*. Edited by Wayland D. Hand, Anna Casetta, and Sondra B. Thiederman. 3 vols. Boston: G. K. Hall, 1981.

# Mistletoe (*Viscum album*)

Traditionally believed to have been a sacred plant of the druids, this plant has many folkloric beliefs associated with it. It has been suggested that one reason why the plant was regarded as sacred was that it never touches the ground; it is a parasitic plant, growing on the bark of various trees, such as oak, apple and poplar, hawthorn, and lime. Birds eat the berries and brush the sticky seeds from their beaks, leaving them on the bark, where they may grow to form new plants. Both the druid name for the plant and the present-day Gaelic name translate as "all-heal," indicating widespread use of this plant in the past. In the eighteenth century Thomas Pennant reported on the practice in Scotland of keeping mistletoe all year round to use for fevers and other troubles. There is a nineteenth-century record of a woman in Inverness-shire, Scotland, using the plant to treat palpitations of the heart (Beith 1995: 227–228).

These records from Scotland are of particular interest since the plant rarely occurs there in the wild and so was presumably deliberately grown for use, or imported. Mistletoe is commonest in the south and west of Britain, and not surprisingly most of the records of its use in folk medicine are from these regions. An infusion was drunk for measles in Somerset (Plant Lore Notes and News 1992: 112), while in Essex a leaf soaked in milk has been eaten to prevent a stroke (Hatfield 1994: 91). It was widely used to treat St. Vitus's dance (chorea)—for example, in Wiltshire (Macpherson MSS) and in Sussex (Arthur 1989: 45). Epilepsy was treated with it in East Anglia and in Herefordshire (Jobson 1959: 144; Bull 1907: 335 fn). The types of mistletoe grown on different species have been ascribed different powers. The mistletoe for treating measles in Somerset was gathered from the hawthorn (Vickery 1995: 243). In Hereford, the mistletoe growing on hawthorn was favored for treating epilepsy (Leather 1912: 79). Similar uses are recorded in Ireland. There is an interesting record from seventeenth-century Essex of its use in cleansing cows of the afterbirth (Vickery 1995: 243). In Herefordshire too the plant was given to cows and to sheep after giving birth (Grigson 1955: 202). These varied surviving medical uses for mistletoe suggest a significant role indeed for the plant in the past.

*Viscum album* is not native to North America. In North American folk medicine there are records of the use of mistletoe for curing headache, either by chewing the leaves or simply wearing them in a hat (UCLA Folklore Archives 1_5397). An infusion of mistletoe has been drunk for high blood pressure (Puckett 1981: 367), for dizziness (Wilson 1968: 323), and for hives (Browne 1958: 20). An infusion made from the berries has been used to treat epilepsy (Long 1961: 80). Alternatively, mistletoe has been worn as an amulet against epilepsy (Puckett 1981: 367). Instructions for gathering mistletoe sometimes specify that the plant must not touch human hands or the ground (Walker 1955: 10).

In Native American medicine the related native genera *Arceuthobium* and *Phoradendron,* also called mistletoe, have been used to treat a large number of conditions—for instance, hemorrhage, rheumatism, high blood pressure, warts, and sores (Moerman 1998: 84, 393–394). An echo of the English veterinary use of mistletoe is found in the Zuni use of *Phoradendron juniperum* to prevent postpartum bleeding in humans (Stevenson 1915: 55). This same species is used by Native American herbal healers today to treat diarrhea and stomach problems, as well as baldness. Epilepsy, palsy, strokes, and tuberculosis are also treated with this species and the related *Phoradendron flavescens* (Kavasch and Baar 1999: 163).

Both European and North American mistletoes have magical associations and are traditionally believed to protect against poison, witchcraft, and lightning (Notes and Queries, 4 (1857) 506; Vickery 1995: 242–243; Whiting 1939: 72, Elmore 1944: 41).

*See also* **Amulet, Baldness, Diarrhea, Epilepsy, Fevers, Headache, Heart trouble, Hives, Warts.**

**References**

Arthur, Dave, (ed.). *A Sussex Life. The Memories of Gilbert Sargent, Countryman.* London: Barrie and Jenkins, 1989.

Beith, Mary. *Healing Threads: Traditional Medicines of the Highlands and Islands.* Edinburgh: Polygon, 1995.

Browne, Ray B. *Popular Beliefs and Practices from Alabama.* Folklore Studies 9. Berkeley and Los Angeles: University of California Publications, 1958.

Bull, H. G. "The Mistletoe in Herefordshire." Trans. Woolhope Naturalists' Field Club (1852–65): 312–47. Reprint 1907.

Elmore, Francis H. *Ethnobotany of the Navaho.* Santa Fe, NM: School of American Research, 1944.

Grigson, Geoffrey. *The Englishman's Flora.* London: Phoenix House, 1955.

Hatfield, Gabrielle. *Country Remedies: Traditional East Anglian Plant Remedies in the Twentieth Century.* Woodbridge: Boydell, 1994.

Jobson, Allan. *In Suffolk Borders.* London: Robert Hale, 1967.

Kavasch, E. Barrie, and Karen Baar. *American Indian Healing Arts: Herbs, Rituals and Remedies for Every Season of Life.* New York: Bantam Books, 1999.

Leather, Ella Mary. *The Folk-Lore of Herefordshire Collected from Oral and Printed Sources.* Hereford and London: Jakeman and Carver 1912.

Long, Grady M. "Folk Customs in Southeast Tennessee." *Tennessee Folklore Society Bulletin* 27 (1961): 76–84.

Macpherson MSS. Collection of folk medicines compiled by J. Harvey Macpherson, in the archives of the Folklore Society, University College London.

Moerman, Daniel E. *Native American Ethnobotany.* Portland, OR: Timber Press, 1998.

Notes and Queries, 4 (1857).

*Plant Lore Notes and News,* no. 24 (1992): 112.

Puckett, Newbell Niles. *Popular Beliefs and Super-*

*stitions: A Compendium of American Folklore from the Ohio Collection of Newbell Niles Puckett.* Edited by Wayland D. Hand, Anna Casetta, and Sondra B. Thiederman. 3 vols. Boston: G. K. Hall, 1981.

Stevenson, Matilda Coxe. *Ethnobotany of the Zuni Indians.* Bureau of American Ethnology Annual Report 30. Washington, DC: Smithsonian Institution, 1915.

Vickery, Roy. *A Dictionary of Plant Lore.* Oxford: Oxford University Press, 1995.

Walker, John. "A Sampling of Folklore from Rutherford County, North Carolina." *North Carolina Folklore* 3(2) (December 1955): 6–16.

Whiting, Alfred F. "Ethnobotany of the Hopi." *Museum of Northern Arizona Bulletin* 15 (1939).

Wilson, Gordon. "Local Plants in Folk Remedies in the Mammoth Cave Region." *Southern Folklore Quarterly* 32 (1968): 320–327.

# Molds

Long before the official Western "discovery" of antibiotics, the value of molds in healing had been realized and used by folk medicine for a wide variety of conditions. There are records of the use of moldy soya beans to treat wounds in China three thousand years ago (Bickel 1972: 60–61) and of a moldy corn mash in the Jewish Talmud (Townend 1944: 158–159); the properties of molds are referred to in ancient Egyptian writings of about 1500 B.C. (Kamel 1960: 487–488). In much more recent times, molds have featured in folk medicine. One of the best known and best-documented examples in Britain is that of "Good Friday Bread." Traditionally a small loaf from a baking on Good Friday was preserved, sometimes for many years, for use in first aid. When a family member became injured, small pieces were cut off, made into a mash, and plastered on the injury. In Devon and Cornwall, this procedure was used to treat animals as well as humans (Townend 1944: 158–159). The practice

has been used within living memory in East Anglia (Hatfield MS). In Ireland, the blue mold from bread was used to prevent cuts from festering (Foster 1951: 62).

Molds on other foodstuffs were used in folk medicine. On the Scottish island of Mull, milk was kept until it went moldy and the mold used to treat ulcerated legs (Beith 1995: 179). In Sussex, in the twentieth century, mold from jam was applied to cuts before bandaging (Prince 1991: 113). In Yorkshire, moldy curd tarts were saved from Christmas baking and used to treat cuts (Prince 1991: 95). In Essex, the cloth from around a cheese "with the mold still adhering" was used to heal wounds (Hatfield MSS). A seventeenth-eighteenth century household book from Norfolk records the use of a poultice of rotten apple to treat sore eyes. The same manuscript contains the recipe for an ointment for treating "green wounds or any swellings." It consists of Agrimony *(Agrimonia eupatoria)* beaten in butter, then left in a cellar to go moldy (Gunton Household Book). Moldy apples have been used in the twentieth century to treat stys (Anon. 1959: 343). The mold from leather was used similarly (Wainwright 1989: 163) in Cambridge, right up to the twentieth century. A letter in the *Daily Express* in 1943 describes how a Suffolk lady used to smear copper pennies with lard and leave them in a damp place to grow mold; the mold was then scraped off into pots. The resulting ointment was much in demand locally (Wainwright 1989: 163). In Herefordshire, the fungus from around the bottom of beech trees was collected and mixed with vaseline and used for "septic places" (Prince 1991: 119). In the Highlands of Scotland, the molds growing on the sides of caves were used in wound treatment, especially for damaged limbs (Beith 1995: 179).

In North American folk medicine, molds were used in much the same way. Meade records the use of moldy bread and milk to treat infections (Meade 1965: 823–828). In the UCLA folk medicine archives there are records of the use of moldy bread applied to wounds (Schedler 1971: 13). Moldy bread also features in an ointment used to treat animal bites (UCLA Folklore Archives 11_5260). From the western South, there is a record of using cheese mold to heal a sore (UCLA Folklore Archives 1_5474). From Missouri, there is a record of the use of wet tree mold to treat wounds (UCLA Folklore Archives 24_5574). Meyer records the use of pork rind "well molded" placed between bandages and applied to a wound to draw out infection. The informant adds that the pork rind is kept in the cellar for use when needed (Meyer 1985: 278).

See also **Cuts, Eye problems, Poultice, Wounds.**

### References

Anonymous. "Gypsies' Penicillin." *Folklore* 70 (1959): 343–344.

Beith, Mary. *Healing Threads: Traditional Medicine of the Highlands and Islands.* Edinburgh: Polygon, 1995.

Bickel, L. *Rise Up to Life.* London: Angus and Robertson, 1972.

Foster, Jeanne Cooper. *Ulster Folklore.* Belfast: H. R. Carter, 1951.

Gunton Household Book, Manuscript Seventeenth/Eighteenth Century. Church of St. Peter Mancroft, Norwich.

Hatfield, Gabrielle. Manuscript Notes in Her Personal Possession.

Kamel, H. "Antibiotics, Vitamins and Hormones in History." *Egyptian Medical Association Journal* 43 (1960).

Meade, G. M. "Home Remedies in Rural America." *Annals of the New York Academy of Science* 120 (1965): 823–828.

Meyer, Clarence. *American Folk Medicine.* Glenwood, IL: Meyerbooks, 1985.

Prince, Dennis. *Grandmother's Cures: An A–Z Of Herbal Remedies.* London: Fontana, 1991.

Schedler, Paul W. "Folk Medicine in Denton County Today: Or, Can Dermatology Dis-place Dishrags?" *Publications of the Texas Folklore Society* 35 (1971): 11–17.

Townend, B. R. "Penicillin in Folk Medicine." *Notes and Queries* 186 (1944).

Wainwright, Milton. "Moulds in Folk Medicine." *Folklore* 100(2) (1989): 162–166.

# Moon

The moon has been regarded as a cause of mental illness by a very wide variety of different cultures, and over a great time span, and the word "lunacy," of course, derives from this belief. Insanity was thought to be worse at the time of a full moon, an idea that is still controversial today. Sleeping in moonlight was considered dangerous, causing madness or blindness (Radford and Radford 1974: 239). The phase of the moon at the time of a child's birth was believed to control the child's destiny and health, even the sex of the next child to be born in the family (Black 1883: 128). A child born under a waning moon would be unlucky, and in the Orkneys it was believed that a marriage celebrated at the time of a waning moon would not be fruitful (Radford and Radford 1961: 239). At least until the mid-nineteenth century it was traditional to curtsey to a new moon and unlucky to point at the moon. It was also unlucky to see the new moon through trees or other obstacles (Radford and Radford 1961: 237, 238). Moonlight plays a part in several wart cures: blowing on warts at the time of a full moon was one such cure. "Bathing" the warts in moonbeams in a metal dish was a folk remedy made famous by Sir Kenelm Digby in the seventeenth century. A cure for whooping cough was to take afflicted children outside and let them look at the moon while their stomachs were rubbed and a charm recited (Radford and Radford 1961: 239). In Scotland it is suggested that medicine for treating worms is best administered at full moon, for at that

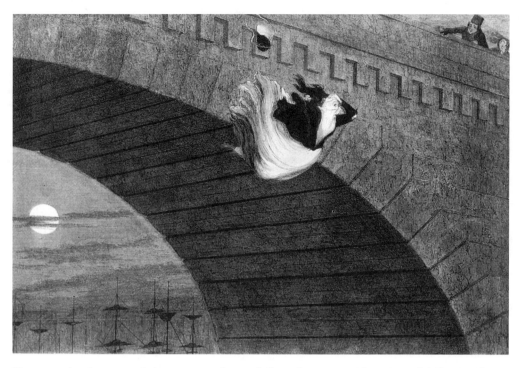

The moon has been regarded as a cause of mental illness by a very wide variety of different cultures. Insanity was thought to be worse at the time of a full moon, an idea which is still controversial today. (National Library of Medicine)

time the worms are more likely to come out (Buchan 1994: 107).

In North American folk medicine there is a belief that conception is more likely to occur at the time of a full moon (Parler 1962, 3: 14). A child born at full moon was destined to become a lunatic (Cannon 1984: 34). Stomach ailments are under the control of the moon (Brown 1952–1964, 6: 293). Sleeping in moonlight will make one go crazy (Brown 1952–1964, 6: 356), a belief evidently held on both sides of the Atlantic. Sitting under a full moon was reckoned to be a cure for freckles (Puckett 1981: 383). The phase of the moon, it was believed, could alter the outcome of a remedy. The rabbit skins used for treating frostbite should be from rabbits killed in the dark of the moon (Thomas and Thomas 1920: 103); hysteria can be cured by dipping the sufferer in an icy stream at the same phase of the moon (Neal 1955: 291);

hair cut at full moon will grow faster (UCLA Folklore Archives 1_5657). Many records document the idea that it is unlucky to view the moon through obstacles (including glass windows) and lucky to view it in other ways (Brown 1952–1964, 7: 184–189), and that it was bad luck to point at the moon (Brown 1952–1964, 7: 189), both beliefs found in Britain.

Among the Native Americans the lunar cycle was the basis of the calendar; the moon played an important role in their religious as well as healing ceremonies. It was thought to control subconscious activity, and one's personality was affected by the phase of the moon at one's birth. The moon could indicate when the birth of a baby was imminent (Frankel 1970: 76). Boys who learned to walk at new moon would be fast runners (Parler 1962, 3: 166). It was unlucky to point at the moon—the finger would rot off (Cannon 1984: 108).

*See also* **Freckles, Frostbite, Warts, Whooping cough, Worms.**

### References

Black, William George. *Folk-Medicine: A Chapter in the History of Culture.* London: Folklore Society, 1883.

Brown, Frank C. *Collection of North Carolina Folklore.* 7 vols. Durham, NC: Duke University Press, 1952–1964.

Buchan, David (ed.). *Folk Tradition and Folk Medicine in Scotland: The Writings of David Rorie.* Edinburgh: Canongate Academic, 1994.

Cannon, Anthon S. *Popular Beliefs and Superstitions from Utah.* Edited by Wayland D. Hand and Jeannine E. Talley. Salt Lake City: University of Utah Press, 1984.

Frankel, Barbara. *Childbirth in the Ghetto: Folk Beliefs of Negro Women in a North Philadelphia Hospital Ward.* M.A. thesis, Temple University, 1970.

Neal, Janice C. "Grandad: Pioneer Medicine Man." *New York Folklore Quarterly* 11 (1955): 277–291.

Parler, Mary Celestia, and University Student Contributors. *Folk Beliefs from Arkansas.* 15 vols. Fayetteville: University of Arkansas, 1962.

Puckett, Newbell Niles. *Popular Beliefs and Superstitions: A Compendium of American Folklore from the Ohio Collection of Newbell Niles Puckett.* Edited by Wayland D. Hand, Anna Casetta, and Sondra B. Thiederman. 3 vols. Boston: G. K. Hall, 1981.

Radford, E., and M. A. Radford. *Encyclopaedia of Superstitions.* Edited and revised by Christina Hole. London: Book Club Associates 1974.

Thomas, Daniel Lindsay, and Lucy Blayney Thomas. *Kentucky Superstitions.* Princeton, NJ: Princeton University Press, 1920.

# Moss

Apart from Sphagnum moss, in British folk medicine different types of moss were often not distinguished, and the term frequently covered some of the lichens as well. In general, moss was used as an absorbent dressing and as a styptic. "Moss" from a dead man's skull was famously used in both folk medicine and official medicine for curing bleeding and headaches (Black 1883: 96–97). In Ireland, wounds were treated with moss from human skulls (Logan 1972: 89). Such moss was sometimes a constituent of the so-called weapon salve, which was popular in the seventeenth century (Radford and Radford 1974: 368). Perhaps as an extension of this idea, the moss from tombstones was carried as a protective amulet against agues and rheumatism (Souter 1995: 35). These so-called mosses may well have been species of lichens, such as *Usnea.* Other mosses in a general sense have been used in British folk medicine for treating insect bites and stings (Hatfield MS) and to staunch bleeding (Allen and Hatfield, in press).

In North American folk medicine moss from a human skull was similarly recommended for treating a wound, either directly (Brown 1952–1964, 6: 123) or via the instrument causing the wound (Spicer 1937: 154). Among the Pennsylvania Germans it was also used, combined with marigold water, for treating vomiting (Brendle and Unger 1935: 177).

*See also* **Amulet, Bleeding, Headache, Insect bites and stings, Skull, Sphagnum moss, Sympathetic magic, Wounds.**

### References

Allen, David, and Gabrielle Hatfield. *Medicinal Plants in Folk Tradition.* Portland, OR: Timber Press, in press.

Black, William George. *Folk-Medicine: A Chapter in the History of Culture.* London: Folklore Society, 1883.

Brendle, Thomas R., and Claude W. Unger. "Folk Medicine of the Pennsylvania Germans: The Non-Occult Cures." *Proceedings of the Pennsylvania German Society* 45 (1935).

Brown, Frank C. *Collection of North Carolina Folklore.* 7 vols. Durham, NC: Duke University Press, 1952–1964.

Logan, Patrick. *Making the Cure: A Look at Irish Folk Medicine.* Dublin: Talbot Press, 1972.

Radford, E., and M. A. Radford. *Encyclopaedia of Superstitions.* Edited and revised by Christina Hole. London: Book Club Associates, 1974.

Souter, Keith. *Cure Craft: Traditional Folk Remedies and Treatment from Antiquity to the Present Day.* Saffron Walden: C. W. Daniel, 1995.

Spicer, Dorothy Gladys. "Medicine and Magic in the New England Colonies." *Trained Nurse* 99 (1937): 153–156.

# Mouse

The use of fried mouse for treating whooping cough is a folk remedy that, surprisingly, persisted in Scotland and parts of England well into the twentieth century (Prince 1991: 104). The dish apparently tastes similar to chicken (Hatfield MSS). In Sussex roast or stewed mouse was used as a treatment for consumption and diphtheria, as well as for whooping cough (Allen 1995: 114). The origin of the remedy is obscure, but it is known that mouse was regarded by Eastern medicine as a remedy for a child *in extremis,* and it has been found in the alimentary canal of children's remains dating to the fourth millennium B.C. at Naqada in Egypt (Beith 1995: 179). Four thousand years later, a mother in Cromarty, Scotland, gave her seriously ill child the liver of a mouse. The child recovered (Beith 1995: 8). In ancient Egypt, roast mouse was also considered a cure for bed-wetting, and an amulet consisting of a mouse bladder was used in the Scottish Highlands for the same purpose (Souter 1995: 137). This remedy has also been reported from England (Prince 1991: 12). Roast mouse has also been used in Aberdeenshire for treating jaundice (Black 1883: 159). A Sussex variant is to bake the mouse to a cinder and powder it. The powder, mixed with jam, was fed to a child to cure bedwetting. It was also used to treat diabetes (Allen 1995: 114). Reputedly, the milk in which a mouse has been boiled was used to procure barrenness in women in Ireland (Black 1883: 159 footnote). Roast mouse has been used to treat croup in children (Gutch 1912: 69).

In North America, there are records of fried mice given for bedwetting, and fried rat has also been recorded for the same purpose (Brown 1952–1964, 6: 47, 48). Roast mouse has been eaten for measles (Welsch 1966: 363) and for fever (Whitney and Bullock 1925: 85). A mixture of mouse meat and lard has been given to children to rid them of worms (Cannon 1984: 38). For infant colic the head of a freshly killed mouse was hung around the neck of the child (UCLA Folklore Archives 21_5889), and wearing a dead mouse was a recommended treatment for warts (Parler 1962, 3: 1076). Ashes of mouse mixed with honey were rubbed on the teeth for bad breath (UCLA Folklore Archive 15_2196). Mouse broth was given, more generally for "illness" (Koch 1980: 128). For pain, squeezing a mouse to death was suggested (Browne 1958: 123).

To put all these strange remedies into perspective, it should be remembered that the official materia medica of Western medicine contained many animal products right up to the eighteenth century. At least some of these mouse remedies can be found in official Western medicine. Salmon's *English Physician,* published in 1693, included a chapter on mice. The whole mouse, burned to ashes, is the basis of an ointment to treat baldness. The flesh of the mouse is recommended for consumption, palpitations, and faintings, as well as for bites and removing splinters; the fat treats tumors; the blood is to be used for warts and to clear the eyes; and the liver is given for fever, the gall for eyesight, the urine for gout, the dung for worms in children (Salmon 1693: 393–397).

Mice also figure in a quite different aspect of folk medicine. From all over the world there are reports similar to the practice in the Highlands of Scotland of placing a child's milk tooth at the entrance to a mouse hole, and asking for a strong new tooth in return (Beith 1995: 179). Frazer in the *Golden Bough* reports similar practices from Germany and from the Pacific island of Raratonga (Frazer 1923: 39). In North America there are records of other associations between mice and teeth; a cure for toothache is to eat a crust that the mice have gnawed (Wintemberg 1899: 48). A string used to hang three mice was placed around a child's neck to assist in teething (Brendle and Unger 1935: 120).

*See also* **Amulet, Bad breath, Bed-wetting, Colic, Croup, Diabetes, Fevers, Jaundice, Teething, Toothache, Tuberculosis, Warts, Whooping cough, Worms.**

### References

Allen, Andrew. *A Dictionary of Sussex Folk Medicine.* Newbury: Countryside Books, 1995.

Beith, Mary. *Healing Threads: Traditional Medicines of the Highlands and Islands.* Edinburgh: Polygon, 1995.

Black, William George. *Folk-Medicine: A Chapter in the History of Culture.* London: Folklore Society, 1883.

Brendle, Thomas R., and Claude W. Unger. "Folk Medicine of the Pennsylvania Germans: The Non-Occult Cures." *Proceedings of the Pennsylvania German Society* 45 (1935).

Brown, Frank C. *Collection of North Carolina Folklore.* 7 vols. Durham, NC: Duke University Press, 1952–1964.

Browne, Ray B. *Popular Beliefs and Practices from Alabama.* Folklore Studies 9. Berkeley and Los Angeles: University of California Publications, 1958.

Cannon, Anthon S. *Popular Beliefs and Superstitions from Utah.* Edited by Wayland D. Hand and Jeannine E. Talley. Salt Lake City: University of Utah Press, 1984.

Frazer, Sir J. G. *The Golden Bough: A Study in Magic and Religion.* Abridged edition, London: Macmillan, 1923.

Gutch, Mrs. (Eliza). *Examples of Printed Folk-Lore Concerning the East Riding of Yorkshire.* County Folk-Lore 6, Printed Extracts 8. London: Folklore Society, 1912.

Hatfield MSS. Manuscript notes in personal possession of Gabrielle Hatfield.

Koch, William E. *Folklore from Kansas: Beliefs and Customs.* Lawrence, KS: Regent Press, 1980.

Parler, Mary Celestia, and University Student Contributors. *Folk Beliefs from Arkansas.* 15 vols. Fayetteville: University of Arkansas, 1962.

Prince, Dennis. *Grandmother's Cures: An A–Z of Herbal Remedies.* London: Fontana, 1991.

Salmon, William, M.D. *The Compleat English Physician.* London, 1693.

Souter, Keith. *Cure Craft: Traditional Folk Remedies and Treatment from Antiquity to the Present Day.* Saffron Walden: C. W. Daniel, 1995.

Welsch, Roger L. *A Treasury of Nebraska Pioneer Folklore.* Lincoln: University of Nebraska Press, 1966.

Whitney, Annie Weston, and Caroline Canfield Bullock. "Folk-Lore from Maryland." *Memoirs of the American Folklore Society* 18 (1925).

Wintemberg, W. J. "Items of German-Canadian Folk-Lore." *Journal of American Folklore* 12 (1899): 45–50.

## Mugwort (*Artemisia vulgaris*)

This is one of the nine sacred herbs described in the Anglo-Saxon *Lacnunga,* and in British folk medicine it has filled a dual role of protection and therapy (Grigson 1955: 382). As recently as the early years of the twentieth century a Somerset man claimed that if the plant is picked right, there is nothing one cannot wish for (Tongue 1965: 33). Smoking the dried herb was found to prevent tiredness and increase appetite (Beith 1995: 229). Placed inside shoes, mugwort gave one the ability "to run all day" (Tongue 1965: 33). It was also considered to keep away evil spirits. In folk medicine one of its main uses in Britain has been as a woman's herb, regulating the menstrual cycle and assisting in childbirth.

This reputation was held in official medicine too: according to the thirteenth-century physicians of Myddvai, to induce childbirth all that was necessary was to strap the herb mugwort to the left thigh (Chevallier 1996: 171). In a seventeenth-century kitchen book kept by successive generations of the Harbord family in Gunton, England, there is an entry headed, "For a poor country woman in labor." It consists of an infusion of mugwort; a footnote adds that the plant can be dried and kept for use all through the year, suggesting that this may have been a remedy that was actually used rather than merely recorded (Gunton Household Book). There is a proverb in Scotland, "Wad ye let the bonny may die in your hand, And the mugwort flowering in the land?" It has a Welsh counterpart. Until the twentieth century some gardens grew a clump of mugwort for use by the woman of the house (Hatfield 1999: 22).

The plant was brought to the New World by European settlers and was reputedly used in frontier medicine to cure tics and twitches, the hands being bathed in water in which the plant had soaked overnight (Souter 1995: 192). Meyer records the use of mugwort to regulate menstrual function (Meyer 1985: 176). It was also used in North American folk medicine to counteract plant poisoning (Meyer 1985: 200). Among the Pennsylvania Germans, the plant was used for treating edema, to induce sweating (Brendle and Unger 1935: 90, 189) and for women's complaints (Lick and Brendle 1922: 39). In the 1920s the plant was still to be found growing in Pennsylvania "around very old gardens" (Lick and Brendle 1922: 298). There are numerous species of Artemisia native to North America, and these have been used in a wide variety of disorders. Confusingly, Artemisia vulgaris is known as common wormwood in North America, the name "mugwort"

usually being applied to other species of Artemisia.

In Native American practice Artemisia vulgaris has been used for a number of conditions, notably for afterpains of childbirth (Schenck and Gifford 1952: 390) and for the treatment of rheumatism (Barrett and Gifford 1933: 167). Various other species of Artemisia were used similarly for these and many other complaints (Moerman 1998: 92–103). According to Lévi-Strauss, the reputation of Artemisia in North America was similar to that in British folk medicine: it was primarily an herb for women (Lévi-Strauss 1966: 46). Several different species have been used in New Mexico to treat dysmenorrhea, difficult childbirth and retained afterbirth and to prevent infection of the umbilical cord (Kay 1996: 71). A. ludoviciana, native to North America, was used by the Cheyenne to drive away evil spirits (Coffey 1993: 245). The same plant, known in Mexico as estafiate or western mugwort, is used for intestinal spasm and for treating diabetes (Kay 1996: 106). It was so highly valued that there is a Mexican saying, "God may fail, but estafiate never" (Campa 1950: 341). Artemisia tridentata, the sagebrush, is very widely used by various Native American tribes for a variety of ailments, including rheumatism, fever, pain, and as an aid to delivery (Moerman 1998: 101–102). Another species of Artemisia, A. tilesii, has been called the panacea of the Eskimo peoples (Fortuine 1988: 215).

See also **Childbirth, Rheumatism.**

**References**
Barrett, S. A., and E. W. Gifford. "Miwok Material Culture." *Bulletin of the Public Museum of the City of Milwaukee* 2(4) (1933).
Beith, Mary. *Healing Threads: Traditional Medicines of the Highlands and Islands.* Edinburgh: Polygon, 1995.
Brendle, Thomas R., and Claude W. Unger. "Folk Medicine of the Pennsylvania Germans:

The Non-Occult Cures." *Proceedings of the Pennsylvania German Society* 45 (1935).

Campa, Arthur L. "Some Herbs and Plants of Early California." *Western Folklore* 9 (1950): 338–347.

Chevallier, Andrew. *The Encyclopedia of Medicinal Plants.* London: Dorling Kindersley, 1996.

Coffey, Timothy. *The History and Folklore of North American Wildflowers.* New York: Facts On File, 1993.

Fortuine, Robert. "The Use of Medicinal Plants by the Alaska Natives." *Alaska Medicine* 30 (1988): 185–226.

Grigson, Geoffrey. *The Englishman's Flora.* London: Phoenix House, 1955.

Gunton Household Book. Seventeenth/eighteenth century manuscript, Church of St. Peter Mancroft, Norwich.

Hatfield, Gabrielle. *Memory, Wisdom and Healing: The History of Domestic Plant Medicine.* Phoenix Mill: Sutton, 1999.

Kay, Margarita Artschwager. *Healing with Plants in the American and Mexican West.* Tucson: University of Arizona Press, 1996.

Lévi-Strauss, Claude. *The Savage Mind (La Pensée Sauvage).* London: Weidenfeld and Nicolson, 1966.

Lick, David E., and Thomas R. Brendle. "Plant Names and Plant Lore among the Pennsylvania Germans." *Proceedings and Addresses of the Pennsylvania German Society* 33 (1922).

Meyer, Clarence. *American Folk Medicine.* Glenwood, IL: Meyerbooks, 1985.

Moerman, Daniel E. *Native American Ethnobotany.* Portland, OR: Timber Press, 1998.

Schenck, Sara M., and E. W. Gifford. "Karok Ethnobotany." *Anthropological Records* 13(6) (1952): 377–392.

Souter, Keith. *Cure Craft: Traditional Folk Remedies and Treatment from Antiquity to the Present Day.* Saffron Walden: C. W. Daniel, 1995.

Tongue, Ruth L. *Somerset Folklore.* Edited by Katherine Briggs. County Folklore 8. London: Folklore Society, 1965.

# Mullein (*Verbascum thapsus*)

This plant has been used as long as records can be traced, in both official and folk medicine, particularly for treating respiratory troubles. A cough mixture is made from the leaves (Newman 1945: 356); in Sussex, this has been used to treat whooping cough (Allen 1995: 46). In Ireland, the plant has been specially valued for treating tuberculosis; the leaves have been dried and smoked for the treatment of consumption and asthma (Vickery 1995: 251). The plant has also been used to treat colds, bronchitis, and catarrh. The soft flannelly leaves of mullein have been used in Ireland to treat running sores, stings, and goiter; the juice has been used as a rub for the pain of rheumatism (Allen and Hatfield, in press). At least since the seventeenth century, the plant has also been used to treat warts (Allen 1995: 178). One of its old English names is "hagtaper," or hedgetaper, from the use of the plant in the past as a wick. One of its names in Ireland, Mary's candle, also reflects this use.

The plant was introduced in North America and has been widely used in folk medicine there in much the same way as in Britain. Meyer records its use for treating asthma and coughs (Meyer 1985: 33–35, 83). As in Ireland, it has also been used to treat tuberculosis; an infusion of the flowers was recommended for consumption (Anon. 1939: 210). The plant has also been used to treat bedwetting, diarrhea, sore feet, as a drink to soothe flu, and for treating hay fever (Meyer 1985: 36, 91, 120, 132, 136). An infusion of the seeds has been used to treat headache, and to control suppression of urine or loss of control of urination (Meyer 1985: 138, 155, 156). The juice of the fresh leaves has been snuffed up to stop nosebleeds, and as "Adam's flannel" the leaves have been used as toilet paper and to treat piles (Meyer 1985: 189, 194). Even carrying the leaves in a pocket is said to prevent piles (Brendle and Unger 1935: 184). As in Ireland, the leaves have been used as a poultice for treating swellings, sprains, and inflammation. A tea made from the flowers has been recommended for stomach upsets (Meyer 1985: 202, 236). Diarrhea has been treated with mullein tea, and the same infusion has been used as a lotion for swollen limbs in dropsy (Brown 1952–1964, 6: 170, 173). Eczema has been treated with glycerine and mullein leaf tea (Browne 1958: 60). Diabetes has also been treated with mullein leaf tea (Wintemberg 1925: 621).

In Native American medicine, the plant has been used to treat a wide range of ailments, including teething, rheumatism, cuts, fevers, piles, and respiratory troubles of all kinds (Moerman 1998: 590–591). The dried leaves have been smoked to treat fits, hiccups, and "craziness," as well as asthma.

*See also* **Asthma, Bed-wetting, Colds, Coughs, Cuts, Diabetes, Diarrhea, Dropsy, Eczema, Fevers, Hay fever, Headache, Nosebleed, Piles, Poultice, Rheumatism, Sore feet, Tuberculosis, Warts, Whooping cough.**

## References

Allen, Andrew. *A Dictionary of Sussex Folk Medicine.* Newbury: Countryside Books, 1995.

Allen, David, and Gabrielle Hatfield. *Medicinal Plants in Folk Tradition.* Portland, OR: Timber Press, in press.

Anonymous. *Idaho Lore.* Caldwell, ID: AMS Press Incorporated, 1939.

Brendle, Thomas R., and Claude W. Unger. "Folk Medicine of the Pennsylvania Germans: The Non-Occult Cures." *Proceedings of the Pennsylvania German Society* 45 (1935).

Brown, Frank C. *Collection of North Carolina Folklore.* 7 vols. Durham, NC: Duke University Press, 1952–1964.

Browne, Ray B. *Popular Beliefs and Practices from Alabama.* Folklore Studies 9. Berkeley and Los Angeles: University of California Publications, 1958.

Meyer, Clarence. *American Folk Medicine.* Glenwood, IL: Meyerbooks, 1985.

Moerman, Daniel E. *Native American Ethnobotany.* Portland, OR: Timber Press, 1998.

Newman, Leslie F. "Some Notes on Folk Medicine in the Eastern Counties." *Folk-Lore* 56 (1945): 349–360.

Vickery, Roy. *A Dictionary of Plant Lore.* Oxford: Oxford University Press, 1995.

Wintemberg, W. J. "Some Items of Negro-Canadian Folk-Lore." *Journal of American Folklore* 38 (1925): 621.

# N

## Native American tradition

Spirituality is the single outstanding characteristic of Native American healing. Religion and medicine are so closely intertwined that most religious ceremonies are associated with either healing or maintenance of health. Health is regarded as a state of balance, illness as a loss of this balance. Native American knowledge of the healing properties of plants is probably unsurpassed, but the plants themselves are regarded as only agents in the healing process. Of equal importance is the empowerment of the herbs, which can be done only by the doctor and the treatment that he provides, including the traditional songs that he sings over the patient (Snow and Stans 2001: xv). The medicine man, who may or may not be a doctor himself, is the keeper of the medicine bundles used in the most sacred healing ceremonies, such as the Green Corn Dance of the Seminole Indians, or the Nightway ceremony of the Navajo. To the rationalist Western mind, it is all too easy to dismiss the spiritual and magical elements in Native American healing; if we do this, we are ignoring a whole dimension of the healing process, a dimension well represented in Lyon's fascinating study (Lyon 1996). Not only do the ceremonies vary from one tribe to another, but the plants used in healing also vary, as a glance at Moerman's index of tribes will quickly demonstrate (Moerman 1998: 625–764).

*See also* **Concepts of disease, Medicine man.**

### References

Lyon, William S. *Encyclopedia of Native American Healing.* Santa Barbara, CA: ABC-CLIO, 1996.

Moerman, Daniel E. *Native American Ethnobotany.* Portland, OR: Timber Press, 1998.

Snow, Alice Micco, and Susan Enns Stans. *Healing Plants: Medicine of the Florida Seminole Indians.* Gainesville: University Press of Florida, 2001.

## Nausea

In British folk medicine for morning sickness during pregnancy, raspberry leaves have been eaten (CECTL MSS). For general nausea, an infusion of balm *(Melissa officinalis)* has been used (Lafont 1984: 11). Various mints *(Mentha* spp.) were used in herbalism for treating nausea and indigestion, and sometimes these were used in folk medicine too. In one remedy, a mixture of mint and ginger was used (F.C.W., pers. com., 1988).

For travel sickness, jellied eel and pigeon pie have been recommended. Carrying a caul was thought to protect sailors against seasickness (Souter 1995: 40, 193).

In North American folk medicine an infusion of goldenrod (*Solidago* sp.) was used to treat nausea (Clark 1970: 11). Chamomile tea was used for nausea as well as indigestion (UCLA Folklore Archives 3_5431). Willow ashes in water were another recommendation (Smith 1929: 72), as was an infusion of dried chicken gizzards (UCLA Folklore Archives 4_5431). Other remedies include egg white and lemon, wormwood tincture (*Artemisia* sp.), cayenne pepper, strong green tea, chamomile tea, peppermint essence (from *Mentha piperita*), or chewing a leaf of mint (*Mentha* sp.) or sage (*Salvia* sp.) (Meyer 1985: 184).

It was suggested that nausea in pregnancy could be prevented by ensuring that the husband sampled everything that the wife drank (UCLA Folklore Archives 2_6048). For general nausea, a dishrag on the throat or a red string tied around the waist are other suggestions (Brown 1952–1964, 6: 236). For trainsickness, a piece of stationery placed on the chest is believed to be a preventative (Brown 1952–1964, 6: 307).

Among the Native Americans, plants used to treat nausea include yarrow (Welch 1964: 84), spearmint (*Mentha* sp.) (Macdonald 1959: 222), and ragweed (*Ambrosia* spp.) (Larson 1953: 246). Indian cup-plant *(Silphium perfoliatum)* was used to alleviate pregnancy sickness (Meyer 1985: 208).

*See also* **Caul, Cayenne, Chamomile, Indigestion, Willow, Yarrow.**

### References

Brown, Frank C. *Collection of North Carolina Folklore.* 7 vols. Durham, NC: Duke University Press, 1952–1964.
CECTL MSS. Manuscript notes in the Centre for English Cultural Tradition and Language, University of Sheffield.
Clark, Joseph D. "North Carolina Popular Beliefs and Superstitions." *North Carolina Folklore* 18 (1970): 1–66.
Lafont, Anne-Marie. *Herbal Folklore.* Bideford: Badger Books, 1984.
Larson, John A. "Medicine among the Indians." *Quarterly Bulletin of NorthWestern Medical School* 27 (1953): 246–249.
Macdonald, Elizabeth. "Indian Medicine in New Brunswick." *Canadian Medical Association Journal* 80(3) (1959): 220–224.
Meyer, Clarence. *American Folk Medicine.* Glenwood, IL: Meyerbooks, 1985.
Smith, Walter R. "Animals and Plants in Oklahoma Folk Cures." In *Folk-Say: A Regional Miscellany.* Edited by B. A. Botkin. Norman: Oklahoma Folk-Lore Society, 1929, 69–78.
Souter, Keith. *Cure Craft: Traditional Folk Remedies and Treatment from Antiquity to the Present Day.* Saffron Walden: C.W. Daniel, 1995.
Welch, Charles E., Jr. "Some Drugs of the North American Indian: Then and Now." *Keystone Folklore Quarterly* 9(3) (1964): 83–99.

# Nettle

*See* **Stinging nettle.**

# Nosebleed

Folklore has provided some novel ways of stopping nosebleeds, many of them based on coldness, such as sliding a cold key down the sufferer's back, or holding a cold flannel on the forehead. The cold-key remedy has been claimed to be the remnant of an old Norse ritual connected with Thor (Black 1883: 183). A ceremonial treatment recorded from Worcestershire involves the "healer" bowing to the sufferer and touching his right forefinger if the bleeding is from the left nostril, and vice versa (Black 1883: 191). A shock tactic recorded from the Scottish Highlands was to hold a live toad in front of the sufferer's face (Beith 1995: 187). More drastically, in Northamptonshire a toad was killed and hung around the person's neck to stop nosebleed

(Black 1883: 62). In the seventeenth century, Boyle recorded how he had cured his own nosebleeds by using moss from a human skull (Black 1883: 96). A skein of scarlet thread tied around the neck with nine knots was suggested to prevent nosebleeds in the nineteenth century. The knots were to be tied by a man for a woman patient, and vice versa (Black 1883: 111). In Norfolk in the twentieth century it was recommended to take a large marble with a hole in it and thread this onto a red thread, tying a knot every three inches. This was worn as a necklace to cure nosebleeds (Mundford Primary School project, 1980, unpub.).

Yarrow *(Achillea millefolium),* sometimes called "nosebleed," had an ambivalent role. It was used to stop bleeding from the nose taken as an infusion, but the leaves stuffed up the nose could provoke a nosebleed, leading to the superstition that if a girl wanted to know whether her boyfriend loved her, she could put the leaves up her nose: if her nose bled, then her love would be reciprocated (Page 1983: 41). This was surely preferable to the remedy recorded in Orkney and Shetland, which was to plug the nose with fresh pig dung to stop it bleeding (Markwick 1975: 130). In the seventeenth century yew berries were apparently used to treat nosebleed (Wright 1912: 233). A slice of cold raw potato held on the back of the neck, or a bunch of broom *(Cytisus scoparius)* around the neck, were Scottish remedies for a nosebleed (Beith 1995: 209, 235). A green seaweed applied to the temples was another remedy used in the nineteenth century in the Scottish Highlands (Beith 1995: 239).

Meyer records a variety of North American folk treatments for nosebleeds, many of them the same as those recorded in Britain. Two of interest seem like "sanitized" versions of the Orkney remedy above—stuffing a wedge of salt pork, or ground beef, up the nose. Raising one or both arms above the head is suggested. Soaking the feet in hot water is an alternative (Meyer 1985: 188–189). Putting a piece of newspaper between the upper lip and the gum (Killion and Waller 1972), tying a red thread around the thumb (similar to Britain, above) (Thomas and Thomas 1920: 95), or snuffing up ashes from a burned goose feather (Roy 1955: 79) are further suggestions for stopping a nosebleed. Allowing the blood to drip onto twigs placed in the form of a cross or onto the place where a brick lay, then replacing the brick, or inserting into the nostril an odd number of hairs plucked from the underarm, are further nosebleed remedies (Brown 1952–1964, 6: 239, 243, 247).

Herbal suggestions include snuffing up powder of horsetail (*Equisetum* spp.) or juice of mullein or witch hazel *(Hamamelis mollis),* all of which are known to staunch bleeding in general. Chewing the roots of nettles is suggested as a preventative for nosebleeds. It has been maintained that drinking an infusion of yarrow for three days will prevent nosebleeds for a year (Meyer 1985: 188–189). In the Spanish Southwest, the blue-green alga that forms slime on ponds was applied to the back of the neck and left to turn yellow as a preventative for nosebleeds (Micheletti 1998: 252). A few drops of dragon's blood from the dragon tree (*Arisaema* sp.) simply held in the hand are maintained to stop a nosebleed (Wilson 1908: 70).

In Native American practice, among the Blackfoot, pieces of puffball were held to the nose for nosebleeds (Hellson 1974: 84). A large variety of other plants have been used to stem a nosebleed, including woodland pinedrops *(Pterospora andromeda).* The stem and berries are used to make an infusion, which is snuffed up the nose (Grinnell 1905: 39).

*See also* **Bleeding, Color, Moss, Mullein, Puffball, Stinging nettle, Toads and frogs, Yarrow, Yew.**

## References

Beith, Mary. *Healing Threads: Traditional Medicines of the Highlands and Islands.* Edinburgh: Polygon, 1995.

Black, William George. *Folk-Medicine: A Chapter in the History of Culture.* London: Folklore Society, 1883.

Brown, Frank C. *Collection of North Carolina Folklore.* 7 vols. Durham, NC: Duke University Press, 1952–1964.

Grinnell, George Bird. "Some Cheyenne Plant Medicines." *American Anthropologist* 7 (1905): 37–43.

Hellson, John C. *Ethnobotany of the Blackfoot Indians.* Mercury Series 19. Ottawa: National Museums of Canada, 1974.

Killion, Ronald G., and Charles T. Waller. *A Treasury of Georgia Folklore.* Atlanta: Cherokee, 1972.

Markwick, Ernest. *The Folklore of Orkney and Shetland.* London: Batsford, 1975.

Meyer, Clarence. *American Folk Medicine.* Glenwood, IL: Meyerbooks, 1985.

Micheletti, Enza (ed.). *North American Folk Healing: An A–Z Guide to Traditional Remedies.* New York and Montreal: Reader's Digest Association, 1998.

Mundford Primary School Project, Norfolk, England, 1980, unpublished.

Page, Robin. *The Country Way of Love.* London: Penguin, 1983.

Roy, Carmen. *La Littérature Orale en Gaspésie.* Bulletin 134, 36 de la Serie Anthropologique. Ottawa: Ministre de Nord Canadien et des Ressources Nationales, (1955): 61–105, 107–136.

Thomas, Daniel Lindsey, and Lucy Blayney Thomas. *Kentucky Superstitions.* Princeton, NJ: Princeton University Press, 1920.

Wilson, Charles Bundy. "Notes on Folk-Medicine." *Journal of American Folklore* 21 (1908): 68–73.

Wright, A. R. "Seventeenth Century Cures and Charms." *Folk-Lore* 23 (1912): 230–236, 490–497.

## Onion (Allium cepa)

The origin of the cultivated onion is obscure, but it is known that both onion and garlic were cultivated in ancient Egypt (Harrison, Masefield, and Wallis 1985: 166). The onion vividly illustrates the overlap between food and medicine in folk practice. A particularly dramatic example of this is described in the ninth-century *Saga of King Harald*. Warriors with severe abdominal injuries were given a meal of onions and herbs; if their injuries shortly afterward smelt of onions, this indicated internal organs were damaged, and they were given up for dead (Beith 1995: 34). Less drastically, onion gruel was regarded as a good cure for colds and fevers, right up to the twentieth century. A Scottish Highland remedy for pneumonia was to place a boiled onion in each armpit (Beith 1995: 231). Onions were cut open and placed in the sickroom, where it was thought that they attracted the infection to themselves, an example of transference. The fact that a cut onion left exposed to the air soon goes black may have supported the idea that it attracts infection.

A Scotsman living in England has related the story, told to him by his grandmother, and to her by her grandmother, of a village in the Scottish Highlands where all but her own family were wiped

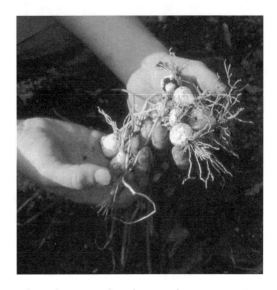

Like garlic, onions have been used to protect against infection. They have treated a wide range of conditions from earache to frostbite. (Sarah Boait)

out by an epidemic fever. The reason given for her family's survival was that the house was "all hung about with onions" (Hatfield pers. com.). A much more modern story concerns a farm in Cheshire that escaped the 1988 foot-and-mouth epidemic. This was attributed to the farmer's wife having placed cut onions along the sills and lintels of the cowsheds (Vickery 1995: 266). Another very widespread folk use for onion was in the treatment of earache: a small piece of roasted onion was placed in the ear. Onions also featured in cough medicine. Sliced and sprinkled with sugar, they provided a thick cough syrup. Raw onion was also used to treat minor burns, and to treat insect bites and stings (Hatfield 1994: 29, 23; Hatfield MS). An onion poultice was used in the Scottish highlands for treating toothache (Beith 1995: 231). Onion has been rubbed on bruises and on chilblains (Vickery 1995: 267), and an onion has been carried in the pocket to ward off rheumatism. Onion has even been used by schoolchildren, rubbed onto the palm of the hand, to lessen the pain of caning (Opie and Opie 1959: 375).

European settlers in North America used onions in folk medicine in many of the same ways. Meyer records its use in treating wasp stings, earache, boils. Raw, they were recommended for catarrh, cooked as gruel for colds. An onion poultice was applied externally for chest colds. Syrup made from onions and honey or sugar was used to treat coughs in adults, whooping cough in children, and croup in infants (Meyer 1985: 39, 43, 65, 67, 78, 86, 100, 266, 558). Onions soaked in vinegar, or roasted and made into an ointment with soap, were used to soften and remove corns. Cooked onions were applied to sore feet (Meyer 1985: 118, 120). For a fever, sliced onions were applied to the soles of the feet. Roast onion applied to the wrist on the opposite side of the body from the aching tooth was suggested as a cure for toothache, while a poultice of salt pork and raw onion was recommended for a sore throat (Meyer 1985: 129, 247, 253). Cooked onions with cayenne pepper were recommended for insomnia (Meyer 1985: 145). Onions were also used to treat gravel and stone. A Baptist minister in Virginia was given a recipe for gravel by a slave; it consisted of horsemint tea (Monarda punctata) and red onion juice. The minister was cured by this, bought the slave, and gave him his freedom (Meyer 1985: 161). The

UCLA Folklore Archive contains more than two thousand records for folk medicinal uses of onion. Many of these are for coughs, colds, and fevers. In addition, onions have been used to treat falling hair (UCLA Folklore Archives 5_1872), worms (Puckett 1981: 503), warts (Stout 1936: 178), burns (as in Britain, see above) (UCLA Folklore Archives 11_5304), diphtheria (Puckett 1981: 362), asthma (UCLA Folklore Archives 10_6176), pneumonia (Browne 1958: 85), and snake bite (Koch 1980: 112).

There are twentieth-century records from the Shinnecock Indians of garden onion placed in the sickroom to draw out a fever (Carr and Westey 1945: 120). Onions were not cultivated by the Native Americans in the remote past, but in their medicine they used a number of related native species, such as wild onion (Allium cernuum) and ramp (Allium tricoccum). A. cernuum, the nodding onion, was used as a poultice applied to the feet for fever by the Cherokee, and its juice was taken, after horsemint tea, for gravel and dropsy. An infusion was taken for colic, and the plant was fried and put on the chest for treating croup (Hamel and Chiltoskey 1975: 47). Among the Isleta, a poultice was applied for infections and for sore throats (Jones 1931: 20). The soaked bulbs were used to treat sores and swellings by the Southern Kwakiutl Indians (Turner and Bell 1973: 272), while among the Quinault, in western Washington, the plant was chewed and applied to the chest for pleurisy pains (Gunther 1973: 24). Bee stings were treated with wild onion by the Native Americans (Vogel 1970: 306).

See also **Amulet, Asthma, Bruises, Burns, Chilblains, Colds, Colic, Corns, Coughs, Croup, Dropsy, Earache, Fevers, Garlic, Gravel and stone, Insect bites and stings, Poultice, Sleeplessness, Snake bite, Sore**

feet, Toothache, Transference, Warts,
Whooping cough, Worms.

## References

Beith, Mary. *Healing Threads: Traditional Medicines of the Highlands and Islands.* Edinburgh: Polygon, 1995.

Browne, Ray B. *Popular Beliefs and Practices from Alabama.* Folklore Studies 9. Berkeley and Los Angeles: University of California Publications, 1958.

Carr, Lloyd G., and Carlos Westey. "Surviving Folktales and Herbal Lore among the Shinnecock Indians." *Journal of American Folklore* 58 (1945): 113–123.

Gunther, Erna. *Ethnobotany of Western Washington.* Rev. ed. Seattle: University of Washington Press, 1973.

Hamel, Paul B., and Mary U. Chiltoskey. *Cherokee Plants and Their Uses: A 400 Year History.* Sylva, NC: Herald, 1975.

Harrison, S. G., G. B. Masefield, and Michael Wallis. *The Oxford Book of Food Plants.* London: Peerage, 1985.

Hatfield, Gabrielle. *Country Remedies: Traditional East Anglian Plant Remedies in the Twentieth Century.* Woodbridge: Boydell, 1994.

Jones, Volney H. *The Ethnobotany of the Isleta Indians.* M.A. thesis, University of New Mexico, 1931.

Koch, William E. *Folklore from Kansas: Beliefs and Customs.* Lawrence, KS: Regent Press, 1980.

Meyer, Clarence. *American Folk Medicine.* Glenwood, IL: Meyerbooks, 1985.

Opie, Iona, and Peter Opie. *The Lore and Language of Schoolchildren.* London: Oxford University Press, 1959.

Puckett, Newbell Niles. *Popular Beliefs and Superstitions: A Compendium of American Folklore from the Ohio Collection of Newbell Niles Puckett.* Edited by Wayland D. Hand, Anna Casetta, and Sondra B. Thiederman. 3 vols. Boston: G. K. Hall, 1981.

Stout, Earl J. "Folklore from Iowa." *Memoirs of the American Folklore Society* 29 (1936).

Turner, Nancy Chapman, and Marcus A. M. Bell. "The Ethnobotany of the Southern Kwakiutl Indians of British Columbia." *Economic Botany* 27 (1973): 257–310.

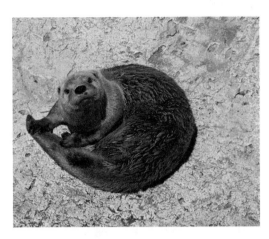

In the Native American tradition, the otter was valued for its healing powers and medicine bags were often made from otter skin. In the Scottish Highlands, licking the liver of a newly killed otter was thought to give a person the power to cure burns. (Library of Congress)

Vickery, Roy. *A Dictionary of Plant Lore.* Oxford: Oxford University Press, 1995.

Vogel, Virgil J. *American Indian Medicine.* Norman: University of Oklahoma Press, 1970.

# Otter

In the Highlands of Scotland, the skin of the otter was used as an amulet during childbirth, as well as being dried and powdered and taken as medicine for smallpox and fevers (Beith 1995: 180). Licking the liver of a newly killed otter was thought to give a person the power to cure burns (Goodrich-Freer 1902: 56).

In the Native American tradition too the otter is valued for its healing powers. Medicine bags were made from otter skin (Skinner 1925: 433). Illness brought on by ingratitude to water animals on the part of a hunter could be cured by an otter medicine man (Vogel 1970: 15). Among the Cheyenne, difficult childbirth was attended by the otter medicine man (UCLA Folklore Archives 20_5807). For lung trouble, otter brains and the water from a rock fissure was used by the Cherokee (Mellinger 1967: 20).

*See also* **Amulet, Burns, Childbirth, Fevers.**

## References

Beith, Mary. *Healing Threads: Traditional Medicines of the Highlands and Islands.* Edinburgh: Polygon, 1995.

Goodrich-Freer, A. "More Folklore from the Hebrides." *Folk-Lore* 13 (1902): 29–62.

Mellinger, Marie B. "Medicine of the Cherokees." *Foxfire* 1(3) (1967): 13–20, 65–72.

Skinner, Alanson. "Traditions of the Iowa Indians." *Journal of American Folklore* 38 (1925): 425–506.

Vogel, Virgil J. *American Indian Medicine.* Norman: University of Oklahoma Press, 1970.

# P

## Palsy

This is the old-fashioned term for paralysis, but in folk medicine it also covered illnesses that caused trembling and shaking. In Irish folk medicine there were a number of plant remedies used to treat it. The cowslip *(Primula veris)* was known as "palsy-wort" in some parts of Ireland and was used to treat the condition. The powdered root of cuckoo pint *(Arum maculatum)* placed under the tongue and swallowed with saliva was another Irish folk cure for palsy. Woodsorrel *(Oxalis acetosella)* was also used. Paralyzed limbs have been rubbed with stinging nettles (Allen and Hatfield, in press). Fasting spittle, ingested, was recommended as a cure for palsy in Yorkshire (Gutch 1901: 177–178). A very ancient remedy for paralysis (as well as lameness) was to place a live mouse or shrew in a box around the neck; when the animal died, the patient was, ideally, cured (Souter 1995: 40). The animal was sometimes plugged into a hole in an ash tree; such trees became known as "shrew ashes" (Radford and Radford 1974: 308).

In North American folk medicine jimson weed was sometimes used to treat palsy (Peattie 1943: 118). The leaves of aspen *(Populus tremula)* were also used, because they tremble in the wind. This is an example of like curing like. Leeches were also used in palsy treatment (Clark 1970: 26,

27). An African American suggestion was to tie a rope around each ankle to prevent the shaking of palsy (Parler 1962, 3: 809). Fowl have been associated in folk medicine with palsy. A bundle of their feathers at the head of the patient's bed was thought to cure palsy (Parler 1962, 3: 808). On the other hand, to hold a dying chicken or other bird in the hand was thought to cause palsy (Brown 1952–1964, 6: 247). In the Native American tradition the songs sung to treat a patient with palsy had a specially steady rhythm (Densmore 1954: 110).

*See also* **African tradition, Ash, Native American tradition, Spit, Stinging nettle, Sympathetic magic, Thornapple.**

### References

Allen, David E., and Gabrielle Hatfield. *Medicinal Plants in Folk Tradition.* Portland, OR: Timber Press, in press.

Brown, Frank C. *Collection of North Carolina Folklore.* 7 vols. Durham, NC: Duke University Press, 1952–1964.

Clark, Joseph D. "North Carolina Popular Beliefs and Superstitions." *North Carolina Folklore* 18 (1970): 1–66.

Densmore, Frances. "Importance of Rhythm in Songs for the Treatment of the Sick by American Indians." *Scientific Monthly* 79(2) (August 1954): 109–112.

Gutch, Eliza. *County Folklore, Vol. II. Printed Extracts Concerning the North Riding of Yorkshire, York and Ainsty.* London: Folklore Society, 1901.

Parler, Mary Celestia, and University Student Contributors. *Folk Beliefs from Arkansas.* 15 vols. Fayetteville: University of Arkansas, 1962.

Peattie, Roderick, ed. *The Great Smokies and the Blue Ridge.* New York: Vanguard Press, 1943.

Radford, E., and M. A. Radford. *Encyclopaedia of Superstitions.* Edited and revised by Christina Hole. London: Book Club Associates, 1974.

Souter, Keith. *Cure Craft: Traditional Folk Remedies and Treatment from Antiquity to the Present Day.* Saffron Walden: C. W. Daniel, 1995.

# Peach (*Prunus persica*)

This plant is thought to have originated in China and is one of the world's most widely grown trees. Although it has been grown in Britain since the sixteenth century and used in official medicine, particularly for treating worms in children (Black 1883: 199), it does not appear to have had a role in British folk medicine. In contrast, its uses in North American folk medicine are widespread. In China, the plant had magical associations and was used ceremonially. The peach stones, or pits, were carried as amulets and believed to confer longevity. Asian immigrants to North America brought this belief with them (Dwyer 1967). In the African tradition, it is believed that mixing semen with peach sap will prevent a man being unfaithful to his wife (Hyatt 1978, 5: 415). Apart from these semimagical beliefs, the practical uses to which it has been put in folk medicine are impressively varied. It has treated thrush (Browne 1958: 27), erysipelas (Brown and Ledford 1967: 28), poison ivy and poison oak (UCLA Folklore Archives 2_6461), rashes in general (Puckett 1981: 430), itching (Clark 1970: 24), insect bites and stings (Killion and Waller 1972: 104), and snake bite (Browne 1958: 95). A poultice of peach tree leaves has been used for removing splinters (Hudson 1928: 154) and treating boils (Mason 1957: 30). Mixed with buttermilk the leaves have been used to lighten the complexion (Parler 1962: 548), and the water in which the leaves have been boiled reputedly prevents baldness (Puckett 1981: 315). Dandruff has been treated with a tea made from peach leaves and sulphur (Clark 1970: 22).

Another major use has been in pain relief. A peach leaf poultice was regarded as a good general standby for pain relief (Rogers 1941: 27). It has treated sore muscles (UCLA Folklore Archives 21_5432) and relieved stone bruises (Long 1962: 1). Pain in the neck has been treated using a young twig tied around the neck (Brown 1952–1964, 6: 237), and burns have been soothed with a compress of peach leaves (Puckett 1981: 334). Gall stones (Brendle and Unger 1935: 192) and jaundice (Parler 1962: 735) have both been treated using peach (the kernels and a leaf tea, respectively). The water in which peach leaves have been boiled has been used as a hot compress to treat appendicitis (Parler 1962: 433). Dried and powdered and mixed with chalk, the leaves and the seeds were used to treat heartburn (Meyer 1985: 234), and the bark was used for an upset stomach (Meyer 1985: 241), while a tea made from the leaves has been used for stomach ailments in general (Woodhull 1930: 66). Indigestion has been treated by chewing the kernels (Koch 1980: 90); vomiting, including pregnancy sickness, has been stopped using a tea made from peach leaves (Browne 1958: 111). Colic was treated with a tea prepared from the bark of the peach tree scraped downward (Rogers 1941: 14). Dysentery (Puckett 1981: 363), diarrhea (Clark 1970: 19), and constipation (Lick and Brendle 1922: 277) have all been treated with peach. Hiccups have apparently been cured by drinking juice from canned peaches (Hand 1966: 144). Rheumatism has been averted by wearing peach leaves in the hat as an amulet

(Wilson 1968: 65). The peach has had gynecological uses too in folk medicine. Labor has been hastened by drinking tea made from peach tree bark: again, according to tradition, the bark should be scraped downward (Hyatt 1965: 135). As a poultice, it treated caked breasts (Meyer 1985: 48). Eating peach kernels has been claimed to shorten change of life (Parler 1962: 1110). Both bleeding (Guerin 1953: 55) and blood poisoning (*Los Angeles News* 1869) have been treated with peach leaves. Worms have been treated with peach-leaf tea (Randolph 1947: 106) or with an infusion of the flowers (Meyer 1985: 270), a use echoed in official medicine and herbalism in Britain. The "meat" of the peach stone was a nineteenth-century remedy for a sick headache (Meyer 1985: 138). Sore throat (UCLA Folklore Archives 6_6500) and gum ailments (UCLA Folklore Archives 6–6545) have both been poulticed with peach leaves. A syrup made from peach kernels has been dripped into sore ears (Parler 1962: 610), and peach kernels have been rubbed onto the forehead for a headache (UCLA Folklore Archives 3_1939). Various infections have been treated using peach leaves. These included cholera (Cadwallader and Wilson 1965: 222, 225), scarlet fever (UCLA Folklore Archives 1_5466), mumps (Anderson 1970: 52), typhoid (Saxon 1945: 535), and malaria (Parler 1962: 763). Peach has been used for a number of respiratory illnesses: for bronchitis (Clark 1970: 14), asthma (McWhorter 1966: 13), pneumonia (Hall 1960: 52) and tuberculosis (Browne 1958: 110). A cure for whooping cough from Randolph County involves passing the child through the fork of a peach tree (Richmond and Van Winkle 1958: 134). A wart cure from Kentucky involves cutting notches in a peach tree equal in number to the warts (Pope 1965: 46). Eating both leaves and bark was recommended for nervousness (UCLA Folklore Archives 22_6416). Peach stones were a constituent of a tonic prescribed by Samuel Thomson (Meyer 1985: 257). In the 1950s a tea was still being made, as a tonic, from peach-tree bark (Browne 1958: 121).

In Native American practice, peach seeds have been eaten to relieve swellings from bruises (Speck 1942: 46). The leaves (Tantaquidgeon 1972: 31) and the seeds (Hamel and Chiltoskey 1975: 47–48) have been used to treat worms. The plant has in addition been used in many of the ways described above, including the treatment of vomiting, constipation, fever (Hamel and Chiltoskey 1975: 47), and kidney trouble (Speck, Hassrick, and Carpenter 1942: 33).

*See also* **African tradition; Amulet; Asthma; Baldness; Bleeding; Boils; Breast problems; Childbirth; Colic; Constipation; Diarrhea; Erysipelas; Headache; Hiccups; Indigestion; Insect bites and stings; Jaundice; Menopause; Poison ivy, Poison oak; Poultice; Rheumatism; Snake bite; Sore throat; Thomson, Samuel; Tonic; Tuberculosis; Warts; Whooping cough; Worms.**

## References

Anderson, John. *Texas Folk Medicine.* Austin, TX: Encino Press, 1970.

Black, William George. *Folk-Medicine: A Chapter in the History of Culture.* London: Folklore Society, 1883.

Brendle, Thomas R., and Claude W. Unger. *Folk Medicine of the Pennsylvania Germans: The Non-Occult Cures.* Proceedings of the Pennsylvania German Society 45 (1935).

Brown, Frank C. *Collection of North Carolina Folklore.* 7 vols. Durham, NC: Duke University Press, 1952–1964.

Brown, Judy, and Lizzie Ledford. "Superstitions." *Foxfire,* 1(2) (1967): 25–28.

Browne, Ray B. *Popular Beliefs and Practices from Alabama.* Folklore Studies 9. Berkeley and Los Angeles: University of California Publications, 1958.

Cadwallader, D. E., and F. J. Wilson. "Folklore Medicine among Georgia's Piedmont Negroes after the Civil War." *Collections of the Georgia Historical Society* 49 (1965): 217–227.

Clark, Joseph D. "North Carolina Popular Beliefs and Superstitions." *North Carolina Folklore* 18 (1970): 1–66.

Dwyer, Philip M. *Herbalism and Ritual: Folk Medical Practices Among Asian Immigrants in Southern California.* Unpublished dissertation, UCLA Folklore and Mythology Studies Center, 1967.

Guerin, Wayne. "Some Folkways of a Stewart County Community." *Tennessee Folklore Society Bulletin* 19 (1953): 49–58.

Hall, Joseph S. *Smoky Mountain Folks and Their Lore.* Gatlinburg, TN: Great Smoky Mountains Natural History Association, 1960.

Hamel, Paul B., and Mary U. Chiltoskey. *Cherokee Plants and Their Uses: A 400 Year History.* Sylva, NC: Herald, 1975.

Hand, Wayland D. "More Popular Beliefs and Superstitions from Pennsylvania." In *Two Penny Ballads and Four Dollar Whiskey,* edited by Robert H. Byington and Kenneth S. Goldstein. Hatboro, PA: Folklore Associates, 1966, 137–164.

Hudson, Arthur Palmer. *Specimens of Mississippi Folk-Lore.* Ann Arbor, MI: Edwards Brothers, 1928.

Hyatt, Harry Middleton. *Folklore from Adams County Illinois.* 2nd rev. ed. New York: Memoirs of the Alma Egan Hyatt Foundation, 1965.

Hyatt, Harry Middleton, M.A. *Hoodoo, Conjuration, Witchcraft, Rootwork.* 5 vols. New York: Memoirs of the Alma Egan Hyatt Foundation, 1978.

Killion, Ronald G., and Charles T. Waller. *A Treasury of Georgia Folklore.* Atlanta: Cherokee, 1972.

Koch, William E. *Folklore from Kansas: Beliefs and Customs.* Lawrence, KS: Regent Press, 1980.

Lick, David E., and Thomas R. Brendle. "Plant Names and Plant Lore among the Pennsylvania Germans." *Proceedings and Addresses of the Pennsylvania German Society* 33 (1922).

Long, Grady M. "Folk Medicine in McMinn, Polk, Bradley, and Meigs Counties, Tennessee, 1910–1927." *Tennessee Folklore Society Bulletin* 28 (1962): 1–8.

*Los Angeles News,* April 14, 1869.

Mason, James. "Home Remedies in West Virginia." *West Virginia Folklore* 7 (1957): 27–32.

McWhorter, Bruce. "Superstitions from Russell County, Kentucky." *Kentucky Folklore Records* 12 (1966): 11–14.

Meyer, Clarence. *American Folk Medicine.* Glenwood, IL: Meyerbooks, 1985.

Parler, Mary Celestia, and University Student Contributors. *Folk Beliefs from Arkansas.* 15 vols. Fayetteville: University of Arkansas, 1962.

Pope, Genevieve. "Superstitions and Beliefs of Fleming County." *Kentucky Folklore Records* 11 (1965): 41–51.

Puckett, Newbell Niles. *Popular Beliefs and Superstitions: A Compendium of American Folklore from the Ohio Collection of Newbell Niles Puckett.* Edited by Wayland D. Hand, Anna Casetta, and Sondra B. Thiederman. 3 vols. Boston: G. K. Hall, 1981.

Randolph, Vance. *Ozark Superstitions.* New York: Columbia University Press, 1947.

Richmond, W. Edson, and Elva Van Winkle. "Is There a Doctor in the House?" *Indiana History Bulletin* 35 (1958): 115–135.

Rogers, E. G. *Early Folk Medical Practices in Tennessee.* Murfreesboro, TN: Rogers, 1941.

Saxon, Lyle. *Gumbo Ya-Ya.* Boston: Houghton and Mifflin, 1945.

Speck, Frank G., R. B. Hassrick, and E. S. Carpenter. "Rappahannock Herbals, Folk-Lore and Science of Cures." *Proceedings of the Delaware County Institute of Science* 10 (1942): 7–55.

Speck, Frank G. "Catawba Herbals and Curative Practices." *Journal of American Folklore* 57 (1944): 37–50.

Tantaquidgeon, Gladys. "Folk Medicine of the Delaware and Related Algonkian Indians." *Pennsylvania Historical Commission Anthropological Papers,* no. 3 (1972).

Wilson, Gordon, Sr. "Folklore of the Mammoth Cave Region." *Kentucky Folklore Series,* no. 4 (1968).

Woodhull, Frost. "Ranch Remedios." *Publications of the Texas Folklore Society* 8 (1930): 9–73.

# Piles

A number of simple first-aid suggestions for treating piles included bathing them in fresh morning dew (the equivalent of today's ice pack) (Hatfield 1994: 44). As preventative measures, avoiding constipation and eating plenty of vegetables were recommended in British folk medicine (Prince 1991: 40). There were a number of plant remedies used in the treatment of piles, the best-known being lesser celandine, also known as pilewort *(Ranunculus ficaria)*. An ointment was made from the bulbils (small tubers in the leaf axils). This has been used both in folk medicine and official herbalism and continues in use. In the east of England a number of other plants were used, including red nettle *(Lamium purpureum)*, ground elder *(Aegopodium podagraria)*, and scabious *(Knautia arvensis)* (Hatfield 1994: 42–44). In Lincolnshire, the berries of mezereon *(Daphne mezereum)* were swallowed like pills to cure piles (Rudkin 1936: 26). In Devon, plantain juice was used to soothe piles (Lafont 1984: 68). In Sussex, an infusion of elder flowers has been used (Vickery 1995: 124).

Both garlic and onion have been used (Hatfield 1994: 43; Vickery 1995: 268) in treatment of piles. Figwort and puffball were both used in the Scottish Highlands in treating piles (Beith 1995: 216, 235). In Devon, various species of figwort were known as "poor man's salve" (Britten and Holland 1878–1886). An ointment for treating piles was made from lard and the ground-up roots. In Scotland, a remedy for piles involved sitting over a pail containing smouldering leather (Simpkins 1914: 409). Carrying a rose-hip in the pocket as an amulet was thought to prevent piles (Hatfield 1994: 42–44). A horse chestnut *(Aesculus hippocastanum)* has similarly been carried (Vickery 1995: 196).

In North American folk medicine, a number of plant and animal products have been carried as amulets to prevent piles. These include chestnut (buckeye) *(Aesculus sp.)*, as in Britain (Welsch 1966: 342), nutmeg *(Myristica fragrans)* (Hyatt 1965: 250), potato (Fogel 1915: 305), elderberry leaves (Hyatt 1965: 250), oakum (UCLA Folklore Archives 5_7593), and the rattles of rattlesnakes (Hyatt 1965: 250). Dietary recommendations for piles include whole black pepper (Hyatt 1965: 250), Epsom salts and sulphur (Hyatt 1965: 250), lemons (Hyatt 1965: 250), brown sugar and walnuts (UCLA Folklore Archives 5_7593), a tea made from the leaves of wild currant bushes *(Ribes sp.)* (UCLA Folklore Archives 21_6836), roasted onions (Parler 1962: 811), and raw potato and castor oil (Hyatt 1965: 250).

Some folk remedies were taken internally for piles. These include milk of sulphur (Meyer 1985: 192), a decoction of yellow dock root, or of wild lettuce *(Lactuca canadensis)*, the fresh juice of mountain ash berries *(Sorbus aucuparia)* (Meyer 1985: 193, 194), essence of fir and tar water (Meyer 1985: 196), or the roots of ironweed *(Vernonia sp.)* infused and mixed with honey (Hohman 1930: 24). However, the great majority of piles remedies were applied externally. Rubbing with burned cork has been suggested (Puckett 1981: 423). Sitting on mullein leaves apparently soothes piles (Fogel 1915: 305), and using these velvety leaves in lieu of toilet paper is also recommended. Sitting on a pine board sounds less comfortable (UCLA Folklore Archives 12_7595). Crouching over steam (Puckett 1981: 423) or over a pot of boiling rattlesnake broom (UCLA Folklore Archives 16_5445) are further suggestions. Some remedies were used in enema form, such as hot water and flaxseed (Meyer 1985: 192), or the juice of pokeberries) (Meyer 1985: 195), or an infusion of raspberry, witch hazel or sumac leaves *(Rhus glabra)* (Meyer 1985: 195), or a warm solution of alum (Browne 1958: 84).

A great variety of ointments have been employed in the folk treatment of piles. Many forms of grease have been used: olive oil (UCLA Folklore Archives 78_6438), lard and gunpowder (Puckett 1981: 423), mutton tallow (Puckett 1981: 423), rabbit fat (Brendle and Unger 1935: 184), buffalo tallow (Welsch 1966: 342), axle grease (Wilson 1968: 77), coal oil (UCLA Folklore Archives 13_6438), and lard mixed with white droppings from a dog (Hyatt 1965: 250). Numerous ointments were prepared using plants. These include peach (Browne 1958: 84), red oak bark (*?Quercus robur*) (Browne 1958: 84), frankincense (Gaine 1796: 19), cinnamon (UCLA Folklore Archives 4_6438), pokeberries (Clark 1970: 27), persimmon bark (*Diospyros* sp.) (McLean 1972: 26), cheese plant *(Malva rotundifolia)* (Browne 1958: 84), the flowers of butter and egg *(Linaria vulgaris)* (Lick and Brendle 1922: 130), the bark of white pine *(Pinus strobus)* (Meyer 1985: 192), jimson weed, balm of Gilead (Brown 1952–1964, 6: 249), the leaves of fireweed *(Erechtites hieracifolia)* (Meyer 1985: 196), or of celandine *(Ranunculus ficaria)* (as used in Britain too) (Meyer 1985: 195), Solomon's seal root *(Polygonatum multiflorum),* or slippery elm bark (Meyer 1985: 194). Chestnuts *(Aesculus* sp.) were made into an ointment for piles (Meyer 1985: 193), as well as being carried as a preventative. A complex ointment was prepared from the barks of witch hazel *(Hamamelis virginiana),* black cherry *(Prunus serotina),* white oak, apple tree, and the leaves of sage (*?Salvia* sp.) (UCLA Folklore Archives 19_6532). A recommendation from the African tradition was to wipe the piles with a banana skin (Puckett 1981: 423). A remarkable recipe was to cook a wasp nest in honey, to produce a salve (Hyatt 1965: 250).

In Native American practice, a very large number of different plants have been employed in the treatment of piles (Moerman 1998: 802). Oak, sumac, buckeye, mullein, persimmon are all used in Native American practice, and their use in general North American folk practice may have originated here.

*See also* **African tradition, Amulet, Apple, Balm of Gilead, Dew, Dock, Elder, Elm, Figwort, Flax, Mullein, Oak, Onion, Peach, Plantain, Poke, Potato, Puffball, Thornapple.**

## References

Beith, Mary. *Healing Threads: Traditional Medicines of the Highlands and Islands.* Edinburgh: Polygon, 1995.

Brendle, Thomas R., and Claude W. Unger. "Folk Medicine of the Pennsylvania Germans: The Non-Occult Cures." *Proceedings of the Pennsylvania German Society* 45 (1935).

Britten, James, and Holland, Robert. *A Dictionary of English Plant Names.* London: Trübner for English Dialect Society, 1878–1886.

Brown, Frank C. *Collection of North Carolina Folklore.* 7 vols. Durham, NC: Duke University Press, 1952–1964.

Browne, Ray B. *Popular Beliefs and Practices from Alabama.* Folklore Studies 9. Berkeley and Los Angeles: University of California Publications, 1958.

Clark, Joseph D. "North Carolina Popular Beliefs and Superstitions." *North Carolina Folklore* 18 (1970): 1–66.

Fogel, Edwin Miller. "Beliefs and Superstitions of the Pennsylvania Germans." *Americana Germanica* 18 (1915).

Gaine, Hugh. *The Journals of Hugh Gaine.* New York, 1796.

Hatfield, Gabrielle. *Country Remedies: Traditional East Anglian Plant Remedies in the Twentieth Century.* Woodbridge: Boydell, 1994.

Hohman, John George. *Long Lost Friend, or Book of Pow-Wows: A Collection of Mysterious and Invaluable Arts and Remedies for Man as Well as Animals.* Edited by A. Monroe Aurand, Jr., Harrisburg, PA: The Aurand Press, 1930.

Hyatt, Harry Middleton. *Folklore from Adams*

*County Illinois.* 2nd rev. ed. New York: Memoirs of the Alma Egan Hyatt Foundation, 1965.

Lafont, Anne-Marie. *A Herbal Folklore.* Bideford: Badger Books, 1984.

Lick, David E., and Thomas R. Brendle. "Plant Names and Plant Lore among the Pennsylvania Germans." *Proceedings and Addresses of the Pennsylvania German Society* 33 (1922).

McLean, Patricia S. "Conjure Doctors in Eastern North Carolina." *North Carolina Folklore* 20 (1972): 21–29.

Meyer, Clarence. *American Folk Medicine.* Glenwood, IL: Meyerbooks, 1985.

Moerman, Daniel E. *Native American Ethnobotany.* Portland, OR: Timber Press, 1998.

Parler, Mary Celestia, and University Student Contributors. *Folk Beliefs from Arkansas.* 15 vols. Fayetteville: University of Arkansas, 1962.

Prince, Dennis. *Grandmother's Cures: An A–Z of Herbal Remedies.* London: Fontana, 1991.

Puckett, Newbell Niles. *Popular Beliefs and Superstitions: A Compendium of American Folklore from the Ohio Collection of Newbell Niles Puckett.* Edited by Wayland D. Hand, Anna Casetta, and Sondra B. Thiederman. 3 vols. Boston: G. K. Hall, 1981.

Rudkin, E. *Lincolnshire Folklore.* London: Gainsborough, 1936.

Simpkins, John Ewart. *Examples of Printed Folk-Lore Concerning Fife, with Some Notes on Clackmannan and Kinross-shire.* County Folk-Lore 7. London: Publications of the Folklore Society, 1914.

Vickery, Roy. *A Dictionary of Plant Lore.* Oxford: Oxford University Press, 1995.

Welsch, Roger L. *A Treasury of Nebraska Pioneer Folklore.* Lincoln: University of Nebraska Press, 1966.

Wilson, Gordon, Sr. "Folklore of the Mammoth Cave Region." *Kentucky Folklore Series,* no. 4 (1968).

# Pine (*Pinus* spp.)

In Britain the only native pine is *Pinus sylvestris,* the Scots pine, and the populations of this have declined over the centu-

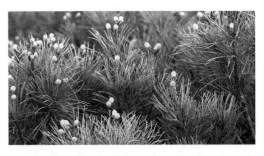

In Scotland, pine bark has been used for treating fevers and a plaster for treating boils and sores has been made from pine resin. The number of native pine species is large in North America, and pine has been extensively used in North American folk medicine. (North Wind Picture Archive)

ries, leaving only small areas of natural pine forest in the Scottish Highlands. The folk medicine surrounding the tree has probably similarly declined, but there are remnants, especially in Scotland, of its former use. The bark has been used for treating fevers (Beith 1995: 233), and a plaster for treating boils and sores has been made from the resin (McCutcheon 1919: 235). In England too the resin was used to heal cuts (Hatfield 1999: 101). The young shoots were made into a cough syrup (Hatfield 1999: 169). In the seventeenth century, pine tree "pineapples" (presumably the young flowering shoots) were used to treat lice (Wright 1912: 230–236). There are large numbers of planted pines, especially in East Anglia, and even their smell has been considered therapeutic; there is a record of a child suffering from a polio-like illness being taken to the pine woods (Hatfield MS), and a similar record from Wales of an ill child being taken for a holiday to an area where pines were planted in order inhale the smell (Vickery 1995: 283).

In North America, in contrast, the number of native pine species is large, and pines have been very extensively used in folk medicine. A remedy very similar to the Scottish one for a plaster uses the pitch pine *(Pinus palustris)*; the pitch or resin is extracted and mixed with beeswax to form a plaster for dressing sore areas. Sometimes the plaster was prepared with hemlock gum and sulphur (Meyer 1985: 197). The white pine, *Pinus strobus,* has been extensively used in folk medicine, as well as for timber; it was so important that the white pine is the emblem on the first flag of the American revolution. It is said that in the sixteenth century the lives of many colonists suffering from scurvy were saved by Native Americans treating them with pine needle tea (Micheletti 1998: 261). A sweetened brew of the needles was used for treating colds and coughs (Meyer 1985: 65, 81). The inner bark of white pine was boiled in milk and used to treat diarrhea and dysentery (Meyer 1985: 91, 96). A plaster of white pine turpentine was used to treat corns (Meyer 1985: 119). A poultice for treating piles was prepared from white pine bark, and a tea made from the same was drunk at the same time (Meyer 1985: 192). For rheumatism, pitch from a white pine log was mixed with sulphur, honey, and brandy to make a liniment to be used hot. This was also taken internally (Meyer 1985: 217). For burns and sores, a poultice was prepared from the bark of the white pine (Meyer 1985: 229). Pine tar, distilled from the wood, formed the basis of many wound salves and cough syrups.

The importance of pine in folk medicine is indicated by the huge number of records for it, more than a thousand, contained in the UCLA Folklore Archives. In addition to the ailments already mentioned, these records show that pine has been used to treat insomnia, by sleeping on a pillow filled with the needles (Lathrop 1961: 18). Spider bites have been treated with pine sap (Hendricks 1980: 98). Heartburn has been treated by chewing pine needles (Parler 1962: 685). A solution from boiled pine cones has been used in New Mexico to treat sore eyes (Moya 1940: 69). Pine tree tea has been used to cure worms (Puckett 1981:

503). Some pine remedies involve ritual. For biliousness, the sufferer is advised to bore a hole in a pine tree and walk three times around the tree, telling the biliousness to go away (Hyatt 1965: 276). For toothache, the advice is to take two pine splinters, push them into the gum surrounding the aching tooth, then bury the splinters in a hole on the north side of a dogwood tree (Waller and Killion 1972: 74). For nosebleed, pine splinters dipped in the blood were driven into a tree (Parler 1962: 804). For fever, the patient is advised to break a pine branch while facing into the setting sun (Fitchett 1936: 360). Another suggestion for fever is to tie a string to a pine tree (Cannon 1984: 98). For backache, the roots of pine from a road where no corpse has passed by should be burned and the rosin applied to the back (Brown 1952–1964, 6: 121). Finally, there is a suggestion that mental troubles can be cured simply by walking in pine woods and inhaling the smell (Brown 1952–1964, 6: 357).

Impressive though the list of uses in folk medicine generally may be, it reflects only a fraction of the ways in which Native Americans used different species of pine. Moerman has records for *Pinus strobus* alone that cover thirteen tribes and more than twenty different ailments (Moerman 1998: 411–412), including tuberculosis, coughs and colds, rheumatism, broken bones, venereal disease, and many others. Twenty-six species of pine have been recorded in Native American use (Moerman 1998: 403–414). Ponderosa pine *(Pinus ponderosa)* was used extensively, as well as the singleleaf pinyon *(Pinus monophylla)* and the lodgepole pine *(Pinus contorta).* Even a pine-tree fungus has been used medicinally. Scraped into whisky, it was given as a remedy for colic (Chamberlain 1888: 156).

*See also* **Backache, Boils, Burns, Colds, Colic, Corns, Coughs, Cuts, Diarrhea,**

Dysentery, Eye problems, Fevers,
Indigestion, Nosebleed, Piles, Poultice,
Rheumatism, Scurvy, Sleeplessness,
Toothache, Worms.

## References

Beith, Mary. *Healing Threads: Traditional Medicines of the Highlands and Islands.* Edinburgh: Polygon, 1995.

Brown, Frank C. *Collection of North Carolina Folklore.* 7 vols. Durham, NC: Duke University Press, 1952–1964.

Cannon, Anthon S. *Popular Beliefs and Superstitions from Utah.* Edited by Wayland D. Hand and Jeannine E. Talley. Salt Lake City: University of Utah Press, 1984.

Chamberlain, A. F. "Notes on the History, Customs and Beliefs of the Mississagua Indians." *Journal of American Folklore* 1 (1888): 150–160.

Fitchett, E. Horace. "Superstitions in South Carolina." *Crisis* 43 (1936): 360–361, 370.

Hatfield, Gabrielle. Manuscript notes, in her personal possession.

Hatfield, Gabrielle. *Memory, Wisdom and Healing: The History of Domestic Plant Medicine.* Phoenix Mill: Sutton, 1999.

Hendricks, George D. *Roosters, Rhymes and Railroad Tracks: A Second Sampling of Superstitions and Popular Beliefs in Texas.* Dallas, TX: Southern Methodist University Press, 1980.

Hyatt, Harry Middleton. *Folklore from Adams County, Illinois.* 2nd rev. ed. New York: Memoirs of the Alma Egan Hyatt Foundation, 1965.

Lathrop, Amy. "Pioneer Remedies from Western Kansas." *Western Folklore* 20 (1961): 1–22.

McCutcheon, Alexander. "Some Highland Household Remedies." *Pharmacology Journal* 19 (April 1919): 235.

Meyer, Clarence. *American Folk Medicine.* Glenwood, IL: Meyerbooks, 1985.

Micheletti, Enza (ed.). *North American Folk Healing: An A–Z Guide to Traditional Remedies.* New York and Montreal: Reader's Digest Association, 1998.

Moerman, Daniel E. *Native American Ethnobotany.* Portland, OR: Timber Press, 1998.

Moya, Benjamin S. *Superstitions and Beliefs among the Spanish-Speaking People of New Mexico.* Master's thesis, University of New Mexico, 1940.

Parler, Mary Celestia, and University Student Contributors. *Folk Beliefs from Arkansas.* Vol. 3. Fayetteville: University of Arkansas, 1962.

Puckett, Newbell Niles. *Popular Beliefs and Superstitions: A Compendium of American Folklore from the Ohio Collection of Newbell Niles Puckett.* Edited by Wayland D. Hand, Anna Casetta, and Sondra B. Thiederman. 3 vols. Boston: G. K. Hall, 1981.

Vickery, Roy. *A Dictionary of Plant Lore.* Oxford: Oxford University Press, 1995.

Waller, Tom, and Gene Killion. "Georgia Folk Medicine." *Southern Folklore Quarterly* 36 (1972): 71–92.

Wright, A. R. "Seventeenth Century Cures and Charms." *Folk-Lore* 23 (1912): 230–236.

# Plague

Bubonic plague is caused by the bacillus *Yersinia pestis* and spread by flea bites as well as in breath and clothing. Rats form a reservoir for the disease. It is thought to have wiped out a quarter of the Roman Empire in the sixth century (Porter 1996: 28). A second wave of the disease at the beginning of the fourteenth century devastated much of Europe, Asia, the Middle East, and North Africa. Ancient talismans against the plague include nailing a horseshoe above the door, a practice inherited from the Romans (Souter 1995: 30), and the well-known magic word "abracadabra," recorded in the second century A.D. by a Roman physician (Souter 1995: 36). In Britain, the plague arrived during the fourteenth century and disappeared during the eighteenth and nineteenth centuries. Between those dates it was naturally one of the most feared illnesses, wiping out entire communities.

Folk medicine, probably powerless in the face of such epidemics, seems to have concentrated on what it was hoped were pre-

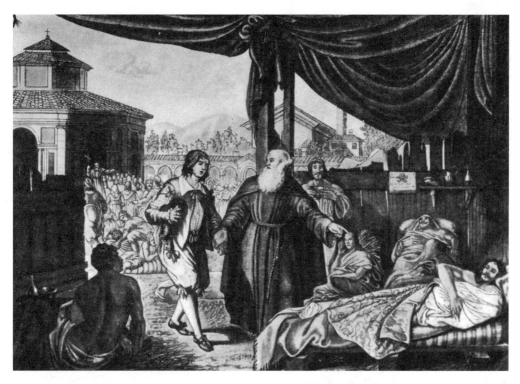

In Britain, the plague arrived during the fourteenth century and disappeared during the eighteenth and nineteenth centuries. Between those dates it was naturally one of the most feared illnesses, wiping out entire communities. (National Library of Medicine)

ventive measures, as had the Romans. In Sussex in the sixteenth century the vicar of Rye recorded that many people in the area used toad poison to protect themselves against the plague; it caused blistering, which, unlike the plague, could be cured (Souter 1995: 124). Vinegar was regarded as a preservative against the plague. It featured both in remedies (Smith and Randall 1987: 42) and as an antiseptic for the coins placed, in return for food supplied to victims, on the "plague stones" (Allen 1995: 124). In Scotland, loaves were hung up on poles to "catch" the plague; when they became discolored they were burned (Simpkins 1912: 134). Wealthier people could afford so-called plague drinks, which often contained expensive imported spices, such as ginger and nutmeg (Souter 1995: 123). Herbal prescriptions against the plague were often complex, and it is impossible to

know how widely they were used by the majority. In Cornwall, butterbur (*Petasites hybridus*) is known as "plaguewort" (Vickery 1995: 284), suggesting that it might have been used in folk medicine. The German name for this plant is *pestilenzwurz*. It was certainly recommended in official medicine for treating "pestilential fevers" (Pechey 1694: 33). Angelica featured in a number of plague remedies and was credited with both preserving people against and curing the plague (Pechey 1694: 5). However, this was probably the garden-grown angelica (*Angelica archangelica*), and it was again a prescription for the relatively wealthy.

Plague reached parts of the Americas with European colonizers, but in most of North America it did not reach the epidemic proportions seen in Europe. It was reintroduced, from Asia, in the middle of the eighteenth century (Porter 1996: 28). Given that plague was not the mass killer in North America that it had been in Europe, it is not surprising to find a relative lack of folk remedies for the plague there. One remedy, a clear example of sympathetic magic is to catch the rat that bit one, cook it, and eat it (Puckett 1981: 332).

*See also* **Sympathetic magic, Toads and frogs, Vinegar.**

**References**

Allen, Andrew. *A Dictionary of Sussex Folk Medicine.* Newbury: Countryside Books, 1995.

Pechey, John. *The Compleat Herbal of Physical Plants.* London: 1694.

Porter, Roy (ed.). *The Cambridge Illustrated History of Medicine.* Cambridge: Cambridge University Press, 1996.

Puckett, Newbell Niles. *Popular Beliefs and Superstitions: A Compendium of American Folklore from the Ohio Collection of Newbell Niles Puckett.* Edited by Wayland D. Hand, Anna Casetta, and Sondra B. Thiederman. 3 vols. Boston: G. K. Hall, 1981.

Simpkins, John Ewart. *Fife. County Folk-Lore Series.* Vol. 7. London: Folk-Lore Society, 1912.

Smith, Janet, and Thea Randall. *Kill or Cure: Medical Remedies of the 16th and 17th Centuries from the Staffordshire Record Office.* Staffordshire: Record Office, 1987.

Souter, Keith. *Cure Craft: Traditional Folk Remedies and Treatment from Antiquity to the Present Day.* Saffron Walden: C. W. Daniel, 1995.

Vickery, Roy. *A Dictionary of Plant Lore.* Oxford: Oxford University Press, 1995.

# Plantain (*Plantago major*)

Still known in country areas in Britain by its Anglo-Saxon name of "waybread," this was one of the nine healing herbs mentioned in the *Lacnunga,* and is still used in folk medicine today. In British folk medicine its main uses are for treating minor cuts and wounds (Vickery 1995: 285), as well as for sores and ulcers (Hatfield 1994: 52), rashes, nettle stings (Tongue 1965: 41), insect bites and stings (Lafont 1984: 68), and varicose veins (Evans 1940: 98). In both Scotland (Goodrich-Freer 1902: 205) and Ireland (Allen and Hatfield, in press), there has been a belief that the upper side of the leaf is for healing whereas the lower side draws out the poison. Plantain has also been used to treat burns and piles (Lafont 1984: 68). In Ireland it has also been used to treat jaundice, headache, chapped skin, and gout (Allen and Hatfield, in press). Its leaves have been carried as an amulet against snake bite (Souter 1995: 186). *Plantago major* follows where humans go and is highly resistant to trampling, which explains its commonness in gateways and beside footpaths. When introduced into North America by the early settlers (deliberately or accidentally) it became known by Native Americans as "white man's footsteps" (Coffey 1993: 212).

It is used in North American folk medicine in much the same way as in Britain—for minor wounds, bites and stings, burns (Meyer 1985: 39, 272, 54). In addition, it has been used to treat swollen feet, neuralgia, and toothache (Meyer 1985: 119, 187, 248). An infusion of plantain leaves has treated diarrhea (UCLA Folklore Archives 12_5361). It has been used for treating the rash caused by poison ivy (Micheletti 1998: 264). The crushed salted leaves have been used to soothe headache (Curtin 1930: 190). The leaves have also been used for treating rheumatism (Puckett 1981: 433), sore throat (Musick 1948: 6), varicose veins (Stout 1936: 186), liver complaints, and epilepsy (Lick and Brendle 1922: 218). They have been rubbed onto the chest for tuberculosis (Puckett 1981: 468) and made into a salve for treating cancer (Puckett 1926: 387–388). They have been smoked for asthma (Relihan 1946: 158). The seeds have been given on bread and butter for treating worms in children (Bomberger 1950: 7).

Mexican Americans use plantain for treating dysentery (Kay 1995: 216). Native Americans chew plantain root for toothache (Willard 1992: 187), a use echoed by that recorded by Meyer, in which the fibrous strings of the plantain leaves are chewed for toothache (Meyer 1985: 248). A number of different species of plantain native to North America have been used medicinally, in addition to *Plantago major*. Native Americans in Mexico use various species of plantain for treating diarrhea, fever, constipation, headache, loss of appetite, as a tonic and diuretic, as well as for sore feet (Kay 1996: 215–216). Other Native American uses include treatment of snake and insect bites (Tantaquidgeon 1972: 74), sores and ulcers (Turner et al. 1983: 115), burns (Raymond 1945: 130), and wounds (Murphey 1990: 43). Both the Chippewa (Densmore 1928: 376) and the Ojibwa (Smith 1932: 341) carried powdered roots as an amulet against snake bite (cf. folk remedy above).

*See also* **Amulet, Asthma, Burns, Cancer, Chapped skin, Constipation, Cuts, Diarrhea, Dysentery, Epilepsy, Fever, Gout, Headache, Insect bites and stings, Jaundice, Piles, Poison ivy, Rheumatism, Snake bite, Sore feet, Sore throat, Tonic, Toothache, Tuberculosis, Worms, Wounds.**

## References

Allen, David E., and Gabrielle Hatfield. *British and Irish Plants in Folk Medicine.* Portland, OR: Timber Press, in press.

Bomberger, C. M. "Almanacs and Herbs." *Pennsylvania Dutchman* 2(2) (May 15, 1950): 1, 7.

Coffey, Timothy. *The History and Folklore of North American Wildflowers.* New York: Facts On File, 1993.

Curtin, L. S. M. "Pioneer Medicine in New Mexico." *Folk-Say* (1930): 186–196.

Densmore, Frances. "Uses of Plants by the Chippewa Indians." *Smithsonian Institution—*

*Bureau of American Ethnology Annual Report* 44 (1928): 273–379.

Evans, John. "Folk-Medicines." *Collections. Montgomeryshire* 46 (1940): 98–99.

Goodrich-Freer, A. *Outer Isles.* London: Constable, 1902.

Hatfield, Gabrielle. *Country Remedies: Traditional East Anglian Plant Remedies in the Twentieth Century.* Woodbridge: Boydell, 1994.

Kay, Margarita Artschwager. *Healing with Plants in the American and Mexican West.* Tucson: University of Arizona Press, 1996.

Lafont, Anne-Marie. *Herbal Folklore.* Bideford: Badger Books, 1984.

Lick, David E., and Thomas R. Brendle. "Plant Names and Plant Lore among the Pennsylvania Germans." *Proceedings and Addresses of the Pennsylvania German Society* 33 (1922).

Meyer, Clarence. *American Folk Medicine.* Glenwood, IL: Meyerbooks, 1985.

Micheletti, Enza (ed.). *North American Folk Healing: An A–Z Guide to Traditional Remedies.* New York and Montreal: Reader's Digest Association, 1998.

Murphey, Edith Van Allen. *Indian Uses of Native Plants.* Glenwood, IL: Meyerbooks, 1990.

Musick, Ruth Ann. "West Virginia Folklore." *Hoosier Folklore* 7 (1948): 1–14.

Puckett, Newbell Niles. *Folk Beliefs of the Southern Negro.* Chapel Hill, NC: Greenwood Press, 1926.

Puckett, Newbell Niles. *Popular Beliefs and Superstitions: A Compendium of American Folklore from the Ohio Collection of Newbell Niles Puckett.* Edited by Wayland D. Hand, Anna Casetta, and Sondra B. Thiederman. 3 vols. Boston: G. K. Hall, 1981.

Raymond, Marcel. "Notes Ethnobotaniques sur les Tête-de-Boules de Manouan." *Contributions de l'Institut Botanique de l'Université de Montréal* 55 (1945): 113–134.

Relihan, Catherine. "Farm Lore: Herbal Remedies." *New York Folklore Quarterly* 2:2 (1946): 156–158.

Smith, Huron H. "Ethnobotany of the Ojibwe Indians." *Bulletin of the Public Museum of the City of Milwaukee* 4 (1932): 327–525.

Souter, Keith. *Cure Craft: Traditional Folk Rem-*

*edies and Treatment from Antiquity to the Present Day.* Saffron Walden: C. W. Daniel, 1995.

Stout, Earl J. "Folklore from Iowa." *Memoirs of the American Folklore Society* 29 (1936).

Tantaquidgeon, Gladys. "Folk Medicine of the Delaware and Related Algonkian Indians." *Pennsylvania Historical Commission Anthropological Papers,* no. 3 (1972).

Tongue, Ruth L. *Somerset Folklore.* Edited Katharine Briggs. County Folklore 8. London: Folklore Society, 1965.

Turner, Nancy J., John Thomas, Barry F. Carlson, and Robert T. Ogilvie. *Ethnobotany of the Nitinaht Indians of Vancouver Island.* Victoria: British Columbia Provincial Museum, 1983.

Vickery, Roy. *A Dictionary of Plant Lore.* Oxford: Oxford University Press, 1995.

Willard, Terry. *Edible and Medicinal Plants of the Rocky Mountains and Neighbouring Territories.* Calgary, ALTA: Wild Rose College of Natural Healing, 1992.

# Poison ivy, Poison oak

These names are used interchangeably for *Rhus toxicodendron* and *Rhus radicans.* Both species are native to North America; neither occur in Britain. They both cause contact dermatitis, for which a number of folk medical cures have been developed. These include bathing in very hot water and applying a paste of powdered chalk or a lotion composed of glycerine and carbolic acid, or of quicklime or alum. Other washes include a strong solution of alum, a mixture of calomel and water, or a solution of gum shellac in sulphuric ether (Meyer 1985: 198–199). Copperas water has been used to soothe the rash (Parler 1962: 826), as has chlorinated water (UCLA Folklore Archives 5_6460) or even bleach (UCLA Folklore Archives 19_6460). Liquid shoe polish, or the water in which an old shoe has been boiled, has been applied (Parler 1962: 826, 828). Pennies boiled in vinegar have been rubbed on (Musick 1964: 38). Bathing

with bicarbonate of soda is also said to bring relief, as will application of wood ashes. Kerosene rubbed in or olive oil applied are alternatives. Mud from the river bottom has been used (Parler 1962: 826), or a mixture of red clay and water (UCLA Folklore Archives 6_6460).

Animal products too have found a use. Heavily salted milk or sour milk beaten until thick (UCLA Folklore Archives 7_6460) have been suggested; alternatives are calf slobber (Parler 1962: 830) and the water used to scald a chicken (Parler 1962: 827). Crayfish meat has been applied (Koch 1980: 109).

Numerous plant products have been employed. These include cornstarch, rubbed on (UCLA Folklore Archives 8_5453), and the inside of a banana skin (Anon. 1968: 116). The smoke from cedar boughs has been recommended (Parler 1962: 826). Wild nasturtiums rubbed on (UCLA Folklore Archives 7_6430), a tea from plantain leaves (Puckett 1981: 426), fig leaf juice *(Ficus carica)* (Parler 1962: 833), hollyhock leaves *(Alcea rosea)* (Clark 1970: 27), sycamore bark *(Platanus* sp.) (Parler 1962: 834), and Indian tobacco *(? Lobelia inflata)* boiled in milk (Koch 1980: 109) have all been tried. Other applications include fresh tomatoes (Parler 1962: 829), string bean leaves (UCLA Folklore Archives 20_7595), and squashed melon flowers (Parler 1962: 630), as well as an infusion of sweet fern *(Comptonia peregrina)* (Browne 1958: 86). Poplar *(Populus* sp.) bark has been made into a lotion (Bruton 1948: no. 29), as have eucalyptus leaves *(Eucalyptus* sp.). An infusion of wormwood *(Artemisia* sp.) (UCLA Folklore Archives 23_5451) or of Manzanita leaves *(Arctoctaphylos* sp.) (UCLA Folklore Archives 23_6460) has been tried. Other plant remedies include oil of goldenrod *(Solidago odora),* mouse-ear herb *(Gnaphalium uliginosum)* in milk, green leaves of nightshade *(Solanum nigrum)* mashed in milk, and green tansy *(Tanace-*

tum vulgare) leaves crushed in buttermilk. Fresh leaves of jewel weed (Impatiens sp.) or of fireweed (Erechtites hieracifolia) or catnip have all been used; in addition, the root of wild Indian turnip, also known as Jack-in-the-Pulpit (Arisaema triphyllum), has been scraped and applied (Meyer 1985: 198–200).

There has been a belief that the plant itself could help cure the itch of poison ivy. Drinking water from a stream flowing past the plant has been suggested, as has eating honey made in the locality where the plant grows (Herrera 1972: 43). In a practice reminiscent of the English cure for nettle sting using nettle juice, it has been suggested that rubbing the affected area deliberately with more of the plant can bring about relief, or that eating a small piece of the root of the plant can do so (Brown 1961, 6: 251).

Carrying a wild cherry or elderberry in the pocket was thought to confer protection against poison ivy (Parler 1962: 825). Other amulets worn to protect against its effects include a string worn around the thumb and big toe (UCLA Folklore Archives 18_6461) and a fishing sinker worn around the neck (Black 1935: 33). Finally, if all else fails, the sufferer can simply curse the plant! (UCLA Folklore Archives 7_5453).

Among Native American remedies for poison ivy are the root of Jack-in-the-Pulpit (Arisaema triphyllum), eaten (MacDonald 1959: 223); the bark of red oak (Quercus sp.) boiled to make a lotion; and the root of graybeard (Cladastris lutea) (Speck 1944: 30). A powder of the stems and leaves of the milk vetch Astragalus adsurgens var. robustior has been used by the Cheyenne (Grinnell 1905: 40). Another species of Solanum, S. carolinense, is used by the Cherokee for treating poison ivy (Hamel and Chiltoskey 1975: 46). Impatiens capensis is used by them also (Hamel and Chiltoskey 1975: 41) and by the Potawatomi (Smith

1933: 42), while another species, Impatiens pallida, is used by the Cherokee (Hamel and Chiltoskey 1975: 41) and by the Iroquois (Herrick 1977: 379).

See also **Catnip, Cherry, Elder, Plantain, Soda, Stinging nettle.**

## References
Anon. Home Remedies. Foxfire 2: 3–4 (1968).

Black, Pauline Monette. Nebraska Folk Cures. University of Nebraska Studies in Language Literature and Criticism 15. Lincoln, NE: University of Nebraska Press, 1935.

Brown, Frank C. Collection of North Carolina Folklore. 7 vols. Durham, NC: Duke University Press, 1952–1964.

Browne, Ray B. Popular Beliefs and Practices from Alabama. Folklore Studies 9. Berkeley and Los Angeles: University of California Publications, 1958.

Bruton, Hoyle S. "Medicine." North Carolina Folklore 1 (1948): 23–26.

Clark, Joseph D. "North Carolina Popular Beliefs and Superstitions." North Carolina Folklore 18 (1970): 1–66.

Grinnell, George Bird. "Some Cheyenne Plant Medicines." American Anthropologist 7 (1905): 37–43.

Hamel, Paul B., and Mary U. Chiltoskey. Cherokee Plants and Their Uses: A 400 Year History. Sylva, NC: Herald, 1975.

Herrera, Mary Armstrong. "The Miseries and Folk Medicine." North Carolina Folklore 20 (1972): 42–46.

Herrick, James William. Iroquois Medical Botany. Ph.D. thesis, State University of New York, Albany, 1977.

Koch, William E. Folklore from Kansas: Beliefs and Customs. Lawrence, KS: Regent Press, 1980.

MacDonald, Elizabeth. "Indian Medicine in New Brunswick." Canadian Medical Association Journal 80(3) (1959): 220–224.

Meyer, Clarence. American Folk Medicine. Glenwood, IL: Meyerbooks, 1985.

Musick, Ruth Ann (ed.). "Superstitions." West Virginia Folklore 14 (1964): 38–52.

Parler, Mary Celestia, and University Student Contributors. Folk Beliefs from Arkansas. 15 vols. Fayetteville: University of Arkansas, 1962.

Puckett, Newbell Niles. *Popular Beliefs and Superstitions: A Compendium of American Folklore from the Ohio Collection of Newbell Niles Puckett.* Edited by Wayland D. Hand, Anna Casetta, and Sondra B. Thiederman. 3 vols. Boston: G. K. Hall, 1981.

Smith, Huron H. "Ethnobotany of the Forest Potawatomi Indians." *Bulletin of the Public Museum of the City of Milwaukee* 7 (1933): 1–230.

Speck, Frank G. "Catawba Herbals and Curative Practices." *Journal of American Folklore* 57 (1944): 37–50.

# Poke (*Phytolacca americana*)

This shrub, native to eastern North America and California, has in folk medicine a particular reputation for treating rheumatism. It is also eaten as a vegetable, the young greens being parboiled and the water discarded because of the toxicity of the raw plant. There are a large number of other subsidiary uses for the plant in folk medicine. It has a reputation for treating skin cancer (Crellin and Philpott 1990: 350) as well as various other skin complaints, including "itch." In Meyer's collection of American folk medicine there are numerous remedies that include poke. The fresh juice of pokeberries was used for treating burns, chilblains, eczema, and erysipelas (Meyer 1985: 54, 62, 105, 108). The roasted root was used for treating felons (infected finger sores); the fresh root applied to soles of the feet was a suggested cure for a headache; and the powdered root mixed with lard provided an ointment for treating itch (Meyer 1985: 122, 139, 149). The young shoots, parboiled, were claimed to prevent typhoid fever (Meyer 1985: 130). For treating rheumatism, both the berries, steeped in brandy, and the root have been used as a decoction (Meyer 1985: 213). For treating ulcers, freshly sliced root was used; for tonsillitis the fresh root was roasted, mashed, and applied warm (Meyer 1985: 230, 253). In Alabama, poke root in whisky was used to treat thrush in children (Browne 1958: 28). In Carolina, the juice of pokeberry has been used to treat tumors (Clark 1970: 22).

In Native American practice, at least six different tribes used poke as an antirheumatic (Moerman 1998: 397–398). In addition, all the uses listed above appear in Native American records, as do other uses of the plant, such as for "building blood" among the Cherokee (Hamel and Chiltoskey 1975: 50); for chest colds, and for sprains and bruises among the Iroquois (Herrick 1977: 316, 317); for severe pain among the Mahuna (Romero 1954: 65); and for dysentery among the Rappahannock (Speck, Hassrick, and Carpenter 1942: 29).

The plant is not native to Britain, and though used by medical herbalists (Chevallier 1996: 245) it has no role in British folk medicine.

*See also* **Bruises, Burns, Cancer, Chilblains, Eczema, Erysipelas, Felons, Headache, Rheumatism, Sprains.**

**References**

Browne, Ray B. *Popular Beliefs and Practices from Alabama.* Folklore Studies 9. Berkeley and Los Angeles: University of California Publications, 1958.

Chevallier, Andrew. *The Encyclopedia of Medicinal Plants.* London: Dorling Kindersley, 1996.

Clark, Joseph D. "North Carolina Popular Beliefs and Superstitions." *North Carolina Folklore* 18 (1970): 1–66.

Crellin, John K., and Jane Philpott. *A Reference Guide to Medicinal Plants.* Durham, NC: Duke University Press, 1990.

Hamel, Paul B., and Mary U. Chiltoskey. *Cherokee Plants and Their Uses: A 400 Year History.* Sylva, NC: Herald, 1975.

Herrick, James William. *Iroquois Medical Botany.* Ph.D. thesis, State University of New York, Albany, 1977.

Meyer, Clarence. *American Folk Medicine.* Glenwood, IL: Meyerbooks, 1985.

Moerman, Daniel E. *Native American Ethnobotany.* Portland, OR: Timber Press, 1998.

Romero, John Bruno. *The Botanical Lore of the California Indians.* New York: Vantage Press, 1954.

Speck, Frank G., R. B. Hassrick, and E. S. Carpenter. "Rappahannock Herbals, Folk-Lore and Science of Cures." *Proceedings of the Delaware County Institute of Science* 10 (1942): 7–55.

# Poppy (*Papaver spp.*)

Both the native wild poppy (*Papaver rhoeas)* and the imported opium poppy *(Papaver somniferum)* have been widely used in folk medicine for the relief of pain and as a sedative. There are records of the native red poppy being used to treat toothache (Allen 1995: 43), earache (Tongue 1965: 39), neuralgia (Evans 1940), and swollen glands (Dacombe 1935). The wild poppy has also been used to treat headaches, especially hangover headaches, for which the seeds were chewed. Infused in a baby's milk, poppy seeds were used to calm fretful babies; they were especially used by the Land Girls (women seconded to work on the land to replace the men who were fighting) during World War II, when they had to work long hours in the fields (Hatfield 1994: 40). Sometimes a dummy was dipped in poppy seeds and given to a baby who was teething. In the Highlands of Scotland, the juice from wild poppies was put into children's food to make them sleep, and the flowers were infused to make a liquid to help with teething (Beith 1995: 234). The wild poppy was used in official medicine in Britain right up to the mid-twentieth century (it is included in the *British Pharmacopoeia Codex* for 1949), and it continues to be used by herbalists as a gentle sedative. Though it contains alkaloids known to affect the central nervous system, it does not appear to be addictive. In marked contrast, the opium poppy—widely grown, for example, in the fens during the eighteenth and nineteenth centuries—became an everyday panacea. Its extract was so cheap that many families bought a large Winchester container of "laudanum" every week for sixpence. Doubtless it brought relief from the rheumatic pains and fevers common in the fens, but it also brought addiction. It has been claimed that the stunted stature of the fen population was attributable to this practice. In the 1920s, a general practitioner in Lincolnshire remarked that a fenman would not thank a person for a pint of beer unless it was spiked with laudanum, nor for a pipe unless it contained opium as well as tobacco (letter to Dr. Mark Taylor, Taylor MSS). Although the opium poppy is a native of much warmer Asian climates, it has been known in Britain at least since the Bronze Age. It does not appear to have been grown on a commercial scale but was grown in many cottage gardens. Failing this, the liquid extract, known as laudanum, was cheap and easily accessible.

The related yellow horned poppy *(Glaucium flavum),* a less common plant of coastal areas of Britain, has had a different use. It is known as "squatmore" in the southwest of England (Grigson 1955: 50) and was used to treat bruises. "Squat" is a local dialect word for bruise probably derived from the Anglo-Saxon. In the Isles of Scilly it was also used to treat pain in the lungs or intestines, and the root was scraped upward to form an emetic, downward to form a purge (Notes and Queries, 10 [1854], 181). The yellow poppies burned to drive away evil spirits in the Highlands of Scotland (Beith 1995: 234) presumably belong to this species.

The red poppy *(Papaver rhoeas)* is not native to North America, although it has become widely naturalized there. In general North American folk medicine there are a

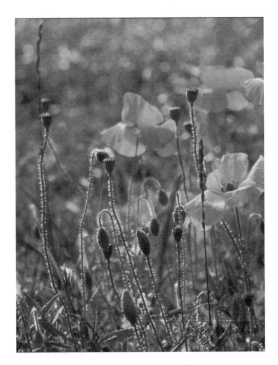

Both wild and cultivated poppies have been widely used for pain relief and for their sedative properties. (Sarah Boait)

few records of the use of poppies as a sedative; usually it is unclear what type of poppy was used. In California, poppy flowers under the pillow were recommended for insomnia (Clark 1970: 24). In Mexico, poppy tea was recommended as a general sedative (UCLA Folklore Archives 2_6372). As in Britain, poppies have been useful in soothing crying babies (UCLA Folklore Archives 10_6146). Even holding the flower under a baby's nose was sufficient to induce sleep (Parler 1962, 3: 217). A poultice of poppy seed was used for pain relief (Creighton 1968: 225).

It is mainly other members of the poppy family, such as the prickly poppy (*Argemone mexicana*), that have been used in Native American folk medicine. This species has been used to treat cataract, while the California poppy (*Escholtzia californica*) has been used for toothache, headache, sores, and as an emetic (Coffey 1993: 27, 29).

The flowers of California poppy laid under the bed have been used to help children sleep (Bocek 1984: 9), an interesting parallel with the use of red poppy in England. The seed pods of *Escholtzia* have been used to dry up a nursing mother's milk (Goodrich and Lawson 1980: 94). The opium poppy has been used for pain and as a sedative by the Cherokee (Hamel and Chiltoskey 1975: 51).

*See also* **Earache, Headache, Sleeplessness, Teething, Toothache.**

### References

Allen, Andrew. *A Dictionary of Sussex Folk Medicine.* Newbury: Countryside Books, 1995.

Beith, Mary. *Healing Threads: Traditional Medicine of the Highlands and Islands.* Edinburgh: Polygon, 1995.

Bocek, Barbara R. "Ethnobotany of Costanoan Indians, California: Based on Collections by John P. Harrington." *Economic Botany* 38(2) (1984): 240–255.

Clark, Joseph D. "North Carolina Popular Beliefs and Superstitions." *North Carolina Folklore* 18 (1970): 1–66.

Coffey, Timothy. *The History and Folklore of North American Wildflowers.* New York: Facts On File, 1993.

Creighton, Helen. *Bluenose Magic, Popular Beliefs and Superstitions in Nova Scotia.* Toronto: Ryerson Press, 1968.

Dacombe, Marianne R. (ed.). *Dorset Up Along and Down Along.* Dorchester: Dorset Federation of Women's Institutes, 1935.

Evans, John. "Folk-Medicines." *Collections. Montgomeryshire* 46 (1940): 98–99.

Goodrich, Jennie, and Claudia Lawson. *Kashaya Pomo Plants.* Los Angeles: American Indian Studies Center, University of California, Los Angeles, 1980.

Grigson, Geoffrey. *The Englishman's Flora.* London: Phoenix House, 1955.

Hamel, Paul B., and Mary U. Chiltoskey. *Cherokee Plants and Their Uses: A 400 Year History.* Sylva, NC: Herald, 1975.

Hatfield, Gabrielle. *Country Remedies: Traditional East Anglian Plant Remedies in the Twentieth Century.* Woodbridge: Boydell, 1994.

*Notes and Queries,* 10:181. London, 1854.

Parler, Mary Celestia, and University Student Contributors. *Folk Beliefs from Arkansas.* 15 vols. Fayetteville: University of Arkansas, 1962.

Taylor MSS. Manuscript notes of Mark R. Taylor in the Norfolk Record Office, Norwich. MS4322.

Tongue, Ruth L. *Somerset Folklore.* Edited by K. M. Briggs. London: Folklore Society, 1965.

# Potato (*Solanum tuberosum*)

Introduced from South America to Britain, probably via Spain, in the latter half of the sixteenth century (Harris et al. 1969: 176), the potato has become one of the world's most important food sources. A large number of ancillary uses for it have been developed, including folk medical ones. In Scotland and in Ireland it has been used to treat rheumatism, either by poulticing the afflicted area or by immersing sore joints in water in which potatoes have been cooked (Grieve 1931: 655). Raw potato has also been used to treat severe back pain. Presumably derived from these empirical uses, the practice of carrying a potato as an amulet to ward off rheumatism is widespread in Britain (Grieve 1931: 655; Black 1883: 182; Vickery 1994: 291–292). A similar use, but for warding off cramp, has been reported from Suffolk (Vickery 1995: 292).

Cooked potatoes have been used, hot, as a chest poultice to relieve asthma (Hatfield MS). Hot potatoes have also been applied to corns (Black 1883: 193). Raw, they have been used to treat minor burns (Black 1883: 193; Allen 1995: 46). For frostbite, cooked potato mixed with sweet oil has been used (Grieve 1931: 655). In Wales the potato has been used within living memory to treat boils, sore throat, and chilblains as well as rheumatism (Jones 1980: 61). In Ireland, as in Wales, sore throat was treated with a poultice of boiled potatoes in a sock; raw potato was an Irish treatment for ulcers (Vickery 1995: 292). The belief is widespread that the water in which potatoes have been cooked can cause warts on the hands, and yet potatoes are, paradoxically, used in the *treatment* of warts (Allen 1995: 179; Tongue 1965: 43).

In North American folk medicine, all the uses for potato described above have been recorded in folk medicine, and many more besides. The wide array of conditions treated is unusual. Rheumatism and warts are the two ailments most commonly treated using potatoes, and as in Britain, the potato was sometimes applied or ingested, sometimes used as an amulet. A potato in the pocket was used to treat chills (Hyatt 1965: 213), to cure lumbago (Cannon 1984: 93), and to prevent rheumatism (Mississippi State Guide 1938: 14), gall stones (UCLA Folklore Archives 1_6305), and nosebleed (UCLA Folklore Archives 5_5441), as well as, more generally, to protect against illness (UCLA Folklore Archives 1_6353). A belief has been reported that keeping a potato under the bed aids conception (UCLA Folklore Archives 6_6689), and is a good remedy for night sweats (Hyatt 1965: 271). Three potatoes in the pocket are suggested as a cure for piles (Fogel 1915: 305); alternatively, the potatoes are eaten with castor oil, on three consecutive nights (Hyatt 1965: 250). Worn around the neck, a potato is suggested as a cure for neuritis (UCLA Folklore Archives 3_5436).

Other conditions treated using potatoes include mumps (UCLA Folklore Archives 18_6410), blood poisoning (Creighton 1968: 199), earache (Welsch 1966: 331), headache (UCLA Folklore Archives 1_5396), tonsillitis (Puckett 1981: 466), appendicitis (treated, unusually, with potato leaves rather than the tuber) (Saxon 1945: 170), and even ruptured appendix (Randolph 1947: 118). A potato poultice on the feet was used as a cure for colds (UCLA Folklore Archives 2_6792) and, placed over the nose, for sinusitis (Clark 1970: 29). Raw potatoes were applied to the stomach for cramps (Cannon 1984: 103), and applied as well to cuts, sores, and wounds (Anderson 1970: 25).

As in Ireland, cooked potatoes in a sock were used to poultice a sore throat (UCLA Folklore Archives 3_5479). Potatoes were either eaten (Hyatt 1965: 237) to cure hiccups or applied as a poultice to the abdomen (Wilson 1968: 323). Bruises were treated using potatoes (Puckett 1981: 370; Cannon 1984: 108), and even fractures (UCLA Folklore Archives 5_5487). Tired muscles were relieved by soaking in water in which peeled potatoes had been standing (Neal 1955: 277). For indigestion or travel sickness potatoes were either eaten (Lathrop 1961: 17) or worn (Stair 1966: 45). Potato scrapings were laid on an aching tooth (UCLA Folklore Archives 9_5514) and used to treat conjunctivitis (Puckett 1981: 370), snow blindness (UCLA Folklore Archives 14_6476), and even cataract (Puckett 1981: 338). Potato peelings have been eaten for diarrhea (UCLA Folklore Archives 18_6474). A poultice of raw potato (Musick 1964: 48), or a drink of water in which peeled potatoes have been standing (Clark 1970: 21), has been used to reduce fever. In addition, potatoes have been used to treat a very wide range of skin conditions, including heat rash (Street 1959: 78), frostbite (Browne 1958: 67), chilblains (UCLA Folklore Archives 10_5312), eczema (Puckett 1981: 367), boils (UCLA Folklore Archives 1_5314), stys (Puckett 1981: 456), ringworm (Anderson 1970: 62), and moles and skin blemishes in general (UCLA Folklore Archives 1_5615). There are very numerous records for the treatment of warts using potatoes (see, for example, McAtee 1958: 152). The juice of potatoes has been applied to insect bites (Wilson Sr. 1968: 72) and to poison ivy rash (UCLA Folklore Archives 1_7614). The water in which potatoes have been boiled is recommended for falling hair (Doering 1945: 153) and for preventing rickets (Puckett 1981: 114). Eating potatoes is recommended for a hangover (Paulsen 1961: 154) and for treating scurvy (Puckett 1981: 438), while for gallstones, the water in which potatoes have been boiled should be drunk (Allison 1950: 313). A potato poultice has been used to treat caked breasts (Mason 1957: 30), chest congestion (Baker 1948: 191), and pneumonia (Cannon 1984: 119). A tea made from boiling potato peelings has been drunk for tuberculosis (Puckett 1981: 468). Potatoes have even been used to treat tumors, either directly as a poultice (Puckett 1981: 468; UCLA Folklore Archives 12_6189) or symbolically by cutting the potato into three pieces and throwing it away (Creighton 1968: 235).

This very wide array of uses is not reflected in Native American usage, where there are records only of its use in treating warts (Speck, Hassrick, and Carpenter 1942: 27), eye inflammation (Herrick 1977: 431), and loneliness due to bereavement (Hamel and Chiltoskey 1975: 51). This suggests that most North American folk medical uses have been reimported, like the potato, from European and other sources.

See also **Amulet, Asthma, Backache, Boils, Breast problems, Bruises, Burns, Cancer, Chilblains, Colds, Corns, Cuts, Diarrhea, Earache, Eczema, Eye problems, Fevers, Fractures, Frostbite, Hiccups, Indigestion, Insect bites and stings, Nausea, Piles, Poison ivy, Poultice, Rheumatism, Rickets, Ringworm, Scurvy, Sore throat, Tuberculosis, Warts, Wounds.**

### References

Allen, Andrew. *A Dictionary of Sussex Folk Medicine.* Newbury: Countryside Books, 1995.

Allison, Lelah. "Folk Beliefs Collected in Southeastern Illinois." *Journal of American Folklore* 63 (1950): 309–324.

Anderson, John. *Texas Folk Medicine.* Austin, TX: Encino Press, 1970.

Baker, Pearl, and Ruth Wilcox. "Folk Remedies in Early Green River." *Utah Humanities Review* 2 (1948): 191–192.

Black, William George. *Folk-Medicine: A Chapter in the History of Culture.* London: Folklore Society, 1883.

Browne, Ray B. *Popular Beliefs and Practices from Alabama.* Folklore Studies 9. Berkley and Los Angeles: University of California Publications, 1958.

Cannon, Anthon S. *Popular Beliefs and Superstitions from Utah.* Edited by Wayland D. Hand and Jeannine E. Talley. Salt Lake City: University of Utah Press, 1984.

Clark, Joseph D. "North Carolina Popular Beliefs and Superstitions." *North Carolina Folklore* 18 (1970): 1–66.

Creighton, Helen. *Bluenose Magic, Popular Beliefs and Superstitions in Nova Scotia.* Toronto: Ryerson Press, 1968.

Doering, J. Frederick. "More Customs from Western Ontario." *Journal of American Folklore* 58 (1945): 150–155.

Fogel, Edwin Miller. "Beliefs and Superstitions of the Pennsylvania Germans." *Americana Germanica* 18 (1915).

Grieve, Mrs. M. *A Modern Herbal.* Edited by Mrs. C. F. Leyel. London: Jonathan Cape, 1931.

Hamel, Paul B., and Mary U. Chiltoskey. *Cherokee Plants and Their Uses: A 400 Year History.* Sylva, NC: Herald, 1975.

Harris, S. G., G. B. Masefield, and Michael Wallis. *The Oxford Book of Food Plants.* Oxford: Oxford University Press, 1969.

Herrick, James. *William Iroquois Medical Botany.* Ph.D. thesis, State University of New York, Albany, 1977.

Hyatt, Harry Middleton. *Folklore from Adams County Illinois.* 2nd rev. ed. New York: Memoirs of the Alma Egan Hyatt Foundation, 1965.

Jones, Anne E. "Folk Medicine in Living Memory in Wales." *Folk Life* 18 (1980): 58–68.

Lathrop, Amy. "Pioneer Remedies from Western Kansas." *Western Folklore* 20 (1961): 1–22.

Mason, James. "Home Remedies in West Virginia." *West Virginia Folklore* 7 (1957): 27–32.

McAtee, W. L. "Medical Lore in Grant Country, Indiana, in the Nineties." *Midwest Folklore* 8 (1958): 151–153.

*Mississippi State Guide.* New York: Federal Writers Project, 1938.

Musick, Ruth Ann (ed.). "Superstitions." *West Virginia Folklore* 14 (1964): 38–52.

Neal, Janice C. "Grandad: Pioneer Medicine Man." *New York Folklore Quarterly* 11 (1955): 277–291.

Paulsen, Frank M. "A Hair of the Dog and Some Other Hangover Cures from Popular Tradition." *Journal of American Folklore* 74 (1961): 152–168.

Puckett, Newbell Niles. *Popular Beliefs and Superstitions: A Compendium of American Folklore from the Ohio Collection of Newbell Niles Puckett.* Edited by Wayland D. Hand, Anna Casetta, and Sondra B. Thiederman. 3 vols. Boston: G. K. Hall, 1981.

Randolph, Vance. *Ozark Superstitions.* New York: Columbia University Press, 1947.

Saxon, Lyle. *Gumbo Ya-Ya.* Boston: Houghton Mifflin, 1945.

Speck, Frank G., R. B. Hassrick, and E. S. Carpenter. "Rapphannock Herbals, Folk-Lore and the Science of Cures." *Proceedings of the Delaware County Institute of Science* 10 (1942): 7–55.

Speck, Frank G., R. B. Hassrick, and E. S. Carpenter. "Rappahanock Herbals, Folk-Lore and Science of cures." *Proceedings of the Delaware County Institute of Science* 10 (1942): 27.

Stair, Madalyn. "Superstitions in Hawkins County." In *A Collection of Folklore by Undergraduate Students of East Tennessee State University,* edited by Thomas G. Burton and Ambrose N. Manning. Institute of Regional Studies Monograph 3. Johnson City: East Tennessee State University, 1966.

Street, Anne C. "Medicine populaire des Iles Saint-Pierre et Miquelon." *Arts et Traditions Populaires* 7 (January–June 1959): 75–85.

Tongue, Ruth L. *Somerset Folklore.* Edited Katharine Briggs. County Folklore 8. London: Folklore Society, 1965.

Vickery, Roy. *A Dictionary of Plant Lore.* Oxford: Oxford University Press, 1995.

Welsch, Roger L. *A Treasury of Nebraska Pioneer Folklore.* Lincoln: University of Nebraska Press, 1966.

Wilson, Gordon, Sr. *Folklore of the Mammoth Cave Region.* Kentucky Folklore Series No. 4, 1968.

Wilson, Gordon. "Local Plants in Folk Remedies in the Mammoth Cave Region." *Southern Folklore Quarterly* 32 (1968): 320–327.

# Poultice

Defined as a mass of healing material externally applied, the poultice is a common method of treatment in folk medicine. Today it is rarely used in orthodox medicine, though it is sometimes still employed in herbalism. In addition to its soothing and healing properties, a poultice was thought to "draw" out any infection or badness from a sore or injury. In Britain, bread poultices were a familiar method of treatment well into the twentieth century. They were applied to boils, cut and grazed knees, and many other minor injuries. Less pleasantly, poultices were often made from cow dung; these were used for drawing out splinters (Hatfield 1994: 11) and for easing swollen knees (Prince 1991: 111–112), as well as for inflamed breasts and as a treatment for a swollen throat (Beith 1995: 172–173). Poultices were often applied warm.

A large number of healing herbs were applied in folk medicine as poultices. Sometimes the fresh herb was lightly crushed and wrapped in muslin; alternatively, dried herbs or herbal extracts were added to a basic poultice—made, for example, of flour or flaxseed. Mallow and houseleek were frequently used as poultices. Vegetables too were used as poultices, especially the potato. Potato poultices have been applied particularly to respiratory ailments, such as pneumonia, asthma, and croup. Carrot poultices were used to treat external cancers. Onion poultices were used to treat chest colds and earache. Cabbage leaves were used, heated and crushed, to heal abscesses.

Colonists settling in North America would have brought with them the tradition of using poultices, and the picture in North American folk medicine is similar to that in Britain. Bread poultices were used as in Britain (Koch 1980: 72). Vegetable poultices were much used, and red beet seems to have been particularly used (Brown 1952–1964, 6: 25). Cabbage leaves have been used to poultice swellings and abscesses (Robertson 1960: 30). In addition, many plants gathered from the wild have been used, lightly crushed, as poultices. As in Britain, mallow (*Malva* spp.) has been used in this way to poultice swellings and treat insect stings (Robertson 1960: 29). Slippery elm was a much-used basis for a poultice (Meyer 1985: 204).

Native Americans also used poultices, though these were sometimes composed of different ingredients; for instance, burns were treated with a poultice of prickly pear, and swellings and strains with a poultice of alder bark (Crellin and Philpott 1989: 356, 42). Nine-bark (*Physocarpus opulifolius*) roots mixed with corn meal formed another much-used poultice of Native American origin, adopted into general North American folk medicine (Meyer 1985: 204).

*See also* **Alder, Cabbage, Cancer, Concepts of disease, Elm, Flax, Houseleek, Insect bites and stings, Mallow, Onion, Potato.**

## References
Beith, Mary. *Healing Threads: Traditional Medicines of the Highlands and Islands.* Edinburgh: Polygon, 1995.

Brown, Frank C. *Collection of North Carolina Folklore.* 7 vols. Durham, NC: Duke University Press, 1952–1964.

Crellin, John K., and Jane Philpott. *A Reference Guide to Medicinal Plants.* Durham, NC: Duke University Press, 1989.

Hatfield, Gabrielle. *Country Remedies: Traditional East Anglian Plant Remedies in the Twentieth Century.* Woodbridge: Boydell, 1994.

Koch, William E. *Folklore from Kansas: Beliefs*

*and Customs.* Lawrence, KS: Regent Press, 1980.

Meyer, Clarence. *American Folk Medicine.* Glenwood, IL: Meyerbooks, 1985.

Prince, Dennis. *Grandmother's Cures: An A–Z of Herbal Remedies.* London: Fontana, 1991.

Robertson, Marion. *Old Settlers' Remedies.* Barrington, NS: Cape Sable Historical Society, 1960.

# Pregnancy

Relatively little appears in the literature about folk medical aids during pregnancy and childbirth, but this is more likely to be due to a reticence surrounding the subject and under-recording rather than a lack of remedies. In Britain right up to the advent of the National Health Service, the village midwife frequently doubled as health advisor to pregnant women. Remedies were also handed down from one generation to the next, usually through the women, but little was written down. In the days of persecution of witches, there was another strong reason to keep such knowledge quiet and so not be answerable to charges of witchcraft. We do know that raspberry tea was one of the staples of folk medicine in pregnancy. It was recommended (and still is) during the last three months of pregnancy, to strengthen the uterine muscles and ensure a speedy delivery. This use is widespread throughout Britain, though rarely recorded from Ireland (Allen and Hatfield, in press). In East Anglia hawthorn leaves were used similarly (Newman and Wilson 1951). During pregnancy there were various restrictions to be observed. In Scotland, for example, a pregnant woman was advised not to cross her legs or her arms (Buchan, ed. 1994: 72). Abnormalities in a baby were often ascribed to experiences of the mother during pregnancy. Birthmarks too were ascribed to an incident during pregnancy, and it was thought they could be removed by licking (Radford and Radford 1974: 54).

Colonial women must have had an even harder time than their European counterparts when it came to surviving pregnancy and childbirth. Divorced from their extended families and even from the native plant remedies they might have used, they must have had to depend on newly acquired knowledge of the local flora. Meyer cites examples of plants used during pregnancy as learned from the Native Americans. They include black snakeroot (*Cimicifuga racemosa*), used to relieve sickness and heartburn during pregnancy, and a decoction of the roots of Indian cup-plant *(Silphium perfoliatum)*, also used to allay pregnancy sickness (Meyer 1985: 207–208). Peach was used to treat pregnancy sickness. Raspberry tea was used, as in Britain, and was recommended by the herbalist Samuel Thomson (Meyer 1985: 207). In North American folk belief, as in British, numerous superstitions surround pregnancy. Birthmarks are attributed to a shock during pregnancy or an unfulfilled craving (Brown 1952–1964, 6: 17–22).

Pregnancy among Native Americans, as among the Scots, was accompanied by certain restrictions. Among the Seminole, the pregnant woman was not allowed to step over anything or to run. The downy milk-pea (*Galactea volubile*) was used as medicine to protect the unborn baby and to ease labor (Snow and Stans 2001: 83). Raspberry was used by a number of Native American tribes to ease childbirth (Moerman 1998: 488).

*See also* **Childbirth; Hawthorn; Midwife; Peach; Thomson, Samuel; Witches.**

### References
Allen, David E., and Gabrielle Hatfield. *British and Irish Plants in Folk Medicine.* Portland, OR: Timber Press, in press.

Brown, Frank C. *Collection of North Carolina*

*Folklore.* 7 vols. Durham, NC: Duke University Press, 1952–1964.

Buchan, David, ed. *Folk Tradition and Folk Medicine in Scotland: The Writings of David Rorie.* Edinburgh: Canongate Academic, 1994.

Meyer, Clarence. *American Folk Medicine.* Glenwood, IL: Meyerbooks, 1985.

Moerman, Daniel E. *Native American Ethnobotany.* Portland, OR: Timber Press, 1998.

Newman, L. F., and E. M. Wilson. "Folk-Lore Survivals in the Southern 'Lake Counties' and in Essex: A Comparison and Contrast. Part I." *Folk-Lore* 62 (1951): 252–266.

Radford, E., and M. A. Radford. *Encyclopaedia of Superstitions.* Edited and revised by Christina Hole. London: Book Club Associates 1974.

Snow, Alice Micco, and Susan Enns Stans. *Healing Plants: Medicine of the Florida Seminole Indians.* Gainesville: University Press of Florida, 2001.

# Prickly ash (*Zanthoxylum spp.*)

This genus does not occur in Britain and has not been used in folk medicine there. In North American folk medicine, prickly ash has been used as a tonic and to treat rheumatism, fevers, and toothache. During the nineteenth century it was marketed by the Shakers, as an herb valuable for all these ailments and for colic and diarrhea as well (Crellin and Philpott 1990: 355). Meyer records its use as a tonic and as an infusion for washing carbuncles. Cloths soaked in a decoction of prickly ash bark and cayenne were applied for renal colic. For stomachache both the berries and the bark have been used. For toothache, the bark was chewed, or poulticed around the aching tooth (Meyer 1985: 40, 57, 71, 158, 216, 236, 238, 247). This use has led to the name of "toothache tree" as an alternative to prickly ash. A tea from the buds of prickly ash has been used to treat measles

(Puckett 1981: 413). Boils have been treated with a decoction of the bark (UCLA Folklore Archives 20_6185). In the Mexican tradition the bark has also provided a cough medicine (Dodson 1932: 88). The burned ashes of the plant have been sprinkled on cancers (Rogers 1941: 28).

All these uses, and others besides, are recorded in Native American usage (Moerman 1998: 610).

*See also* **Boils, Cancer, Colic, Coughs, Diarrhea, Fevers, Mexican tradition, Rheumatism, Shakers, Toothache.**

### References
Crellin, John K., and Jane Philpott. *A Reference Guide to Medicinal Plants.* Durham, NC: Duke University Press, 1990.

Dodson, Ruth. "Folk Curing among the Mexicans." *Publications of the Texas Folklore Society* 10 (1932): 82–98.

Meyer, Clarence. *American Folk Medicine.* Glenwood, IL: Meyerbooks, 1985.

Moerman, Daniel E. *Native American Ethnobotany.* Portland, OR: Timber Press, 1998.

Puckett, Newbell Niles. *Popular Beliefs and Superstitions: A Compendium of American Folklore from the Ohio Collection of Newbell Niles Puckett.* Edited by Wayland D. Hand, Anna Casetta, and Sondra B. Thiederman. 3 vols. Boston: G. K. Hall,1981.

Rogers, E. G. *Early Folk Medical Practices in Tennessee.* Murfreesboro, TN: 1941.

# Puffball (*Lycoperdon spp.; Bovista spp.*)

There are numerous British country names for this fungus (bulfer, Norfolk; devil's soot bag, Suffolk; Smoky Jo, Norfolk; blindball, Ireland), but there was one principal use for it in British folk medicine, and this was to staunch bleeding. Either the spores were dusted onto a wound, or a poultice was made from the whole fungus and applied. This use occurs throughout Europe and is evidently an ancient practice. In the prehistoric village of Skara Brae, Orkney, a group of fruit bodies was found accumulated in such a way as to suggest deliberate harvesting, probably for medicinal use (Watling and Seaward 1976). Nearly two thousand years later, in the seventeenth century, Parkinson reported their use for chafed skin as well as for staunching bleeding (Parkinson 1640: 1324). In much more recent times, well into the twentieth century, they were so commonly used in East Anglia that most farmers kept one hanging in the shed or the kitchen, for use on humans and farm animals; barbers frequently kept them for emergency use on cuts they inflicted on customers, and butchers likewise kept them handy in case of accidents (Vickery 1995: 298). In the Highlands of Scotland they were used similarly for treating wounds, and also piles, burns, and scalds (Beith 1995: 235). Their use for burns is also reported from East Anglia (Evans 1966: 90). In Norfolk, the spores were claimed to prevent tetanus (Wigby 1976: 67). The plant was burned and the fumes smoked into bee hives to sedate the bees while honey was collected. It was believed in Scotland that the spores were injurious to eyes, and it has been claimed that, inhaled in large amounts, the spores have an anesthetic effect on humans (Beith 1995: 236).

In North American folk medicine, the same principal use of the puffball appears, but not extensively. It has been claimed that the spores can stop the bleeding even from an amputated limb (Meyer 1985: 277). There are records from Carolina of the use of spores to stop bleeding (Clark 1970: 19). Snuffing up the spores has been recommended for nosebleeds (Brown 1952–1964, 6: 240).

Among Native Americans the plants were used much as in East Anglia, to treat cuts on humans and animals (Carr and Westez 1945: 121). In addition the spores,

mixed with water, were used to treat internal bleeding (Hellson 1974: 84, 89). Puffballs featured in Native American legend, too (Moerman 1998: 323). Interestingly, the spores had a reputation among Native Americans for their poisonous quality, and, as in Scotland, they were considered especially harmful to the eyes (Compton 1993: 134). Just as in seventeenth-century Britain, several Native American tribes used puffballs as baby powder to prevent chafing (Vogel 1970: 236).

*See also* **Bleeding, Burns, Nosebleed, Piles, Poultice.**

## References

Beith, Mary. *Healing Threads: Traditional Medicines of the Highlands and Islands.* Edinburgh: Polygon, 1995.

Brown, Frank C. *Collection of North Carolina Folklore.* 7 vols. Durham, NC: Duke University Press, 1952–1964.

Carr, Lloyd G., and Carlos Westez. "Surviving Folktales and Herbal Lore among the Shinnecock Indians of Long Island." *Journal of American Folklore* 58 (1945): 113–121.

Clark, Joseph D. "North Carolina Popular Beliefs and Superstitions." *North Carolina Folklore* 18 (1970): 1–66.

Compton, Brian Douglas. *Upper North Wakashan and Southern Tsimshian Ethnobotany: The Knowledge and Usage of Plants.* Ph.D. dissertation, University of British Columbia, Vancouver, 1993.

Evans, George Ewart. *The Pattern under the Plough.* London: Faber, 1966.

Hellson, John C. *Ethnobotany of the Blackfoot Indians.* Mercury Series 19. Ottawa: National Museums of Canada, 1974.

Meyer, Clarence. *American Folk Medicine.* Glenwood, IL: Meyerbooks, 1985.

Moerman, Daniel E. *Native American Ethnobotany.* Portland OR: Timber Press, 1998.

Parkinson, John. *Theatrum Botanicum.* London: Thomas Cotes, 1640.

Vickery, Roy. *A Dictionary of Plant Lore.* Oxford: Oxford University Press, 1995.

Vogel, Virgil J. *American Indian Medicine.* Norman, Okla.: University of Oklahoma Press, 1970.

Watling, R., and M. R. D. Seaward. "Some Observations on Puff-balls from British Archaeological Sites." *Journal of Archaeological Science,* 3 (1976): 165–172.

Wigby, Frederick C. *Just a Country Boy.* Wymondham: Geo. R. Reeve, 1976.

# Q

## Quinsy

This term was used in both official and folk medicine to denote swelling and inflammation of the throat, with an abscess on or near the tonsils. Unsurprisingly, many of the remedies overlapped with those used for sore throats. Many folk medical remedies involved the use of poultices, often hot, which could burst the abscess and bring relief. In the Scottish Highlands a poultice of cow dung applied externally was recommended (Beith 1995: 173). The leaves of greater plantain were also applied as a poultice (Beith 1995: 234). A baked potato placed in a sock and applied hot was another remedy of modern times (Prince 1991: 98). A piece of fat bacon tied onto the throat was also used (Prince 1991: 105). Fried mouse was eaten for quinsy, as well as for whooping cough (Billson 1895: 55). In one Cambridgeshire village in the 1930s there was a man renowned for his ability to cure quinsy. His method was to dip a long, black, satin ribbon in hartshorn oil and give it to the sufferer to wear next to the skin (Porter 1974: 44).

In North American folk medicine, wearing gold beads was claimed to prevent quinsy. Treatments included wearing red flannel around the neck and swallowing whole figs that had been boiled in milk (Brown 1952–1964, 6: 252–253). Other suggestions include smoking dried catnip in a pipe, or drinking an infusion of slippery elm (Puckett 1981: 429), or inhaling the fumes from an infusion of hops (Jack 1964: 36). Gargling with sage tea (UCLA Folklore Archive 9_7613), with a tea of burdock root (Browne 1958: 87), or, more drastically, with a mixture of gunpowder and glycerin (Black 1935: 14) have all been recommended. Poultices were widely used, as in Britain. They include poke root and flaxseed (Puckett 1981: 429). Hot pancakes could be applied to the throat (UCLA Folklore Archive 3_6478) or live earthworms bound on with a cloth (Puckett 1981: 429). Toads, frogs or snails were applied to the throat (Puckett 1981: 429). A poultice of hog manure was sometimes used, echoing the use in Scotland of a cow manure poultice (Fogel 1915: 133). One reported remedy involved holding each of three frogs in turn in the affected throat; the frogs were reputedly poisoned, a clear example of a remedy using transference (Ballard 1956: 167–168).

The native Americans used a number of plant remedies for treating quinsy, including wild cherry, sumac (*Rhus* spp.), and elder (Edgar 1960: 1038).

*See also* **Burdock, Catnip, Cherry, Elder, Elm, Excreta, Flax, Gold, Hops, Mouse, Plantain, Poke, Potato, Poultice, Snail, Sore throat, Toads and frogs, Transference, Whooping cough.**

## References

Ballard, Hattie R. "The Year We Were Sick." *New York Folklore Quarterly* 12 (1956): 164–170.

Beith, Mary. *Healing Threads: Traditional Medicines of the Highlands and Islands.* Edinburgh: Polygon, 1995.

Billson, C. J. *Leicestershire and Rutland: County Folklore.* London: Folklore Society, 1895.

Black, Pauline Monette. *Nebraska Folk Cures.* Studies in Language, Literature and Criticism 15. Lincoln: University of Nebraska, 1935.

Brown, Frank C. *Collection of North Carolina Folklore.* 7 vols. Durham, NC: Duke University Press, 1952–1964.

Browne, Ray B. *Popular Beliefs and Practices from Alabama.* Folklore Studies 9. Berkeley and Los Angeles: University of California Publications, 1958.

Edgar, Irving I. "Origins of the Healing Art." *The Journal of the Michigan State Medical Society* 59(7) (1960): 1035–1039.

Fogel, Edwin Miller. "Beliefs and Superstitions of the Pennsylvania Germans." *Americana Germanica* 18 (1915).

Jack, Phil R. "Folk Medicine from Western Pennsylvania." *Pennsylvania Folklife* 14(1) (October 1964): 35–37.

Porter, Enid. *The Folklore of East Anglia.* London: Batsford, 1974.

Prince, Dennis. *Grandmother's Cures: An A–Z of Herbal Remedies.* London: Fontana, 1991.

Puckett, Newbell Niles. *Popular Beliefs and Superstitions: A Compendium of American Folklore from the Ohio Collection of Newbell Niles Puckett.* Edited by Wayland D. Hand, Anna Casetta, and Sondra B. Thiederman. 3 vols. Boston: G. K. Hall, 1981.

# R

## Renal colic

*See* **Colic.**

## Rheumatism and arthritis

The number and variety of folk remedies for these conditions are indicative of their frequency and of the fact that no really successful cure has been or is available.

In Norfolk, fastening a stone with a hole in it under the bed was one suggestion, or placing a thick glass under one leg of the bed (Taylor MSS, Cringleford W.I., Norfolk, 1925). Liniments composed of turpentine, vinegar, and eggs have been used right up to the present day (L.H., Norwich, 1985, pers. com.). Epsom salts have been found helpful, as has old draft cider turning to vinegar (T.W., Gwent, Wales, 1980, pers. com.). The herbal treatments used in British folk medicine include oak (Hatfield 1994: 46), celery seed *(Apium graveolens)* (Taylor MSS, Cringleford W.I., Norfolk, 1925), bogbean (Vickery 1995: 441), wormwood *(Artemisia absinthium),* agrimony *(Agrimonia eupatoria),* chicory *(Cichorium intybus),* yarrow, willow, stinging nettle, parsley *(Pterselinum crispum),* horseradish *(Armoracia rusticana),* cabbage water, potato water (Hatfield 1994: 46–47), and white deadnettle *(lamium album)* (Taylor MSS, Cringleford W.I., Norfolk, 1925). In the fenlands of East Anglia, poppy tea prepared from white opium poppies grown in gardens was a standby for rheumatism and ague (Porter 1974: 52). Dandelion was widely used in Ireland for rheumatism, and burdock was also used there (Allen and Hatfield, in press). Among the more unusual rheumatism treatments, recorded from the Highlands of Scotland, is poulticing with molehill earth, as hot as possible, and then with seaweed (Beith 1995: 178). The burst vesicles of bladder-wrack, a type of seaweed *(Fucus vesiculosus),* were sometimes added to the bath to relieve the pain of bunions and stiff joints (Hatfield MS). Eating an apple that has been halved and wrapped around a cobweb was recommended in Norfolk in recent times. An alternative was to eat a spider and wash it down with cider! (Mundford Primary School project, 1980 unpub.).

Various plants have been carried to ward off rheumatism; these include acorns (R. H., Brandon, Suffolk, 1990), horse chestnuts *(Aesculus hoppocastanum)* made into a necklace (Mundford Primary School project, Norfolk 1980, unpub.), potato, nutmeg *(Myristica fragrans)* (Vickery 1995: 291, 259), hazel nut *(Corylus avellana)* (Foster 1951: 60), and white bryony (Taylor 1929: 117). Animal-derived amulets worn against rheumatism include the legs of a mole—the front legs if the arms were

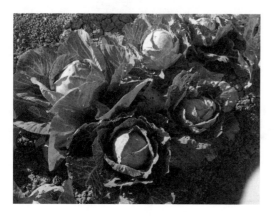

Cabbage water was among the many herbal treatments used for rheumatism in British folk medicine. Many of the other British folk uses of cabbage relate to its large cooling leaves. These have been used as a compress for breast abscesses and ulcers, as well as for reducing fever. (Library of Congress)

affected, the back ones for sore legs (Emerson 1887).

Another category of folk remedies for rheumatism depend on counter-irritation; "rubs" of oil of wintergreen (from *Gaultheria* sp., or from *Betula lenta*), hot mustard poultices (from *Brassica* spp.), chilli peppers, even beating with stinging nettles (a remedy attributed to the Romans in Britain and still practiced in parts of East Anglia) (Hatfield MS), or with holly (Tongue 1965: 42) all produce local heat and sometimes comfort. Interestingly, there is increasing evidence for a more directly therapeutic action for some of these, and chilli pepper extract has recently been endorsed as a painkiller by the orthodox medical profession, while stinging nettle is undergoing clinical trials in Germany.

Other counter-irritants were produced from animal sources. In Sussex folk medicine, both bee stings and wood-ant stings were used (Allen 1995: 86–87), and these practices were probably far more widespread than the written records might suggest.

The oil from the liver of the sting-ray was another treatment for rheumatism used by Suffolk fishermen in the nineteenth century (Emerson: 1887) and reflected in the more modern use of cod-liver-oil, which is widespread and currently fashionable. "Oil" of earthworms, made by burying a bottle of worms in a dung heap until they became liquefied, was similarly used (Lowestoft Journal 1.2.1957). This last remedy may have been "borrowed" from conventional medicine. It appears, for example, in Salmon's *English Physician* of 1693 (Salmon 1693: 698). In Fife, a preparation of black slugs was used (Simpkins 1914: 411). On the now-uninhabited island of St. Kilda, fulmar oil was used as a rub and during the seventeenth century was exported to London, where it was used similarly for rheumatism (Beith 1995: 165).

In folk medicine, damp is often regarded as a cause of rheumatism, perhaps because inflamed joints are often more painful in damp conditions. It is interesting to find, then, that water animals seem to be associated with rheumatism cures. Garters made from eelskin were a Suffolk folk remedy, used both for prevention and cure of rheumatism well into the nineteenth century (Lowestoft Journal: 1.2.1957). The association with water is paralleled in Native American medicine, where the beaver was considered a cause of rheumatism (Lyon 1996: 18). The use of sea water for bathing rheumatic joints and of water from special healing wells in the Scottish Highlands (Beith 1995: 136, 140) and elsewhere could be extensions of this association.

In Britain there is a superstition that cutting the green boughs of elder will cause rheumatism in later years (Hatfield MS).

Some individuals were famed for their ability to treat rheumatism. In the Scottish Highlands one such healer was a seventh son. He treated sore backs by walking along them (Beith 1995: 94, 97–98).

In North American folk medicine there are innumerable rheumatism treatments. Like those in Britain, they can be categorized into counter-irritant "rubs," healing herbs, amulets, and other superstitions. Numerous plants have been used by different cultures at different times for the treatment of rheumatism and arthritis. Celery seed was used as in Britain (and continues to be used by herbalists), but many of the other plants used are natives of North America and, until relatively recently, were not generally available in Britain. Some of them, such as black cohosh (*Cimicifuga racemosa*), were originally folk remedies but have now reached official herbalism on both sides of the Atlantic. As its common name of squaw root suggests, this plant was originally a Native American remedy. Wild yam (*Dioscorea villosa*), a native plant of North and Central America, is sometimes called "rheumatism root," indicating its use by early colonial settlers. This remedy too has been imported into official herbalism in Europe (Chevallier 1996: 89). Willow, the plant from which salicylic acid, and hence aspirin, was developed, was used in folk medicine on both sides of the Atlantic, the white willow (*Salix alba*) in Britain and various species, including black willow (*Salix nigra*), in North America. Creosote bush (*Larrea tridentata*) was used by Indians, Mexicans, and Spanish of the southwestern states; an infusion was made from the leaves (Meyer 1985: 214). All these varied herbal treatments were used for their painkilling or diuretic properties. Poke was widely used for treating rheumatism. Both the berries and the roots have been used (Brown 1952–1964, 6: 261). Other plants used in the treatment of rheumatism include horseradish and cayenne pepper (Brown 1952–1964, 6: 259, 260). Dandelion tea has been recommended (UCLA Folklore Archives 4_6465), as has a poultice of burdock leaves (UCLA Folklore Archives 4_6838), both remedies familiar also in Ireland. Both catnip and prickly ash have been used in rheumatism treatment. A poultice of mullein leaves has also been used (Puckett 1981: 433). In Newfoundland, an infusion of alder buds has been drunk (Bergen 1899: 837). Lying down and covering oneself with elm leaves is another suggestion (Parler 1962: 838). In New Mexico, adding boiled cedar leaves to the bath has been recommended (Moya 1940: 47). In Pennsylvania, a rub has been made from hemp seed (*Cannabis sativa*) and chicken fat (Rupp 1946: 254).

As in Britain, numerous amulets have been carried to protect against rheumatism. These include acorns, horse chestnuts, nutmegs, and potato (all familiar in British folk medicine too). Both snakeskin and eelskin (Brown 1952–1964, 6: 256, 258) have been worn, and carrying a rabbit's foot has been practiced (Brown 1952–1964, 6: 257)—again, remedies similar to those in Britain. A leather strip has been worn, a remedy from the African tradition (Brown 1952–1964, 6: 265). Flannel, especially red flannel, has been used to bandage affected parts (Brown 1952–1964, 6: 264) or has been worn as an amulet. Threads of various kinds have also been used, tied around the wrist, around a toe, or around the waist (Brown 1952–1964, 6: 265–266). Coins, rings, bracelets, and anklets of copper, brass, lead, and pewter have been widely worn as amulets against rheumatism (Brown 1952–1964, 6: 266–268). Other amulets used are the feather of a buzzard and a fin-bone of the haddock (Brown 1952–1964, 6: 255, 257).

Transferring rheumatism to a cat was a folk remedy in North America taken from the German tradition (Meyer 1985: 218). Sleeping with a dog has been widely recommended (Brown 1952–1964, 6: 255).

Rheumatism has even been "transferred" to a tree, by rubbing against it after a hog has rubbed there (Brown 1952–1964, 6: 257). Live toads bound to an aching limb, or split frogs applied to the feet, are further examples of transference (Brown 1952–1964, 6: 256, 258).

Animal-derived remedies for rheumatism also bear a striking resemblance to British folk remedies. An oil derived from angleworms or grubworms has been used (Brown 1952–1964: 254, 257). Bee stings are recommended (Brown 1952–1964, 6: 254). Grease derived from goat, dog, or buzzard (Brown 1952–1964, 6: 255, 256) has been used as a rub. Walking through cow manure and then through wet grass has been suggested (UCLA Folklore Archive 2_6464), or applying hard, dry horse dung (Browne 1958: 89). Drinking one's early-morning urine has been recommended (Puckett 1981: 431). The blood of a black hen applied to the sore areas has also been suggested (Pickard and Buley 1945: 84).

Miscellaneous remedies from the North American folk medicine include bathing in a cold stream where the ice has broken (Wilson 1968: 302) or using the mineral waters of St. Louis, Michigan (Michigan State Guide 1964: 446). The association between water and rheumatism is also illustrated in a common "cure" involving placing water under the bed of the sufferer (Hendricks 1956: 10).

As in Britain, certain individuals were credited with the ability to cure rheumatism. A posthumous son or a seventh daughter (Puckett 1926: 363) was thought to have this ability, as was a widow who had given birth to twins (Neal 1955: 284).

Folk medicine emphasizes the role of diet in rheumatism, and numerous special diets have been suggested as helpful. One of the best-known such diets in recent times is the cider vinegar diet propounded by Jarvis, whose books based on folk medicine in Vermont have run into numerous editions and become widely popular in North America and Britain (Jarvis 1961).

In Native American medicine a very large number of plants, belonging to several hundred different genera, have been used to treat rheumatism (Moerman 1998: 772–774). Among these, nettle (*Urtica* spp.), wormwood (*Artemisia* spp.), yarrow (*Achillea millefolium* sp.) and juniper (*Juniperus* spp.) have been particularly widely used, all of them as external applications.

*See also* **African tradition, Alder, Amulet, Apple, Bogbean, Bryony, Burdock, Cabbage, Catnip, Cayenne, Dandelion, Elder, Holly, Mullein, Poke, Poppy, Potato, Prickly ash, Seventh son, Spider, Stinging nettle, Toads and frogs, Transference, Urine, Yarrow.**

### References
Allen, Andrew. *A Dictionary of Sussex Folk Medicine.* Newbury: Countryside Books, 1995.
Allen, David E., and Gabrielle Hatfield. *Medicinal Plants in Folk Tradition.* Portland, OR: Timber Press, in press.
Beith, Mary. *Healing Threads: Traditional Medicines of the Highlands and Islands.* Edinburgh: Polygon, 1995.
Bergen, Fanny D. "Animal and Plant Lore Collected from the Oral Tradition of English Speaking Folk." *Memoirs of the American Folk-Lore Society* 7 (1899).
Brown, Frank C. *Collection of North Carolina Folklore.* 7 vols. Durham, NC: Duke University Press, 1952–1964.
Browne, Ray B. *Popular Beliefs and Practices from Alabama.* Folklore Studies 9. Berkeley and Los Angeles: University of California Publications, 1958.
Chevallier, Andrew. *The Encyclopedia of Medicinal Plants.* London: Dorling Kindersley, 1996.
Emerson, P. H. *Pictures of East Anglian Life.* London: Sampson Low, 1887.
Foster, Jeanne Cooper. *Ulster Folklore.* Belfast: H. R. Carter, 1951.
Hatfield, Gabrielle. *Country Remedies: Traditional East Anglian Plant Remedies in the Twentieth Century.* Woodbridge: Boydell, 1994.

Hendricks, George D. "Superstitions Collected in Denton, Texas." *Western Folklore* 15 (1956): 1–18.

Jarvis, D. C. *Folk Medicine.* London: Pan Books, 1961. Originally published W. H. Allen, 1960.

Lyon, William S. *Encyclopedia of Native American Healing.* Santa Barbara, CA: ABC-CLIO, 1996.

Meyer, Clarence. *American Folk Medicine.* Glenwood, IL: Meyerbooks, 1985.

*Michigan State Guide.* 8th ed. New York: Federal Writers Project, 1964.

Moerman, Daniel E. *Native American Ethnobotany.* Portland, OR: Timber Press, 1998.

Moya, Benjamin S. *Superstitions and Beliefs among the Spanish-Speaking People of New Mexico.* Master's thesis, University of New Mexico, 1940.

Mundford Primary School, Norfolk, England. School project, 1980, unpublished.

Neal, Janice G. "Grandad: Pioneer Medicine Man." *New York Folklore Quarterly* 11 (1955): 277–291.

Parler, Mary Celestia, and University Student Contributors. *Folk Beliefs from Arkansas.* 15 vols. Fayetteville: University of Arkansas, 1962.

Pickard, Madge E., and R. Carlyle Buley. *The Midwest Pioneer, His Ills, Cures and Doctors.* Crawfordsville, IN: R. E. Banta, 1945.

Porter, Enid. *The Folklore of East Anglia.* London: Batsford, 1974.

Puckett, Newbell Niles. *Folk Beliefs of the Southern Negro.* Chapel Hill, NC: Greenwood Press, 1926.

Puckett, Newbell Niles. *Popular Beliefs and Superstitions: A Compendium of American Folklore from the Ohio Collection of Newbell Niles Puckett.* Edited by Wayland D. Hand, Anna Casetta, and Sondra B. Thiederman. 3 vols. Boston: G. K. Hall, 1981.

Rupp, William J. "Bird Names and Bird Lore of the Pennsylvania Germans." *Pennsylvania German Society Proceedings and Addresses* 52 (1946).

Salmon, William, M.D. *The Compleat English Physician.* London: 1693.

Simpkins, John Ewart. *Examples of Printed Folk-Lore Concerning Fife, with Some Notes on Clackmannan and Kinross-shires.* County Folklore 7. London: Folklore Society, 1914.

Taylor, Mark R. "Norfolk Folklore." *Folk-Lore* 40 (1929): 113–133.

Taylor MSS. Manuscript notes by Mark R. Taylor in the Norfolk Record Office, Norwich. MS4322.

Tongue, Ruth L. *Somerset Folklore.* Edited Katharine Briggs. County Folklore 8. London: Folklore Society, 1965.

Vickery, Roy. *A Dictionary of Plant Lore.* Oxford: Oxford University Press, 1995.

Wilson, Gordon, Sr. *Folklore of the Mammoth Cave Region.* Bowling Green, KY: Kentucky Folklore Series 4, 1968.

# Rickets

In British folk medicine snail slime was used as a treatment for rickets (Prince 1991: 104). In parts of Scotland, snails in vinegar were eaten for rickets (Beith 1995: 185). Alternatively, the child could be passed three times through a split ash tree or willow tree. The tree was then bound up, and as it healed, so the child would recover (Radford and Radford 1974: 21, 365). Another version of this passing-through ceremony involved stones with huge holes in them, such as Men-an-Tol in Cornwall. The child was passed nine times through the hole (Souter 1995: 37). Lime-containing springs were also used to treat rickets (Souter 1995: 95). There seem to have been few plant remedies used for rickets. In Ireland, the Royal Fern (*Osmunda regalis*) had a reputation for healing rickets (Page 1988: 22), and Shepherd's Purse (*Capsella bursa-pastoris*) was also used (Ó Súilleabháin 1942: 313).

In North American folk medicine, advice for rickets included washing in cold water, administering cod liver oil or bone and lime water, or sarsaparilla (Brown 1952–1964, 6: 269). The grease from dishwater rubbed on the child was another recommendation (Puckett 1981: 437), as was washing the child's legs with cow's milk (Saxon 1945:

532) or with the water in which potatoes have been boiled (Puckett 1981: 114). A New England remedy was to bury some of the child's hair at a crossroads, preferably at full moon (Black 1883: 125). Dipping the child nine times in a spring was another suggestion (Levine 1941: 489) or, as in Britain, passing it three times through a split in a young tree (Brown 1952–1964, 6: 56). Sunshine and fat meat (Ross 1934: 59) were obviously sound recommendations, as both increase the vitamin D necessary to correct rickets. There was a belief that a child under a few months old should not be allowed to see itself in a mirror, otherwise it would develop rickets (Parler 1962, 3: 209).

The Native Americans of the Pacific north coast used oolachan fish oil, a natural source of vitamin D equivalent to the cod liver oil officially recommended today (Fiddes 1965: 401).

*See also* **Ash, Moon, Sarsaparilla, Snail.**

### References

Beith, Mary. *Healing Threads: Traditional Medicines of the Highlands and Islands.* Edinburgh: Polygon, 1995.

Black, William George. *Folk-Medicine: A Chapter in the History of Culture.* London: Folklore Society, 1883.

Brown, Frank C. *Collection of North Carolina Folklore.* 7 vols. Durham, NC: Duke University Press, 1952–1964.

Fiddes, G. W. J. "He Took Down His Shingle (A Backward Look at the Indian Medicine Man)." *Canadian Journal of Public Health* 56 (1965): 400–401.

Levine, Harold D. "Folk Medicine in New Hampshire." *New England Journal of Medicine* 224 (1941): 487–492.

Ó Súilleabháin, Seán. *A Handbook of Irish Folklore.* Wexford: Educational Company of Ireland, 1942.

Page, Christopher N. *Ferns: Their Habitats in the British and Irish Landscape.* London: Collins, 1988.

Parler, Mary Celestia, and University Student Contributors. *Folk Beliefs from Arkansas.* 15 vols. Fayetteville: University of Arkansas, 1962.

Prince, Dennis. *Grandmother's Cures: An A–Z of Herbal Remedies.* London: Fontana, 1991.

Puckett, Newbell Niles. *Popular Beliefs and Superstitions: A Compendium of American Folklore from the Ohio Collection of Newbell Niles Puckett.* Edited by Wayland D. Hand, Anna Casetta, Sondra B. Thiederman. 3 vols. Boston: G. K. Hall, 1981.

Radford, E., and M. A. Radford. *Encyclopaedia of Superstitions.* Edited and revised by Christina Hole. London: Book Club Associates 1974.

Ross, R. A. "Granny Grandiosity." *Southern Medicine and Surgery* 96 (February 1934): 57–59.

Saxon, Lyle. *Gumbo Ya-Ya.* Boston: Houghton Mifflin, 1945.

Souter, Keith. *Cure Craft: Traditional Folk Remedies and Treatment from Antiquity to the Present Day.* Saffron Walden: C.W. Daniel, 1995.

# Ringworm

This fungal skin complaint was also known in the past as "tetter," or "tetters," and was thought to be caused by a worm. In British folk medicine, there were a number of semi-magical ways of curing it. Fossil belemnites were thought to help heal ringworm (Blakeborough 1898: 141). In Ireland, a priest who is a seventh son can cure ringworm by breathing on the affected area three times and blessing it; this procedure is repeated three times in an eight-day period (Huttson 1957: 57). In Shetland, a person suffering from ringworm took a pinch of ashes between forefinger and thumb, and recited a suitable charm each morning before eating on three successive mornings (Black 1883: 42). Tracing a finger around the child's face three times, each day for three days, was supposed to cure a child of ringworm (Addy 1895: 91). Rubbing the patient's head with a silver watch was recommended, or measuring the dis-eased area and then rubbing it with a shilling (Black 1883: 182).

As in the treatment of warts, fasting spittle was thought to be effective, but a shilling treated first with fasting spittle was more so (Black 1883: 184). Rubbing with a gold ring was also suggested in the Scottish Highlands (Beith 1995: 159). An Irish remedy was to rub the affected area with golden syrup (Hatfield MS). Herbal remedies include an infusion of chickweed (Prince 1991: 123), or of houseleek (Vickery 1995: 199). In Ireland boiled garlic was used (Vickery 1995: 151) or the juice of laurel leaves *(Prunus laurocerasus)* mixed with un-salted butter (Logan 1972: 74), or water in which oak leaves have been boiled (Vickery 1995: 264). A poultice of burdock leaves is another Irish cure. It was recommended that this should be prepared on the opposite side of a river from the patient, so the "worm" would not smell the remedy and change position (Wellborn 1963: 161). In Suffolk, an ointment to heal ringworm was made from lard and the leaves of primroses *(Primula vulgaris)* (Vickery 1995: 297). Walnut tree bark *(Juglans* sp.) and sunspurge *(Euphorbia helioscopia)* have also been used to treat ringworm (Thiselton Dyer 1889: 210, 296). In Wales, ringworm was treated with rotten apples or rotten pears, or with an infusion of coltsfoot leaves *(Tussilago farfara).* Wood tar collected on an axe held in the flame was also used in Wales to treat ringworm. The fat of fried bacon was another ringworm treatment from Wales (Jones 1980: 62). In Suffolk coal oil was used with apparent success to treat ringworm (Hatfield MS).

In North American folk medicine there is a similar mixture of practical and magical treatments for ringworm. The touch of a posthumous child has been suggested as effective (Puckett 1981: 379). One very simple method was to scratch the surface of the skin around the affected area, which stopped it from spreading. Copper coins dipped in vinegar were a common cure (and, given that copper salts are toxic to fungi in general, one that may have a scientific basis). Iodine solution was used to paint the affected area of skin. Butter and sulphur, and gunpowder and vinegar, were also used. A widespread folk treatment for ringworm was the ash of paper. This was burned on an axe (just as in the Welsh remedy described for wood above), and the resulting oily ash was rubbed onto the ringworm (Cannon 1984: 122). Rubbing the affected area with a sowbug is a remedy from Mexico (UCLA Folklore Archives 4_6482), while in Louisiana the blood of a black hen was claimed to be effective (Boudreaux 1971: 127). Blood from the tail of a black cat has been suggested, as a remedy that will prevent the ring of ringworm closing up, which could presage death of the patient (Bergen 1899: 68). Allowing flies to crawl over the affected area is perhaps an example of transference (Puckett 1981: 437). Rubbing with one's mother's wedding ring nine times a day for nine days is a remedy from Texas (Hendricks 1980: 94). Urine has been used to treat ringworm, especially the first urine in the morning (Puckett 1981: 437). Fasting spittle was another cure. In Alabama, the spit of a black-eyed person is specified. Calf slobber has been suggested too (Puckett 1981: 379). Wash-day blueing was also used (Browne 1958: 90, 91). In Maine, placing a salt pickle on the area of ringworm was suggested (UCLA Folklore Archives 1_7602), and in Nebraska, a mixture of egg yolk, turpentine, coal oil, vinegar, and salt was rubbed on (Welsch 1966: 362). In Ohio, ringworm on the head was treated with sour buttermilk (Puckett 1981: 437).

Herbs used to treat ringworm include burdock (as in Britain), yellow dock, and bloodroot, as well as tobacco or the green rind of a walnut *(Juglans* sp.) (Meyer 1985: 220–221). Garlic has been used in Arkansas

(Parler 1962: 864), as has the root of may-apple *(Podophyllum peltatum)* (Dennie 1956: 278). Another suggestion is to eat fig leaves *(Ficus carica)* and milk (Puckett 1981: 437), or to rub on the juice of fig leaves (Cadwallader 1965: 221, 225). Rubbing with a carrot has been successful in Indiana (Halpert 1950: 6). Other herbal treatments include an ointment made from pokeberries, or the root of the rain lily *(Zephyranthes* sp.) rubbed on (Woodhull 1930: 45, 64). Aralia roots *(Aralia* sp.) have been used (Pickard and Buley 1945: 45), as has oil of corn (Neal 1955: 289). Green gourd tea, thickened into a paste with cornmeal, is a remedy from Alabama (Browne 1958: 91).

Native American herbals for ringworm treatment include a poultice of poison ivy leaves *(Toxicodendron* sp.), the sap of the red mulberry *(Morus rubra)* (Vogel 1970: 220, 350), and a salve made from yellow birch buds *(Betula nigra)* (Speck 1944: 43). Pine tar (from *Pinus virginiana)* is used by the Cherokee for treating "tetterworm" (Hamel and Chiltoskey 1975: 49).

Miscellaneous ringworm cures included immersing the head (where the head is affected) in a horse trough (Puckett 1981: 437) and applying a thimble to the opposite side of the hand from that affected by ringworm (Parler 1962: 861). A seventh son was thought to have the power to cure ringworm, but only if a nurse had put a worm in his hand at birth (Puckett 1981: 438).

*See also* **Apple, Bloodroot, Burdock, Chickweed, Corn, Dock, Garlic, Gold, Houseleek, Poke, Poultice, Seventh son, Spit, Tobacco, Transference, Urine, Vinegar, Warts.**

### References
Addy, Sidney Oldall. *Household Tales with Other Traditional Remains Collected in the Counties of York, Lincoln, Derby and Nottingham.* London: 1895.

Beith, Mary. *Healing Threads: Traditional Medicines of the Highlands and Islands.* Edinburgh: Polygon, 1995.

Bergen, Fanny D. "Animal and Plant Lore Collected from the Oral Tradition of English Speaking Folk." *Memoirs of the American Folk-Lore Society* 7 (1899).

Black, William George. *Folk-Medicine: A Chapter in the History of Culture.* London: Folklore Society, 1883.

Blakeborough, Richard. *Yorkshire Wit, Character, Folklore and Customs.* London: 1898.

Boudreaux, Anna M. "Les Remèdes du Vieux Temps: Remedies and Cures of the Kaplan Area in Southwestern Louisiana." *Southern Folklore Quarterly* 35 (1971): 121–140.

Browne, Ray B. *Popular Beliefs and Practices from Alabama.* Folklore Studies 9. Berkeley and Los Angeles: University of California Publications, 1958.

Cadwallader, D. E., and F. J. Wilson. "Folklore Medicine among Georgia's Piedmont Negroes after the Civil War." *Collections of the Georgia Historical Society* 49 (1965): 217–227.

Cannon, Anthon S. *Popular Beliefs and Superstitions from Utah.* Edited by Wayland D. Hand and Jeannine E. Talley. Salt Lake City: University of Utah Press, 1984.

Dennie, Charles C. "Old Doc." *Virginia Medical Monthly* 83 (1956): 278–284.

Halpert, Violetta. "Folk Cures from Indiana." *Hoosier Folklore* 9 (1950): 1–12.

Hamel, Paul B., and Mary U. Chiltoskey. *Cherokee Plants and Their Uses: A 400 Year History.* Sylva, NC: Herald, 1975.

Hendricks, George D. *Roosters, Rhymes and Railroad Tracks: A Second Sampling of Superstitions and Popular Beliefs in Texas.* Dallas, TX: Southern Methodist University Press, 1980.

Huttson, Arthur E. "Folklore in the News: Other Treatments." *Western Folklore* 16 (1957): 56–58.

Jones, Anne E. "Folk Medicine in Living Memory in Wales." *Folk Life* 18 (1980): 58–68.

Logan, Patrick. *Making the Cure: A Look at Irish Folk Medicine.* Dublin: Talbot Press, 1972.

Meyer, Clarence. *American Folk Medicine.* Glenwood, IL: Meyerbooks, 1985.

Neal, Janice C. "Grandad: Pioneer Medicine Man." *New York Folklore Quarterly* 11 (1955): 277–291.

Parler, Mary Celestia, and University Student Contributors. *Folk Beliefs from Arkansas.* 15 vols. Fayetteville: University of Arkansas, 1962.

Pickard, Madge E., and R. Carlyle Buley. *The Midwest Pioneer, His Ills, Cures and Doctors.* Crawfordsville, IN: R. E. Banta, 1945.

Prince, Dennis. *Grandmother's Cures: An A–Z of Herbal Remedies.* London: Fontana, 1991.

Puckett, Newbell Niles. *Popular Beliefs and Superstitions: A Compendium of American Folklore from the Ohio Collection of Newbell Niles Puckett.* Edited by Wayland D. Hand, Anna Casetta, Sondra B. Thiederman. 3 vols. Boston: G. K. Hall, 1981.

Speck, Frank G. "Catawba Herbals and Curative Practices." *Journal of American Folklore* 57 (1944): 37–50.

Thiselton Dyer, T. F. *The Folk-Lore of Plants.* London: 1889.

Vickery, Roy. *A Dictionary of Plant Lore.* Oxford: Oxford University Press, 1995.

Vogel, Virgil J. *American Indian Medicine.* Norman: University of Oklahoma Press, 1970.

Wellborn, Grace Pleasant. "Plant Lore and the Scarlet Letter." *Southern Folklore Quarterly* 27 (1963): 160–167.

Welsch, Roger L. *A Treasury of Nebraska Pioneer Folklore.* Lincoln: University of Nebraska Press, 1966.

Woodhull, Frost. "Ranch Remedios." *Publications of the Texas Folklore Society* 8 (1930): 9–73.

# Rose

The wild roses native to Britain have been used to a limited extent in folk medicine. The crushed leaves were used in the twentieth century in Essex for treatment of cuts. The juice has been used in treating colds and sore throats in both England and Ireland (Allen and Hatfield, in press). The gall growing on rose, known as a "robin's pincushion," has been used in treatment of whooping cough (Taylor MSS) and carried as an amulet to prevent toothache (Leather 1912: 82). Rose-hip syrup, a rich source of vitamin C, has traditionally been given to babies and was a valued source of vitamins during the Second World War. Cultivated roses were more widely used in official medicine, especially the so-called apothecaries rose, *Rosa gallica.*

In North American folk medicine, roses have featured in a number of remedies, the type of rose not usually being specified. Rose petals have been chewed to sweeten the breath (Traux 1957: 48), and rose petal tea has been used to soothe sore eyes ) (Levine 1941: 491) or an upset stomach (Creson, D.L., et al. 1969: 265). The dew from rose petals has been used to remove freckles (UCLA Folklore Archives 7_5963). Rose leaves have been used to treat sores (Puckett 1981: 449) and diarrhea (Hendricks 1980: 82) as well as fever (Parler 1962: 635). Breathing the fumes from burning rose leaves has been used for rheumatism (Koch 1980: 65). A belief has been reported that red roses cure anemia (UCLA Folklore Archives 15_6742), a possible example of sympathetic magic.

The native species *Rosa acicularis* has been used in many ways among the Native Americans, for treating cuts, stings, labor pains, dysentery, muscle pain, indigestion, and colic. The galls have been used for treating burns (Willard 1992: 118–119). A wash for sore eyes is prepared by the Pawnee from the roots of wild roses (Nebraska State Guide 1947: 110). Other rose species have been used by the Native Americans in numerous ways (Moerman 1998: 482–486).

*See also* **Amulet, Anemia, Bad breath, Burns, Childbirth, Colds, Colic, Cuts, Dew, Diarrhea, Dysentery, Eye problems, Fevers, Freckles, Indigestion, Insect bites and stings, Rheumatism, Sore throat, Sympathetic magic, Toothache, Whooping cough.**

## References

Allen, David E., and Gabrielle Hatfield. *Medicinal Plants in Folk Tradition.* Portland, OR: Timber Press, in press.

Creson, D. L., et al. "Folk Medicine in Mexican-American Sub-Culture." *Diseases of the Nervous System* 30 (April 1969): 264–266.

Hendricks, George D. *Roosters, Rhymes and Railroad Tracks: A Second Sampling of Superstitions and Popular Beliefs in Texas.* Dallas, TX: Southern Methodist University Press, 1980.

Koch, William E. *Folklore from Kansas: Beliefs and Customs.* Lawrence, KS: Regent Press, 1980.

Leather, Ella Mary. *The Folk-Lore of Herefordshire Collected from Oral and Printed Sources.* Hereford and London: Jakeman and Carver, 1912.

Levine, Harold D. "Folk Medicine in New Hampshire." *New England Journal of Medicine* 224 (1941): 497–492.

Moerman, Daniel E. *Native American Ethnobotany.* Portland, OR: Timber Press, 1998.

*Nebraska State Guide.* New York: Federal Writers Project, 1947.

Parler, Mary Celestia, and University Student Contributors. *Folk Beliefs from Arkansas.* 15 vols. Fayetteville: University of Arkansas, 1962.

Puckett, Newbell Niles. *Popular Beliefs and Superstitions: A Compendium of American Folklore from the Ohio Collection of Newbell Niles Puckett.* Edited by Wayland D. Hand, Anna Casetta, and Sondra B. Thiederman. 3 vols. Boston: G. K. Hall, 1981.

Taylor MSS. Taylor, Mark R. Manuscript notes in the Norfolk Records Office. MS4322.

Traux, Grace H. "Down Our Way, Our Daily Bread." *Kentucky Folklore Record* 3 (1957): 45–48.

Willard, Terry. *Edible and Medicinal Plants of the Rocky Mountains and Neighbouring Territories.* Calgary, ALTA: Wild Rose College of Natural Healing, 1992.

# Rowan (*Sorbus aucuparia*)

The role of this tree (also known as mountain ash) in British folklore is primarily a protective one. The tree was thought to confer protection against the forces of evil, and it is still frequently planted near a house. Even a stick of rowan kept near the home can be useful. In Devon in the late twentieth century one lady kept a piece of rowan near her cottage to protect but also to cure minor ailments; she treated her own eczema by rubbing with this stick (Lafont 1984: 55). The herbal remedies prepared from rowan mainly come from the Celtic areas of Britain, where the tree is most common. The berries were used in the seventeenth century in Wales to treat scurvy (Ray 1670: 290). In the eighteenth century in Scotland the bark was used to treat constipation, and in the nineteenth century a toothache remedy was obtained from rowan (Pennant 1771: 311). The berries were boiled in the Scottish Highlands as a cure for sore throat; mixed with apples, they were also used for whooping cough (Beith 1995: 237). In Ireland, an infusion of the leaves was used to treat rheumatism, and the dried leaves were smoked to treat asthma (Moloney 1919: 22). The leaves were also used to treat sore eyes. The bark was boiled to form a cough mixture, and was included in a remedy for scrofula. The berries were eaten raw as a blood tonic and were also eaten to get rid of worms (Allen and Hatfield in press).

A piece of rowan was carried as an amulet to protect against rheumatism (Hawke 1973: 28). Another semi-magical use was for whooping cough; hair from the sufferer was plugged into a rowan tree (Radbill 1955: 48).

Rowan is not native to North America but has been introduced there. A stick of rowan, or "wicken" as it is also known, was used in a protective role, as in Britain (Brown 1952–1964, 7: 154). The fresh juice of mountain ash berries has been drunk to treat piles (Meyer 1985: 194), and jelly made from them has been used to treat asthma (Neal 1955: 283). The British

mountain ash has been used by the Potawatomi as an emetic to treat pleurisy, pneumonia, and croup (Smith 1933: 78). Other
related species of Sorbus are native to North
America, and these have been used in Native American medicine as a tonic, analgesic, emetic, and for treating rheumatism, as
well as for bed-wetting, stomach problems,
and head lice (Moerman 1998: 538–539).

*See also* **Amulet, Apple, Asthma,
Bed-wetting, Constipation, Coughs,
Croup, Eczema, Eye problems, Hair
problems, Piles, Rheumatism, Scurvy,
Sore throat, Tonic, Toothache,
Tuberculosis, Whooping cough, Worms.**

## References

Allen, David E., and Gabrielle Hatfield. *Medicinal Plants in Folk Tradition.* Portland, OR: Timber Press, in press.

Beith, Mary. *Healing Threads: Traditional Medicines of the Highlands and Islands.* Edinburgh: Polygon, 1995.

Brown, Frank C. *Collection of North Carolina Folklore.* 7 vols. Durham, NC: Duke University Press, 1952–1964.

Hawke, Kathleen. *Cornish Sayings, Superstitions and Remedies.* Redruth, Cornwall: Dyllanson Truran, 1973.

Lafont, Anne-Marie. *Herbal Folklore.* Bideford: Badger Books, 1984.

Meyer, Clarence. *American Folk Medicine.* Glenwood, IL: Meyerbooks, 1985.

Moerman, Daniel E. *Native American Ethnobotany.* Portland, OR: Timber Press, 1998.

Moloney, M. F. *Irish Ethnobotany and the Evolution of Medicine in Ireland.* Dublin: M. H. Gill and Son, 1919.

Neal, Janice C. "Granddad: Pioneer Medicine Man." *New York Folklore Quarterly* 11 (1955): 277–291.

Pennant, Thomas. *A Tour in Scotland 1769.* London: John Monk, 1771.

Radbill, Samuel X. "Whooping Cough in Fact and Fancy." *Bulletin of History of Medicine* 11 (1955): 277–291.

Ray, John. *Catalogus Plantarum Angliae, et Insularum Adjacentium.* London: John Martyn, 1670.

Smith, Huron H. "Ethnobotany of the Forest Potawatomi Indians." *Bulletin of the Public Museum of the City of Milwaukee* 7 (1933): 1–230.

# S

## St. John's wort
## (*Hypericum perforatum*)

In European folk medicine this plant was used above all in the treatment of wounds. The flowers infused in oil yield a bright orange liquid, which has formed the basis for many healing ointments. Among its country names is "rosin rose," a name recorded in Yorkshire, England, as well as in North America (Grigson 1955: 75). A related species *Hypericum androsaemum* is known as tutsan, from the French "toute-saine" (all healthy). St. John's wort was recommended in many of the herbals and was a constituent of official wound-healing salves. In British folk medicine such salves were used for treating wounds (one of its Gaelic names translates as "bloodwort") and burns, as well as being used internally for treating diarrhea (Allen and Hatfield, in press). Though the herbals recommended it as a soothing herb for nervous conditions including melancholy, in folk medicine this has been a relatively minor use.

The other major use for the plant was as protection against evil spirits. Whether the plant was used in this way in pre-Christian days is difficult to know, but it certainly became associated with the Christianized midsummer night bonfires held on the feast of St. John, June 24. A French proverb, to have "all the herbs of St. John," is used to imply that one is ready for anything! (Grigson 1955: 76).

The plant was reputedly introduced into Philadelphia in 1696 by pilgrims, and it was popular among the Pennsylvania Dutch as the basis of a salve. It first appeared in California in 1900 and became a troublesome weed there for the next half-century. It became known there as "Klamath Weed" and was eventually controlled by introduction of a European beetle that eats it (Coffey 1993: 66); now it is extensively grown for herbalists and has become world renowned for its treatment of depression. Meanwhile, in rural folk medicine, the plant had a reputation in North America similar to that in Britain. Pioneers hung sprigs of the plant over doorways to keep away evil spirits (Micheletti 1998: 286). It was used to treat wounds, including, during the American Civil War, gunshot wounds (Micheletti 1998: 286). In addition it has been used for healing scalds and burns, in a salve to reduce swellings, as a liver tonic, to treat inflamed bowels, and to cure bed-wetting in children (Meyer 1985: 36, 45, 55, 167, 244).

In Native American usage, the Cherokee used it to treat bloody flux and bowel complaints as well as sores, nosebleed, snake bite, diarrhea, and to promote menstruation (Hamel and Chiltoskey 1975: 53). Other species of *Hypericum* have been used by the Native Americans for a wide range of ailments, including tuberculosis (Smith 1923: 37) (Moerman 1998: 272–273).

*See also* **Bed-wetting, Burns, Depression, Diarrhea, Nosebleed, Snake bite, Tuberculosis, Wounds.**

## References

Allen, David E., and Gabrielle Hatfield. *Medicinal Plants in Folk Tradition.* Portland, OR: Timber Press, in press.

Coffey, Timothy. *The History and Folklore of North American Wildflowers.* New York: Facts On File, 1993.

Grigson, Geoffrey. *The Englishman's Flora.* London: Phoenix House, 1955.

Hamel, Paul B., and Mary U. Chiltoskey. *Cherokee Plants and Their Uses: A 400 Year History.* Sylva, NC: Herald, 1975.

Meyer, Clarence. *American Folk Medicine.* Glenwood, IL: Meyerbooks, 1985.

Micheletti, Enza (ed.). *North American Folk Healing: An A–Z Guide to Traditional Remedies.* New York and Montreal: Reader's Digest Association, 1998.

Moerman, Daniel E. *Native American Ethnobotany.* Portland, OR: Timber Press, 1998.

Smith, Huron H. "Ethnobotany of the Menomini Indians." *Bulletin of the Public Museum of the City of Milwaukee* 4 (1923): 1–174.

# Sarsaparilla (*Smilax* spp.)

This woody climber is a native of eastern North America and Central America and the rain forests of South America. It does not occur in Europe but is currently used there by medical herbalists, since its introduction into their materia medica in the sixteenth century. Originally it was hailed as a cure for syphilis, but subsequently it was used mainly as a tonic and blood purifier to treat skin conditions and rheumatism, and these are its main uses in North American folk medicine (see, for example, Meyer 1985: 41, 215). Sarsaparilla mead was drunk in nineteenth-century North America to treat indigestion, fever, headache, and

diarrhea (Pickard and Buley 1945: 267). Sarsaparilla tea was taken for gravel (Browne 1958: 69). At the present time it is sold in proprietary form as a laxative and used as a flavoring for soft drinks (Kay 1996: 255).

Native American uses for species of *Smilax* include treatment of burns, cuts, sores, rheumatism (Hamel and Chiltoskey 1975: 37) and leg ulcers (Taylor 1940: 7). The Aztecs used it for treating joint pain (Kay 1996: 254).

Wild Sarsaparilla (*Aralia nudicaulis*) belongs to another botanical family (Araliaceae). It is native to North America and has been used by Native Americans for burns, wounds, sores, and as a cough medicine (Willard 1992: 148). Because of the confusion surrounding the name "sarsaparilla," it is not always clear to which plant a particular record refers. An infusion of the roots of *Aralia nudicaulis* has been used in folk medicine in the treatment of tuberculosis (Roy 1955: 85). An infusion of the plant has also been used as a tonic (UCLA Folklore Archive 2_5634).

*See also* **Burns, Cuts, Diarrhea, Fevers, Gravel and stone, Headache, Indigestion, Rheumatism, Tonic, Tuberculosis.**

## References

Browne, Ray B. *Popular Beliefs and Practices from Alabama.* Folklore Studies 9. Berkeley and Los Angeles: University of California Publications, 1958.

Hamel, Paul B., and Mary U. Chiltoskey. *Cherokee Plants and Their Uses: A 400 Year History.* Sylva, NC: Herald, 1975.

Kay, Margarita Artschwager. *Healing with Plants in the American and Mexican West.* Tucson: University of Arizona Press, 1996.

Meyer, Clarence. *American Folk Medicine.* Glenwood, IL: Meyerbooks, 1985.

Pickard, Madge E., and R. Carlyle Buley. *The Midwest Pioneer, His Ills, Cures and Doctors.* Crawfordsville, IN: R. E. Banta, 1945.

Roy, Carmen. *La Littérature Orale en Gaspésie.* Bulletin 134, 36 de la Serie Anthropolo-

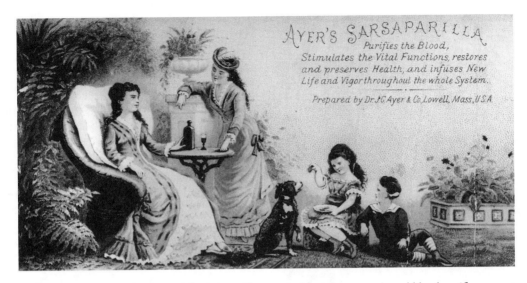

Originally hailed as a cure for syphilis, sarsaparilla was used mainly as a tonic and blood purifier to treat skin conditions and rheumatism. (National Library of Medicine)

gique. Ottawa: Ministre de Nord Canadien et des Ressources Nationales (1955): 61–105, 107–136.

Taylor, Linda Averill. *Plants Used as Curatives by Certain Southeastern Tribes.* Cambridge, MA: Botanical Museum of Harvard University, 1940.

Willard, Terry. *Edible and Medicinal Plants of the Rocky Mountains and Neighbouring Territories.* Calgary, ALTA: Wild Rose College of Natural Healing, 1992.

## Sassafras (*Sassafras albicum*)

Native throughout North America, this shrub was "discovered" by French, Spanish, and later English colonists in the sixteenth century. It had been used by the Native Americans as a tonic and a treatment for syphilis and was greeted as a panacea for the ills of the New World, becoming of great commercial value. As it became evident that it did not in fact cure syphilis, it began to fall from fashion in European medicine, but it has continued to be widely used in domestic medicine in both the New and the Old Worlds. Early colonists used it for treating fevers and for rheumatic pain, and as a general tonic. It is still known by the name "ague tree" in New England (Micheletti 1998: 293). Combined with other herbs, it was drunk as a "blood purifier." With slippery elm and corn meal, it formed a poultice for treating boils and ulcers; a decoction of sassafras root and burdock was claimed to prevent boils (Meyer 1985: 40, 44, 58, 204). Oil of sassafras was used for treating chilblains as well as earache, corns, and sprains (Meyer 1985: 101, 118, 233). A decoction of the twigs, mixed with mare's milk, was used as an eye wash (Meyer 1985: 110). The pith from the stalk, mixed with warm water, was similarly used to bathe sore eyes (Meyer 1985: 114). Chewing the bark was recommended to prevent a feeling of faintness (Meyer 1985: 115).

In addition, sassafras was a component of many rheumatism remedies (Meyer 1985: 215, 217, 219). The UCLA Folklore Archives contain more than five hundred remedies involving sassafras and show that it has been used for almost every conceivable ailment. In addition to those already mentioned, the plant has been used to treat kidney disease, sore throat (Halpert 1950:

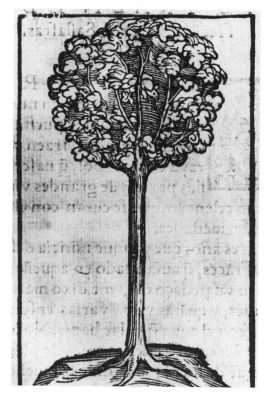

Sassafras is a shrub native to North America. As it became evident that sassafras did not cure syphilis, it began to fall from fashion in European medicine, but it has continued to be widely used in domestic medicine in both the New and the Old Worlds. (National Library of Medicine)

3, 4), pain (Lick and Brendle 1922: 282), measles (UCLA Folklore Archive 1_6407), poison ivy rash (Mullins 1973: 40), head lice (Miller 1959: 7), colic (Long 1962: 4), croup (Browne 1958: 18), high blood pressure (Caroland 1962: 44), and asthma (Clark 1961: 11). Sassafras tea was widely drunk, especially in the Appalachian region, until recent times (Crellin and Philpott 1990: 363). It was considered pleasant as a drink, hot or cold, and with lemon added. It was even claimed to aid weight reduction (Meyer 1985: 264), a claim reflecting one of its uses by the Cherokee (Hamel and Chiltoskey 1975: 54). Faith in its healing powers has extended to wearing the plant too, as an amulet; a necklace of pieces of

sassafras root was claimed to help teething (Parler 1962: 277), while a bag of sassafras around the neck could prevent illness (UCLA Folklore Archives 1_6728).

In Native American usage, sassafras has been used for treating dysentery (Meyer 1985). Its main uses have been in the treatment of fevers and of rheumatism (Hamel and Chiltoskey 1975: 54), as a wash for sore eyes, and as a general tonic (Tantaquidgeon 1928: 266). It has also been used by the Cherokee for aiding a difficult labor.

Recent scares concerning its possible toxicity have banned sassafras from official medicinal use in North America.

*See also* **Amulet, Asthma, Boils, Burdock, Chilblains, Childbirth, Colic, Corn, Corns, Croup, Dysentery, Earache, Elm, Eye problems, Fevers, Hair problems, Hunger, Poison ivy, Rheumatism, Sore throat, Sprains, Teething, Tonic.**

## References

Browne, Ray B. *Popular Beliefs and Practices from Alabama.* Folklore Studies 9. Berkeley and Los Angeles: University of California Publications, 1958.

Caroland, Emma Jean, ed. "Popular Beliefs and Superstitions Known to Students of Clarksville High School." *Tennessee Folklore Society Bulletin* 28 (1962): 37–47.

Clark, Joseph D. "Superstitions from North Carolina." *North Carolina Folklore* 9(2) (1961): 4–22.

Crellin, John K., and Jane Philpott. *A Reference Guide to Medicinal Plants.* Durham, NC: Duke University Press, 1990.

Halpert, Violetta. "Folk Cures from Indiana." *Hoosier Folklore* 9 (1950): 1–12.

Hamel, Paul B., and Mary U. Chiltoskey. *Cherokee Plants and Their Uses: A 400 Year History.* Sylva, NC: Herald, 1975.

Lick, David E., and Thomas R. Brendle. "Plant Names and Plant Lore among the Pennsylvania Germans." *Proceedings and Addresses of the Pennsylvania German Society* 33 (1922).

Long, Grady M. "Folk Medicine in McMinn, Polk, Bradley and Meigs Counties, Tennessee, 1910–1937." *Tennessee Folklore Society Bulletin* 28 (1962): 1–8.

Meyer, Clarence. *American Folk Medicine.* Glenwood, IL: Meyerbooks, 1985.

Micheletti, Enza (ed.). *North American Folk Healing: An A–Z Guide to Traditional Remedies.* New York and Montreal: Reader's Digest Association, 1998.

Miller, Genevieve. "The Sassafras Tree." *Bulletin of the Cleveland Medical Library* 6(1) (January 1959): 3–7.

Mullins, Gladys. "Herbs of the Southern Islands and their Medicinal Uses." *Kentucky Folklore Record* 19 (1973): 36–41.

Parler, Mary Celestia, and University Student Contributors. *Folk Beliefs from Arkansas.* 15 vols. Fayetteville: University of Arkansas, 1962.

Tantaquidgeon, Gladys. "Mohegan Medicinal Practices, Weather-Lore and Superstitions." *Smithsonian Institution-Bureau of American Ethnology Annual Report* 44 (1928): 264–270.

# Scrofula

*See* **Tuberculosis.**

# Scurvy

In British folk medicine a number of native wild plants were eaten to prevent and cure scurvy. In Scotland cuckoo flower *(Cardamine pratense),* dock, and scurvygrass *(Cochlearia* spp.) were among them. The latter, as its name suggests, was widely recognized for its value in treating scurvy, and the plant was taken by fishermen and sailors on voyages; its Gaelic name translates as "the sailor." It has been suggested that the Vikings may have used this plant (Beith 1995: 239). Sailors off the Welsh coast used to disembark to collect alexanders *(Smyrnium olusatrum)* to prevent scurvy (Quelch 1941: 200). In the south of England, sea bindweed *(Calystegia soldanella)* also went by the country name of "scurvy-grass." Watercress *(Rorippa nasturtium-aquaticum)* has

also been used to prevent scurvy—for example, in the Isle of Mull (Vickery 1995: 384). The berries of rowan were eaten for scurvy in Wales in the seventeenth century (Ray 1670: 290). In both Scotland and Ireland, the seaweed dulse *(Palmaria palmata)* was used for scurvy (Allen and Hatfield, in press). Many plants today regarded as weeds were eaten in the past to supplement a poor diet, and some of these, such as goosegrass *(Galium aparine),* were rich in vitamin C and would have helped prevent scurvy (Lafont 1984: 39). In Norfolk there was a belief that drinking one's own urine, fasting, was good for scurvy (Taylor 1929: 120); in the North of England, fasting spittle was recommended (Gutch 1899: 177).

In North American folk medicine, raw potatoes sliced in vinegar have been recommended for scurvy, or a mixture of salt and charcoal (Brown 1952–1964, 6: 271). As in Britain, an infusion of scurvy grass, or eating the plant fresh was another suggestion (Meyer 1985: 224). Also as in Britain, watercress has been used to treat and prevent scurvy (Parler 1962, 3: 866). Spruce beer (from *Picea* spp.) was used as a scurvy preventive by Captain Cook in the eighteenth century, and a century later an infusion of spruce was used in the Californian Gold Rush (Vogel 1970: 249). Fir tops (from *Abies* spp.) were another remedy (Bergen 1899: 111). As in Britain, various "weeds" were used, eaten raw, to prevent scurvy. They include dandelion (as in Britain) (Clark 1970: 29) and winter cress (*Barbarea* sp.) (Lick and Brendle 1922: 158). Strawberries were found to be useful (Pickard and Buley 1945: 45). Nonplant remedies include burying one's legs in dirt (Lawson and Porter 1951: 163) and drinking rum (UCLA Folklore Archives 25_6466).

In the Native American tradition, cranberries, now known to be a rich source of vitamin C, were used to prevent and treat scurvy (Cobb 1917: 103). Various types of cranberry were eaten raw in the summer and dried for winter use (Moerman 1998: 583), and this knowledge was used by settlers in New England. Sea captains there took supplies of cranberries on their voyages to prevent scurvy (UCLA Folklore Archives 4_5467). Also in the Native American tradition, the bark, leaves, and stems of white spruce *(Picea glauca)* have been used (Chandler, Freeman, and Hooper 1979: 59). Many wild plants were eaten raw as dietary aids; the Alaskans ate raw dandelion leaves (Heller 1953: 71). Wild garlic *(Allium reticulatum)* was used to treat scurvy. At Camp Missouri in the early nineteenth century, soldiers were cured of scurvy using this plant (Vogel 1970: 109). Jacques Cartier's crew were treated for scurvy by the Iroquois using a preparation of hemlock spruce (Edgar 1960: 1038). Eating the adrenal glands of the moose and the walls of its second stomach was said to prevent scurvy among Native Americans (Vogel 1970: 250).

*See also* **Dandelion, Dock, Garlic, Hemlock spruce, Rowan, Spit, Urine.**

## References

Allen, David E., and Gabrielle Hatfield. *Medicinal Plants in Folk Tradition.* Portland, OR: Timber Press, in press.

Beith, Mary. *Healing Threads: Traditional Medicines of the Highlands and Islands.* Edinburgh: Polygon, 1995.

Bergen, Fanny D. "Animal and Plant Lore Collected from the Oral Tradition of English Speaking Folk." *Memoirs of the American Folk-Lore Society* 7 (1899).

Brown, Frank C. *Collection of North Carolina Folklore.* 7 vols. Durham, NC: Duke University Press, 1952–1964.

Chandler, R. Frank, Lois Freeman, and Shirley N. Hooper. "Herbal Remedies of the Maritime Indians." *Journal of Ethnopharmacology* 1 (1979): 49–68.

Clark, Joseph D. "North Carolina Popular Beliefs and Superstitions." *North Carolina Folklore* 18 (1970): 1–66.

Cobb, Carolus M. "Some Medical Practices among the New England Indians and Early Settlers." *Boston Medical and Surgical Journal* 177(4) (1917): 97–105.

Edgar, Irving I. "Origins of the Healing Art." *The Journal of the Michigan State Medical Society* 59(7) (1960): 1035–1039.

Gutch, Mrs. (Eliza). *Examples of Printed Lore Concerning the North Riding of Yorkshire, York and the Ainsty.* County Folk-Lore 2, *Publications of the Folk-Lore Society* 45 (1899). Printed Extracts 4. London: 1901.

Heller, Christine A. *Edible and Poisonous Plants of Alaska.* College, AK: Cooperative Agricultural Extension Service, 1953.

Lafont, Anne-Marie. *Herbal Folklore.* Bideford: Badger Books, 1984.

Lawson, O. C., and Kenneth W. Porter. "Texas Poltergeist, 1881." *Journal of American Folklore* 64 (1951): 371–382.

Lick, David E., and Thomas R. Brendle. "Plant Names and Plant Lore among the Pennsylvania Germans." *Proceedings and Addresses of the Pennsylvania German Society* 33 (1922).

Meyer, Clarence. *American Folk Medicine.* Glenwood, IL: Meyerbooks, 1985.

Moerman, Daniel E. *Native American Ethnobotany.* Portland, OR: Timber Press, 1998.

Parler, Mary Celestia, and University Student Contributors. *Folk Beliefs from Arkansas.* 15 vols. Fayetteville: University of Arkansas, 1962.

Pickard, Madge E., and R. Carlyle Buley. *The Midwest Pioneer, His Ills, Cures and Doctors.* Crawfordsville, IN: R. E. Banta, 1945.

Quelch, Mary Thorne. *Herbs for Daily Use.* London: Faber, 1941.

Ray, John. *Catalogus Plantarum Angliae, et Insularum Adjacentium.* London: John Martyn, 1670.

Taylor, Mark R. "Norfolk Folklore." *Folk-Lore* 40 (1929): 113–133.

Vickery, Roy. *A Dictionary of Plant Lore.* Oxford: Oxford University Press, 1995.

Vogel, Virgil J. *American Indian Medicine.* Norman: University of Oklahoma Press, 1970.

# Seventh son

In traditional healing the seventh son, or, better still, the seventh son of a seventh son, was often credited with powers of healing. The origin of this tradition is unclear, but it appeared in England during the sixteenth century and was common during the seventeenth century. When such an individual claimed to cure scrofula, also known as the "king's evil," he was seen as a threat to the monopoly of the king in this respect and was liable to punishment (Thomas 1973: 237). Sometimes such power was seen as a threat to the church, as in the case of a seventh son who claimed to cure the deaf, blind, and lame, and was investigated in 1607 by the bishop of London (Thomas 1973: 239). In the Celtic tradition there are many documented examples of a seventh son believed to have special healing powers (Napier 1879: 90). In some parts of Ireland and Scotland, a seventh daughter was credited with similar powers.

Scrofula in particular was often treated by a seventh child; in Caithness and Sutherland, a seventh daughter treated a man for scrofula, a seventh son treated a woman. The seventh son of a seventh son was particularly gifted and thought to be able to cure many diseases. In Ireland a famous healer, Finbarr Nolan, based his claims upon being the seventh son of a seventh son. Such a claim could be tested by putting an earthworm on the palm of the hand. If the claimant was genuine, the worm would die immediately (Beith 1995: 93, 188). It has been suggested that the seventh son in Scotland should have worms put into his hand before baptism, to confirm his healing powers. In Ireland, such a child was rubbed, before baptism, with an object that he would in future use to heal with—a silver coin, or a piece of his father's hair. This object had then to be worn by his parents throughout his life (Black 1883: 136).

Sometimes the healer gave the patient a coin with a hole through it, which must then be worn by the patient throughout his life (Henderson 1879: 306). Although scrofula was the commonest disease to be treated by a seventh child, sometimes thrush was cured too. The healer blew three times into the sufferer's mouth (Jones 1908: 315–319). In the twentieth century in Cavan, Ireland, sore throat was still being healed by a seventh son (Westropp 1911: 57).

These same beliefs appear in North American folk medicine. A seventh son was believed to have the power to heal (Brown 1952–1964, 6: 38). A seventh son of a seventh son was able to cure warts, burns, bleeding and other conditions (Rayburn 1941: 162), and the seventh daughter of a seventh daughter was believed to have second sight (Puckett 1981: 1049). From Pennsylvania there is a report of the hair of a seventh son preventing whooping cough (Phillips 1892: 248). Goiter could be cured by the touch of the seventh son of a seventh son (Brown 1952–1964, 6: 201). Bleeding could be stopped by a seventh son (Brown 1952–1964, 6: 212). Thrush was cured, as in Britain, by a seventh son blowing into the patient's mouth (Lassiter 1947: 32).

The belief in the healing powers of a seventh son is to be found among Native Americans too. Among the Cherokee a seventh son is regarded as a prophet, with the power of healing by touch (Bourke 1892: 457).

*See also* **Bleeding, Burns, Sore throat, Tuberculosis, Warts, Whooping cough.**

### References
Beith, Mary. *Healing Threads: Traditional Medicines of the Highlands and Islands.* Edinburgh: Polygon, 1995.
Black, William George. *Folk-Medicine: A Chapter in the History of Culture.* London: Folklore Society, 1883.

Bourke, John G. *Medicine Men of the Apache.* Ninth Annual Report of the Bureau of Ethnology, 1887–1888. Washington, DC: 1892, 443–603.

Brown, Frank C. *Collection of North Carolina Folklore.* 7 vols. Durham, NC: Duke University Press, 1952–1964.

Henderson, William. *Notes of the Folk-Lore of the Northern Counties of England and the Borders.* London: Folklore Society, 1879.

Jones, B. H. "Folk-Medicine." *Folk-Lore* 19 (1908): 315–319.

Lassiter, W. R. "Why I'm an Old Bachelor." *Tennessee Folklore Society Bulletin* 13 (1947): 27–35.

Napier, James. *Folk Lore or Superstitious Beliefs in the West of Scotland within this Century.* Paisley: 1879.

Phillips, Henry, Jr. "Second Contribution to the Study of Folk-Lore in Philadelphia and Vicinity." *Proceedings of the American Philosophical Society* 31 (1892): 246–249.

Puckett, Newbell Niles. *Popular Beliefs and Superstitions: A Compendium of American Folklore from the Ohio Collection of Newbell Niles Puckett.* Edited by Wayland D. Hand, Anna Casetta, and Sondra B. Thiederman. 3 vols. Boston: G. K. Hall, 1981.

Rayburn, Otto Ernest. *Ozark Country.* New York: Duell, Sloan, and Pearce, 1941.

Thomas, Keith. *Religion and the Decline of Magic.* Penguin University Books, 1973.

Westropp, Thomas. "A Folklore Survey of County Clare." *Folk-Lore* 22 (1911): 49–60.

# Shakers

Founded in 1746 by immigrants from Manchester, England, this community, like other groups of colonists, was forced by not only the scarcity of official medical aid but also their own creed of self-sufficiency to be largely self-reliant for medical treatment. They brought with them their own knowledge of herbs but in their new home encountered many medicinal plants that were unknown to them. The detailed records that they kept show that they not only learned from Native American Indians about the uses of some of these but employed local Indians to gather the herbs for which they became famous. A large and profitable industry in the production of herbs, seeds, and herbal preparations was built up by the Shaker communities and finally ended in only 1947. Their products supplied the pharmaceutical trade all over North America and were eventually distributed worldwide. They had self-appointed "doctors" within their communities, some of whom, like "Doctor" Barnabas Hinkley (1808–1861), went on to train as recognized orthodox medical practitioners (Miller 1998: 35). The school of herbalism that the Shaker physicians followed was that of Eclectics. The Shakers illustrate the impossibility of defining the boundaries between folk medicine and orthodoxy: their materia medica was virtually indistinguishable from that of the recognized and officially qualified doctors of the day.

**Reference**

Miller, Amy Bess. *Shaker Medicinal Herbs: A Compendium of History, Lore and Uses.* Pownal: Storey Books, 1998.

# Shingles

This painful affliction has attracted diverse remedies in British folk medicine. In the Isle of Wight an ointment was made from the verdigris scraped off church bells (Prince 1991: 100). In Dorset, the source of the verdigris was the pump (Udal 1922: 220). In the seventeenth century, the blood of a cat was recommended for shingles (Newman 1948: 135). Blood taken from the tail of a black cat was a cure in Ireland (Black 1883: 116). On the island of Lewis, in the Scottish Highlands, the blood of a black cock was recommended, or the blood of a person named Munro (Beith 1995: 166). In Devon, the leaves of the blackberry were applied as a soothing poultice (Lafont 1984: 17). In the Scottish Highlands, the juice of the houseleek was particularly recommended for shingles (Beith 1995: 224). The same plant was used similarly in Essex (Taylor MSS). In Wales, stonecrop *(Sedum acre)* has been used within living memory in the treatment of shingles. Another Welsh cure for shingles is egg yolk and linseed oil (Jones 1980: 59). In Gloucestershire, wheat has been used in shingles treatment (Burne 1911: 238). Dried primrose leaves *(Primula vulgaris)* soaked in sweet oil are a remedy from East Anglia (Taylor 1929: 116).

A nineteenth-century example of transference of shingles comes from Hartland, in Devon. The patient was taken to running water, where seven rushes were picked and stroked across the shingles. The rushes were then thrown into the river. The process was repeated three mornings in succession (Lafont 1984: 74).

There is a widespread belief that if the rash of shingles reaches right around the body, the patient will die (Thiselton Dyer 1878: 147).

Sometimes individuals were credited with the power to heal shingles. In Wales, it was believed that a person who had eaten the flesh of an eagle had this ability, and so did his descendants (Jones 1980: 67).

In New England, the blood of a completely black hen was said to be a cure for shingles (Black 1883: 117), and this cure and variants on it appear frequently in North American folk medicine. A variation from Illinois is to split open a black hawk and lay it on the affected area. This remedy is said to be Native American in origin. In Adams County (Illinois) the skin of a snake wrapped around the sufferer has also been used to relieve shingles (Hyatt 1965: 240). The blood of a black cat is a frequently recorded remedy for shingles (see, for example, Roberts 1927: 167). Wearing a cord around the waist with either seven or nine knots in it is a remedy collected in Ohio. Another from the same region is to make a cross on the shingles with moistened mud from a dirt dauber's nest (Puckett 1981: 439). In Newfoundland, a child with shingles was passed under the belly of a jackass to cure shingles, another example of transference (Patterson 1897: 215). Some individuals in Nova Scotia were credited with the power to "charm" shingles (Creighton 1968: 212). In North America, as in Britain, there was a belief that if the shingles encompassed the body completely, the patient would die (Browne 1958: 93). One way to prevent this was to wear an eelskin around the waist (UCLA Folklore Archives 22_7597).

Substances topically applied to shingles include gunpowder (Hendricks 1980: 96) and black ink (Browne 1958: 93). Oat straw fried in lard has been drunk for shingles and applied to the rash (always with a circular motion, to avoid the blisters closing up inside, which would mean death) (Hyatt 1965: 240). As in England's Gloucestershire, wheat has been used to treat shingles. A poultice of burned wheat straw has been used in Alabama (Browne 1958: 93). Cotton wool soaked in castor oil (Puckett 1981: 439), ashes of a hickory log applied (Brown 1952–1964, 6: 273), and a salve of cranberries and sulphur or of currants (Puckett 1981: 439) are other applications that have been used to treat shingles. Drawing a circle around the affected area with the juice from an old pipe stem is claimed to prevent them from spreading and with bringing about a cure (Hyatt 1965: 240). Asafoetida *(Ferula* sp.) and whisky taken internally has been used (Puckett 1981: 439). Finally, wearing a string soaked in turpentine around the neck will reputedly prevent the wearer from getting shingles (Puckett 1981: 439).

*See also* **Blackberry, Houseleek, Poultice, Transference.**

## References

Beith, Mary. *Healing Threads: Traditional Medicines of the Highlands and Islands.* Edinburgh: Polygon, 1995.

Black, William George. *Folk-Medicine: A Chapter in the History of Culture.* London: Folklore Society, 1883.

Brown, Frank C. *Collection of North Carolina Folklore.* 7 vols. Durham, NC: Duke University Press, 1952–1964.

Browne, Ray B. *Popular Beliefs and Practices from Alabama.* Folklore Studies 9. Berkeley and Los Angeles: University of California Publications, 1958.

Burne, Margaret. "Parish Gleanings from Upton St. Leonard's, Gloucestershire." *Folk-Lore* 22 (1911), 236–239.

Creighton, Helen. *Bluenose Magic, Popular Beliefs and Superstitions in Nova Scotia.* Toronto: Ryerson Press, 1968.

Hendricks, George D. *Roosters Rhymes and Railroad Tracks: A Second Sampling of Superstitions and Popular Beliefs in Texas.* Dallas, TX: Southern Methodist University Press, 1980.

Hyatt, Harry Middleton. *Folklore from Adams County Illinois.* 2nd rev. ed. New York: Memoirs of the Alma Egan Hyatt Foundation, 1965.

Jones, Anne E. "Folk Medicine in Living Memory in Wales." *Folk Life* 18 (1980): 58–68.

Lafont, Anne-Marie. *Herbal Folklore.* Bideford: Badger Books, 1984.

Newman, Leslie F. "Some Notes on the Pharmacology and Therapeutic Value of Folk-Medicine." *Folk-Lore* 59 (1948): 118–135.

Patterson, George. "Folk-Lore in Newfoundland." *Journal of American Folklore* 10 (1897): 214–215.

Prince, Dennis. *Grandmother's Cures: An A–Z of Herbal Remedies.* London: Fontana, 1991.

Puckett, Newbell Niles. *Popular Beliefs and Superstitions: A Compendium of American Folklore from the Ohio Collection of Newbell Niles Puckett.* Edited by Wayland D. Hand, Anna Casetta, and Sondra B. Thiederman. 3 vols. Boston: G. K. Hall, 1981.

Roberts, Hilda. "Louisiana Superstitions." *Journal of American Folklore* 40 (1927): 144–208.

Robertson, Marion. *Old Settlers' Remedies.* Barrington, NS: Cape Sable Historical Society, 1960.

Taylor, Mark R. Manuscript notes in Norfolk Records Office, Norwich MS4322.

Taylor, Mark R. "Norfolk Folk Lore." *Folk-Lore* 40 (1929).

Thiselton Dyer, T. F. *English Folk-Lore.* London: Hardwicke and Bogue, 1878.

Udal, John Symonds. *Dorsetshire Folk-Lore.* Hartford (privately published), 1922.

# Silverweed (*Potentilla anserina*)

In British folk medicine, this plant has been used consistently over a number of centuries for two principal uses. As a cosmetic, it was reported in use in the sixteenth century by Pena and De l'Obel (Pena and De l'Obel 1571), and it was still used to remove freckles and suntan in the Highlands in the nineteenth century (Pratt 1857, 1: 32). Traditionally, according to Black, the silverweed should be steeped for nine days in buttermilk (Black 1883: 119). It was used specifically to treat the scars of smallpox in Leicestershire (Friend 1883–1884, 2: 371). Its second major use was to relieve soreness of the feet. Reputedly used by the Roman soldiers on long marches, its leaves were later placed in the shoes of pilgrims and of eighteenth-century carriers (Deering 1738: 162). This custom persisted among schoolboys in Yorkshire into the nineteenth century (Allen and Hatfield, in press), and in East Anglia it has been used within living memory (Newman 1945; Hatfield MS). The Irish uses of the plant have been different. Here it has been used to treat diarrhea, bleeding piles (Moore MS), and heart troubles (Gregory 1920).

Though the plant is native in North America too, it does not appear to have been widely used there in folk medicine.

Other species of *Potentilla*, such as *P. canadensis*, seem to have been used instead. There is an eighteenth-century record of the use of an infusion of *Potentilla erecta* or *Potentilla canadensis* to treat fever (Meyer 1985: 127). During the nineteenth century, various species of *Potentilla* were used in domestic medicine for treating diarrhea (Crellin and Philpott 1990: 212). In Native American practice, various *Potentilla* species have been used, especially in the treatment of diarrhea (Moerman 1998: 435).

*See also* **Diarrhea, Heart trouble, Piles, Smallpox, Sore feet.**

### References

Allen, David E., and Gabrielle Hatfield. *Medicinal Plants in Folk Tradition*. Portland, OR: Timber Press, in press.

Black, William George. *Folk-Medicine: A Chapter in the History of Culture*. Folklore Society, London, 1883.

Crellin, John K., and Jane Philpott. *A Reference Guide to Medicinal Plants*. Durham, NC: Duke University Press, 1990.

Deering, G. C. *Catalogus Stirpium; or a catalogue of plants.. more especially about Nottingham*. Nottingham: privately published, 1738.

Friend, Hilderic. *Flowers and Flower Lore*. 2 vols. London: Swan Sonnenschein, 1883–1884.

Gregory, (Isabella Augusta), Lady. *Visions and Beliefs in the West of Ireland*. First Series. New York and London: Putnam, 1920.

Meyer, Clarence. *American Folk Medicine*. Glenwood, IL: Meyerbooks, 1985.

Moerman, Daniel E. *Native American Ethnobotany*. Portland, OR: Timber Press, 1998.

Moore MS. *Botany of the County of Londonderry 1834–1835*. Unpublished report produced by David Moore for the Irish Ordnance Survey. Herbarium Library, National Botanic Gardens, Dublin.

Newman, Leslie F. "Some Notes on Folk Medicine in the Eastern Counties." *Folk-Lore* 56 (1945): 349–360.

Pena, Pierre, and De l'Obel, Mathias. *Stirpium Adversaria Nova*. London: Thomas Purefoy, 1571.

Pratt, Anne. *Wild Flowers*. London: Society for Promoting Christian Knowledge, 1857.

# Skull

The human skull, unsurprisingly, has held symbolic significance in folk medicine, but in addition it has been used as a physical remedy, in both official (Salmon 1693: 290) and folk medicine. A much-quoted story from a small town in Wales concerned a miner's wife in the mid-nineteenth century who asked a local sexton for a small portion of human skull, which was then powdered and given for epilepsy (Grendon 1909: 123). In Scotland, where the same remedy was used, it was stipulated that the skull should be that of a man for treating a female patient, and vice versa (Black 1883: 96). Part of an epilepsy cure from the Scottish Highlands involved the patient's drinking water from a human skull (Beith 1995: 101). Elsewhere in Scotland, drinking from a suicide's skull was particularly recommended for epilepsy and for insanity. Grated skull was also ingested, as in Wales (Beith 1995: 183). A tooth from a dead man's mouth was sometimes worn as an amulet against toothache (Black 1883: 98).

In North American folk medicine an amulet of a piece of human skull was worn against epilepsy (Brown 1952–1964, 6: 178). The "distillate" of a human skull was used in the past to produce a sweat (Brown 1952–1964, 6: 298). Among the Native American Nooka, scrapings from inside a skull were used as a contraceptive (Peacock 1896: 277).

*See also* **Amulet, Epilepsy, Moss, Toothache.**

### References

Beith, Mary. *Healing Threads: Traditional Medicines of the Highlands and Islands*. Edinburgh: Polygon, 1995.

Black, William George. *Folk-Medicine: A Chap-*

ter in the History of Culture. London: Folk-lore Society, 1883.

Brown, Frank C. Collection of North Carolina Folklore. 7 vols. Durham, North Carolina: Duke University Press, 1952–1964.

Grendon, Felix. "The Anglo-Saxon Charms." Journal of American Folklore 22 (1909): 105–237.

Peacock, Mabel. "Executed Criminals and Folk Medicine." Folk-Lore 7 (1896): 268–283.

Salmon, William. The Compleat English Physician. London, 1693.

# Sleeplessness

A variety of native plants were used in British folk medicine to treat insomnia, including agrimony (Agrimonia eupatoria). This was said to be so effective that if the sufferer put a sprig under the pillow, he would sleep until it was removed! (Souter 1995: 172). In Scotland, chickweed tea was taken for insomnia (Beith 1995: 211), while cowslip is used in Devon (Lafont 1984: 29) as well as in Ireland (see, for example, Moloney 1910: 32). In the Highlands of Scotland, heather (Calluna vulgaris) was recommended as bedding to ensure a good sleep. It was also used as a poultice for the head and drunk as an infusion to counter insomnia (Beith 1995: 222). Syrup of white poppies was widely used and abused for procuring oblivion, and laudanum was so cheap in Victorian Britain that every household had access to it. The milder and nonaddictive native red poppy was also used as a gentler alternative in East Anglia. Hops were also thought to be helpful in ensuring a good sleep (Vesey-Fitzgerald 1944: 25). The commonest method of use was to fill a pillow with dried hops; such pillows are, of course, still available in health food shops.

Dietary advice in both Britain and North America included having a light supper, having a milky drink before retiring, eating bananas, or roasted apple, and eating honey (Jarvis 1961: 105). Onions were recommended too, and even rubbing the soles of a child's feet with garlic has been suggested (Meyer 1985: 145). Pumpkin (Cucurbita sp.) was thought to help sleep. Lettuce (Lactuca sativa) (both wild and cultivated) and chamomile were used in orthodox Western medicine and in herbalism to promote sleep, but their inclusion in Beatrix Potter's The Tale of the Flopsy Bunnies has enshrined them in the annals of folk medicine. Here, as is so often the case, it is hard or impossible to draw a clear distinction between folk and official remedies. The water from boiled lettuces was used in recent times to procure sleep in Essex, where saffron tea (Crocus sativus) was also used (E.M., Barking Essex, 1985, pers. com.).

As in Europe, hops were used to aid sleep by settlers in North America as well as by Native Americans. Sleeping on a hop-filled pillow is still recommended in folk medicine. A tea made from catnip is also recommended. For a sleepless baby, onion juice is suggested (Browne 1958: 22, 93, 94). A preparation of the roots of purple boneset is another recommendation (Long 1962: 3). The root of species of Lady's slipper (Cypripedium acaule, C. pubescens) was used as a sedative by the Indians, and early settlers named it "American valerian." The yellow lady's slipper occurs throughout Europe as well as in North America, but its use as a sedative seems to have been learned by Europeans from the Native Americans. Valerian (Valeriana officinalis), on the other hand, was originally a Western sedative, praised in the herbals, and introduced and now naturalized in North America. In Britain it is used for insomnia in herbalist practice (Chevallier 1996: 146), but not in folk medicine, which has found other uses for the plant. In North America valerian has been adopted by folk medicine for a number of uses, but in Meyer's book, for example, the only instance of its use for insomnia is quoted from a physician's recommendation (Meyer 1985: 146). The opium poppy was used by the Cherokee to promote sleep (Hamel and Chiltoskey 1975: 50).

Miscellaneous advice for treating insomnia includes taking a glass of hot water (Gruber 1894) and putting a pan of water (Frazier 1936: 35) or salt (Hyatt 1965: 270) under the bed. Keeping a bedroom window open is another suggestion. The tooth of a dead dog or a dead jackal is said to be a cure for sleeplessness (Puckett 1981: 292).

The idea of counting sheep to help one to fall asleep is a widespread one, and all kinds of other repetitive mental activities have been suggested. Lullabies, with their simple repetitive tunes and words, fall into this category too.

*See also* **Apple, Boneset, Catnip, Chamomile, Chickweed, Cowslip, Garlic, Honey, Hops, Onion, Poppy, Poultice, Valerian.**

### References

Beith, Mary. *Healing Threads: Traditional Medicines of the Highlands and Islands.* Edinburgh: Polygon, 1995.

Browne, Ray B. *Popular Beliefs and Practices from Alabama.* Folklore Studies 9. Berkeley and Los Angeles: University of California Publications, 1958.

Chevallier, Andrew. *The Encyclopedia of Medicinal Plants.* London: Dorling Kindersley, 1996.

Frazier, Neal. "A Collection of Middle Tennessee Superstitions." *Tennessee Folklore Society Bulletin* 2 (1936): 33–48.

Gruber, John. *Hagerstown Town and Country Almanac.* Hagerstown, MD: John Gruber, 1852–1914.

Hamel, Paul B., and Mary U. Chiltoskey. *Cherokee Plants and Their Uses: A 400 Year History.* Sylva, NC: Herald, 1975.

Hyatt, Harry Middleton. *Folklore from Adams County Illinois.* 2nd rev. ed. New York: Memoirs of the Alma Egan Hyatt Foundation, 1965.

Jarvis, D. C. *Folk Medicine.* London: Pan Books, 1961.

Lafont, Anne-Marie. *Herbal Folklore.* Bideford: Badger Books, 1984.

Long, Grady M. "Folk Medicine in McMinn, Polk, Bradley and Meigs Counties, Tennessee 1910–1927." *Tennessee Folklore Society Bulletin* 28 (1962): 1–8.

Meyer, Clarence. *American Folk Medicine.* Glenwood, IL: Meyerbooks, 1985.

Moloney, M. F. *Irish Ethnobotany.* Dublin: M. H. Gill, 1910.

Parler, Mary Celestia, and University Student Contributors. *Folk Beliefs from Arkansas.* 15 vols. Fayetteville: University of Arkansas, 1962.

Potter, Beatrix. *The Tale of the Flopsy Bunnies.* Frederick Warne, reissue edition 1987.

Puckett, Newbell Niles. *Popular Beliefs and Superstitions: A Compendium of American Folklore from the Ohio Collection of Newbell Niles Puckett.* Edited by Wayland D. Hand, Anna Casetta, and Sondra B. Thiederman. 3 vols. Boston: G. K. Hall, 1981.

Souter, Keith. *Cure Craft: Traditional Folk Remedies and Treatment from Antiquity to the Present Day.* Saffron Walden: C. W. Daniel, 1995.

Vesey-Fitzgerald, B. "Gypsy Medicine." *Journal of the Gypsy Lore Society* 23 (1944): 21–33.

## Smallpox

The disease was known early in ancient India and China, but it does not seem to have reached Europe until the sixteenth century. For Europeans the illness, though serious, was not always fatal, and those who survived it presumably passed on a degree of immunity to their children. Little information seems to be available concerning folk treatments for smallpox. This may indicate that in domestic medicine, as in the best of orthodox practice, survival depended more on good nursing and good luck, than on any specific treatment. In seventeenth-century England, a pupil of Sydenham was fortunate to be nursed through the disease by his master, to whom he clearly felt he owed his survival (Nixon 1941, 2: 774). Both John Wesley, in his book *Primitive Physic,* and William Buchan in his *Domestic Medicine* recommend a light diet, with milk (or milk and water) to drink, apples to eat, and fresh air in the patient's room.

In Britain, smallpox epidemics were particularly prevalent in the seventeenth and eighteenth centuries. Even those wealthy enough to turn to physicians for advice sometimes chose domestic medicine instead. In Scotland, Lady Clerk of Penicuik wrote to her husband in 1699 telling him that their son Jamie had smallpox. She had given him marigold posset *(Calendula officinalis)* to drink and sent for some saffron *(Crocus sativus),* which she would bind about his neck to prevent the soreness, and also give him as medicine (SRO GD18/5219). These items would have been too expensive for most people to afford, unlike the boiled sheep's droppings used in the Highlands of Scotland or the mice or the potion made from otter's skin (Beith 1995: 173, 179, 180). Wood lice in a small bag were used as a "charm" against smallpox up to the nineteenth century (Brown 1951: 337). Ground cinders of toads were administered for smallpox in the nineteenth century (N & Q 1849: 426). The green hellebore *(Helleborus viridis)* apparently had a reputation as a prophylactic against smallpox. This is mentioned by Gerard in his herbal, but whether it was used in folk practice is unknown. In the eighteenth century, an infusion of vetch seeds *(Vicia sativa)* was used to treat smallpox (Lightfoot 1777: 396).

Those who did survive smallpox were often left disfigured, and kitchen books and medical books alike contain numerous recipes for ointments to heal the scarring. To what extent these were actually used in folk medicine is unknown. One plant that was used in folk medicine to heal the scarring of smallpox is silverweed (Friend 1884, 2: 371). An East Anglian smallpox remedy that has survived up to recent times is to

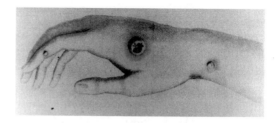

The real breakthrough in controlling smallpox nationally came when Jenner discovered the practice of vaccinating with cow pox which was practiced in folk medicine in rural Gloucestershire. Jenner's interest and hard work ultimately led to the adoption of a vaccination in Britain. Pictured here is the hand Jenner used as a source of his vaccine. (National Library of Medicine)

put an apple beside the bed. The spots will be transferred to the apple, which is then buried (Mundford 1980).

The story of vaccination against smallpox is a curious blend of folk and orthodox medicine. We know that inoculation (deliberately introducing a small dose of the disease) was practiced in ancient China and in India in the fifth century. During the early eighteenth century Lady Mary Montagu was responsible for introducing the practice from Turkey to Britain, although there is evidence that the practice of giving a "kindly pock" was already in use in part of the Highlands of Scotland (Kennedy 1715). The real breakthrough in controlling the disease nationally came when Jenner discovered the practice of vaccinating with cow pox as practiced in folk medicine in rural Gloucestershire. His interest and hard work ultimately led to the adoption of vaccination in Britain (Guthrie 1945: 248).

Smallpox reached the New World during the sixteenth century, when it was brought to the Caribbean and spread with devastating results throughout South and later North America. Waves of the disease arrived with settlers throughout the sixteenth and seventeenth centuries, and the Native Americans died in thousands, evidently having no natural resistance to the disease. Though not quite so devastating for Europeans, it nevertheless caused thousands of deaths among them as well.

In North American folk medicine there were several prophylactic remedies against smallpox. Onion (Brown 1952–1964, 6: 275), garlic (Brendle and Unger 1935: 97), or asafoetida (*Ferula* sp.) (Brown 1952–1964, 6: 275) were carried as amulets. Wearing a necklace of three kidney beans (UCLA Folklore Archive 5_5472) or of rattlesnake rattles (Cannon 1984: 122) was another protective measure. Cutting off the tongue of a heifer, rubbing the smallpox sores with the still-warm tongue, throwing it over the head three times, and finally giving it to a black cat to eat is a remedy that is an example of transference, and one that smacks of desperation (Brown 1952–1964, 6: 275).

There were some practical measures adopted by folk medicine for treating smallpox. Saltpeter and brandy were recommended, as was cream of tartar (Hendricks 1980: 97). An alternative was a steam bath followed by jumping into ice cold water (Brown 1952–1964, 6: 275). Skunk oil rubbed on was another suggestion (Stout 1936: 184). Buzzard grease was said to be a cure (Puckett 1926: 389). As in Scotland, a tea made from sheep manure was used (Cannon 1984: 122). The blood of a black dog was recommended (Randolph 1933: 4).

Plant remedies used to treat smallpox include a tea made from pokeberry leaves (Pickard and Buley 1945: 41), an ointment made from alder bark (Lick and Brendle 1922: 234), a preparation of foxglove (Gruber 1881: 15), watermelon juice *(Citrullus lanatus)* (Hendricks 1966: 52), and a drink made from barley (*Hordeum* sp.) and pumpkin (*Cucurbita* sp.) stem (Bourke 1894). A salve made from yarrow and tallow was also used (Long 1962: 5). Mormon midwives used a mixture of cornmeal gruel and whisky, which was applied with a feather (Noall 1944: 112). Among slaves, two remedies used were black pepper tea and cornshuck tea (Saxon 1945: 248).

There were a number of remedies used for treating or preventing the scars of smallpox. These include sweet oil and lemon juice (Brown 1952–1964, 6: 275) and a salve made from golden seal (Long 1962: 3). Rue (*Ruta* sp.) hung around the neck was thought to prevent damage to the eyes from smallpox (Brendle and Unger 1935: 97). In New Mexico an infusion of logwood (*Haemotoxylon* sp.) was used (Curtin 1930: 195).

The introduction of smallpox to the Native Americans proved so devastating that in seventeenth-century New England the settlers were able to take over empty Indian farms, whose owners had all died of smallpox (Johnson 1997: 31). Gumweed (*Grindelia* spp.) was apparently used by the Nevada Indians during smallpox epidemics (Willard 1992: 215). Other plants used by the Native Americans to treat the disease include a mixture of princess pine (*Chimaphila* sp.), black cherry *(Prunus serotina)*, and wild turnip *(Brassica napus)* (Wallis 1922: 29). Snakeroot *(Aristolochia serpentaria)* was also used (Vogel 1970: 51), as was an infusion of the stems and leaves of rabbitbrush (*Chrysothamnus* sp.) (Welch 1964: 88). However, even the extensive herbal knowledge of the Indians was inadequate in the face of this invading illness.

There is evidence that inoculation was practiced in folk medicine in Africa and that knowledge of it was brought by the slaves to North America (Farmer 1958: 600). After a century of controversy surrounding both inoculation and vaccination, the latter was finally approved by orthodox medicine. The first North Americans to be vaccinated were in fact slaves, and it was not until early in the nineteenth century that a program of vaccination among the white population began (Bassett 1940: 18).

*See also* **Alder, Amulet, Apple, Corn, Foxglove, Garlic, Golden seal, Onion, Poke, Silverweed, Transference, Yarrow.**

## References

Bassett, Victor H. "Plantation Medicine." *Journal of the Medical Association of Georgia* 29 (1940): 112–122.

Beith, Mary. *Healing Threads: Traditional Medicines of the Highlands and Islands.* Edinburgh: Polygon, 1995.

Bourke, John G. "Popular Medicine, Customs and Superstitions of the Rio Grande." *Journal of American Folklore* 7 (1894): 119–146.

Brendle, Thomas R., and Claude W. Unger. "Folk Medicine of the Pennsylvania Germans: The Non-Occult Cures." *Proceedings of the Pennsylvania German Society* 45 (1935).

Brown, Frank C. *Collection of North Carolina Folklore.* 7 vols. Durham, NC: Duke University Press, 1952–1964.

Brown, P. W. F. "Correspondence: Another Variation of Lucky Pig Charm." *Folk-Lore* 62 (1951): 337.

Buchan, William. *Domestic Medicine.* Edinburgh, 1769.

Cannon, Anthon S. *Popular Beliefs and Superstitions from Utah.* Edited by Wayland D. Hand and Jeannine E. Talley. Salt Lake City: University of Utah Press, 1984.

Curtin, L. S. M. "Pioneer Medicine in New Mexico." *Folk-Say* (1930): 186–196.

Farmer, Laurence. "The Smallpox Inoculation Controversy and the Boston Press 1721–1722." *Bulletin of the New York Academy of Medicine* 34(9) (1958): 599–608.

Friend, Hilderic. *Flowers and Flower Lore.* 2 vols. London: Swan Sonnenschein, 1884.

Gerard, John. *The Herball or Generall Historie of Plantes.* London: John Norton, 1597.

Gruber, John. *Hagerstown Town and Country Almanac.* 1852–1914.

Guthrie, Douglas. *A History of Medicine.* London: Thomas Nelson, 1945.

Hendricks, George D. *Mirrors, Mice and Mustaches: A Sampling of Superstitions and Popular Beliefs in Texas.* Austin: Texas Folklore Society, 1966.

Hendricks, George D. *Roosters, Rhymes and Railroad Tracks: A Second Sampling of Superstitions and Popular Beliefs in Texas.* Dallas, TX: Southern Methodist University Press, 1980.

Johnson, Paul. *A History of the American People.* London: Weidenfeld and Nicolson, 1997.

Kennedy, P. *Essay on External Remedies.* 1715. Quoted in H. G. Tait, *Edinburgh Medical Journal* 58 (1951): 182.

Lick, David E., and Thomas R. Brendle. "Plant Names and Plant Lore among the Pennsylvania Germans." *Proceedings and Addresses of the Pennsylvania German Society* 33 (1922).

Lightfoot, John. *Flora Scotica.* 2 vols. London: Benjamin White, 1777.

Long, Grady M. "Folk Medicine in McMinn, Polk, Bradley and Meigs Counties, Tennessee, 1910–1927." *Tennessee Folklore Society Bulletin* 28 (1962): 1–8.

Mundford Primary School Project, Norfolk, 1980, unpublished.

N&Q Notes and Queries, London.

Nixon, J. A. "Salt-Water Surgeons." *Lancet* 2 (1941): 774.

Noall, Claire. "Superstitions, Customs and Prescriptions of Mormon Midwives." *California Folklore Quarterly* 3 (1944): 102–144.

Pickard, Madge E., and R. Carlyle Buley. *The Midwest Pioneer, His Ills, Cures and Doctors.* Crawfordsville, IN: R. E. Banta, 1945.

Puckett, Newbell Niles. *Folk Beliefs of the Southern Negro.* Chapel Hill, NC: Greenwood Press, 1926.

Randolph, Vance. "Ozark Superstitions." *Journal of American Folklore* 46 (1933): 1–21.

Saxon, Lyle. *Gumbo Ya-Ya.* Boston: Houghton Mifflin, 1945.

SRO. Scottish Record Office, Edinburgh.

Stout, Earl J. "Folklore from Iowa." *Memoirs of the American Folklore Society* 29 (1936).

Vogel, Virgil J. *American Indian Medicine.* Norman: University of Oklahoma Press, 1970.

Wallis, Wilson D. "Medicines Used by the MicMac Indians." *American Anthropologist* 24 (1922): 24–30.

Welch, Charles E., Jr. "Some Drugs of the North American Indian: Then and Now." *Keystone Folklore Quarterly* 9(3) (1964): 83–99.

Wesley, John. *Primitive Physic.* London, 1755.
Willard, Terry. *Edible and Medicinal Plants of the Rocky Mountains and Neighbouring Territories.* Calgary, ALTA: Wild Rose College of Natural Healing, 1992.

# Snail

The snail was a recognized part of the official English materia medica, used especially to treat consumption (see, for example, Salmon 1693: 693). This recipe was also used in domestic medicine. Nathan Coward, of Dersingham, in Norfolk, England, writing in 1778, records how a broth made from "dodmans" (Norfolk word for snails) removed from their shells cured his wife when doctors had failed. The recipe had been given to him by his grandmother, Tabitha (Coward 1800: 24). The reputation of snail broth for treating consumption survived in England at least into the twentieth century (Taylor 1929: 115). "Disguised with herbs and other condiments," it was said to be not unpalatable (Gerish 1920). In the mid-twentieth century there is a record of a woman, then aged seventy-four, who remembered from her childhood a longshoreman of Weymouth harbor who had been cured of consumption by a diet of snails (EFS Record Number 342).

In folk medicine, snail slime also had a reputation for helping straighten deformed limbs in children (Prince 1991: 104). To strengthen the spine, it was recommended to rub with grey snails (Addy 1893: 91). Froth from a pricked snail was a Worcestershire cure for earache (Black 1883: 158), and it was used similarly in Ireland (Logan 1972: 34). Swallowing live snails was recommended for asthma in Yorkshire (Rolleston 1944: 8). In Somerset, raw limpets and snails were recommended for bronchitis (Tongue 1965: 37). An eighteenth-century cure for a cough was snails boiled in barley water (Black 1883: 157). Snail

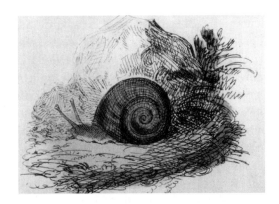

The snail was a recognized part of the official English Materia Medica, used especially to treat consumption. In folk medicine, snail slime also had a reputation for helping straighten children's deformed limbs, and in Yorkshire, swallowing live snails was recommended for asthma. (National Library of Medicine)

slime mixed with brown sugar was a recommendation for whooping cough (Radford and Radford 1974: 312). In Sussex, snail juice as a cough remedy survived into the twentieth century (Allen 1995: 150). In Scotland, snails figured in a wide variety of folk remedies, for treating rheumatism, rickets, cold sores and swellings (especially tubercular tumors) (Beith 1995: 185). Snails have frequently been used, within living memory, throughout Britain to treat warts; the snail was encouraged to walk over the wart and was then impaled on a thorn; as it withered, so the wart disappeared.

In North American folk medicine, the commonest ailments treated with snails are consumption (Brown 1952–1964, 6: 159) and warts (see, for example, Wintemberg 1918: 127). Various other ailments have been treated with snails. Snail slime has been rubbed on thrush (Puckett 1981: 118) and on erysipelas (Foster 1953: 212). Cooked snails soaked in raisin wine have been applied as a poultice for a sore throat (UCLA Folklore Archive 4_2615). A snail's head has been wrapped and worn on the neck to treat headache (UCLA Folklore Archive 11_1907). Ashes of snail shells have treated a sore scalp (UCLA Folklore Archive 10_2611) and, mixed with honey, have been used on sore gums (UCLA Folklore Archive 2_1875). For rheumatism, an amulet consisting of a snail soaked in vinegar and rolled in meal has been worn around the neck (Puckett 1926: 362). Snails and their shells, ground up and warmed, have been applied to neck swelling (UCLA Folklore Archive 1_2236). For dizziness, it has been recommended to eat large ground-up snails, warmed (UCLA Folklore Archive 1_1481).

In the Native American tradition, snails have also been used in healing. Among the Kwakiutl, a snail has been placed in the throat for tonsillitis and diphtheria. A poultice of snail bodies has been applied to cuts (Boas 1932: 193).

*See also* **Amulet, Asthma, Coughs, Cuts, Dizziness, Earache, Erysipelas, Headache, Poultice, Rheumatism, Rickets, Sore throat, Tuberculosis, Warts, Whooping cough.**

### References

Addy, Sidney Oldall. *Household Tales with Other Traditional remains Collected in the Counties of York, Lincoln, Derby and Nottingham.* London: 1893.

Allen, Andrew. *A Dictionary of Sussex Folk Medicine.* Newbury: Countryside Books, 1995.

Beith, Mary. *Healing Threads: Traditional Medicines of the Highlands and Islands.* Edinburgh: Polygon, 1995.

Black, William George. *Folk-Medicine: A Chapter in the History of Culture.* London: Folklore Society, 1883.

Boas, Franz. "Current Beliefs of the Kwakiutl Indians." *Journal of American Folklore* 45 (1932): 177–260.

Brown, Frank C. *Collection of North Carolina Folklore.* 7 vols. Durham, NC: Duke University Press, 1952–1964.

Coward, Nathan. *Quaint Scraps and Sudden Cog-*

*itations.* Lynn, Norfolk: Wm. Turner, 1800.

EFS. English Folklore Survey. Manuscript notes at University College London.

Foster, George M. "Relationships between Spanish and Spanish-American Folk Medicine." *Journal of American Folklore* 66 (1953): 201–217.

Gerish, W. B. *Norfolk Beliefs.* 1920. Manuscript notes in Yarmouth Public Library.

Logan, Patrick. *Making the Cure: A Look at Irish Folk Medicine.* Dublin: Talbot Press, 1972.

Prince, Dennis. *Grandmother's Cures: An A–Z of Herbal Remedies.* London: Fontana, 1991.

Puckett, Newbell Niles. *Folk Beliefs of the Southern Negro.* Chapel Hill, NC: Greenwood Press, 1926.

Puckett, Newbell Niles. *Popular Beliefs and Superstitions: A Compendium of American Folklore from the Ohio Collection of Newbell Niles Puckett.* Edited by Wayland D. Hand, Anna Casetta, and Sondra B. Thiederman. 3 vols. Boston: G. K. Hall, 1981.

Radford, E., and M. A. Radford. *Encyclopaedia of Superstitions.* Edited and revised by Christina Hole. London: Book Club Associates, 1974.

Rolleston, J. D. "Respiratory Folk-Lore." *Tubercle* 25 (1944): 7–12.

Salmon, William. *The Compleat English Physician.* London: 1693.

Taylor, Mark R. "Norfolk Folklore." *Folk-Lore* 40 (1929): 113–133.

Tongue, Ruth L. *Somerset Folklore.* Edited Katharine Briggs. County Folklore 8. London: Folklore Society, 1965.

Wintemberg, W. J. "Folk-Lore Collected in Toronto and Vicinity." *Journal of American Folklore* 31 (1918): 125–134.

## Snake

The symbolism of the snake as a healing agent stretches back at least to the time of the ancient Greeks, whose god of healing, Aesculapius, was represented by a snake. The same symbolism has been adopted by the British Medical Association, the badge of which includes a snake. In folk medicine, parts of the snake have been used in practical ways to treat a wide variety of ailments. The sloughed-off skin of a snake, in particular, has been credited with healing powers. In the middle to late nineteenth century there was a man who sat on the steps of King's College Chapel in Cambridge and made his living selling the cast skins of snakes as a remedy for headache (Black 1883: 156). They were also used against infection right up to the twentieth century. A lady from Devon recalls her sister's septic finger being cured by a piece of snakeskin wrapped around it (Prince 1991: 101). The whole snake was regarded as a cure for snake bite, an example of sympathetic magic. In Sussex, one treatment for a swollen neck was to draw a snake along the swelling, then put the snake in a bottle and bury it; as the snake rotted, so the swelling would disappear, a clear example of transference (Black 1883: 58). Snakeskin was used to remove splinters—it was rubbed on the skin opposite the thorn and was believed to repel it, so that it fell out (Notes and Queries, 3 [1851] 258; Black 1883: 156). The oil from melted adder fat was used in Sussex as a cure for deafness as recently as the twentieth century, and the sloughed skin was used similarly. Soaked in wine, it was eaten to treat toothache (Allen 1995: 164).

In the official materia medica of the sixteenth and seventeenth centuries, the flesh of "vipers" was regarded as a panacea and was used for ailments as diverse as leprosy and poor eyesight. Snake blood had a reputation as a cosmetic. The price of such items put them out of reach of ordinary people, unless they prepared their own. Sir Kenelm Digby, famous for his "powder of sympathy" in the seventeenth century, had a very beautiful wife who ate capons fed with viper flesh (Allen 1995: 168). In Elizabethan Sussex a snakeskin was worn to prevent backache and rheumatism (Allen 1995: 169).

In North American folk medicine there was a much wider range of snakes available

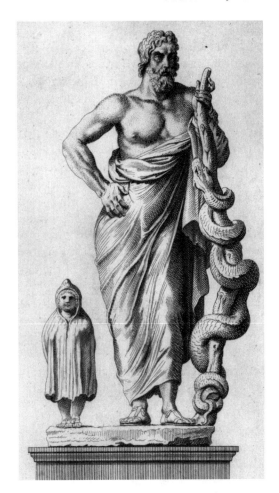

Aesculapius, the Greek god of healing (pictured here), was represented by a snake. In folk medicine, parts of the snake have been used in a practical way to treat a wide variety of ailments. (National Library of Medicine)

for use. Many of the medicinal uses are similar to those in Britain. In New England in the nineteenth century either keeping a pet snake or wearing a snakeskin around the neck was thought to prevent rheumatism (Black 1883: 156). Snake oil was used for gout in colonial Virginia (Eggleston 1899: 204). In Kansas snakeskin was worn as a hatband to cure headache (Davenport 1898: 132). Snakeskin soaked in vinegar was used to treat a wound (UCLA Folklore Archives 1_5578). A live snake's belly was rubbed on warts to remove them (UCLA

Folklore Archives 24_5542). The rattle-snake features in a large number of North American remedies. Much as in Britain with the adder skin, a rattlesnake skin was worn to prevent rheumatism (Thomas and Thomas 1920: 113) and backache (Bergen 1899: 76). Rattlesnake oil has been used to treat rheumatism (Puckett 1981: 431) and baldness (UCLA Folklore Archives 13_5277), as well as earache (Parler 1962, 3: 613). The gall of the rattlesnake was used to treat eye disorders (a remedy originating from China) (UCLA Folklore Archives 24_5372) and biliousness (UCLA Folklore Archives 8_6737). Even the bite of the rattlesnake found its uses. The venom was claimed to cure cramp-colic (Porter 1894: 112). A bite from a rattlesnake was said to cure tuberculosis (Pound 1946: 166).

In the Native American tradition it was believed that gently biting along the body of a living green snake would cure tooth-ache (Speck 1923: 278).

*See also* **Backache, Baldness, Colic, Deafness, Earache, Gout, Headache, Rheumatism, Snake bite, Sympathetic magic, Toothache, Transference, Tuberculosis, Warts, Wound.**

## References
Allen, Andrew. *A Dictionary of Sussex Folk Medicine.* Newbury: Countryside Books, 1995.
Bergen, Fanny D. "Animal and Plant Lore Collected from the Oral Tradition of English Speaking Folk." *Memoirs of the American Folk-Lore Society* 7 (1899).
Black, William George. *Folk-Medicine: A Chapter in the History of Culture.* London: Folklore Society, 1883.
Davenport, Gertrude C. "Folk-Cures from Kansas." *Journal of American Folklore* 11 (1898): 129–132.
Eggleston, Edward. "Some Curious Colonial Remedies." *American Historical Review* 5 (1899): 199–206.
*Notes and Queries*, 3: 258. London, 1851.
Parler, Mary Celestia, and University Student Contributors. *Folk Beliefs from Arkansas.* 15 vols. Fayetteville: University of Arkansas, 1962.
Porter, J. Hampden. "Notes on the Folklore of the Mountain Whites of the Alleghenies." *Journal of American Folklore* 7 (1894): 105–117.
Pound, Louise. "Nebraska Snake Lore." *Southern Folklore Quarterly* 10 (1946): 163–176.
Prince, Dennis. *Grandmother's Cures: An A–Z of Herbal Remedies.* London: Fontana, 1991.
Puckett, Newbell Niles. *Popular Beliefs and Superstitions: A Compendium of American Folklore from the Ohio Collection of Newbell Niles Puckett.* Edited by Wayland D. Hand, Anna Casetta, and Sondra B. Thiederman. 3 vols. Boston: G. K. Hall, 1981.
Speck, Frank G. "Reptile Lore of the Northern Indians." *Journal of American Folklore* 36 (1923): 273–280.
Thomas, Daniel Lindsay, and Lucy Blayney Thomas. *Kentucky Superstitions.* Princeton, NJ: Princeton University Press, 1920.

# Snake bite

Various amulets were used in British folk medicine to protect against snake bite, the commonest of these being fossil ammonites, popularly called "snake-stones." So-called adder stones, thought to be fossilized secretions from the adder, were similarly used in the Scottish Highlands (Beith 1995: 157). Agate had a dual role; worn as an amulet it was thought to protect against snake bite, while rubbed on a snake bite it was said to absorb the poison (Souter 1995: 186, 187). The leaf of the plantain was carried as an amulet against snake bite (Souter 1995: 66).

In British folk medicine, treatments for snake bite were varied and strange. Goat-shorn shavings in goat's milk was an Anglo-Saxon remedy (Cockayne 1864, 1: 351, 353). The milk of a one-colored cow (preferably white), when churned into butter, formed a cure for bites of snakes, especially adders, in the Highlands of Scotland (Beith

1995: 174). More recent nineteenth- and twentieth-century remedies are no less strange. The entrails of a newly killed hen were recommended as an application to a snake bite in Wiltshire (Black 1883: 46); in a Devonshire variation of this remedy, the wound should be thrust into the stomach of a newly killed chicken—if the flesh of the chicken turned dark, the cure had been achieved (Thiselton Dyer 1880: 137). Dried adder heads were valued in the Scottish Highlands as a cure for adder bite, an example of sympathetic magic. In the island of Skye adder heads were collected in a bag. When needed, they were dipped in a stream at a place where it divided two crofts. The water dripping from the bag when it was removed from the stream was used to treat adder bite (Matheson, 1949: 391). Much more simply, application of salt immediately after the animal had been bitten was an East Anglian treatment for cows bitten by an adder (Lilias Rider Haggard, ed., 1974: 129). In the Highlands of Scotland, baking soda was used similarly for treating snake bites (Beith 1995: 185).

Among plants used to treat snake bite in British folk medicine are ground ivy *(Glechoma hederacea)* and juniper *(Juniperus communis)*. In the latter case, the berries were crushed and placed on the wound (Beith 1995: 221, 225). Ash leaves were sometimes used as a poultice to treat snake bites (Beith 1995: 203).

In North America, the variety of indigenous venomous snakes is much greater than in Britain. It is therefore unsurprising that the range of plants used in their treatment is correspondingly greater. It is reported that in 1690 a woman in Virginia treated a victim of a rattlesnake bite by giving him ground-up bezoar (the concretion from the stomach of various animals, including goat—this was an item popular in the official pharmacopeia of the day), followed by an infusion of dittany (Eggleston

1899: 206). American dittany *(Cunila origanoides)* was a popular herb among early colonists, drunk usually as a tea for colds. The country names of some species indicate their former use; snakeroot *(Aristolochia serpentaria)* and snakebutton *(Liatris squarrosa)* were both used to treat snake bites, the latter especially for the rattlesnake bite (Grieve 1931: 746). Rattlesnake weed *(Lycopus sp.)*, as its name implies, was used too (Jeffrey 1955: 255). As in Britain, ash was used. A tea made from white ash bark mixed with corn meal was applied as a poultice to snake bites (Puckett 1981: 442). Rubbing ash wood over the wound was another recommendation. The ash has been associated with the power to deter snakes since the time of Pliny. Dock leaves have also been used to poultice snake bite wounds (Clark 1970: 30). In the African American tradition *Aralia spinosa* was used to treat snake bite (Vogel 1970: 273).

A plethora of nonplant remedies have been used for snake bite. They include (as in Britain) the application of parts of a snake, or of a split chicken. Alternatives were mouse flesh, or a toad. Salt, whisky, turpentine, tobacco, and kerosene were among other applications (Brown 1952–1964, 6: 275–282).

In the Native American tradition a large number of different plants have been used for the treatment of snake bite. Moerman gives more than ninety different genera (Moerman 1998: 819–820). They include ash *(Fraxinus* spp.), used by several tribes, including the Iroquois, and *Aristolochia,* again used by several tribes. Different species of milkweed *(Asclepias* spp.) were widely used. Peyote was chewed and poulticed onto snake bites in northern Mexico (Vogel 1970: 166).

*See also* **Amulet, Ash, Colds, Dock, Mouse, Plantain, Poultice, Soda, Sympathetic magic, Toads and frogs, Wounds.**

## References

Beith, Mary. *Healing Threads: Traditional Medicines of the Highlands and Islands.* Edinburgh: Polygon, 1995.

Black, William George. *Folk-Medicine: A Chapter in the History of Culture.* London: Folklore Society, 1883.

Brown, Frank C. *Collection of North Carolina Folklore.* 7 vols. Durham, NC: Duke University Press, 1952–1964.

Clark, Joseph D. "North Carolina Popular Beliefs and Superstitions." *North Carolina Folklore* 18 (1970): 1–66.

Cockayne, Rev. O. *Leechdoms, Wortcunning and Starcraft of Early England.* 3 vols. London: Rolls Series, 35, 1864.

Eggleston, Edward. "Some Curious Colonial Remedies." *American Historical Review* 5 (1899): 199–206.

Grieve, Mrs. M. *A Modern Herbal.* London: Jonathan Cape, 1931.

Jeffrey, Lloyd N. "Snake Yarns of the West and Southwest." *Western Folklore* 14 (1955): 246–258.

Matheson, Neil. "Highland Healers." *Scots Magazine* Feb. 1949, 391.

Moerman, Daniel E. *Native American Ethnobotany.* Portland, OR: Timber Press, 1998.

Puckett, Newbell Niles. *Popular Beliefs and Superstitions: A Compendium of American Folklore from the Ohio Collection of Newbell Niles Puckett.* Edited by Wayland D. Hand, Anna Casetta, and Sondra B. Thiederman. 3 vols. Boston: G. K. Hall, 1981.

Rider Haggard, Lilias (ed.). *I Walked by Night.* Woodbridge: Boydell Press, 1974.

Souter, Keith. *Cure Craft: Traditional Folk Remedies and Treatment from Antiquity to the Present Day.* Saffron Walden: C. W. Daniel, 1995.

Thiselton Dyer, T. F. (ed.). *English Folk-lore.* London: Bogue, 1880.

Vogel, Virgil J. *American Indian Medicine.* Norman: University of Oklahoma Press, 1970.

# Snow

A British folk remedy for chilblains is to rub them with snow or to run through the snow (Porter 1974: 44). Rubbing a baby's feet in the first snow of the season was thought to prevent it from getting chilblains (Leather 1912: 78). Water from melted snow was saved and used for treating burns (Mundford Primary School project, unpublished).

In North American folk medicine these remedies and others are found. Again, walking barefoot in snow is recommended for chilblains (Anon. 1939: 208). Running around the house three times in the snow was recommended for frostbite (Brown 1952–1964, 6: 199). Washing the hands in the first snow would prevent chapped hands during the winter (Farr 1935: 15). March snow water was held to be good for the complexion (Allen 1963: 68) and for the hair (Brown 1952–1964, 6: 204). Running barefoot in snow or ice was suggested for a sore throat (Anderson 1970: 67). Placing a baby's feet in the first snow prevented it from having croup or pneumonia (Parler 1962, 3: 238, 260). Eating some of the first snow prevented toothache (Hyatt 1965: 285). March snow was credited with removing warts (Browne 1958: 115) and freckles (Hyatt 1965: 267). Snow held on the back of the neck was recommended for nosebleed (Gardner 1937: no. 36). A cure for headache was to wash in snow water on Good Friday (Hyatt 1965: 235). As in Britain, water from melted snow was bottled and used for treating burns (Mason 1957: 29). In addition, snow water was used for sore or weak eyes (Hyatt 1965: 243). Catching the first snow in the mouth and swallowing it would ensure good health all year (Hyatt 1965: 196).

In the Native American tradition, ice and snow were invoked to heal sunburn (Mellinger 1967: 20).

*See also* **Burns, Chilblains, Croup, Freckles, Frostbite, Headache, Nosebleed, Sore throat, Sunburn, Toothache, Warts.**

## References

Allen, John W. *Legends and Lore of Southern Illinois*. Carbondale, IL: Southern Illinois University, 1963.

Anderson, John. *Texas Folk Medicine*. Austin: Encino Press, 1970.

Anon. *Idaho Lore*. Caldwell, ID: AMS Press Incorporated, 1939.

Brown, Frank C. *Collection of North Carolina Folklore*. 7 vols. Durham, North Carolina, 1952–1964.

Browne, Ray B. *Popular Beliefs and Practices from Alabama*. Berkeley and Los Angeles: University of California Publications, Folklore Studies 9, 1958.

Farr, T. J. "Tennessee Superstitions and Beliefs." *Tennessee Folklore Society Bulletin* 1(2) (1935): 13–27.

Gardner, Emelyn Elizabeth. *Folklore from the Schoharie Hills, New York*. Ann Arbor: University of Michigan Press, 1937.

Hyatt, Harry Middleton. *Folklore from Adams County Illinois*. 2nd rev. ed. New York: Memoirs of the Alma Egan Hyatt Foundation, 1965.

Leather, Ella Mary. *The Folk-Lore of Herefordshire Collected from Oral and Printed Sources*. Hereford and London: Jakeman and Carver, 1912.

Mason, James. "Home Remedies in West Virginia." *West Virginia Folklore* 7 (1957): 27–32.

Mellinger, Marie B. "Medicine of the Cherokees." *Foxfire* 1(3) (1967): 13–20.

Mundford Primary School project, Norfolk, 1980. Unpublished.

Parler, Mary Celestia, and University Student Contributors. *Folk Beliefs from Arkansas*. 15 vols. Fayetteville: University of Arkansas, 1962.

Porter, Enid. *The Folklore of East Anglia*. London: Batsford, 1974.

## Soda

Sodium bicarbonate is one of a small number of household ingredients that have been widely used in folk medicine. In Britain it has been used to treat insect bites and stings, indigestion, and heartburn, and as a soak for tender feet (Prince 1991: 27, 32, 33). It has also been used in Scotland for snake bites and for treating chilblains (Beith 1995: 185, 188).

In North America soda has been used in very similar ways, to treat insect stings and indigestion (Micheletti 1998: 43) as well as hiccups and snake bites (Brown 1952–1964, 6: 215, 281).

*See also* **Chilblains, Hiccups, Indigestion, Insect bites and stings, Snake bite.**

## References

Beith, Mary. *Healing Threads: Traditional Medicines of the Highlands and Islands*. Edinburgh: Polygon, 1995.

Brown, Frank C. *Collection of North Carolina Folklore*. 7 vols. Durham, NC: Duke University Press, 1952–1964.

Micheletti, Enza (ed.). *North American Folk Healing: An A–Z Guide to Traditional Remedies*. New York and Montreal: Reader's Digest Association, 1998.

Prince, Dennis. *Grandmother's Cures: An A–Z of Herbal Remedies*. London: Fontana, 1991.

## Sore feet

Rubbing feet with deer tallow or with a mixture of oatmeal and butter to prevent soreness was practiced in the Highlands of Scotland (Beith 1995: 174). An English equivalent was to rub the feet with melted candle wax and spirits (*The Daily Express Enquire Within* 1934: 439). Urine was used to treat sore feet—for example, in Wales (Jones 1980: 61). Fresh alder leaves placed in the shoes were claimed to prevent feet becoming sore (Beith 1995: 202). Silverweed leaves were used similarly. An ointment made from the roots of mallow, or a foot bath prepared by steeping the flowers of marigolds (*Calendula officinalis*) in hot water, were both remedies in Somerset (Tongue 1965: 40, 43). A rub for tired feet in the Scottish Highlands was the water in which Sphagnum moss had been boiled (Beith 1995: 244). The water in which houseleeks had been boiled was used in Norfolk for sore feet (Mundford Primary School project, 1980, unpub.). Cabbage leaves were recommended for tired and sweaty feet, and were used by soldiers during the Second World War to counter "trench foot" (Hatfield MS). Bladder wrack *(Fucus vesiculosus)* was used in Ireland for treating sore and sweaty feet (Allen and Hatfield, in press). The bark of oak has been added to the bath water to relieve sore and sweaty feet in Donegal (McGlinchey 1986: 84). Mugwort leaves inside the shoes have been claimed to prevent a traveler from becoming weary (Lafont 1984: 6). Dock leaves have been used inside the shoes to treat sore feet (EFS 241Sr) or sweaty feet (CECTL MSS). Excessive sweating of the feet has been checked by beating with holly, a procedure better known as a chilblain treatment (EFS 107 Ch). Plantain leaves have been use to relieve rubbing (Shaw 1955: 49).

In North American folk medicine, there were a number of suggestions for sore and aching feet. These include oatmeal or bran in the socks, or fuller's earth, mixed with powdered starch and zinc. A foot bath of wheat bran and soda was another recommendation, as was hot water or warm moist sand, or vinegar. Herbal soothers included a poultice of plantain leaves, a decoction of the bark of white oak or red oak, or the large leaf of horseradish *(Armoracia rusticana),* burdock or cabbage, with the main vein removed, warmed and applied to the foot. A poultice of mashed roast onions was also suggested (Meyer 1985: 119–120). Raw potato (Puckett 1981: 374) and dried turnip (UCLA Folklore Archives 7_6185) have also been used to relieve sore feet and blisters. Foot soaks have been prepared from weeping willow leaves *(Salix ?babylon-*

*ica)* (Puckett 1981: 374), jimson weed *(Datura* sp.*)* (UCLA Folklore Archives 20_5377), elderberry bark (Parler 1962: 631), hemlock bark (Browne 1958: 63), or violet *(Viola* sp.*)* (Cadwallader and Wilson 1965: 223). Grape leaves *(Vitis* spp.) have been recommended worn in the shoes to prevent sore feet (Hyatt 1965: 222).

A thin slice of salt pork bound onto sore feet overnight was recommended in Maine (UCLA Folklore Archives 18_7590). Washing sore feet in dishwater is a suggestion from Kentucky (Thomas and Thomas 1920: 103). During the Civil War, whisky was put in the shoes to prevent sore feet (Hyatt 1965: 222). Among the Pennsylvania Germans, a cure for sore feet was to cut out a foot-sized piece of turf and replace it upside down, then rest the sore foot on it (Brendle and Unger 1935: 75). Perhaps the most poetic cure for sore feet comes from Illinois, where the recommendation is to walk barefoot in the early morning dew (Hyatt 1965: 222).

In Native American practice, a number of plants were used to relieve sore feet, including princess pine *(Chimaphila umbellata)* (UCLA Folklore Archives 17_7610). Steam from a hot infusion of tansy *(Tanacetum vulgare)* was also used (Speck 1944: 45). Pine needles *(Pinus lasiocarpa)* were placed in the moccasins as a foot deodorant; sagewort leaves *(Artemisia ludoviciana)* were used similarly, as well as for treating blisters (Hellson 1974: 75, 123, 124). Aspen leaves *(Populus tremuloides)* were also used as a foot deodorant and antiperspirant (Turner, Bouchard, and Kennedy 1980: 134).

*See also* **Alder, Burdock, Cabbage, Chilblains, Dew, Dock, Earth, Elder, Hemlock spruce, Holly, Houseleek, Mallow, Mugwort, Onion, Pine, Plantain, Potato, Silverweed, Soda, Sphagnum moss, Urine.**

## References

Allen, David E., and Gabrielle Hatfield. *Medicinal Plants in Folk Tradition.* Portland, OR: Timber Press, in press.

Beith, Mary. *Healing Threads: Traditional Medicines of the Highlands and Islands.* Edinburgh: Polygon, 1995.

Brendle, Thomas R., and Claude W. Unger. "Folk Medicine of the Pennsylvania Germans: The Non-Occult Cures." *Proceedings of the Pennsylvania German Society* 45 (1935).

Browne, Ray B. *Popular Beliefs and Practices from Alabama.* Folklore Studies 9. Berkeley and Los Angeles: University of California Publications, 1958.

Cadwallader, D. E., and F. J. Wilson. "Folklore Medicine among Georgia's Piedmont Negroes after the Civil War." *Collections of the Georgia Historical Society* 49 (1965): 217–227.

CECTL MSS. Manuscript material at the Centre for English Cultural Tradition and Language, University of Sheffield.

*The Daily Express Enquire Within.* London: Daily Express, 1934.

EFS. English Folklore Survey. Manuscript material at University College London.

Hellson, John C. *Ethnobotany of the Blackfoot Indians.* Mercury Series 19. Ottawa: National Museums of Canada, 1974.

Hyatt, Harry Middleton. *Folklore from Adams County Illinois.* 2nd rev. ed. New York: Memoirs of the Alma Egan Hyatt Foundation, 1965.

Jones, Anne E. "Folk Medicine in Living Memory in Wales." *Folk Life* 18 (1980): 58–68.

Lafont, Anne-Marie. *Herbal Folklore.* Bideford: Badger Books, 1984.

McGlinchey, Charles. *The Last of the Name.* Edited by Brian Friel. Belfast: Blackstaff Press, 1986.

Meyer, Clarence. *American Folk Medicine.* Glenwood, IL: Meyerbooks, 1985.

Mundford Primary School, Norfolk. School project 1980, unpublished.

Parler, Mary Celestia, and University Student Contributors. *Folk Beliefs from Arkansas.* 15 vols. Fayetteville: University of Arkansas, 1962.

Puckett, Newbell Niles. *Popular Beliefs and Superstitions: A Compendium of American Folklore from the Ohio Collection of Newbell Niles Puckett.* Edited by Wayland D. Hand, Anna Casetta, Sondra B. Thiederman. 3 vols. Boston: G. K. Hall, 1981.

Shaw, Margaret Fay. *Folkways and Folklore of South Uist.* London: Routledge, 1955.

Speck, Frank G. "Catawba Herbals and Curative Practices." *Journal of American Folklore* 57 (1944): 37–50.

Thomas, Daniel Lindsey, and Lucey Blayney Thomas. *Kentucky Superstitions.* Princeton, NJ: Princeton University Press, 1920.

Tongue, Ruth L. *Somerset Folklore.* County Folklore. Edited by K. M. Briggs. Vol. 8. London: Folklore Society, 1965.

Turner, Nancy J., R. Bouchard, and Dorothy I. D. Kennedy. *Ethnobotany of the Okanagan-Colville Indians of British Columbia and Washington.* Victoria: British Columbia Provincial Museum, 1980.

# Sore throat

The many and varied causes of sore throat have not been clearly distinguished in folk medicine in the past, but obviously it has been observed that this condition sometimes led to serious and even fatal illness. Even in domestic medicine, it was not therefore taken lightly, and this is reflected in the very wide variety of folk remedies. The various plant infusions, such as black currant *(Ribes nigra)* (both the leaves and the fruit) (see, e.g., Hatfield 1994 appendix), raspberry, lemon, and honey (often with whisky added) are all readily understandable to the modern reader. Other plants used to make a gargle were sloe berries *(Prunus spinosa),* berries of rowan, and sage *(Salvia officinalis).* In the Scottish Highlands, a fungus growing on the bark of elder was made into a gargle for a sore throat, as were the leaves and flowers of hawthorn and an infusion made from the powdered bark of oak (Beith 1995: 215,

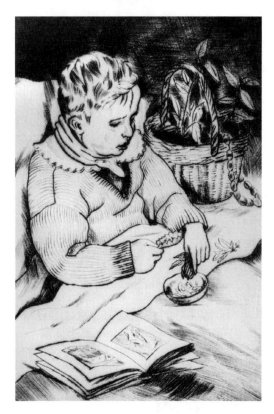

Wrapping up warmly and going to bed made obvious sense for those who suffered from a sore throat. Much more obscure in its origin is the practice, widespread in England up to the twentieth century, of wrapping one of the sufferer's worn socks around the throat. (National Library of Medicine)

221, 230, 237). The root of comfrey *(Symphytum officinale)* was chewed for a sore throat (Hatfield 1994: 30). A poultice for a sore throat was made from cooked potatoes. In Ireland, cabbage leaves tied around the throat were used similarly (Black 1883: 192). A decoction of the bark of wild cherry was used in East Anglia (Hatfield 1994: 30).

Wrapping up warmly and going to bed made obvious sense. Much more obscure in its origin is the practice, widespread in England up to the twentieth century, of wrapping one of the sufferer's worn socks around the throat. Similarly, a rasher of bacon worn around the throat overnight was used in Northamptonshire (Prince 1991: 98). In Ireland, salt herring applied to the soles of the feet was a remedy for a sore throat (Black 1883: 182). Wearing a red thread around the neck has also been reported as a traditional cure for a sore throat (Souter 1995: 187).

In general, North American folk medicine treatments for sore throat were similar to those in Britain. A sock worn around the throat was widely used (Brown 1952–1964, 6: 286–287). Bacon and other forms of meat were wrapped around a sore throat (Brown 1952–1964, 6: 284). Herrings were used, as in Scotland (Bergen 1899: 77) and red flannel was also recommended (Brown 1952–1964, 6: 286). Wearing beads of amber or gold were measures recommended to prevent a sore throat (Brown 1952–1964, 6: 288). Plant remedies used include a poultice of navy beans or of jimson leaves, or of roasted onions or slippery elm (Brown 1952–1964, 6: 284, 285). As in Britain, a syrup of sugar and onion was recommended (Brown 1952–1964, 6: 285). Also as in Britain, comfrey roots was used in sore throat treatment (Meyer 1985: 254). Numerous other examples of sore throat treatment are to be found in the UCLA Folklore Archives.

In the Native American tradition, innumerable different plants were used in sore throat treatment, belonging to nearly two hundred different genera (Moerman 1998: 821–823). Among them are some plants recognizable in British folk medicine too—for example, plum and cherry *(Prunus* spp.), oak *(Quercus* spp.), and dock *(Rumex* spp.). The majority, however, are plants unfamiliar to British folk medicine. Spruce *(Picea* spp.), wormwood *(Artemisia* spp.), and biscuitroot *(Lomatium* spp.) are among the most widely used.

*See also* **Amber, Cherry, Coughs, Dock, Elder, Elm, Gold, Hawthorn, Onion, Potato, Poultice, Quinsy, Rowan, Thornapple.**

ialist325

## References

Beith, Mary. *Healing Threads: Traditional Medicines of the Highlands and Islands.* Edinburgh: Polygon, 1995.
Bergen, Fanny D. "Animal and Plant Lore Collected from the Oral Tradition of English Speaking Folk." *Memoirs of the American Folk-Lore Society* 7 (1899).
Black, William George. *Folk-Medicine: A Chapter in the History of Culture.* London: Folklore Society, 1883.
Brown, Frank C. *Collection of North Carolina Folklore.* 7 vols. Durham, NC: Duke University Press, 1952–1964.
Hatfield, Gabrielle. *Country Remedies: Traditional East Anglian Plant Remedies in the Twentieth Century.* Woodbridge: Boydell, 1994.
Meyer, Clarence. *American Folk Medicine.* Glenwood, IL: Meyerbooks, 1985.
Moerman, Daniel E. *Native American Ethnobotany.* Portland, OR: Timber Press, 1998.
Prince, Dennis. *Grandmother's Cures: An A–Z of Herbal Remedies.* London: Fontana, 1991.
Souter, Keith. *Cure Craft: Traditional Folk Remedies and Treatment from Antiquity to the Present Day.* Saffron Walden: C. W. Daniel, 1995.

## Specialist

There are many examples in folk medicine of an individual who is famous for the ability to cure one illness. These individuals may or may not be healers in the general sense. In Ireland and Scotland, often the seventh son was considered to have special healing powers, in particular the power to cure the "evil" (i.e., the King's Evil, scrofula). Wart charmers are a good example of the specialist folk healer, but there are many others. In East Anglia in the twentieth century there was a woman locally famous for her treatment of eczema, another for her ointment for "festered fingers" (Hatfield MS). Irish folk medicine abounds with examples of individuals who had "the power" to cure one particular ailment.

The power was usually of unknown origin, sometimes inherited, and it could usually be deliberately passed to another. In the case of an herbal remedy, this, of course, holds no mystery; however, there are numerous examples of people who themselves had no explanation for their special ability. Often there was an element of secrecy surrounding the way in which the cure was performed; if details were revealed, the power would be lost. In Ulster, Buckley records, the person who has the "cure" may be a seventh daughter, a posthumous child, a woman who marries a man of the same name, or the seventh son of a seventh son (Buckley 1980: 15–34). Given the secrecy surrounding such "cures" and the oral transmission of any knowledge concerning them, it is unsurprising that we have so little knowledge of how the cures were performed. It is unclear whether specialists represent the end-point of a folk medical system of healers or whether they were always a distinct phenomenon. Bone setters are another example of specialist healers. In Celtic areas of Britain they persisted into the twentieth century. A highland bone setter who died in 1902 had learned his skill both from his father and from a cousin. His practice was extensive, and on a Saturday he would see as many as thirty patients. The rest of his time was spent farming (Buchan 1994: 52).

Similar specialists served North American communities. As in Britain, few of them are fully documented, but each would have been well known in the community where they worked. Among the Cajuns of southern Louisiana there were many faith healers, each specializing in treating one particular ailment (Micheletti 1998: 206–207). In Syracuse there was a family of bone setters whose practice spanned seventy years (Jones 1949: 480). As in Britain, many people suffering from warts had recourse to wart charmers. Other specialist healers had the power to "talk the fire" out of burns (Kirkland 1992: 41–52).

## References

Buchan, David, ed. *Folk Tradition and Folk Medicine in Scotland: The Writings of David Rorie.* Edinburgh: Canongate Academic, 1994.

Buckley, Anthony D. "Unofficial Healing in Ulster." *Ulster Folklife* 26 (1980): 15–34.

Jones, Louis C. "Practitioners of Folk Medicine." *Bulletin of the History of Medicine* 23 (1949): 480–493.

Kirkland, James. "Talking Fire Out of Burns: A Magico-Religious Healing Tradition." In *Herbal and Magical Medicine. Traditional Healing Today.* Edited by James Kirkland, Holly F. Matthews, C.W. Sullivan III and Karen Baldwin. Durham, NC: Duke University Press, 1992.

Micheletti, Enza, ed. *North American Folk Healing: An A–Z Guide to Traditional Remedies.* New York and Montreal: Reader's Digest Association, 1998.

# Sphagnum moss (*Sphagnum spp.*)

This remarkable plant can hold many times its own weight of water, and folk medicine has exploited this characteristic. It has been used as a wound dressing as long ago as the Battle of Clontarf in 1014 (Grieve 1931: 553) and as recently as World War I and World War II, where its antiseptic as well as its absorptive qualities proved useful (Chevallier 1996: 26; Beith 1995: 244). It has formed the basis for sanitary towels and babies' nappies, both in rural communities and, more recently, in commercialized form (Willard 1992: 28). As a wound dressing, it was sometimes covered with clay to give added protection, as in Devon (St. Clair 1971). In the Scottish Highlands it has been used as a rub for sore and tired feet (Beith 1995: 244). In Somerset, it has treated sore eyes (Tongue 1965: 39). In Ireland, it has been packed tightly around sprains (Logan 1972) and has been used to treat rashes and burns (Allen and Hatfield, in press).

In North American "frontier medicine" it was used for cuts, grazes, abscesses, and hemorrhoids, sometimes combined with an antiseptic herb such as garlic or witch hazel (*Hamamelis* sp.) (Souter 1995: 170). As a dressing for wounds and sores it has been used in Newfoundland "from earliest times" (Grieve 1931: 553), and knowledge of this usage has persisted to recent times (UCLA Folklore Archive 10_6556). In Native American medicine it was used as a wound dressing, as well as for nappies and sanitary pads. It also served as a disinfectant (Turner et al. 1983: 59), and was used to treat children's sores (Carrier Linguistic Committee 1973: 87).

*See also* **Abscesses, Burns, Cuts, Eye problems, Garlic, Piles, Sore feet, Sprains, Wounds.**

## References

Allen, David E., and Gabrielle Hatfield. *Medicinal Plants in Folk Tradition.* Portland, OR: Timber Press, in press.

Beith, Mary. *Healing Threads: Traditional Medicines of the Highlands and Islands.* Edinburgh: Polygon, 1995.

Carrier Linguistic Community. *Plants of Carrier Country.* Fort St. James, British Columbia: Carrier Linguistic Committee, 1973.

Chevallier, Andrew. *The Encyclopedia of Medicinal Plants.* London: Dorling Kindersley, 1996.

Grieve, Mrs. M. *A Modern Herbal.* London: Jonathan Cape, 1931.

Logan, Patrick *Making the Cure: A Look at Irish Folk Medicine.* Dublin: Talbot Press, 1972.

St. Clair, Sheila. *Folklore of the Ulster People.* Cork: Mercier Press, 1971.

Souter, Keith. *Cure Craft: Traditional Folk Remedies and Treatment from Antiquity to the Present Day.* Saffron Walden: C. W. Daniel, 1995.

Tongue, Ruth L. *Somerset Folklore.* Edited by K. M. Briggs. London: Folklore Society, 1965.

Turner, Nancy J., John Thomas, Barry F. Carl-

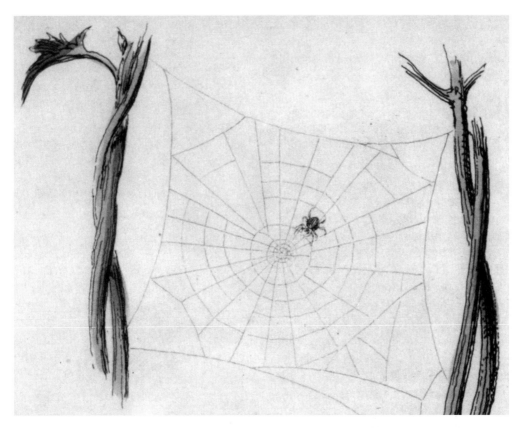

Both the spider and its web have been used in British folk medicine. Rolled in its own web, a spider was often swallowed for whooping cough, fever, and sore throat. (National Library of Medicine)

son, and Robert T. Ogilvie. *Ethnobotany of the Nitinaht Indians of Vancouver Island.* Victoria: British Columbia Provincial Museum, 1983.

Willard, Terry. *Edible and Medicinal Plants of the Rocky Mountains and Neighbouring Territories.* Calgary, ALTA: Wild Rose College of Natural Healing, 1992.

# Spider

Both the spider and its web have been used in British folk medicine. Cobwebs have been a handy first-aid measure for treating cuts for as far back as records extend; and they were used both in official medicine (recommended by Dioscorides) and in folk medicine. They have been used in country areas, with apparent success, within living memory. Especially when someone cut their hand between the thumb and index finger, it was believed that tetanus was a possible outcome; in many rural areas the tetanus bacillus is still endemic in the soil. Surprisingly to modern ears, this type of cut in particular was treated with cobwebs. The effect seems to have been twofold: the web helps blood clotting and therefore stems blood loss; in addition it seems to have reduced the rate of infection. Though there have not been detailed studies of the chemical composition of spiders' webs, from what little is known it seems that there is an anti-infective agent in the cobweb.

The spider itself was used in some folk remedies. Rolled in its own web, it was swallowed for whooping cough, fever, and sore throat. In Sussex, a spider rolled in butter was used as a treatment for fever (Allen 1995: 22). In Norfolk, the spider in its own web was used (Mundford Primary School, Norfolk, 1980, unpub.). Spiders were also used as amulets, to ward off fever. In the seventeenth and eighteenth centuries they were carried in nutshells or muslin bags around the neck (Allen 1995: 23). Elias Ashmole records in his dairy for May 11, 1681, how he took a dose of elixir and hung three spiders about his neck "and they drove my ague away" (Black 1883: 60). In the nineteenth century in West Sussex live spiders rolled in butter were taken for jaundice (Black 1883: 60), while in Norfolk the unfortunate spider was pinned above the mantelpiece as a cure for whooping cough. As it died, the whooping cough would disappear (Thiselton Dyer 1880: 154). In Worcestershire, the spider was worn as an amulet against toothache (Black 1883: 61), while in the Highlands of Scotland it was sealed in a goose-quill and hung around a child's neck as a cure for thrush (Beith 1995: 186). It was, and still is, considered unlucky to kill a spider: "If you want to live and thrive, let a spider run alive" is a well-known proverb (Opie and Opie 1959: 220).

In North American folk medicine the uses of spiders and their webs are similar to those in Britain. In New England, pills were made for treating fever composed of a spider rolled in molasses (Black 1883: 61). Spider webs were used for stemming nosebleeds (Kimmerle and Gelber 1976: 14). Turpentine mixed with spider webs was applied to cuts (UCLA Folklore Archives 1_5356). Spider webs from the north side of a barn were recommended for treating fever (Hendricks 1966: 44). A spider in a nutshell was believed to cure all kinds of illness (Puckett 1981: 271). As in Britain, it was considered unlucky to kill a spider (UCLA Folklore Archives 17–6779).

Native Americans used a compress made

from spider webs for treating cuts and grazes (Souter 1995: 151).

*See also* **Amulet, Cuts, Fevers, Jaundice, Nosebleed, Sore throat, Toothache, Whooping cough.**

### References
Allen, Andrew. *A Dictionary of Sussex Folk Medicine.* Newbury: Countryside Books, 1995.
Beith, Mary. *Healing Threads: Traditional Medicines of the Highlands and Islands.* Edinburgh: Polygon, 1995.
Black, William George. *Folk-Medicine: A Chapter in the History of Culture.* London: Folklore Society, 1883.
Hendricks, George D. *Mirrors, Mice and Mustaches: A Sampling of Superstitions and Popular Beliefs in Texas.* Austin: Texas Folklore Society, 1966.
Kimmerle, Marjorie, and Mark Gelber. *Popular Beliefs and Superstitions from Colorado.* Boulder: University of Colorado, unpublished, 1976.
Mundford Primary School, School project, 1980, unpublished.
Opie, Iona, and Peter Opie. *The Lore and Language of Schoolchildren.* London: Oxford University Press, 1959.
Puckett, Newbell Niles. *Popular Beliefs and Superstitions: A Compendium of American Folklore from the Ohio Collection of Newbell Niles Puckett.* Edited by Wayland D. Hand, Anna Casetta, and Sondra B. Thiederman. 3 vols. Boston: G. K. Hall, 1981.
Souter, Keith. *Cure Craft: Traditional Folk Remedies and Treatment from Antiquity to the Present Day.* Saffron Walden: C. W. Daniel, 1995.
Thiselton Dyer, T. F. *English Folk-lore.* 2nd ed. London: Bogue, 1880.

# Spit

In British folk medicine human and dog saliva have been credited with healing powers. So-called fasting spittle, the first saliva in the mouth on waking, is supposed to have particular virtues in healing warts and ringworm as well as in counteracting the evil eye (Black 1883: 184). In the twenty-first century, there are still plenty of people who claim to have cured warts in this way and minor injuries too, even skin ulcers (E.J., Perthshire, Scotland, pers. com. 2003). The instinct to lick small cuts and wounds has now been "justified" in scientific terms; saliva has been shown to contain antibacterial and antifungal as well as growth-promoting substances (Root-Bernstein and Root-Bernstein 2000: 113–118). In the early years of the twentieth century there was a man in Dorset famous for his cures of cataract, which he performed simply by licking the patient's eye (EFS 342). In Fife, Scotland, eye inflammations and foreign bodies in the eye were treated by licking the eye with fasting spittle (Buchan 1994: 242). Many healers employed spit in their healing methods (Beith 1995: 94). Spit played a part in a cure for hiccups. Some plant remedies involved saliva, too; dock leaves plus spit were recommended to soothe stings (Allen and Hatfield, in press), and ribwort plantain leaves with spittle were used to help heal cuts (Beith 1995: 234).

In North American folk medicine spit has been used in similar ways; for treating warts, to avert bad luck and to treat cuts (Brown 1952–1964, 6: 168, 312, 502). Stys have been treated with spittle, and licking or spitting on burns has been suggested (Cannon 1984: 96, 126). Interestingly, in the Native American tradition, folk tales suggest a similar role for spit, healing sore eyes (Harrington 1908: 335) and arrow wounds (Radin 1931: 151).

*See also* **Burns, Cuts, Dog, Evil eye, Healer, Hiccups, Ringworm, Warts.**

### References

Allen, David E., and Gabrielle Hatfield. *Medicinal Plants in Folk Tradition.* Portland, OR: Timber Press, in press.
Beith, Mary. *Healing Threads: Traditional Medicines of the Highlands and Islands.* Edinburgh: Polygon, 1995.
Black, William George. *Folk-Medicine: A Chapter in the History of Culture.* London: Folklore Society, 1883.
Brown, Frank C. *Collection of North Carolina Folklore.* 7 vols. Durham, NC: Duke University Press, 1952–1964.
Buchan, David, ed. *Folk Tradition and Folk Medicine in Scotland: The Writings of David Rorie.* Edinburgh: Canongate Academic, 1994.
Cannon, Anthon S. *Popular Beliefs and Superstitions from Utah.* Edited by Wayland D. Hand and Jeannine E. Talley. Salt Lake City: University of Utah Press, 1984.
EFS. English Folklore Survey. Manuscript notes at University College London.
Harrington, John Peabody. "A Yuma Account of Origins." *Journal of American Folklore* 21 (1908): 324–348.
Radin, Paul. "The Thunderbird Warclub: A Winnebago Tale." *Journal of American Folklore* 44 (1931): 143–165.
Root-Bernstein, Robert, and Michèle Root-Bernstein. *Honey, Mud Maggots and Other Medical Marvels: The Science behind Folk Remedies and Old Wives' Tales.* London: Pan Books, 2000.

## Spots

*See* **Acne.**

## Sprains

One simple measure for treating sprains has been cold water (Prince 1991: 49), still recommended in official medicine today. Confusingly, hot water was also suggested, or an alternation of cold and hot (Souter 1995: 188). In Scotland, pig fat was used as an embrocation for sprains, as was a liniment prepared from egg white, and eelskin as a bandage (Simpkins 1914: 410, 411). Another household remedy was malt vinegar, rubbed on (Prince 1991: 102). In northeast Scotland, the water in which skate had been boiled (known as "skate bree") was recommended as a lotion for a sprain (Gregor 1881: 46). In Wales, a poultice of warm manure was used for sprains (EFS 221).

A thread tied around the damaged area was a traditional semi-magical cure for a sprain. In Ireland, it was specifically a red thread used in this way (Logan 1972: 124). In the north of Scotland, a linen thread was tied in place while a charm was recited. Nine knots were tied in the thread, the charm being recited as each was secured (Black and Northcote 1903: 144). In the Scottish Highlands, a thread made from a sinew from a rutting stag was regarded as the most efficacious (Beith 1995: 170). In the north of England, individuals who were breech born were credited with the ability to heal sprains by stamping on them; after this, the sprain was wrapped in eelskin (Radford and Radford 1974: 321–322).

A number of native plants have been used in Britain and Ireland to treat sprains. Comfrey was very widely used for this purpose (EFS 277). In the north and west of Britain, where comfrey is relatively uncommon, its place was largely taken by royal fern *(Osmunda regalis)* (Phytologist 5 [1854]: 30; Logan 1972: 124). The bark of various trees was used—wych elm *(Ulmus glabra)* in Ireland, and oak *(Quercus robur)* in England. Withering recorded in the eighteenth century the use of "verjuice," from crab-apple *(Malus sylvestris)* for treating sprains (Withering 1787–1792: 296). St. John's wort was widely used for treating sprains (Tongue 1965: 35). Chickweed was used especially in Ireland (Allen and Hatfield, in press), as was mallow. Elder was used in Scotland and England, and an ointment was made from the root of coltsfoot *(Tussilago farfara)* (Johnston 1853: 129). The petals of Madonna lily soaked in brandy were used to treat sprains as well as cuts and bruises (EFS 195). The jelly-like contents from the vesicles of the seaweed *Fucus vesiculosus* was used to treat sprains (Freethy 1985: 82). A number of other plants were used in sprain treatment in Ire-

land. They include figwort (Hart 1898: 385), foxglove, dandelion, ragwort *(Senecio jacobaea),* broom *(Cytisus scoparius),* ivy, and woodsage *(Teucrium scorodonia)* (Allen and Hatfield, in press). Willow moss *(Fontinalis antipyretica)* was packed around sprains (Logan 1972: 124). In Wales, a cabbage leaf was wrapped around a sprained ankle and held in place with a sock (W.T., Gwent, 1980, pers. com.). In Cambridgeshire, dock leaves were used similarly (D.M.P., 1996, pers. com.).

In North American folk medicine a number of simple household remedies were applied to sprains. As in Britain, both hot water and cold have been recommended. Epsom salts were recommended (UCLA Folklore Archives 17_5487). A poultice of bread, oatmeal, or bran mixed with vinegar has been used. A liniment of egg white, mixed with salt, or salt and honey, has been applied. An alternative was resin and butter (Meyer 1985: 231–232), or hot salted cornmeal (G. Wilson 1968: 322). Mud was sometimes applied to soothe sprains (UCLA Folklore Archives 1_6787), or a dirt-dauber's nest mixed with vinegar (Clark 1970: 31). A crushed wasp nest mixed with vinegar has also been used (UCLA Folklore Archives 2_5490). An unusual embrocation was made from worms and cooking oil (UCLA Folklore Archives 3_5490). Rendered jellyfish were an alternative (Bergen 1899: 73). A number of animal fats were employed to treat sprains, including skunk oil (UCLA Folklore Archives 20_7615), goose grease (Thomas and Thomas 1920: 115), bear oil (UCLA Folklore Archives 7_7590), snake fat (Eggleston 1899: 204), and dog lard (Puckett 1981: 451). Both eelskin and snakeskin were used to bandage sprains (Bergen 1899: 76), as were wet rabbit skins (De Lys 1948: 116). In the African tradition, leather is worn around the wrist to cure a sprain (Brown 1952–1964, 6: 288). As in Britain, a cow-dung poultice was used by the Ozarks

(Randolph 1931: 99). A salve has been made from toads, butter, and arnica (*Arnica* sp.) (Relihan 1947: 169).

Arnica was also used alone for treating sprains (Cannon 1984: 1925), and is still much used today, although nowadays it is commercially available as an ointment. Other plant remedies used in North American folk medicine to treat sprains include agrimony (*Agrimonia* sp.), boiled with vinegar and homemade soap (Lick and Brendle 1922: 179); smartweed (*Polygonum* sp.), cooked in vinegar and packed around the injured part (Puckett 1981: 451); dandelion juice mixed with alcohol (Cannon 1984: 125); lily of the valley (*Maianthemum* sp.) (Clark 1970: 31); whiteflowered boneset with vinegar (*Eupatorium* sp.) (UCLA Folklore Archives 21_7611); and wormwood (*Artemisia* sp.) (Relihan 1946: 157). As in Britain, various tree barks were used: elder (Fogel 1915: 131), smooth alder *(Alnus incana)* (Lick and Brendle 1922: 233), black oak (Randolph 1947: 100). In the Mexican tradition a poultice of sunflower seeds (*Helianthus* sp.) was used (Smithers 1961: 27). Whole leaves were used to comfort sprains. Mullein was used in this way (Parler 1962: 911), as were burdock (Meyer 1985: 233) and jimson weed (Brown 1952–1964: 289).

Eelskin bandages were used in the Native American tradition, just as in Britain (Parsons 1926: 485). Plants used in the Native American tradition include mouse-ear everlasting *(Gnaphalium obtusifolium)* (Welch 1964: 92), juniper balsam *(Juniperus communis)* (Wallis 1922: 28), and water hemlock *(Cicuta maculata)* (Taylor 1967: 279). Various species of jimson weed (Moerman 1998: 1944–1964) were used, as well as the smooth alder mentioned above (Moerman 1998: 60).

*See also* **African tradition, Alder, Bruises, Burdock, Cabbage, Chickweed, Comfrey, Cuts, Dandelion, Dock, Elder, Excreta,** **Figwort, Foxglove, Ivy, Mallow, Mexican tradition, Mullein, St. John's wort, Thornapple, Toads and frogs, Vinegar.**

## References

Allen, David E., and Gabrielle Hatfield. *Medicinal Plants in Folk Tradition.* Portland, OR: Timber Press, in press.

Beith, Mary. *Healing Threads: Traditional Medicines of the Highlands and Islands.* Edinburgh: Polygon, 1995.

Bergen, Fanny D. "Animal and Plant Lore Collected from the Oral Tradition of English Speaking Folk." *Memoirs of the American Folk-Lore Society* 7 (1899).

Black, G. F., collector, and W. Thomas Northcote, editor. "Examples of Printed Folk-Lore Concerning Orkney and Shetland Islands" (County Folklore Printed Extracts 3:5). *Publications of the Folklore Society* 49 (1903).

Brown, Frank C. *Collection of North Carolina Folklore.* 7 vols., Durham, NC: Duke University Press, 1952–1964.

Cannon, Anthon S. *Popular Beliefs and Superstitions from Utah.* Edited by Wayland D. Hand and Jeannine E. Talley. Salt Lake City: University of Utah Press, 1984.

Clark, Joseph D. "North Carolina Popular Beliefs and Superstitions." *North Carolina Folklore* 18 (1970): 1–66.

De Lys, Claudia. *A Treasury of American Superstitions.* New York: Philosophical Library, 1948.

EFS. English Folklore Survey. Manuscript notes at University College London.

Eggleston, Edward. "Some Curious Colonial Remedies." *American Historical Review* 5 (1899): 199–206.

Fogel, Edwin Miller. "Beliefs and Superstitions of the Pennsylvania Germans." *Americana Germanica* 18 (1915).

Freethy, Ron. *From Agar to Zenry.* Marlborough: Crowood Press, 1985.

Gregor, Walter. "Notes on the Folklore of the North East of Scotland." *Publications of the Folklore Society* 7 (1881).

Hart, Henry Chichester. *Flora of the County Donegal.* Dublin: Sealy, Bryers, and Walker, 1898.

Johnston, George. *The Natural History of the East-*

*ern Borders.* Vol. 1, *The Botany.* London: Van Voorst, 1853.

Lick, David E., and Thomas R. Brendle. "Plant Names and Plant Lore among the Pennsylvania Germans." *Proceedings and Addresses of the Pennsylvania German Society* 33 (1922).

Logan, Patrick. *Making the Cure: A Look at Irish Folk Medicine.* Dublin: Talbot Press, 1972.

Meyer, Clarence. *American Folk Medicine.* Glenwood, IL: Meyerbooks, 1985.

Moerman, Daniel E. *Native American Ethnobotany.* Portland, OR: Timber Press, 1998.

Parler, Mary Celestia, and University Student Contributors. *Folk Beliefs from Arkansas.* 15 vols. Fayetteville: University of Arkansas, 1962.

Parsons, Elsie Clews. "Micmac Notes." *Journal of American Folklore* 39(1926): 460–485.

Prince, Dennis. *Grandmother's Cures: An A–Z of Herbal Remedies.* London: Fontana, 1991.

Puckett, Newbell Niles. *Popular Beliefs and Superstitions: A Compendium of American Folklore from the Ohio Collection of Newbell Niles Puckett.* Edited by Wayland D. Hand, Anna Casetta, and Sondra B. Thiederman. 3 vols. Boston: G. K. Hall, 1981.

Radford, E., and M. A. Radford. *Encyclopaedia of Superstitions.* Edited by Christina Hole. London: Book Club Associates, 1974.

Randolph, Vance. *The Ozarks: An American Survival of Primitive Society.* New York: Vanguard Press, 1931.

Relihan, Catherine. "Farm Lore: Herb Remedies." *New York Folklore Quarterly* 2(2) (1946): 156–158.

———. "Folk Remedies." *New York Folklore Quarterly* 3 (1947): 81–84, 166–169.

Simpkins, John Ewart. *Examples of Printed Folk-Lore Concerning Fife, with Some Notes on Clackmannan and Kinross-shire.* County Folk-Lore 7. London: Publications of the Folklore Society, 1914.

Smithers, W. D. "Nature's Pharmacy and the Curanderos." *Sul Ross State College Bulletin* 41 (1961): 3.

Souter, Keith. *Cure Craft: Traditional Folk Remedies and Treatment from Antiquity to the Present Day.* Saffron Walden: C. W. Daniel, 1995.

Taylor, Dorothy Bright. "Indian Medicine Herbs." *New York Folklore Quarterly* 23 (1967): 274–282.

Thomas, Daniel Lindsay, and Lucy Blayney Thomas. *Kentucky Superstitions.* Princeton, NJ: Princeton University Press, 1920.

Tongue, Ruth L. *Somerset Folklore.* Edited Katharine Briggs. County Folklore 8. London: Folklore Society, 1965.

Wallis, Wilson D. "Medicines Used by the Micmac Indians." *American Anthropologist* 24 (1922): 24–30.

Welch, Charles E. "Some Drugs of the North American Indian: Then and Now." *Keystone Folklore Quarterly* 9(2) (1964): 83–89.

Wilson, Gordon. "Local Plants in Folk Remedies in the Mammoth Cave Region." *Southern Folklore Quarterly* 32 (1968): 320–327.

Withering, William. *A Botanical Arrangement of British Plants.* 2nd ed. 3 vols. Birmingham: M. Swinney, 1787–1792.

# Stinging nettle (*Urtica spp.*)

There are two species of nettle probably native to Britain: *Urtica dioica,* which has been present at least since the Bronze Age as a weed of cultivated land, and the smaller annual *Urtica urens.* A third species, *Urtica pilulifera,* occurs in Britain as a casual weed and was reputedly introduced by the Romans as a rheumatism cure for their soldiers. Folk remedies do not generally distinguish between these species.

Nettle is one of the most widely used plants in British folk medicine, its uses ranging from treatment of rheumatism, anemia, and heavy periods, rashes (an example of sympathetic magic), coughs and colds and ear infections to the suppression of sexual excitement (Allen and Hatfield, in press). Rheumatism was treated both with an infusion of nettles and externally by beating the affected area (Vickery 1995: 255). In Suffolk, England, in the twentieth century the use of juice from the stalk to treat a nettle sting was still current (Taylor

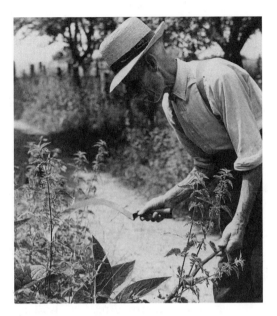

Man scything stinging nettles, Britain, 1941. Nettle is one of the most widely used plants in British folk medicine. (Hulton-Deutsch Collection/CORBIS)

MSS), a remedy mentioned in John Wesley's *Primitive Physic,* first published in 1747. In the Scottish Highlands, uses of nettle include treatment of insomnia and tuberculosis as well as the staunching of minor wounds (Beith 1995: 230). The young tops in springtime are the part of the plant that is used, and tradition seems to have ensured that the older parts of the plant, now known to be toxic, are not included.

The stinging nettle is probably an introduction to North America but is now widespread as a weed of cultivated land. Its first appearance in New England was noted by Josselyn in the seventeenth century (Josselyn 1672). In North American folk medicine, nettle roots have been chewed to cure and prevent nosebleed and nettle tea has been recommended to clear phlegm. Nettles form part of an ointment to treat bleeding hemorrhoids. The juice of nettles was given for a "scall head," while nettle roots dried and powdered and mixed with molasses was a cure for hoarseness (Meyer 1985: 189, 191, 195, 222, 254).

The use of stinging nettles to beat limbs afflicted with rheumatism is still practiced today in England, and the same practice has been followed by many Native American tribes (see, for example, Turner, Thomas et al. 1983: 128; and Gunther 1973: 28). Nettles were also used in a steam bath for treating rheumatism—for example, among the Shushwap (Palmer 1975: 229–251). Other Native American uses for nettles include cold treatment (Train et al. 1941: 146) and the soothing of rashes (Carrier Linguistic Committee 1973: 83) and of bleeding hemorrhoids (Turner et al. 1990: 289). Nettles were used as a hair tonic (Turner et al. 1990: 289) and a general tonic (Gunther 1973: 28). The Nevada Indians used fumes from nettles in sweat lodges to treat pneumonia and flu, while the Salish used an infusion, or the young leaves chewed, to ease labor (Willard 1992: 74). For other Native American uses of nettles, see Moerman (Moerman 1998: 578–582).

Young nettles are still eaten as a vegetable in many parts of the world; they are excellent sources of iron.

*See also* **Anemia, Bleeding, Childbirth, Colds, Coughs, Menstrual problems, Nosebleed, Piles, Rheumatism, Sleeplessness, Sympathetic magic, Tonic, Tuberculosis.**

## References

Allen, David E., and Gabrielle Hatfield. *Medicinal Plants in Folk Tradition.* Portland, OR: Timber Press, in press.

Beith, Mary. *Healing Threads: Traditional Medicines of the Highlands and Islands.* Edinburgh: Polygon, 1995.

Carrier Linguistic Committee. *Plants of Carrier Country.* Fort St. James, BC: Carrier Linguistic Committee, 1973.

Gunther, Erna. *Ethnobotany of Western Washington.* Rev. ed. Seattle: University of Washington Press, 1973.

Josselyn, John. *New England's Rarities Discovered.* London: Widdowes, 1672.

Meyer, Clarence. *American Folk Medicine.* Glenwood, IL: Meyerbooks, 1985.

Moerman, Daniel E. *Native American Ethnobotany.* Portland, OR: Timber Press, 1998.

Palmer, Gary. "Shushwap Indian Ethnobotany." *Syesis* 8 (1975): 29–51.

Taylor MSS. Manuscript notes of Mark R. Taylor, Norfolk Record Office, Norwich. MS4322.

Train, Percy, James R. Heinrichs, and W. Andrew Archer. *Medicinal Uses of Plants by Indian Tribes of Nevada.* Washington, DC: U.S. Department of Agriculture, 1941.

Turner, Thomas, et al. *Ethnobotany of the Nitinaht Indians of Vancouver Island.* Victoria: British Columbia Provincial Museum, 1983.

Turner, Nancy J., Laurence C. Thompson, and M. Terry Thompson et al. *Thompson Ethnobotany: Knowledge and Uses of Plants by the Thompson Indians of British Columbia.* Victoria: Royal British Columbia Museum, 1990.

Vickery, Roy. *A Dictionary of Plant Lore.* Oxford: Oxford University Press, 1995.

Willard, Terry. *Edible and Medicinal Plants of the Rocky Mountains and Neighbouring Territories.* Calgary, ALTA: Wild Rose College of Natural Healing, 1992.

# Sunburn

A number of plants have been used in British folk medicine to treat sunburn. In East Anglia an infusion of vervain *(Verbena officinalis)* or of meadowsweet *(Filipendula ulmaria)* or of sage *(Salvia officinalis)* was used to soothe it (Hatfield 1994: 50). In Devon, an ointment was used made from boiling ivy stalks in butter (Lafont 1984: 49). The berries of black bryony were used in the Isle of Wight (Bromfield 1856: 507). In Scotland, the juice of sundew *(Drosera* sp.) was mixed with milk and applied to sunburn (McNeill 1910: 123), or an infusion of tormentil *(Potentilla erecta)* could be used (Vickery 1995: 373). Honeysuckle *(Lonicera periclymenum)* also provided a sunburn remedy in the Highlands of Scotland (Beith 1995: 223). In Wales dock leaves were wrapped around sunburned areas to soothe them (Vickery 1995: 108). Raw potato juice, a common first-aid remedy for minor burns in general, was also used to treat sunburn, as was the juice from crushed strawberries *(Fragaria vesca)* (Souter 1995: 190).

Sage features in North American folk treatment of sunburn too (Meyer 1985: 228), and so also do strawberries (UCLA Folklore Archives 15_6476). The juice of *Aloe vera* has been used, or a salve prepared from lemon or lime juice mixed with vinegar and olive oil (Meyer 1985: 228). Fresh cream has been recommended, or a salve of buttermilk and tansy *(Tancetum vulgare)* (Brown 1952–1964, 6: 297). Bathing the affected area with strong tea has also been recommended (Koch 1980: 76), as has wrapping with vinegar and brown paper (UCLA Folklore Archives 24_6475). A preparation of witch hazel twigs *(Hamamelis* sp.) has been used (Clark 1970: 32). Nutmeg has been worn as an amulet to protect against sunburn (Brown 1952–1964, 6: 297). Bathing in an easterly flowing stream has been recommended for sunburn (Parler 1962, 3: 947). There was a belief that an aged person could "blow" the fire out of sun blisters (Turner 1937: 168).

Among the Cherokee, sunburn was treated by invoking ice and snow (Mellinger 1967: 20).

*See also* **Aloe vera, Bryony, Burns, Dock, Ivy, Potato.**

## References

Beith, Mary. *Healing Threads: Traditional Medicines of the Highlands and Islands.* Edinburgh: Polygon, 1995.

Bromfield, William Arthur. *Flora Vectensis.* Edited by Sir William Jackson Hooker and Thomas Bell Salter. London: Pamplin, 1856.

Brown, Frank C. *Collection of North Carolina Folklore.* 7 vols. Durham, NC: Duke University Press,1952–1964.

Clark, Joseph D. "North Carolina Popular Beliefs

and Superstitions." *North Carolina Folklore* 18 (1970): 1–66.

Hatfield, Gabrielle. *Country Remedies: Traditional East Anglian Plant Remedies in the Twentieth Century.* Woodbridge: Boydell, 1994.

Koch, William E. *Folklore from Kansas: Beliefs and Customs.* Lawrence, KS: Regent Press, 1980.

Lafont, Anne-Marie. *Herbal Folklore.* Bideford: Badger Books, 1984.

McNeill, Murdoch. *Colonsay: One of the Hebrides.* Edinburgh: David Douglas, 1910.

Mellinger, Marie B. "Medicine of the Cherokees." *Foxfire* 1(3) (1967): 13–20, 65–72.

Meyer, Clarence. *American Folk Medicine.* Glenwood, IL: Meyerbooks, 1985.

Parler, Mary Celestia, and University Student Contributors. *Folk Beliefs from Arkansas.* 15 vols. Fayetteville: University of Arkansas, 1962.

Souter, Keith. *Cure Craft: Traditional Folk Remedies and Treatment from Antiquity to the Present Day.* Saffron Walden: C. W. Daniel, 1995.

Turner, Tressa. "The Human Comedy in Folk Superstitions." *Publications of the Texas Folklore Society* 13 (1937): 146–175.

Vickery, Roy. *A Dictionary of Plant Lore.* Oxford: Oxford University Press, 1995.

# Sympathetic magic

Some folk remedies are derived from the source that caused the ailment in the first place, a treatment described as "sympathetic magic." Examples are the use of a dead snake to cure a snake bite, or of the "hair of the dog that bit you" to cure a dog bite. In the seventeenth century the idea of curing a wound by treating the weapon that caused it was promulgated by Sir Kenelm Digby, adopted by barber surgeons, and then filtered into folk medicine. As recently as the twentieth century it was common in the Cambridgeshire fens for farm workers when they cut themselves to apply salve to both the wound and the instrument that had inflicted it (Porter 1974: 45).

In North American folk medicine, similar practices are to be found (Brown 1952–1964, 6: 229–231). By extension of this idea, substances that produced symptoms similar to the disease were sometimes the basis of remedies. Inducing the symptoms of fever by giving something that caused the patient to sweat is an example of this. Sympathetic magic blends into "imitative magic." Folk remedies involving holed stones as a cure for barrenness or to ease labor are examples of imitative magic (Buchan 1994: 46), as are red substances used to cure nosebleed. Again, numerous examples are to be found in North American folk medicine too, such as the use of strings of toothlike objects in aiding a baby's teething (Gardner 1937: 51). Numerous wart cures involve counting the warts and then cutting a similar number of notches in a stick, or putting the same number of pebbles in a bag. In Native American medicine too the idea can be recognized. Corn grains, themselves resembling warts, were used to treat warts (Vogel 1970: 294).

*See also* **Color; Dog; Fevers; Mad dog, bite of; Nosebleed; Snake bite; Warts; Wound.**

**References**
Brown, Frank C. *Collection of North Carolina Folklore.* 7 vols. Durham, NC: Duke University Press, 1952–1964.

Buchan, David, ed. *Folk Tradition and Folk Medicine in Scotland: The Writings of David Rorie.* Edinburgh: Canongate Academic, 1994.

Gardner, Emelyn Elizabeth. *Folklore from the Schoharie Hills, New York State.* Ann Arbor: University of Michigan Press, 1937.

Porter, Enid. *The Folklore of East Anglia.* London: Batsford, 1974.

Vogel, Virgil J. *American Indian Medicine.* Norman: University of Oklahoma Press, 1970.

# T

## Teething

In British folk medicine many different amulets were recommended to ease teething in infants. A necklace of coral or of nine strands of scarlet silk, or a bag containing wood lice or some hairs from a donkey, were placed around a baby's neck to protect it from the dangers of teething (Radford and Radford 1974: 336). Plants were used as amulets too. They include a necklace of figwort stems (Hatfield 1994: 55) or of dried bittersweet berries *(Solanum dulcamara)* (Taylor 1929: 123), or peony root *(Paeonia* sp.) (Latham 1878: 44) or sea beans. Stems of elder and traveler's joy *(? Clematis vitalba)* were similarly made into teething beads (Bloom 1830: 26). That some of these plants used as amulets were at least originally intended to be chewed by the teething infant is suggested by a seventeenth-century recipe from Sussex for making a necklace from dried roots of the narcotic plant henbane, orpine *(Sedum telephium),* and vervain *(Verbena officinalis),* all soaked in alcohol and dried. Then let the child "wear and chew them" (Allen 1995: 83). In official herbalism ready-made necklaces of imported orris *(Iris x germanica)* were available commercially to aid teething. This usage can be traced back to the fourth century (Radbill 1964: 134).

Various native plants were used topically to ease the pain of teething. They include the wild red poppy *(Papaver rhoeas),* used both in England (Hatfield 1994: 55) and Scotland (Beith 1995: 234). The cultivated opium poppy *(Papaver somniferum)* was used similarly (Porter 1969: 85). Leaves of groundsel *(Senecio vulgaris)* were infused in a baby's milk to soothe teething pains (Jobson 1967: 58).

In North American folk medicine there is a wide array of amulets for teething children. They include a necklace of coral, a mole's foot tied in a piece of cloth, or nine sillybugs, a bone from the head of a hog, rattlesnake bones, a tooth of a bear or a deer, and a frog tied around the neck (Brown 1952–1964, 6: 58–61). At least some of these threaded objects were for the child to chew on; for this purpose a turtle bone was sometimes tied around the neck (Browne 1958: 25). Amber beads were also thought to help in teething (Thomas and Thomas 1920: 118), as was a coin on a thread around the neck (UCLA Folklore Archives 25_5854). A necklace could be made from beans known as Job's tears *(Coix lacryma-jobi)* (Meyer 1985: 248), a remedy evidently learned from the Native American tradition, since it is reported in use by the Cherokee (Moerman 1998: 171). In the African tradition necklaces were made from the stems of horse nettle *(Solanum carolinense),* a species related to the British bittersweet used similarly (Puckett 1981: 346). Beads were also made from pieces of elder stalk, as in Britain, and from Jerusalem root (?*Helianthus tuberosus*) (Brown 1952–1964, 6: 61). Salves were prepared from rabbit's brains or from garlic (Brown 1952–1964, 6: 60, 61) or from the root of butterfly weed (*Asclepias tuberosa*) (Browne 1958: 25). Whisky was rubbed on the gums (UCLA Folklore Archives 4_5871), or melon rinds (Brandon 1955: 97), or tea made from catnip (Stekert 1970: 139), or the juice dripped from burned persimmon twigs (*Diospyros virginiana*) (Browne 1958: 25).

A treatment for teething involving transference was to rub the baby's gums with a live fish, which was then returned to the water (Randolph 1931: 107).

*See also* **African tradition, Amber, Amulet, Beans, Catnip, Elder, Figwort, Native American tradition, Poppy, Transference.**

## References

Allen, Andrew. *A Dictionary of Sussex Folk Medicine.* Newbury: Countryside Books, 1995.

Beith, Mary. *Healing Threads: Traditional Medicines of the Highlands and Islands.* Edinburgh: Polygon, 1995.

Bloom, J. Harvey. *Folk Lore, Old Customs and Superstitions in Shakespeare Land.* London: Mitchell Hughes and Clark, 1830.

Brandon, Elizabeth. *Les Moeurs de la Paroisse de Vermillon en Louisiane.* Ph.D. dissertation, University of Laval, Quebec, 1955.

Brown, Frank C. *Collection of North Carolina Folklore.* 7 vols. Durham, NC: Duke University Press, 1952–1964.

Browne, Ray B. *Popular Beliefs and Practices from Alabama.* Folklore Studies 9. Berkeley and Los Angeles: University of California Publications, 1958.

Hatfield, Gabrielle. *Country Remedies: Traditional East Anglian Plant Remedies in the Twentieth Century.* Woodbridge: Boydell Press Press, 1994.

Jobson, Allan. *In Suffolk Borders.* London: Robert Hale, 1967.

Latham, C. "Some West Sussex Superstitions Lingering in 1868." *Folk-Lore Record* 1 (1878): 1–67.

Meyer, Clarence. *American Folk Medicine.* Glenwood, IL: Meyerbooks, 1985.

Moerman, Daniel E. *Native American Ethnobotany.* Portland, OR: Timber Press, 1998.

Porter, E. M. *Cambridgeshire Customs and Folklore.* London: Routledge, 1969.

Puckett, Newbell Niles. *Popular Beliefs and Superstitions: A Compendium of American Folklore from the Ohio Collection of Newbell Niles Puckett.* Edited by Wayland D. Hand, Anna Casetta, and Sondra B. Thiederman. 3 vols. Boston: G. K. Hall, 1981.

Radbill, Samuel X. "The Folklore of Teething." *Keystone Folklore Quarterly* 9 (1964): 123–143.

Radford, E., and M. A. Radford. *Encyclopaedia of Superstitions.* Edited and revised by Christina Hole. London: Book Club Associates, 1974.

Randolph, Vance. *The Ozarks: An American Survival of Primitive Society.* New York: Vanguard Press, 1931.

Stekert, Ellen J. "Focus for Conflict: Southern Mountain Medical Beliefs in Detroit." *Journal of American Folklore* 83 (1970): 115–147.

Taylor, Mark R. "Norfolk Folklore." *Folk-Lore* 50 (1929): 113–133.

Thomas, Daniel Lindsay, and Lucy Blayney Thomas. *Kentucky Superstitions.* Princeton, NJ: Princeton University Press, 1920.

## Tetters

*See* **Ringworm.**

## Thomson, Samuel

Born in Albany, New Hampshire, into a farming family, Samuel Thomson (1769–1843) inherited a body of oral knowledge of folk medicine. During his childhood, this was supplemented by information from friends and neighbors, especially Mrs. Benton, a local "doctoress" in roots and herbs (Fox 1924: 21). By the time he was sixteen his knowledge was extensive, and he hoped

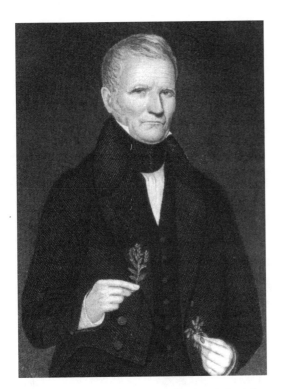

Samuel Thomson devised a system of herbalism that became famous and influential both in North America and in Britain. (National Library of Medicine)

to become a doctor. However, the family decided they could not spare him. At age twenty-two he had a farm and a family of his own, but his interest in medicinal plants continued, and after successfully treating his own children, he decided to become an herbal practitioner. He read extensively, especially the writings of Hippocrates, and devised a system of herbalism that became famous and influential both in North America and in Britain (Griggs 1981: 175). Though the roots of his knowledge belong in folk medicine, "Thomsonianism" became assimilated into official herbalism, both in North America and in Britain.

## References

Fox, William. *Family Botanic Guide.* 23rd ed. Sheffield: William Fox and Son, 1924.

Griggs, Barbara. *Green Pharmacy: A History of Herbal Medicine.* London: Jill Norman and Hobhouse, 1981.

# Thornapple

This genus (*Datura* spp.) is not native to Britain, and it is known to be poisonous. For both these reasons, it is surprising to find that it has a place in British folk medicine. It occurs as a weed of cultivated land throughout the world. The name "Datura" is Sanskrit in origin, and the plant probably originated in India. In England one species, *Datura stramonium,* appears sporadically, especially after a hot summer, and most commonly in East Anglia, and it is from here that the known folk medical uses come. A village midwife who died in the early years of the twentieth century used a burn ointment prepared from this plant in much the same way as Gerard records it in his sixteenth-century herbal. Gerard gives as the source of this remedy a woman from Ipswich who had been badly burned and was helped by this remedy; it may therefore originally have been a folk remedy, "borrowed" by the medical profession (Gerard 1597: 278). Possibly the Norfolk midwife rediscovered the remedy from the pages of Gerard's herbal, an illustration of the interaction throughout the centuries between folk and mainstream medicine. An Essex remedy used thornapple in an unusual way: the top of the fruit was cut off, the inside was pulped, and vinegar was added. Inhaling the fumes brought about pain relief (Hatfield 1994: 40).

The plant sprang into fashion in eighteenth-century North America as an asthma remedy. This use was introduced to Britain by General Gent in 1802, and the dried leaves were still being smoked for asthma by fishermen on the North Norfolk coast at the beginning of the twentieth century (Hatfield MS). More than one species of *Datura* occur in North America. In North American folk medicine thornapple is known as "Jimson weed," or "Jamestown weed," after the colonial settlement of that name. One of its principal uses has been the relief of asthma, with smoked, dried leaves. Sometimes the leaves were mixed with other herbs, such as rosemary (*Rosmarinus* sp.), aniseed (*Pimipinella anisum*), skunk cabbage (*Symplocarpus foetidus*), or lobelia (Meyer 1985: 34–35). The root has been made into a salve for treating piles (Meyer 1985: 194). The green leaves have been applied as a poultice to inflamed bowels (Meyer 1985: 202). The seeds, mixed with elder root and fried in lard, form an ointment used to remove splinters (Meyer 1985: 228).

Some of these uses were probably learned from the Native Americans. A nineteenth-century doctor, J. C. Gunn, recorded that the plant was much used by the Native Americans for bruises, contusions, wounds, ulcerations, and bites of reptiles (Meyer 1985: 272). More recently, Croom has indicated that it was used by the Lumbee Indians to treat external cancers and tick bites (Croom 1982). Moerman gives uses of three different species of Datura (Moerman 1998: 194–196). The desert thornapple, *Datura discolor,* was used by the Pima as an analgesic in childbirth, and as an application to boils, sore eyes, and sore ears (Curtin 1949: 85). *Datura stramonium* has been used by five different tribes, applied as an external application to wounds, piles, and inflammations (Moerman 1998: 194). Among the Cherokee, the leaves were smoked for asthma, just as in Britain (Tantaquidgeon 1972: 37). Another species of thornapple, *Datura wrightii,* the sacred thornapple, has, as its name suggests, been used ceremonially as a hallucinogen among a large number of different tribes, as well as being used for its painkilling properties, and, at least in the past, as a poison (Moerman 1998: 194). Probably such a poisonous plant was used mainly by experts, as in the account given by Stevenson in 1915 of an operation carried out by Nai'uchi, a famous medicine man of the Zuni, who used the powdered root as an anesthetic while operating on a woman's breast (Stevenson 1915).

*See also* **Asthma, Boils, Bruises, Burns, Cancer, Childbirth, Earache, Elder, Eye problems, Lobelia, Medicine man, Midwife, Piles, Poultice, Wounds.**

### References

Croom, E. M. *Medicinal Plants of the Lumbee Indians.* Ph.D. dissertation, North Carolina State University, 1982.

Curtin, L. S. M. *By the Prophet of the Earth.* Santa Fe, NM: San Vincente Foundation, 1949.

Gerard, John. *The Herball or Generall Historie of Plantes.* London: John Norton, 1597.

Hatfield, Gabrielle. *Country Remedies: Traditional East Anglian Plant Remedies in the Twentieth Century.* Woodbridge: Boydell Press, 1994.

Meyer, Clarence. *American Folk Medicine.* Glenwood, IL: Meyerbooks, 1985.

Moerman, Daniel E. *Native American Ethnobotany.* Portland, OR: Timber Press, 1998.

Stevenson, Matilda Coxe. "Ethnobotany of the Zuni Indians." In *Thirtieth Annual Report of the Bureau of American Ethnology.* Washington, D.C.: U.S. Government Printing Office, 1915.

Tantaquidgeon, Gladys. "Folk Medicine of the Delaware and Related Algonkian Indians." *Pennsylvania Historical Commission Anthropological Papers,* no. 3 (1972).

# Thyme (*Thymus spp.*)

In British folk medicine this plant has been used mainly for coughs, colds (Tongue 1965: 38), and sore throats, and as a sedative to help insomnia and prevent nightmares (Jobson 1967: 32). In the Highlands of Scotland, thyme tea was an everyday drink (Beith 1995: 246). The smell of crushed thyme was inhaled for headache in parts of Ireland (Allen and Hatfield, in press). Thyme is primarily a Mediterranean herb, not native to North America but introduced there. It has not been used extensively in folk medicine there, but its uses are similar. It has been used for bronchitis, head cold and sore throat (Meyer 1985: 50, 67, 252). As a sedative, it has been used to relieve menstrual pain (Meyer 1985: 174). It has been used to treat a sore mouth (Lick and Brendle 1922: 157), and bathing in crushed thyme has been recommended for fevers (Campbell 1953: 3). As in Britain, thyme tea has been drunk for insomnia (Browne 1958: 94).

In Native American practice thyme has been little used. Moerman (1998) gives a record for its use in treating chills and fever (Tantaquidgeon 1942: 56, 84).

Thymol, a constituent of thyme, is a component of many proprietary mouthwashes and gargles.

*See also* **Colds, Coughs, Fevers, Headache, Sleeplessness, Sore throat.**

### References

Allen, David E., and Gabrielle Hatfield. *Medicinal Plants in Folk Tradition.* Portland, OR: Timber Press, in press.

Beith, Mary. *Healing Threads: Traditional Medicines of the Highlands and Islands.* Edinburgh: Polygon, 1995.

Browne, Ray B. *Popular Beliefs and Practices from Alabama.* Folklore Studies 9. Berkeley and Los Angeles: University of California Publications, 1958.

Campbell, Marie. "Folk Remedies from Southern Georgia." *Tennessee Folklore Society Bulletin* 19 (1953): 1–4.

Jobson, Allan. *In Suffolk Borders.* London: Robert Hale, 1967.

Lick, David E., and Thomas R. Brendle. "Plant Names and Plant Lore among the Pennsylvania Germans." *Proceedings and Addresses of the Pennsylvania German Society* 33 (1922).

Meyer, Clarence. *American Folk Medicine.* Glenwood, IL: Meyerbooks, 1985.

Moerman, Daniel E. *Native American Ethnobotany.* Portland, OR: Timber Press, 1998.

Tantaquidgeon, Gladys. *A Study of the Delaware Indian Medicine Practice and Folk Beliefs.* Harrisburg: Pennsylvania Historical Commission, 1942.

Tongue, Ruth L. *Somerset Folklore.* Edited by Katharine Briggs. County Folklore 8. London: Folklore Society, 1965.

# Toads and frogs

In British folk medicine these animals have been exploited in a number of different ways. It was believed that to hold a live frog or a toad in the mouth of a child suffering from whooping cough would result in a cure, an example of transference (Notes and Queries, 3 [1851]: 258). In Cheshire, a live frog was held in the mouth of a child suffering from thrush (Black 1883: 35). Drinking the water in which a toad had previously been placed was a variation of this treatment used in the Scottish Highlands (Beith 1995: 143). A live frog or toad bound onto an open wound was said to promote healing. A live toad was worn in a bag to treat fits (Notes and Queries, 11 [1897]: 384), or scrofula (Notes and Queries, 4 [1875]: 83). Sometimes the ashes of a burned frog were used in a similar way (Beith 1995: 174). The powdered ashes of toad were used to treat smallpox (Notes and Queries, 9 [1902]: 426).

The power attributed to frogs and toads, and perhaps their association with witchcraft, has led to a variety of folk beliefs. In the fens of Cambridgeshire the story is told of a pregnant woman who picked up a toad by mistake when collecting potatoes. She shook with fright so much that the baby when it was born had had its fingers shaken off—they were just little stumps (Marshall 1967: 172). In the Scottish Highlands some healers, as recently as the twentieth century, carried a "bag of heads" to help them in their work, and one of these was a toad's head (Matheson 1949: 391). By association, small stones named frog or toad stones in Scotland (probably fossil fish teeth) were used for drawing poison out of wounds and for staunching bleeding (Beith 1995: 158). Land toads were thought to have the power to draw out the poison of cancer (Notes and

Queries. London, 1849 ff. 16: 193). Dropsy was treated in the Scottish Highlands by cutting a frog in half and applying the two halves to the patient's swollen body (Beith 1995: 175–176). It was said that licking a frog's eyes can give a person the power to heal sore eyes, by licking them in turn (Gregor 1881: 144). The practice of licking a person's eye to remove a foreign body was claimed to be more effective if a frog's eye was licked first.

Frogspawn was used in Scotland to treat inflammations of the skin, including erysipelas (Beith 1995: 176). Also in Scotland, a toad was held in front of a person's face suffering from a bleeding nose; whether this was meant to act as shock therapy or developed from association with the healing powers of frogs and toads is debatable (Beith 1995: 187).

Modern pharmacology has confirmed the highly poisonous nature of toad venom, secreted when the animal feels itself under threat. This venom has been used in China as a heart medicine, while Romans are known to have poisoned each other with it. The same poison was used in an attempt to fend off the plague. In nature, it protects the toad from being swallowed by other animals. A strange form of quackery developed in England in the seventeenth and eighteenth centuries, based on the well-known toxicity of the toad. Itinerant quacks hired "toadies," who, as the crowd watched, swallowed a toad, feigned death, and were then miraculously "cured" by their master. Whether they really did swallow the toads is impossible to know with certainty. From this bizarre practice comes the use of the phrase "toadying," used of someone willing to do anything to suck up to another (Allen 1995: 155).

Many of the same beliefs and practices are to be found in North American folk medicine. There are a number of examples of transference of disease, using a frog or a toad. A remedy of African American origin suggests that as a cure for asthma the sufferer should, three nights in succession, find a frog by moonlight and spit into its throat (UCLA Folklore Archives 24_6176). Other examples of transference include wrapping a live toad around the part of the body affected by rheumatism (Brown 1952–1964, 6: 258). Quinsy (Pickard and Buley 1945: 82), goiter (Hyatt 1965: 230), heavy menstruation (Josselyn 1875: 253), and even cancer (De Lys 1948: 316) have all been treated with a live toad bound to the body. Live frogs have been applied to cuts to help them heal (UCLA Folklore Archives 8_6260). They have been applied to stone bruises (Miller 1933: 475) and swollen glands (Jones 1908: 1207), and hung around a child's neck to ease teething (Smiley 1919: 379). Such widespread use of the toad in transference reflects presumably the belief that the toad has the power to absorb illness from the human patient. This belief is reflected in a record from Utah that claims that toads have the power of removing the poison of cancer from the body (Cannon 1984: 98).

It is not just as a victim of transference that the toad or frog has been used in folk medicine, however. The blood of the toad has been used to treat a scar (UCLA Folklore Archives 25_5465). The ashes of a burned frog hung around the neck were claimed to check bleeding (UCLA Folklore Archives 13_5285). Fever could be treated with ground frog heads (Hendricks 1966: 44), and whooping cough with a soup made from nine frogs (Hendricks 1980: 109). Heart trouble was treated with ground-up toad skins (Hendricks 1980: 86).

Among Native Americans there are numerous beliefs concerning the curing power of toads and frogs. The Fox believe that toads have the power to cure sickness (Jones 1911: 215). Among the Penobscot a live toad is worn in a bag and placed at the site of pain, an example of transference, as in British folk medicine above (Speck 1923:

276). Frogs and toads both figure in the lore of the Kwakiutl, especially surrounding pregnancy and childbirth. In order to conceive a child, it is suggested a woman should squat where a frog has been squatting. If a pregnant woman sees a toad, to prevent misfortune the husband should kill and dry it; when the child is born, the dried toad is passed four times over the child's belly. During the last two moons of pregnancy, a woman should drink water in which toads' toes have been rubbed (Boas 1932: 193–196).

The folklore surrounding frogs, toads and warts is extensive, and similar on both sides of the Atlantic. Frogs and toads are credited with both causing warts and being able to cure them. Given these numerous uses of toads and frogs in folklore, it is not surprising that there is thought to be a penalty for damaging them. In Florida it has been suggested that if you pick up a toad and it tries to jump you should release it, otherwise you will have nervous twitching for the rest of your life (UCLA Folklore Archives 23_5602). There is a widespread belief, particularly among children in North America, that if you kill a frog or a toad, you will stub your toe (Puckett 1926: 435).

Modern studies have shown that the toad skin contains cardiac glycosides fifty times more potent than those obtained from the foxglove. It also contains hallucinogens that could have been the basis of witches' "flying" ointment (Allen 1995: 158). Frogs too have been shown to contain some remarkable compounds, called maganins, which provide a protective shield against bacterial and fungal infection (Allen 1995: 76).

*See also* **Asthma, Bleeding, Bruises, Cancer, Childbirth, Cuts, Dropsy, Epilepsy, Erysipelas, Eye problems, Fevers, Heart trouble, Menstrual problems, Plague, Pregnancy, Quinsy, Rheumatism, Smallpox, Teething, Tuberculosis, Warts, Whooping cough, Witch, Wounds.**

# References

Allen, Andrew. *A Dictionary of Sussex Folk Medicine.* Newbury: Countryside Books, 1995.

Beith, Mary. *Healing Threads: Traditional Medicines of the Highlands and Islands.* Edinburgh: Polygon, 1995.

Black, William George. *Folk-Medicine: A Chapter in the History of Culture.* London: Folklore Society, 1883.

Boas, Franz. "Current Beliefs of the Kwakiutl Indians." *Journal of American Folklore* 45 (1932): 177–260.

Brown, Frank C. *Collection of North Carolina Folklore.* 7 vols. Durham, NC: Duke University Press, 1952–1964.

Cannon, Anthon S. *Popular Beliefs and Superstitions from Utah.* Edited by Wayland D. Hand and Jeannine E. Talley. Salt Lake City: University of Utah Press, 1984.

De Lys, Claudia. *A Treasury of American Superstitions.* New York: Philosophical Library, 1948.

Gregor, Walter. *Notes on the Folk-Lore of the North-East of Scotland.* Publication 7. London: Folklore Society, 1881.

Hendricks, George D. *Mirrors, Mice and Mustaches: A Sampling of Superstitions and Popular Beliefs in Texas.* Austin: Texas Folklore Society, 1966.

Hendricks, George D. "Roosters, Rhymes and Railroad Tracks." *A Second Sampling of Superstitions and Popular Beliefs in Texas.* Dallas, TX: Southern Methodist University Press, 1980.

Hyatt, Harry Middleton. *Folklore from Adams County Illinois.* 2nd rev. ed. New York: Memoirs of the Alma Egan Hyatt Foundation, 1965.

Jones, Frank A. "Some Medical Superstitions among the Southern Negroes." *Journal of the American Medical Association* 50 (1908): 1207.

Jones, William. "Notes on the Fox Indians." *Journal of American Folklore* 24 (1911): 209–237.

Josselyn, John. *An Account of Two Voyages to New England Made during the Years 1638, 1663.* Reprint Boston: Veazie, 1875.

Marshall, Sybill. *Fenland Chronicle.* Cambridge: Cambridge University Press, 1967.

Matheson, Neil. "Highland Healers." *Scots Magazine* (February 1949).

Miller, Joseph L. "The Healing Gods or Medical Superstition." *West Virginia Medical Journal* 29 (1933): 465–478.

*Notes and Queries* 4, p. 83. London, 1875.

*Notes and Queries* 11, p. 384. London, 1897.

Pickard, Madge E., and R. Carlyle Buley. *The Midwest Pioneer, His Ills, Cures and Doctors.* Crawfordsville, IN: R. E. Banta, 1945.

Puckett, Newbell Niles. *Folk Beliefs of the Southern Negro.* Chapel Hill, NC: Greenwood Press, 1926.

Smiley, Portia. "Folk-Lore from Virginia, South Carolina, Georgia, Alabama and Florida." *Journal of American Folklore* 32 (1919): 357–383.

Speck, Frank G. "Reptile Lore of the Northern Indians." *Journal of American Folklore* 36 (1923): 273–280.

# Tobacco (*Nicotiana tabacum*)

This plant is a native of tropical America. After its introduction to Britain in the sixteenth century, it was used medicinally as well as recreationally. During outbreaks of the plague there was a belief that smoking tobacco could protect from infection (McMullen 1962: 33). Chewed tobacco was used to treat insect bites and stings, and to kill fleas on humans and domestic animals (R.C., Norton Subcourse, Norfolk, pers. com., 1990). Some insecticides are still manufactured from it. In Ireland, the leaves were chewed for toothache (Vickery 1995: 372), a remedy also reported from Somerset (Tongue 1965: 42). In the Scottish Highlands tobacco leaves were used to stem bleeding (Beith 1995: 246), and in Bedfordshire a slice of shag tobacco was tightly bound onto cuts, using a red handkerchief (EFS 195).

In North American folk medicine, tobacco has been more widely used. A salve prepared from tobacco and butter was used to treat piles (Meyer 1985: 192). Tobacco juice was applied to ringworm (Meyer 1985: 221). The leaves pounded with honey formed a poultice for treating worms (Meyer 1985: 268). A moistened tobacco leaf was applied to soothe bruises (Meyer 1985: 274). Infant colic was treated with tobacco smoke (Brown 1952–1964, 6: 49), and colic in an adult was treated with pills made from tobacco (Brown 1952–1964, 6: 157). Tobacco juice was applied to warts (Brown 1952–1964, 6: 331). As in Britain, wounds were bound with tobacco (Meyer 1985: 277), insect bites were treated with chewed tobacco (Brown 1952–1964, 6: 289, 291), and toothache was treated by chewing tobacco (Brown 1952–1964, 6: 305). Snakebite (Smith 1929: 74), appendicitis (Kell 1965: 109), labor pain (Anderson 1970: 49), and headache (Callahan 1952: 89) were all treated with tobacco as well. The belief in Britain that tobacco could protect against infection was also found in North America, where during the eighteenth century smoking it was thought to protect against smallpox (Long 1956: 274).

In Native American practice, various species of tobacco were extensively used ceremonially. In addition they were used medicinally in a large number of ailments, including insect bites, worms, toothache, earache, bruises, cuts and bleeding, snake bite, fever, fainting, tuberculosis, dropsy, labor pain, and as an emetic (Moerman 1998: 354–357).

*See also* **Bleeding, Bruises, Childbirth, Colic, Cuts, Dropsy, Fevers, Headache, Insect bites and stings, Piles, Plague, Ringworm, Smallpox, Snake bite, Toothache, Tuberculosis, Warts, Worms.**

## References
Anderson, John. *Texas Folk Medicine.* Austin: Encino Press, 1970.

Beith, Mary. *Healing Threads: Traditional Medicines of the Highlands and Islands.* Edinburgh: Polygon, 1995.

Brown, Frank C. *Collection of North Carolina Folklore.* 7 vols. Durham, NC: Duke University Press, 1952–1964.

Callahan, North. *Smoky Mountain Country.* New York: Duell, Sloan, and Pearce, 1952.

EFS. English Folklore Survey. Manuscript notes at University College London.

Kell, Katherine T. "Tobacco in Folk Cures in Western Society." *Journal of American Folklore* 78 (1965): 99–114.

Long, Dorothy. "Medical Care among the North Carolina Moravians." *Bulletin of the Medical Library Association* 44 (1956): 271–284.

McMullen, J. T. "The Tobacco Controversy, 1571–1961." *North Carolina Folklore* 10(1) (1962): 30–35.

Meyer, Clarence. *American Folk Medicine.* Glenwood, IL: Meyerbooks, 1985.

Moerman, Daniel E. *Native American Ethnobotany.* Portland, OR: Timber Press, 1998.

Smith, Walter R. "Animals and Plants in Oklahoma Folk Cures." In *Folk-Say: A Regional Miscellany.* Edited by B. A. Botkin. Norman: Oklahoma Folk-Lore Society, 1929.

Tongue, Ruth L. *Somerset Folklore.* Edited by Katharine Briggs. County Folklore 8. London: Folklore Society, 1965.

Vickery, Roy. *A Dictionary of Plant Lore.* Oxford: Oxford University Press, 1995.

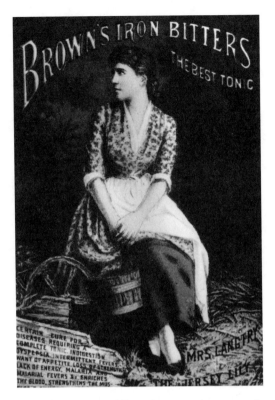

In North American folk medicine, tonics were made from dandelion, dock, elder, burdock, and other native plants. (National Library of Medicine)

# Tonic

A springtime tonic was a familiar feature of country life in Britain right up to the twentieth century. It often included stinging nettles, and a wide variety of other wild plants (Hatfield 1994: 55–56), including goosegrass (*Galium aparine)* and horehound, dandelion, dock, burdock, and elder. Often children receiving the tonic did not know what it contained; one elderly lady described vivid memories of her childhood when every spring an old lady visited the house with a large bucket of unpleasant-tasting medicine, with small green apples bobbing about in it. Every year, despite protests, it was administered! There was evidently a widespread (and probably well founded) idea that everyone, especially children, needed building up after the winter, and these tonics were regarded as "good for the blood." In Fife, Scotland, the water of a particular well was drunk to purge the system in the springtime. Sulphur with cream of tartar was also used as a springtime drink (Buchan 1994: 241).

In North American folk medicine, many of these same plants were similarly used. In addition to dandelion, dock, elder, and burdock, tonics were made from other plants native to North America but not Britain, such as Oregon grape (*Mahonia aquifolium),* mayapple *(Podophyllum peltatum),* spruce (*Picea* spp.), and sassafras (Meyer 1985: 255–259). The naturalized black alder *(Alnus glutinosa)* also features in a tonic in North American folk medicine, where we are told it should be "esteemed as a jewel" (Meyer 1985: 258). Interestingly, it seems to have been used as a tonic in the past in British folk medicine, judging by the eighteenth-century diary of the Rev. James Woodforde. Calamus root *(Acorus calamus)* and cherry bark were also used as tonics (Brown 1952–1964, 6: 115–116). Sulphur, mixed with either molasses or cream of tartar, provided another springtime tonic (Brown 1952–1964, 6: 116), as it did in Scotland.

Among Native Americans, more than 160 genera of plants have been used as tonics! (Moerman 1998: 823). In herbalism a very large number of medicinal plants both in Britain and in North America are regarded as "tonics," a concept that has lingered in folk medicine and herbalist practice long after being discarded by orthodox medicine.

*See also* **Alder, Burdock, Cherry, Dandelion, Dock, Elder, Horehound, Sassafras, Stinging nettle.**

### References

Brown, Frank C. *Collection of North Carolina Folklore.* 7 vols. Durham, NC: Duke University Press, 1952–1964.

Buchan, David, Ed. *Folk Tradition and Folk Medicine in Scotland: The Writings of David Rorie.* Edinburgh: Canongate Academic, 1994.

Hatfield, Gabrielle. *Country Remedies: Traditional East Anglian Plant Remedies in the Twentieth Century.* Woodbridge: Boydell Press, 1994.

Meyer, Clarence. *American Folk Medicine.* Glenwood, IL: Meyerbooks, 1985.

Moerman, Daniel E. *Native American Ethnobotany.* Portland, OR: Timber Press, 1998.

# Toothache

Pliny in the first century A.D. recommended the tooth of a mole as an amulet worn against toothache, and since then various versions of this remedy have been used in folk medicine. In England the foot of a mole was carried as a protection against toothache (Souter 1995: 192). Bizarrely, a tooth from a corpse, worn as an amulet, was said to have been used against toothache

in Northamptonshire (Black 1883: 98). Carrying a double hazelnut *(Corylus avellana)* has also been reported (Porter 1974: 46), while in Cornwall it is said that biting off the first fern that appears in the spring will cure toothache and prevent it for the rest of the year (Black 1883: 202). In Norfolk, a remedy involving transference recorded in the late twentieth century was to cut one's toenails, wrap them in tissue, and place them in a slit in an ash tree (Mundford 1980, unpub.).

Some in Scotland resorted to holy wells for a cure (Notes and Queries, 4 [1851]: 227). Beith reports an interesting example of transference in which an oatmeal bannock is baked with saliva and placed in water under a bridge where the living and dead cross; as it disintegrates, so the toothache will disappear (Beith 1995: 138). In another version of this cure, the sufferer must go between the sun and the sky to a place where the living and dead cross (i.e., a ford) and take a stone from there with his teeth (Black 1883: 182). Also in Scotland, a rusty nail taken from a graveyard and rubbed on the gum of an aching tooth, then buried in the churchyard, was another "cure" involving transference. Simply driving a nail into an oak beam was used as a toothache cure in nineteenth-century Kilmarnock (Black 1883: 39). Cutting toenails while under an ash tree was a cure from Cornwall (Eyre 1902: 173). Interestingly, a caterpillar wrapped in a small piece of red cloth and placed under the aching tooth has also been reported in Scotland (Beith 1995: 167); this could be related to the very ancient and widespread idea that toothache is caused by some kind of worm.

Examples of more understandable toothache remedies include whisky (in Scotland) and the burned bark of ash. In the Isle of Mull (western Scotland) in the eighteenth century, Lightfoot reported the use of a mixture of yellow flag root *(Iris pseudacorus)* and daisies *(Bellis perennis),* poured into the

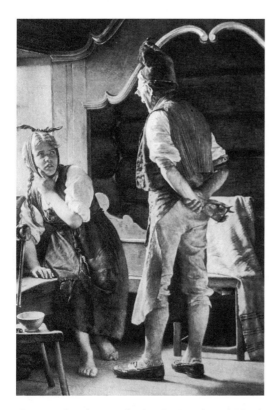

Young girl with a toothache. In British and North American folk medicine, there was a wide array of toothache cures and preventatives. (National Library of Medicine)

nostrils, as a toothache cure (Lightfoot 1777, 2: 1078). A poultice of red onions could be applied to the cheek (Beith 1995: 231), or the root of scabious *(Scabiosa succisa)* applied to the aching tooth (Beith 1995: 238). More drastically, a poultice made from spearwort *(Ranunculus flammula)*, bruised and placed in a limpet shell, was applied to the jaw; presumably the resulting blistering effect was a counter-irritant, similar to the use of horseradish *(Armoracia rusticana)* in Norfolk in the twentieth century. In the latter remedy, the horseradish was tied to the wrist on the opposite side from the toothache. Feverfew *(Tanacetum parthenium)* was used similarly, as were cabbage leaves. Inhalations for toothache in East Anglia include the smoke from burned senna leaves (Taylor MSS).

There is a record of henbane root *(Hyoscyamus niger)* soaked in vinegar being used in a Norfolk village in the early twentieth century for toothache (F.C.W., pers. com., 1990). This remedy is clearly recognizable from Gerard's herbal of 1636. Mixed with acorn meal, henbane was a toothache remedy in Saxon times (Cockayne 1864, 2: 51). Also in East Anglia, the leaves of blackberry were chewed for toothache (E.M., Essex, pers. com., 1985).

Cloves, the flower buds of a tropical tree *(Syzygium aromaticum),* have frequently been used to allay toothache and are still used today as a domestic remedy. Presumably this is, in folk medical terms, a relatively recent remedy, probably derived from book knowledge.

In North American folk medicine, there was a similarly wide array of toothache cures and preventatives, falling into the same broad categories as those in Britain. In the semi-magical category, amulets carried or worn against toothache include a tooth or bone from an animal (Brown 1952–1964, 6: 302), a dime with a hole drilled through it (UCLA Folklore Archives 20_5513), a nutmeg, a pewter ring, carrying a bead or a bullet (Brown 1952–1964, 6: 304, 307), or carrying a double nut (Cannon 1984: 128) (echoing the British remedy of a double hazelnut). The nail-clipping remedies from Britain find their counterparts too in North America. Finger and toenail trimmings, buried in a hole bored in a tree, is a remedy for toothache (Brown 1952–1964, 6: 302). Onion strips worn around the wrist were recommended (Anderson 1968: 198). Inhalations for toothache include tobacco smoke and smoke from the leaves of "life everlasting" *(Gnaphalium* sp.) (Brown 1952–1964, 6: 304). Applications to the sore tooth include salt, soda, ashes, a hot raisin and red pepper (Brown 1952–1964, 6: 304–305).

Oil of cloves and Cajeput oil (derived

from *Melaleuca leucadendron*) were used, neither of these plants being native to North America. (Meyer 1985: 247). A number of poultices were used to provide counter-irritation, such as toast sprinkled with pepper or ginger grated onto vinegar and brown paper. As in Britain, onion poultices were also used. Sometimes a roast onion was applied to the wrist on the opposite side from the aching tooth (cf. horseradish remedy above). Fresh bloodroot inserted into a cavity of an aching tooth was used to give relief (Meyer 1985: 247).

Among the Native Americans many other plants were also used, including the bark of the so-called toothache tree *(Zanthoxylum americanum)*, which was either mashed and applied to the aching tooth or chewed (Herrick 1977: 368). The roots of bull nettle *(Solanum eleagnifolium)* were similarly chewed (Stevenson 1915: 60), as were the leaves of yarrow. The use of tobacco for toothache was widespread; either the smoke was blown onto the aching tooth, the leaves were crushed to form a poultice, or the tooth was plugged with tobacco (Carr and Westez 1945: 113–123). The roots of purple coneflower (*Echinacea* spp.) were chewed for toothache (Hart 1992: 38). Various species of Iris were used for toothache by Native Americans, as in Scotland (Train, Henrichs, and Archer 1941: 89). More than a hundred different genera of plants are known to have been used by the Native Americans to treat toothache (Moerman 1998: 824–825).

Finally, there are several snake-related North American remedies for toothache. From French Canada comes the suggestion that a piece of sloughed-off snakeskin placed in an aching tooth will bring relief (Wintemberg 1908: 362). A Native American cure and preventative for toothache is to bite gently along the length of a living snake.

See also **Amulet, Ash, Blackberry, Bloodroot, Cabbage, Cayenne, Prickly ash, Snake, Soda, Tobacco, Transference, Yarrow.**

## References

Anderson, John Q. "Magical Transference of Disease in Texas Folk Medicine." *Western Folklore* 27 (1968): 191–199.

Beith, Mary. *Healing Threads: Traditional Medicines of the Highlands and Islands.* Edinburgh: Polygon, 1995.

Black, William George. *Folk-Medicine: A Chapter in the History of Culture.* London: Folklore Society, 1883.

Brown, Frank C. *Collection of North Carolina Folklore.* 7 vols. Durham, NC: Duke University Press, 1952–1964.

Cannon, Anthon S. *Popular Beliefs and Superstitions from Utah.* Edited by Wayland D. Hand and Jeannine E. Talley. Salt Lake City: University of Utah Press, 1984.

Carr, Lloyd G., and Carlos Westez. "Surviving Folktales and Herbal Lore among the Shinnecock Indians." *Journal of American Folklore* 58 (1945): 113–123.

Cockayne, Rev. T. O. *Leechdoms, Wortcunning and Starcraft of Early England.* 3 vols. London, 1864.

Eyre, L. M. "Folklore Notes from St. Briavel's." *Folk-Lore* 13 (1902): 170–177.

Hart, Jeff. *Montana Native Plants and Early Peoples.* Helena: Montana Historical Society Press, 1992.

Herrick, James William. *Iroquois Medical Botany.* Ph.D. thesis, State University of New York, Albany, 1977.

Lightfoot, John. *Flora Scotica.* 2 vols. London: Benjamin White, 1777.

Meyer, Clarence. *American Folk Medicine.* Glenwood, IL: Meyerbooks, 1985.

Moerman, Daniel E. *Native American Ethnobotany.* Portland, OR: Timber Press, 1998.

Mundford Primary School Project, Norfolk, 1980, unpub.

*Notes and Queries* 4, p. 227. London, 1851.

Porter, Enid. *The Folklore of East Anglia.* London: Batsford, 1974.

Souter, Keith. *Cure Craft. Traditional Folk Remedies and Treatment from Antiquity to the*

*Present Day.* Saffron Walden: C.W. Daniel Company, 1995.

Stevenson, Matilda Coxe. *Ethnobotany of the Zuni Indians.* Smithsonian Institution-Bureau of American Ethnology Annual Report Number 30, 1915.

Taylor MSS. Manuscript notes of Mark R. Taylor, Norfolk Record Office, Norwich. MS4322.

Train, Percy, James R. Henrichs, and W. Andrew Archer. *Medicinal Uses of Plants by Indian Tribes of Nevada.* Washington, D.C.: U.S. Department of Agriculture, 1941.

Wintemberg, W. J. "Items of French-Canadian Folklore, Essex Co., Ontario." *Journal of American Folklore* 21 (1908): 362–363.

# Tormentil (*Potentilla erecta*)

The main use of this plant in British folk medicine has been to treat diarrhea. Among its less common uses, it has treated cuts in Cumbria (Freethy 1985: 127) and worms in the Scottish Highlands (Beith 1995: 246), and it has served as a general tonic—for example, in the Shetlands (Vickery 1995: 373).

The plant is not native to North America, and its folk usage there is minimal. Meyer records the use of a plaster of tormentil root and vinegar for treating kidney complaints (Meyer 1985: 156). In Native American usage, various species of *Potentilla* that are native to North America have been used in wound treatment, as a tonic, and for treating diarrhea and dysentery (Moerman 1998: 435).

*See also* **Cuts, Diarrhea, Dysentery, Silverweed, Tonic, Worms, Wounds.**

## References

Beith, Mary. *Healing Threads: Traditional Medicines of the Highlands and Islands.* Edinburgh: Polygon, 1995.

Freethy, Ron. *From Agar to Zenry.* Marlborough: Crowood Press, 1985.

Meyer, Clarence. *American Folk Medicine.* Glenwood, IL: Meyerbooks, 1985.

Moerman, Daniel E. *Native American Ethnobotany.* Portland, OR: Timber Press, 1998.

Vickery, Roy. *A Dictionary of Plant Lore.* Oxford: Oxford University Press, 1995.

# Traill, Catherine Parr

Catherine Parr Traill (1802–1899) was one of six daughters of a wealthy Suffolk, England, merchant. She married an army officer and emigrated to Canada, a week after one of her sisters. She wrote two books giving advice to future settlers—*The Backwoods of Canada* in 1836 and *The Canadian Settler's Guide,* 1855. She became an expert on the wildflowers of Canada, and the books she wrote about them brought her fame and recognition from the Canadian government in the form of a hundred pounds and the gift of an island on the Otonabee River (Miller 1994: 77).

## Reference

Miller, Charles. *Early Travellers in North America.* Stroud: Alan Sutton, 1994.

# Transference

The idea of a disease being voluntarily passed to another person, an animal, a plant, or an inanimate object is of great antiquity. Black suggests that it may have arisen from the observation of the spread, by infection, of many diseases from one individual to another. If this happened naturally, could it be made to happen at will? In the simplest examples of transference, the disease is passed directly from the patient to the animal or object. The story in the New Testament of the devils cast out into the Gadarene swine is sometimes interpreted as an example of transference. Pliny gives examples in his writings of transference. At least one of them, involving transfer of colic to a duck, was still practiced in relatively recent times in Yorkshire (Hand 1965: 94). A very explicit example of transference comes from the eighteenth-century writings of Sir John Clerk of Penicuik, Midlothian, in Scotland. For gout, he recommends laying a dog to one's feet—the pain will pass from one's own limbs to his (SRO GD18/2142). Moncrief, in his eighteenth-century book *The Poor Man's Physician,* states that in cases of smallpox, "many keep an Ewe or Wedder in their chamber or upon the bed; because these creatures are easily infected and draw the venom to themselves—by which means some ease may happen to the sick Person" (Moncrief 1731: 60). From this original concept of transference, the idea has been developed to include many ailments that are not contagious.

In both British and North American folk medicine there are countless examples of transference. Although almost every common ailment has its transference "cure," some stand out for the number and frequency of such cures. The majority of wart cures involve transference, but this is sometimes of a more complex kind, involving an intermediate agent of transfer. The wart is rubbed with an object that is then destroyed or placed where someone else will collect it. Snails, slugs, pebbles, grains of wheat, and beans have all been used in this way in both British and North American folk medicine. Snake-bite cures often involve transference—to a snake or a fowl, for example. Whooping cough is another ailment for which transference cures have been widely used. Living frogs, toad, or fish were held in the mouth of the patient and then released. A spider in a nutshell worn around the neck was another cure for whooping cough; in this instance, as the spider died, the cough would fade away. In Gloucestershire, hair from a child suffering from whooping cough was fed to a dog, transferring the disease with it (Notes and Queries 1849: 37). In Ireland, mumps was

transferred to a pig (Rolleston 1943: 298).

Examples of transference of illness to animals abound in North American folk medicine. Epilepsy was "cured" in Pennsylvania by having the patient sleep above a cowshed (Hohman 1930: 69). A child with fits was encouraged to play with a puppy; as the puppy sickened and died, the child recovered (Johnson 1896: 75). Another epilepsy treatment was to trap a grasshopper in a thimble; as it died, the disease would disappear (Relihan 1947: 84). Tuberculosis could be transferred to a cat, just by keeping it company (Puckett 1981: 467). Anderson gives numerous examples taken from Texas folk medicine of transference to animals. They include asthma transferred to a Chihuahua; or to crickets tied on a silken string; red ants in a bag suspended around the patient's neck as a sore throat cure; and wood lice used similarly for teething problems (Anderson 1968: 191–199). For chicken pox, it was apparently necessary only to let a chicken fly over the patient to achieve transference (Anderson 1968: 197). In Georgia, pain could be transferred simply by touching the corresponding part of an animal's body (Killion and Waller 1972: 107).

Sometimes the disease is deliberately transferred to another person, as when warts are rubbed on pebbles that are then placed at a crossroad; whoever picks them up will develop warts. Labor pain was transferred to the husband by crawling over him (Hyatt 1978, 1: 391). Simply wishing the disease onto another person could cure a sufferer (UCLA Folklore Archives 9_5826). The belief that venereal diseases could be cured by communicating them to others has been a cause of much suffering (Randolph 1947: 150).

In other instances, a dead person is the intended recipient, as in the story of an Irishman who attended a wake for a dead neighbor in order to ask him to take away his rheumatism. According to the account, the cure was effective (Black 1883: 43). In another version of this procedure, dressings from an invalid were placed in a coffin and buried with the corpse (Thiselton Dyer 1878: 171).

Water sometimes acted as an agent of transfer. In Scotland, the water used to wash an invalid was poured over a cat, to transfer the illness. It was considered dangerous to cross water that had been used in a cure, as this could mean catching the illness (Dalyell 1835: 90, 104).

Trees were often the recipients of transferred disease. An elm in Bedfordshire was famous at the end of the nineteenth century as a "recipient" for ague (Vickery 1995: 127). Ash trees were used to cure hernia, by splitting a young tree, passing the sufferer through, and binding up the tree again. In this instance the tree, one hoped, mended, and so did the patient. Toothache cures sometimes involved attaching hair or fingernails to a tree; simply driving a nail into an oak tree was believed to take away toothache (Black 1883: 39). From New England there is a story of transference of a fever to an apple tree. In Sussex, nail clippings of the person suffering from fever were placed in a hole in an aspen tree (*Populus tremula*) (Allen 1995: 24). A similar practice is recorded from Newfoundland (Bergen 1899: 66). In Missouri, a complex ritual of transference involved a piece of string equal in length to the circumference of the patient's chest. A knot was tied in it for each fever a patient had suffered. It was then fastened at chest height to a tree, the whole ceremony to be done secretly (Randolph 1947: 134).

Trees near healing wells were sometimes decorated with pieces of clothing or hair from visiting patients. Examples of this are given by Hastings from Ireland (Hastings 1956–1960, 4: 749); these may represent an element of transference, or they may have been votive offerings to the tree or wa-

ter spirits. Either way, this practice is known worldwide.

*See also* **Ash, Asthma, Colic, Fevers, Gout, Snake bite, Sore throat, Spider, Toothache, Tuberculosis, Warts, Whooping cough.**

### References

Allen, Andrew. *A Dictionary of Sussex Folk Medicine.* Newbury: Countryside Books, 1995.

Anderson, John Q. "Magical Transference of Disease in Texas Folk Medicine." *Western Folklore* 27 (1968): 191–199.

Bergen, Fanny D. "Animal and Plant Lore Collected from the Oral Tradition of English Speaking Folk." *Memoirs of the American Folk-Lore Society* 7 (1899).

Black, William George. *Folk-Medicine: A Chapter in the History of Culture.* London: Folklore Society, 1883.

Dalyell, John Graham. *The Darker Superstitions of Scotland.* Glasgow: 1835.

Hand, Wayland D. "The Magical Transference of Disease." *North Carolina Folklore* 13 (1965): 83–109.

Hastings, James, ed. *Encyclopedia of Religion and Ethics.* Reprint ed. 13 vols. New York: 1956–1960. Originally published Edinburgh: Clark, 1908-1926.

Hohman, John George. *Long Lost Friend, or Book of Pow-Wows.* Edited by A. Monroe Aurand, Jr., Harrisburg, PA: Aurand Press, 1930.

Hyatt, Harry Middleton. *Hoodoo, Conjuration, Witchcraft, Rootwork.* Memoirs of the Alma Egan Hyatt Foundation, 5 vols. New York: Hyatt Foundation, 1978.

Johnson, Clifton. *What They Say in New England.* Boston: G. K. Hall, 1896.

Killion, Ronald G., and Charles T. Waller. *A Treasury of Georgia Folklore.* Atlanta: Cherokee, 1972.

Moncrief, John. *The Poor Man's Physician, or the Receits of the Famous John Moncrief of Tippermalloch.* 3rd ed. Edinburgh: 1731.

*Notes and Queries,* p. 37. London, 1849.

Puckett, Newbell Niles. *Popular Beliefs and Superstitions: A Compendium of American Folklore from the Ohio Collection of Newbell Niles Puckett.* Edited by Wayland D. Hand, Anna

Casetta, and Sondra B. Thiederman. 3 vols. Boston: G. K. Hall, 1981.

Randolph, Vance. *Ozark Superstitions.* New York: Columbia University Press, 1947.

Relihan, Catherine M. "Folk Remedies." *New York Folklore Quarterly* 3 (1947): 81–84.

Rolleston, J. D. "The Folklore of Children's Diseases." *Folk-Lore* 54 (1943): 287–307.

SRO. Scottish Record Office, Edinburgh. Papers of Clerk of Penicuik. GD18/2142.

Thiselton Dyer, Rev. T. F. *English Folk-Lore.* London: Hardwick and Bogue, 1878.

Vickery, Roy. *A Dictionary of Plant Lore.* Oxford: Oxford University Press, 1995.

# Tuberculosis

This disease is known from Palaeolithic and Neolithic bones, and from the skeletons of Egyptian mummies (Guthrie 1945: 2, 29). To what extent in folk medicine a link was made between the pulmonary symptoms and the skeletal ones is unclear. In common parlance, "consumption" generally refers to the characteristic cough and wasting, which was readily recognizable. "Scrofula" was the name given to the swollen glands and bones of tuberculosis, but the term probably covered all kinds of other malignant and nonmalignant swellings too. Famously, scrofula was also called the "King's Evil," because there was a widespread belief throughout Europe from the fifth century that it could be cured by the royal touch (Guthrie 1945: 210). For those without access to the royal touch, there were other variations on this "cure." In the Scottish Highlands, scrofula was considered curable by the touch of the hand of a dead criminal (Beith 1995: 170). In parts of Scotland it was believed that a seventh son could cure scrofula in a woman and that a seventh daughter could cure a man. Wearing a silver coin (with the royal image on it) as an amulet was considered protective against tuberculosis (Beith 1995: 161).

In East Anglia there was a belief that tuberculosis could not be passed within a family between members of the opposite sex unless they were husband and wife, so in crowded families it was not seen as a risk for an infant daughter to sleep in the same room as her father with tuberculosis (Taylor MSS). There was also a belief that butchers did not catch consumption.

Sea air was considered helpful to consumptives, while the water of some health spas was recommended for scrofula (Souter 1995: 90, 94–95). A well near Cromarty in the Black Isle, Scotland, was once famous as a cure for consumption (Beith 1995: 141). In the west of Scotland, a cure for tuberculosis consisted of pouring over the patient the tops of nine sea waves, then passing the sufferer through a hole in a sea cliff three times (Rolleston 1941: 63). In Cornwall a holed stone was used to heal children with scrofula, by passing them three times through the hole (Black 1883: 66). In Shropshire, the advice was to rise before the sun and remove a sod of turf, returning to the spot on nine successive mornings to remove it and breathe nine times into the hole (Rolleston 1941: 54). Another rural remedy was to breathe in the air surrounding penned sheep or cattle, a practice mentioned by John Wesley in the eighteenth century (Wesley 1792) and still recommended in Sussex, England, as recently as 1936 (Allen 1995: 39). The water from cow pats was an East Anglian recommendation for tuberculosis (Taylor MSS). Pennant recorded that in the eighteenth century buttermilk was drunk for consumption (Beith 1995: 167). A number of other remedies were animal based, such as the extract of snail slime employed in seventeenth- and eighteenth-century orthodox European medicine, and still used in British folk medicine right up to the twentieth century (Allen 1995: 148–150). Roasted mouse was used for consumption. Stag-horn jelly in whisky was a Scottish Highland remedy for consumption, and a broth made from leeches was also used there (Beith 1995:

170, 178). Wood lice were taken as pills for scrofula in Cornwall (Black 1883: 198).

A number of plant remedies were used in British folk medicine. There is a twentieth-century record of a child being treated with lichen for tuberculosis (EFS, record number 342). For the pulmonary symptoms of tuberculosis, an extract of the root of elecampane *(Inula helenium),* mixed with honey, was a Sussex home remedy (Allen 1995: 67). A decoction of lungwort *(Pulmonaria officinalis)* was used in Norfolk, as was beer made from nettles *(Urtica dioica),* while in Suffolk red roses, crushed with sugar, were used for the spitting of blood that accompanies consumption (Taylor MSS). Other plants used in British folk medicine to treat consumption include bogbean, ground ivy *(Glechoma hederacea),* and the root of nettle as well as the flowering tops of heather *(Erica* spp.) (Beith 1995: 207, 221, 222, 230). The Gaelic name for woodruff *(Asperula odorata)* is *lus na caithimh,* meaning "wasting wort," indicating its use in consumption (Beith 1995: 250). Centaury *(Centaurea nigra)* and dandelion were used to boost appetite in consumptives (Beith 1995: 211, 213). Common sorrel *(Rumex acetosa)* was eaten, and oat gruel was recommended as nutritious (Beith 1995: 231, 243). Martin recorded the use in the eighteenth century in the Scottish Highlands of a lamb broth made with alexanders *(Smyrnium olusatrum)* and lovage *(Ligusticum scoticum)* (Beith 1995: 202). In the eighteenth century in Orkney a drink known as "Arby" was made for consumptives from the roots of thrift *(Armeria maritima)* boiled in milk (Neill 1805: 59). In South Wales, the dew shaken from the flowers of chamomile was a remedy for tuberculosis (Trevelyan 1909: 315). Nettle leaf tea was used to treat consumption. In Ireland, a species of buttercup *(Ranunculus acris)* was applied, pulped, to "suppurating" tuberculosis (Barbour 1897:

388). An alternative was a preparation made from seven stalks of knapweed *(Centaurea nigra),* seven of fairy lint *(Linum catharticum),* and seven of maidenhair *(Adiantum venus-capillaris),* pounded in seven noggins of water from a place where three streams meet (McGlinchey 1986: 87). An eighteenth-century doctor from County Cork, Ireland, made her fortune with a tuberculosis remedy prepared from brooklime *(Veronica beccabunga)* (Ó Clara 1978: 35). For scrofula, wearing a bag of vervain *(Verbena officinalis)* was recommended (Moloney 1919: 37). Burdock was an ancient remedy in Ireland for scrofula (Wilde 1898: 34).

Tuberculosis was introduced by settlers into the New World, with devastating results. It has been suggested that the glandular form of the disease, scrofula, was the predominant one in medieval Europe, whereas the pulmonary form of the disease became epidemic in the nineteenth and early twentieth centuries (Porter 1996: 37). African Americans and Native Americans had less resistance than did the white settlers to either form of the disease. As in Britain, folk remedies were derived from mineral, animal, and plant sources. Staying in the sun was a recommendation for avoiding tuberculosis (Cannon 1984: 129). Eating coal oil and table salt was also thought to prevent the disease (UCLA Folklore Archive 4_5517), as was wearing a dime around the ankle (Saxon 1945: 353) (cf. wearing a silver coin in the Scottish Highlands, above). A pan of water under the bed was thought to help the night sweats of tuberculosis (UCLA Folklore Archive 3_6426). For a tubercular child, a lock of hair was removed and plugged into a tree at a point higher than the child's head; when the child grew to that height, he or she would be cured. Sticking a table fork into the bedhead of the patient was also practiced (Thomas and Thomas 1920: 100). Snail flesh was recommended, as in

Britain (Brown 1952–1964, 6: 159). Another suggestion was eating small frogs (DeLys 1948: 322), a cooked coon (Puckett 1981: 467), or the hind leg of a fat dog (Thomas and Thomas 1920: 100). The blood from the tail of a cat without a white hair was also suggested (Brown 1952–1964, 6: 159). A catskin worn on the chest was used to treat tuberculosis (Cannon 1984: 129), while in the African American tradition, allowing a cat to sleep on the bed was thought to prevent tuberculosis (Hyatt 1965: 252). Drinking turtle fat was recommended in Mexico (UCLA Folklore Archive 4_6543). Alligator fat (UCLA Folklore Archive 3_6543) and rattlesnake grease (UCLA Folklore Archive 2_6543) were other suggestions. Mustang liniment was claimed to be a cure for consumption, and eating a pickled rattlesnake skin was also recommended (Brown 1952–1964, 6: 160, 308). Eating a rat was a suggested cure (UCLA Folklore Archive 3_5519). For scrofula, codfish skins were applied (Meyer 1985: 223). As in Britain, the fumes from a cattle shed or horse stall (Hyatt 1965: 252) were inhaled, or those from the skunk (Reynolds 1950: 13). Drinking warm milk from a red cow was considered helpful (Hyatt 1965: 252), and goat's milk was also recommended (UCLA Folklore Archive 20_6542). As in Britain, the dew from a manure pile was used (Hyatt 1965: 252).

Many different plants were used in North American folk medicine to treat the symptoms of tuberculosis. It is ironic that elecampane *(Inula helenium)*, like the disease, was introduced into North America by colonists (Coffey 1993: 266), and a decoction of the root was used to treat the lung symptoms. In the nineteenth century, the roots were boiled with sugar and licorice *(Glycyrrhiza glabra)*, skunk cabbage *(Symplocarpus foetidus)*, or bloodroot, to form cough lozenges (Micheletti 1998: 139). Nettle leaf tea was used to treat consumption, as in Britain. Pine bark and honey

were recommended (Lick and Brendle 1922: 237), or simply inhaling the air of pine woods (Woodlief 1964: 162). Both bathing in and drinking a preparation of logwood *(Haematoxylon campechianum)* was suggested (Curtin 1930: 195). Mullein tea was used, as in Britain (UCLA Folklore Archive 7_7593). Other plants used in treating scrofula in North American folk medicine include yellow dock, whortle berries *(Vaccinium arboreum)*, hellebore *(Veratrum viride)*, wild lettuce *(Lactuca canadensis)*, and noble liverwort *(Hepatica sp.)* (Meyer 1985: 223). Salves were made from twinleaf root *(Jeffersonia diphylla)*, deer's tongue *(Erythronium americanum)*, or elder *(Sambucus canadensis)* (Meyer 1985: 223). Other plants used include sagebrush *(Artemisia sp.)* (Attebury 1963: 93), red clover *(Trifolium pratense)* (Hyatt 1965: 252), sanicle *(Sanicula sp.)* (Lick and Brendle 1922: 212), and cocklebur *(Xanthium strumarium)* (Parler 1962, 3: 974). Chaparral *(Larrea tridentata)* was used in the Southwest by pioneers (Micheletti 1998: 81), who presumably learned its use from Native Americans. The Pima in Mexico used the plant in this way (Kay 1996: 179). Pine has been known as an antiseptic and expectorant from the time of Pliny; it was recommended by, for example, Gerard as a cure for tuberculosis. In Mexico a similar recommendation was made by a Tucson *curandero* (Kay 1996: 213). There is a Blackfoot story of a beaver that in return for kindness appears in a dream to a woman suffering from tuberculosis and suggests she try the resin of lodge-pole pine, which cures her (Moerman 1998: 404). The buds of this tree *(Pinus contorta)* are made into a decoction for treating tuberculosis (Willard 1992: 39). The Alaskan Athabascan use a tea made from the berries or twigs of Juniper *(Juniperus communis)* in the treatment of tuberculosis (Kay 1996: 171). Interestingly, St. John's wort *(Hypericum perforatum)* was made into a tea by Native

Americans and drunk to treat tuberculosis. Modern research shows that the plant is active against the bacteria causing tuberculosis (Micheletti 1998: 287). More than two hundred genera have been used by the Native Americans in the treatment of tuberculosis (Moerman 1998: 825). Aside from plant remedies, there were dietary recommendations among the Native Americans. Bear liver was eaten (MacNeish 1954: 198). Drinking sour cream was thought to prevent tuberculosis (UCLA Folklore Archive 2_5522). Among the Umatilla, a steam bath followed by immersion in cold water was used for tuberculosis sufferers (UCLA Folklore Archive 1_5521).

*See also* **Amulet, Bloodroot, Bogbean, Burdock, Chamomile, Dandelion, Dew, Dock, Earth, Mouse, Mullein, Pine, St. John's wort, Seventh son, Snail, Stinging nettle.**

## References

Allen, Andrew. *A Dictionary of Sussex Folk Medicine.* Newbury: Countryside Books, 1995.

Attebury, Louie W. "Home Remedies and Superstitions." In *Idaho Reader,* edited by Grace Edgington Jordan. Boise, ID: Syms-York, 1963.

Barbour, John H. "Some Country Remedies and Their Uses." *Folk-Lore* 8 (1897): 386–390.

Beith, Mary. *Healing Threads: Traditional Medicines of the Highlands and Islands.* Edinburgh: Polygon, 1995.

Black, William George. *Folk-Medicine: A Chapter in the History of Culture.* London: Folklore Society, 1883.

Brown, Frank C. *Collection of North Carolina Folklore.* 7 vols. Durham, NC: Duke University Press, 1952–1964.

Cannon, Anthon S. *Popular Beliefs and Superstitions from Utah.* Edited by Wayland D. Hand and Jeannine E. Talley. Salt Lake City: University of Utah Press, 1984.

Coffey, Timothy. *The History and Folklore of North American Wildflowers.* New York: Facts On File, 1993.

Curtin, L. S. M. "Pioneer Medicine in New Mexico." *Folk-Say* (1930): 186–196.

De Lys, Claudia. *A Treasury of American Superstitions.* New York: Philosophical Library, 1948.

EFS. English Folklore Survey. Manuscript notes in University College London.

Guthrie, Douglas. *A History of Medicine.* London: Nelson, 1945.

Hyatt, Harry Middleton. *Folklore from Adams County Illinois.* 2nd rev. ed. New York: Memoirs of the Alma Egan Hyatt Foundation, 1965.

Kay, Margarita Artschwager. *Healing with Plants in the American and Mexican West.* Tucson: University of Arizona Press, 1996.

Lick, David E., and Thomas R. Brendle. "Plant Names and Plant Lore among the Pennsylvania Germans." *Proceedings and Addresses of the Pennsylvania German Society* 33 (1922).

MacNeish, June Helm. "Contemporary Folk Beliefs of a Slave Indian Band." *Journal of American Folklore* 67 (1954): 185–198.

McGlinchey, Charles. *The Last of the Name.* Edited by Brian Friel. Belfast: Blackstaff Press, 1986.

Meyer, Clarence. *American Folk Medicine.* Glenwood, IL: Meyerbooks, 1985.

Micheletti, Enza (ed.). *North American Folk Healing: An A–Z Guide to Traditional Remedies.* New York and Montreal: Reader's Digest Association, 1998.

Moerman, Daniel E. *Native American Ethnobotany.* Portland, OR: Timber Press, 1998.

Moloney, Michael F. *Irish Ethno-Botany and the Evolution of Medicine in Ireland.* Dublin: M. H. Gill and Son, 1919.

"'Ó Clara, Padraig': The Big Mrs. Pearson." *Cork Holly Bough* Christmas (1978): 35.

Neill, Patrick. "Remarks Made in a Tour through Some of the Shetland Islands in 1804." *Scots Magazine* 67 (1805): 347–352, 431–435.

Parler, Mary Celestia, and University Student Contributors. *Folk Beliefs from Arkansas.* 15 vols. Fayetteville: University of Arkansas, 1962.

Porter, Roy, ed. *The Cambridge Illustrated History of Medicine.* Cambridge: Cambridge University Press, 1996.

Puckett, Newbell Niles. *Popular Beliefs and Superstitions: A Compendium of American Folklore from the Ohio Collection of Newbell Niles Puckett.* Edited by Wayland D. Hand, Anna

Casetta, and Sondra B. Thiederman. 3 vols. Boston: G. K. Hall, 1981.

Reynolds, Hubert. "Grandma's Handbook." *Tennessee Folklore Society Bulletin* 16 (1950): 13–14.

Rolleston, J. D. "The Folk-Lore of Pulmonary Tuberculosis." *Tubercle* 22 (1941): 55–65.

Saxon, Lyle. *Gumbo Ya-Ya*. Boston: Houghton Mifflin, 1945.

Souter, Keith. *Cure Craft: Traditional Folk Remedies and Treatment from Antiquity to the Present Day*. Saffron Walden: C. W. Daniel, 1995.

Taylor MSS. Manuscript notes of Mark R. Taylor in the Norfolk Records Office, Norwich. MS4322.

Thomas, Daniel Lindsay, and Lucy Blayney Thomas. *Kentucky Superstitions*. Princeton, NJ: Princeton University Press, 1920.

Trevelyan, Marie. *Folk-Lore and Folk-Stories of Wales*. London: Elliot Stock, 1909.

Wesley, John. *Primitive Physic: Or an Easy and Natural Way of Curing Most Diseases*. London: 1792.

Wilde, Lady (Jane). *Ancient Cures, Charms, and Usages of Ireland*. London: Ward and Downey, 1898.

Willard, Terry. *Edible and Medicinal Plants of the Rocky Mountains and Neighbouring Territories*. Calgary, ALTA: Wild Rose College of Natural Healing, 1992.

Woodlief, Ray. "North Carolina's Mineral Springs." *North Carolina Medical Journal* 25 (1964): 159–164.

# ❧ U ❧

## Urine

Urine has been used as a remedy since ancient times, and its use has persisted in folk medicine right up to the present. Throughout Britain one of the commonest treatments for chilblains was to dip them in the chamber pot, a practice recorded for England, Scotland, and Wales (Hatfield 1999: 102; Beith 1995: 187; Jones 1980: 61). In Scotland, urine has been used as an application to treat thrush, erysipelas, bladder trouble, and gonorrhea (Buchan 1994). For jaundice and dropsy it was recommended that the patient should fast for nine days and drink all the urine produced during this time. In Scotland, urine has also been applied to chapped hands, infected wounds, and leg ulcers. For rheumatism urine was applied to the sore joints and taken internally (Souter 1995: 74–75). In Ireland a mixture of milk and urine was taken for jaundice (Logan 1972: 47). Sometimes stale urine and bran was used to poultice sore joints (Beith 1995: 187). Boils were treated with urine, and washing the skin with a wet nappy (diaper) was recommended to prevent teenage spots (Beith 1995: 188). Warts were frequently treated with urine. Bed-wetting was thought to be cured by urinating on the grave of a person of the opposite sex. An alternative was to urinate on burned ash keys (the fruit of the ash) (Radford and Radford 1974: 22, 347).

In North American folk medicine, urine has been widely used for many of these same ailments and others as well. Skin conditions treated with it include ringworm (Puckett 1981: 437), itching or chapped skin (UCLA Folklore Archives 10_5309), freckles (Bergen 1899: 71), erysipelas (Brown 1952–1964, 6: 179) and felons (Hyatt 1965: 327), as well as acne. Sore eyes have been treated with urine (Brown 1952–1964, 6: 180). Earache was treated with a few drops of warm urine (Parler 1962, 3: 611). It has been given alone or in a mixture, for croup (Creighton 1968: 210), coughs (Riddell 1934: 44), and tuberculosis (Marie-Ursule 1951: 180). Other miscellaneous uses include treatment of malaria (for which cow urine was used) (UCLA Folklore Archives 20_5427), snake bite (Kimmerle and Gelber 1976: 13), poison vine rash (Brown 1952–1964, 6: 252), insect bites and stings (Brown 1952–1964, 6: 289), fright (UCLA Folklore Archives 21_5596), and for childbirth, during which the urine of a young girl was recommended (Creighton 1968: 206).

In the Native American tradition, urine was used to wash the eyes to keep them healthy and to treat diseases of the ear (Boas 1932: 190), including deafness (Van Wart 1948: 576).

Urea is still today a component of many face creams, a "sanitized" version of folk medicine of the past. Modern analysis has justified many of the other folk uses of urine as well (Root-Bernstein and Root-Bernstein 2000: 119–132).

*See also* **Acne, Ash, Bed-wetting, Boils, Chapped skin, Chilblains, Childbirth, Coughs, Croup, Deafness, Dropsy, Earache, Erysipelas, Eye problems, Felons, Insect bites and stings, Jaundice, Poultice, Rheumatism, Ringworm, Snake bite, Tuberculosis, Warts, Wounds.**

## References
Beith, Mary. *Healing Threads: Traditional Medicines of the Highlands and Islands.* Edinburgh: Polygon, 1995.

Bergen, Fanny D. "Animal and Plant Lore Collected from the Oral Tradition of English Speaking Folk." *Memoirs of the American Folk-Lore Society* 7 (1899).

Boas, Franz. "Current Beliefs of the Kwakiutl Indians." *Journal of American Folklore* 45 (1932): 177–260.

Brown, Frank C. *Collection of North Carolina Folklore.* 7 vols. Durham, NC: Duke University Press, 1952–1964.

Buchan, David (ed.). *Folk Traditions and Folk Medicine in Scotland: The Writings of David Rorie.* Edinburgh: Canongate Academic, 1994.

Creighton, Helen. *Bluenose Magic, Popular Beliefs and Superstitions in Nova Scotia.* Toronto: Ryerson Press, 1968.

Hatfield, Gabrielle. *Memory, Wisdom and Healing: The History of Domestic Plant Medicine.* Phoenix Mill: Sutton, 1999.

Hyatt, Harry Middleton. *Folklore from Adams County Illinois.* 2nd rev. ed. New York: Memoirs of the Alma Egan Hyatt Foundation, 1965.

Jones, Anne E. "Folk Medicine in Living Memory in Wales." *Folk Life* 18 (1980): 58–68.

Kimmerle, Marjorie, and Mark Gelber. *Popular Beliefs and Superstitions from Colorado.* Boulder: University of Colorado, 1976 (unpublished).

Logan, Patrick. *Making the Cure: A Look at Irish Folk Medicine.* Dublin: Talbot Press, 1972.

Marie-Ursule, Soeur. "Civilisation traditionelle des Lavalois." *Les Archives de Folklore* 5–6 (1951): 1–403.

Parler, Mary Celestia, and University Student Contributors. *Folk Beliefs from Arkansas.* 15 vols. Fayetteville: University of Arkansas, 1962.

Puckett, Newbell Niles. *Popular Beliefs and Superstitions: A Compendium of American Folklore from the Ohio Collection of Newbell Niles Puckett.* Edited by Wayland D. Hand, Anna Casetta, and Sondra B. Thiederman. 3 vols. Boston: G. K. Hall, 1981.

Radford, E., and M. A. Radford. *Encyclopaedia of Superstitions.* Edited and revised by Christina Hole. London: Book Club Associates, 1974.

Riddell, William Renwick. "Some Old Canadian Folk Medicine." *Canada Lancet and Practitioner* 83 (August 1934): 41–44.

Root-Bernstein, Robert, and Michèle Root-Bernstein. *Honey, Mud Maggots and Other Medical Marvels: The Science behind Folk Remedies and Old Wives' Tales.* London: Pan Books, 2000.

Souter, Keith. *Cure Craft: Traditional Folk Remedies and Treatment from Antiquity to the Present Day.* Saffron Walden: C. W. Daniel, 1995.

Van Wart, Arthur F. "The Indians of the Maritime Provinces: Their Diseases and Native Cures." *Canadian Medical Association Journal* 59(6) (1948): 573–577.

# V

## Valerian (*Valeriana officinalis*)

This is an example of an herb used differently in British folk medicine than it is in official medicine and herbalism. Its folk medical uses have been limited. It has been used for treating cuts (Vickery 1995: 379) and as a general tonic (Palmer 1994: 122). In Scotland it has also been used for treating indigestion (McDonald 1958: 248), and in Ireland it has also been used to treat tuberculosis (Maloney 1972). In official medicine and in herbalism the plant has been used as a sedative, to overcome nervousness and help sleeplessness (Chevallier 1996: 146). This use has not been found in the records of folk medicine, however (Allen and Hatfield, in press). The related garden valerian *(Valeriana pyrenaica),* also known as "setwall," was used in official medicine for treating epilepsy and wounds (Pechey 1694: 188). Gerard quoted in his sixteenth-century herbal the proverb, "They that will have their heal Must put setwall in their keale" (Gerard 1597: 919), suggesting that this plant was more extensively used in his time and may have been used in folk medicine too.

*Valeriana officinalis* is not native to North America, although some other species of valerian are. Its use in North American folk medicine has been slight. The Pennsylvania Germans used valerian for treating fevers, headache, spasm and dysentery (Lick and Brendle 1922: 167). Interestingly, the garden valerian mentioned above as used by British physicians was "brought to us out of Germany" during the seventeenth century, according to William Salmon (Salmon 1693: 794). Other records for folk use of valerian are relatively few. For nervousness, a piece of valerian root under the pillow has been recommended (Saxon 1945: 531), and for removing the pain of bruising a strong decoction of valerian root was used (Meyer 1985: 274).

Related native species of valerian have been used in the Native American tradition; for example, *Valeriana dioica* has been used by the Blackfoot for stomach trouble (McClintock 1909: 275) and by the Thompson for diarrhea (Turner et al. 1990: 290), while rheumatism and wounds have been treated by the Blackfoot and the Menominee with *Valeriana edulis* (Chamberlin 1911: 350; Smith 1923: 57). More than one species of valerian has been used to treat tuberculosis (Vesta 1952: 45). For other uses by the Native Americans, see Moerman (Moerman 1998: 587–588).

A quite unrelated species, *Cypripedium acaule,* sometimes called "American Valerian," is used for treating nervousness (Bergen 1899: 115).

*See also* **Bruises, Cuts, Diarrhea, Dysentery, Epilepsy, Fevers, Headache,**

**Indigestion, Rheumatism, Tonic, Tuberculosis, Wounds.**

## References

Allen, David E., and Gabrielle Hatfield. *Medicinal Plants in Folk Tradition.* Portland, OR: Timber Press, in press.

Bergen, Fanny D. "Animal and Plant Lore Collected from the Oral Tradition of English Speaking Folk." *Memoirs of the American Folk-Lore Society* 7 (1899).

Chamberlin, Ralph. "The Ethno-Botany of the Gosiute Indians of Utah." *Memoirs of the American Anthropological Association* 2(5) (1911): 331–405.

Chevallier, Andrew. *The Encyclopedia of Medicinal Plants.* London: Dorling Kindersley, 1996.

Gerard, John. *The Herball or Generall Historie of Plantes.* London: John Norton, 1597.

Lick, David E., and Thomas R. Brendle. "Plant Names and Plant Lore among the Pennsylvania Germans." *Proceedings and Addresses of the Pennsylvania German Society* 33 (1922).

Maloney, Beatrice. "Traditional Herbal Cures in County Cavan: Part 1." *Ulster Folklife* 18 (1972): 66–79.

McClintock, Walter. "Materia Medica of the Blackfeet." *Zeitschrift für Ethnologie* 11 (1909): 273–276.

McDonald, Allan. *Gaelic Words and Expressions from South Uist and Eriskay.* Edited by J. L. Campbell. Dublin: Dublin Institute for Advanced Studies, 1958.

Meyer, Clarence. *American Folk Medicine.* Glenwood, IL: Meyerbooks, 1985.

Moerman, Daniel E. *Native American Ethnobotany.* Portland, OR: Timber Press, 1998.

Palmer, Roy. *The Folklore of Gloucestershire.* Tiverton: Westcountry Books, 1994.

Pechey, John. *The Compleat Herbal of Physical Plants.* London: 1694.

Salmon, William, M.D. *The Compleat English Physician.* London: 1693.

Saxon, Lyle. *Gumbo Ya-Ya.* Boston: Houghton Mifflin, 1945.

Smith, Huron H. "Ethnobotany of the Menomini Indians." *Bulletin of the Public Museum of the City of Milwaukee* 4 (1923): 1–174.

Turner, Nancy J., Laurence C. Thompson, M. Terry Thompson, and Annie Z. York. *Thompson Ethnobotany: Knowledge and Usage of Plants by the Thompson Indians of British Columbia.* Victoria: Royal British Columbia Museum, 1990.

Vesta, Paul A. "The Ethnobotany of the Ramaho Navaho." *Papers of the Peabody Museum of American Archaeology and Ethnology* 40(4) (1952): 1–94.

Vickery, Roy. *A Dictionary of Plant Lore.* Oxford: Oxford University Press, 1995.

# Vinegar

A vinegar douche was widely used as a contraceptive in British folk medicine. Vinegar was also used to treat insect bites and stings (Prince 1991: 49–50). A small quantity of vinegar dripped into the ear was a cure for nosebleeds; it was used on both sides of the Atlantic (Souter 1995: 180). There were numerous other household remedies involving vinegar. A newly laid egg, complete with shell, was dissolved in vinegar and mixed with melted honey to form a cure for whooping cough (Prince 1991: 115). Vinegar was used to "bring out" a bruise (Porter 1974: 46), and bandages soaked in vinegar were used as a soothing dressing for sprains and bruises (Prince 1991: 102). Vinegar and brown paper, of Jack-and-Jill fame, was used not only as a plaster applied to headaches and bruises, but also as an application for toothache (Prince 1991: 121). Vinegar was sometimes used as a solvent for herbal ingredients, as in a cure for corns that involved soaking an ivy leaf in vinegar (Tongue 1965: 38).

In North American folk medicine the uses of vinegar have been similar. Poultices made from bread and vinegar or clay and vinegar have been used to treat bruising and sprains (Meyer 1985: 232, 274), and the same whooping cough remedy of dissolving an egg in vinegar has been recorded in North America as in Britain (Meyer 1985: 266). A paste of flour and vinegar, or of linen ashes and vinegar, has been applied to wounds to stop bleeding (Meyer 1985: 276). Vinegar has been used as a wash for piles (Meyer 1985: 192). A cloth steeped in hot vinegar has been applied for pain (Meyer 1985: 186). Warm water and vinegar has been used as a vaginal douche for infection (Meyer 1985: 165). Vinegar has been recommended as a soak for swollen feet (Meyer 1985: 119). Vinegar, sugar, and salt has been recommended for dysentery (Meyer 1985: 95). Vinegar has been widely used as a solvent for herbal remedies, as in the ringworm remedy of bloodroot sliced in vinegar (Meyer 1985: 221). Sprains have been treated, as in Britain, with vinegar and brown paper or with chalk and vinegar; hiccups have been treated with sugar and vinegar (Brown 1952–1964, 6: 213, 289). Both poison ivy and warts have been treated with vinegar (Anderson 1970: 55), as has sunburn (Koch 1980: 76). As in Britain, vinegar has also been used as a contraceptive (Puckett 1981: 11). Other examples of the numerous uses of vinegar in North American folk medicine can be found in the UCLA Folklore Archives.

Often the type of vinegar is not specified in folk medicine, but apple cider vinegar has become famous largely through the work of Dr. Jarvis, who recommended it for a wide variety of ailments including rheumatism and a variety of skin conditions (Jarvis 1961: 90, 175–177). His books have been very popular both in North America and in Britain, and cider vinegar is now used in Britain in domestic medicine as well.

*See also* **Bleeding, Bloodroot, Bruises, Contraception, Corns, Dysentery, Headache, Hiccups, Insect bites and stings, Ivy, Nosebleed, Piles, Poison ivy, Poultice, Rheumatism, Sore feet, Sunburn, Toothache, Warts, Whooping cough.**

### References

Anderson, John. *Texas Folk Medicine*. Austin, TX: Encino Press, 1970.

Brown, Frank C. *Collection of North Carolina Folklore*. 7 vols. Durham, NC: Duke University Press, 1952–1964.

Jarvis, D. C. *Folk Medicine*. London: Pan Books, 1961.

Koch, William E. *Folklore from Kansas: Beliefs and Customs*. Lawrence, KS: Regent Press, 1980.

Meyer, Clarence. *American Folk Medicine*. Glenwood, IL: Meyerbooks, 1985.

Porter, Enid. *The Folklore of East Anglia*. London: Batsford, 1974.

Prince, Dennis. *Grandmother's Cures: An A–Z of Herbal Remedies*. London: Fontana, 1991.

Puckett, Newbell Niles. *Popular Beliefs and Superstitions: A Compendium of American Folklore from the Ohio Collection of Newbell Niles Puckett*. Edited by Wayland D. Hand, Anna Casetta, and Sondra B. Thiederman. 3 vols. Boston: G. K. Hall, 1981.

Souter, Keith. *Cure Craft: Traditional Folk Remedies and Treatment from Antiquity to the Present Day*. Saffron Walden: C. W. Daniel, 1995.

Tongue, Ruth L. *Somerset Folklore*. Edited Katharine Briggs. County Folklore 8. London: Folklore Society, 1965.

# ❧ W ❧

## Warts

Every aspect of folk medicine is represented in miniature in the vast array of folk treatments for warts. Why they should have attracted quite so much attention is not clear; perhaps it was observed at an early stage that warts were mysterious, came and went without apparent cause, and succumbed to all kinds of treatments. Perhaps because they do not represent a life-threatening condition, warts provided an ideal ailment for folk experimentation.

In modern medical parlance, warts are caused by a papilloma virus; what in the past were described as warts may have included a variety of other skin complaints, such as corns, calluses, and even malignant lesions of the skin. As is always the case when considering folk categories of disease, we cannot be sure retrospectively of the diagnosis. However, warts are such a commonly recognized complaint that we can safely assume that the majority of wart cures were indeed applied to warts.

Methods used for treating warts both in the past and up to the present time include physical agents that are rubbed on the wart. These for convenience can be divided into plants, products of animal origin, and miscellany. In the first category fall such common plants as dandelion (the white juice is rubbed on the wart); numerous species of spurge (*Euphorbia* spp.) (again, the thick

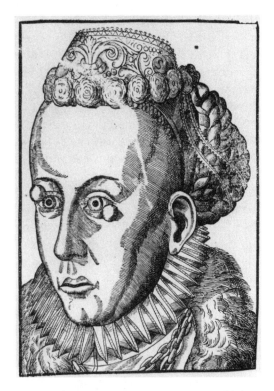

Because they were so common, warts provided an ideal ailment for folk experimentation. Methods used for treating warts both in the past and up to the present include plants and products of animal origin that are applied to the wart. (National Library of Medicine)

white latex is rubbed on); and the greater celandine *(Chelidonium majus)*, which exudes a bright orange latex when the stems and leaves are broken. The use of these plants appears to be purely practical and devoid of ritual, perhaps suggesting the plant juice is itself the effective agent. Other British plant species used as simple applications to warts are too numerous to list individually (Hatfield 1999: 147–159).

Animal products used as wart applications include human saliva, menstrual blood, urine, and the blood of a mole. Miscellaneous agents include soot, ash, coal, and ink.

Wart treatments also include wart "charming," buying and selling warts, and simply counting them. However, there is no hard and fast line between these different methods. Even apparently practical methods, such as rubbing the wart with a slice of apple, are often accompanied by ritual, such as throwing the apple over the shoulder.

One feature common in the treatment of warts is the idea of using a stolen object in the cure. In East Anglia, this has variously been recorded as a stolen piece of beef or of bacon—but its stolen nature is stressed, and the operation must be done secretly (Hatfield 1999: 155). The meat after being rubbed on the wart is then disposed of (usually buried in the garden), and as it rots, so the wart will disappear.

The idea of transference of the disease is taken a step farther in a remedy for warts that consists of placing in a parcel the same number of pebbles as one has warts. The parcel is then placed at a crossroad, and whoever picks it up will acquire the warts. A commonly recorded remedy from East Anglia is to take a slug or a snail, allow it to walk over the warts, and then impale it on a thorn outside. As it withers, so will the warts disappear. Cutting notches in an ash tree, the same number as there are warts, is another example of transference.

It is significant that many folk remedies for warts have built-in time factors. Since warts are often a self-limiting condition, a skeptical view would suggest that the remedy itself is irrelevant—it is simply a matter of time before the warts disappear naturally. A modern dermatologist claims the most effective treatment for warts he has found is to make the patient an appointment at a wart clinic; by the time of the appointment, the warts have often vanished! However, it is difficult to account for reports of warts disappearing literally overnight. Such reports are numerous, and many are of cases of wart "charming." Here we are entering the realm of suggestion and psychotherapy, though it is unconvincing to evoke these as curative mechanisms to explain reported rapid cures of warts in animals (Hatfield 1999: 155).

Why should such a plethora of folk remedies exist for the treatment of warts? One obvious reason could be their commonness in the recent past—a small survey in England in 1999 revealed surprisingly that two-thirds of the informants had had warts at some time in their lives (Hatfield 1998). Another factor may be the observation that warts are susceptible to the power of suggestion. This is underlined by the finding that hypnotherapy can be a useful tool in the official treatment of warts (Ewin 1992: 1).

All the remedies mentioned for warts in British folk medicine, and many more besides, have been recorded in North American folk medicine. To attempt to summarize them is almost impossible. Their wealth and variety is illustrated by the fact that the Brown Collection of North Carolina Folklore contains almost three hundred entries, while the UCLA Folklore Archive contains more than 4,500 records! All the elements noted in British folk medicine are present. Secrecy is often involved, as in stealing a piece of meat, rubbing it on the wart, and hiding it (Brown 1952–1964, 6: 318). Many of the remedies involve transference to an inanimate object, such as a stolen dishcloth (Brown 1952–1964, 6: 337), a plant (Brown 1952–1964, 6: 330), or an animal (Brown 1952–1964, 6: 324). As in Britain, warts are bought or sold or charmed away (Baldwin 1992: 188–189).

*See also* **Apple, Blood, Cricket, Dandelion, Snail, Spit, Sympathetic magic, Transference.**

### References

Baldwin, Karen. "Folk Medical Practices of North Carolinians." In *Herbal and Magical Medicine,* edited by James Kirkland, Holly F. Mathews, C. W. Sullivan III, and Karen Baldwin. Durham, NC: Duke University Press, 1992.

Brown, Frank C. *Collection of North Carolina Folklore.* 7 vols. Durham, NC: Duke University Press, 1952–1964.

Ewin, D. M. "Hypnotherapy for Warts." *American Journal of Clinical Hypnosis* 35(1) (July 1992): 1–10.

Hatfield, Gabrielle. *Warts: Summary of Wart-Cure Survey for the Folklore Society.* London: Folklore Society, 1998.

———. *Memory, Wisdom and Healing. The History of Domestic Plant Medicine.* Phoenix Mill: Sutton. 1999.

# Water

Apart from its obvious symbolism of cleansing, water has played many roles in British folk medicine. Sometimes particular "healing wells" had reputations for healing one sort of ailment. In later times, many such wells were dedicated to a particular saint. Thus when the name "St. Mary's Well" was used, it often applied to a well that in the past had been thought to promote fertility (Buchan 1994: 267). The water of a particular well often had a reputation for curing certain ailments. The historic well at Orton, for example, was believed to cure whooping cough as well as eye and joint diseases (Buchan 1994: 267). In Herefordshire, St. Peter's well had a reputation for curing rheumatism (Leather 1912: 13). During the seventeenth and subsequent centuries the use of healing

wells was rationalized by the medical profession, which pointed to the differing chemical composition of the water from different wells. This led to the fashion of "taking the waters" (Souter 1995: 93–95). Meanwhile, locally famous water sources continued to be used by ordinary people in folk medicine. The so-called chalybeate springs, with iron-rich water, were visited for tuberculosis, as well as for women's diseases (Beith 1995: 132). In Somerset, wells were used to treat a great variety of ailments, including leprosy, rheumatism, epilepsy, and jaundice (Tongue 1965: 218–219). The famous healing well of Holywell was visited by the lowly and the royal, from the time of William the Conqueror onward (Black 1883: 103).

As well as the water from springs, cave water was sometimes attributed with healing powers. Water dripping from a cave on the Black Isle in Scotland was thought to cure ear ailments (Beith 1995: 132). The water of fast-flowing streams was also used in folk medicine, often accompanied by prayers or charms. Rushes from a running stream were placed in the mouth of a child with thrush and then returned to the stream, carrying the disease with them (Black 1883: 104). Mumps was treated in Ireland by drinking three times from a stream (Black 1883: 105–106), while on Exmoor, running water was part of a cure for "boneshave," or sciatica (Black 1883: 107). In Devon for shingles, rushes growing near a stream were laid on the affected area and then thrown into the stream (Lafont 1984: 74).

In North American folk medicine, particular springs have again had individual reputations for healing. Sulphur springs had a reputation for curing boils (Wilson 1968: 68) The White Sulphur Springs of Meagher County were used by Native Americans and later by settlers to help rheumatism (Montana State Guide 1939: 270). For kidney disease and typhoid, Chippewa natural spring water was used until well into the twentieth century (Saul 1949: 58). Thermal water in North Carolina was believed to cure rheumatism and other ailments (Woodlief 1964: 162). There was a general belief in the healthiness of well water. It was considered purer than city water, and the minerals it contained were healthy (UCLA Folklore Archive 9_6776). Rusty well water was good for poison, but green well water was itself a poison (UCLA Folklore Archive 5_5453). Drinking well water was said to make a person grow tall (Cannon 1984: 69).

As in Britain, the curative power of running water was used in North American folk medicine. Water from the Mississippi River was considered to aid fertility (Robinson 1948: 132–133). Bathing in free-flowing water was considered beneficial for rheumatism (Brown 1952–1964, 6: 265). Sometimes the direction of flow was specified. For frost bite bathing the feet in a westward-flowing stream was recommended (UCLA Folklore Archives 3_6834), while water running northward was believed by some to have healing powers (UCLA Folklore Archive 10_6808). Some folk cures used the idea of flowing water carrying away disease. Warts were rubbed with salt, then washed in running water (Puckett 1981: 484). Blood from a hemorrhage was placed in a bottle that was then thrown into running water (Hyatt 1970: 386).

*See also* **Boils, Deafness, Dew, Earache, Epilepsy, Forge water, Frostbite, Jaundice, Rheumatism, Shingles, Snow, Tuberculosis, Whooping cough.**

## References

Beith, Mary. *Healing Threads: Traditional Medicines of the Highlands and Islands.* Edinburgh: Polygon, 1995.

Black, William George. *Folk-Medicine: A Chapter in the History of Culture.* London: Folklore Society, 1883.

Brown, Frank C. *Collection of North Carolina Folklore.* 7 vols. Durham, NC: Duke University Press, 1952–1964.

Buchan, David (ed.). *Folk Tradition and Folk Medicine in Scotland: The Writings of David Rorie.* Edinburgh: Canongate Academic, 1994.

Cannon, Anthon S. *Popular Beliefs and Superstitions from Utah.* Edited by Wayland D. Hand and Jeannine E. Talley. Salt Lake City: University of Utah Press, 1984.

Hyatt, Harry Middleton. *Hoodoo, Conjuration, Witchcraft, Rootwork.* 5 vols. New York: Memoirs of the Alma Egan Hyatt Foundation, 1970.

Lafont, Anne-Marie. *Herbal Folklore.* Bideford: Badger Books, 1984.

Leather, Ella Mary. *The Folk-Lore of Herefordshire Collected from Oral and Printed Sources.* Hereford and London: Jakeman and Carver, 1912.

*Montana State Guide.* New York: Federal Writers Project, 1939.

Puckett, Newbell Niles. *Popular Beliefs and Superstitions: A Compendium of American Folklore from the Ohio Collection of Newbell Niles Puckett.* Edited by Wayland D. Hand, Anna Casetta, and Sondra B. Thiederman. 3 vols. Boston: G. K. Hall, 1981.

Robinson, Lura. *Old New Orleans Custom.* New York: Vanguard Press, 1948.

Saul, F. William. *Pink Pills for Pale People.* Philadelphia: Dorrance, 1949.

Souter, Keith. *Cure Craft: Traditional Folk Remedies and Treatment from Antiquity to the Present Day.* Saffron Walden: C. W. Daniel, 1995.

Tongue, Ruth L. *Somerset Folklore.* Edited by Katharine Briggs. County Folklore 8. London: Folklore Society, 1965.

Wilson, Gordon, Sr. *Folklore of the Mammoth Cave Region.* Kentucky Folklore Series 4. Bowling Green, KY: Kentucky Folklore Society, 1968.

Woodlief, Ray. "North Carolina's Mineral Springs." *North Carolina Medical Journal* 25 (1964): 159–164.

# Whitlows

*See* **Felons.**

# Whooping cough

In British folk medicine this has attracted a very wide range of remedies, some of them seemingly bizarre. In East Anglia, Sussex, and in Scotland, and probably in other parts of Britain too, eating a fried mouse was a popular remedy right up to the twentieth century. Apparently this is a very ancient idea and can be traced back to the ancient Egyptians (Beith 1995: 179). A preparation made from the wood louse, or slater, was also used to treat whooping cough in the Scottish Highlands (Beith 1995: 184). Also among the Gaels, swallowing a live spider was recommended (Beith 1995: 186). Inhaling the tar fumes from roadworks or the fumes from old-fashioned gasworks was also widely believed to be helpful (Hatfield MS). A new-laid egg dissolved in vinegar, shell and all, and mixed with honey, has been used for whooping cough (Prince 1991: 115). In Westmoreland in the 1930s, a moleskin was tied around the necks of children suffering from whooping cough (Prince 1991: 112). Another amulet, used in the west of England, was stranger still: the patient was told to wear, in a silk bag, hair taken from the end of the cross on the donkey's back (Prince 1991: 100). Another cure was to pass the sufferer over the back of a donkey and under its belly (Tongue 1965: 44).

The belief that a child who rode on a bear would never have whooping cough was said to be widespread in England at one time and to have earned a lot of money for bear keepers (Black 1883: 159). The exhaled breath of various animals was held to be beneficial; standing near a horse or cow in an enclosed space and breathing in their breath was practiced in Sussex until quite recent times (Allen 1995: 38), and in Norfolk ferrets have been used similarly (Hatfield MS). Syrup made from sweetened juice of crushed snails was used in Sussex well into the twentieth century (Allen 1995: 149). There are also reports of a broth made from owls being taken for whooping cough in Sussex (Allen 1995: 154). A live spider hung in a bag by the fire until it died (Porter 1974: 50) has been used to treat whooping cough in East Anglia, and in the Scottish Highlands a live spider was swallowed as a cure (Beith 1995: 186).

Any remedy recommended by someone riding a piebald horse was claimed to be successful (Allen 1995: 180). This idea was also prevalent in the Highlands of Scotland. It has been suggested that it could be related to the cult of a Celtic Apollo, often depicted on horseback (Beith 1995: 91). Another Highland remedy was to give the child water to drink in which a toad had been placed (Beith 1995: 143) or giving the child water to drink out of an animal horn that had been taken from a living animal (Beith 1995: 143). Water from a hollowed rock or stone was considered especially useful (Beith 1995: 148). Mare's milk was recommended in the Highlands of Scotland as a soothing drink for a child with whooping cough (Beith 1995: 178).

Numerous whooping cough remedies provide examples of the transference of disease. Particular ash trees were until the nineteenth century revered for their ability to cure various ailments, including whooping cough (Vickery 1995: 19). Passing the suffering child under an arch formed by a bramble *(Rubus fruticosus)* bush rooted at both ends was a popular whooping cough remedy, still in use in Wales in the twentieth century (Simpson 1976: 108). Sometimes an offering of bread and butter was left for the bramble bush (Leather 1912: 82). Passing a child under the belly of a donkey, holding a live fish in the mouth of the sufferer, or a frog or toad (Mundford Primary School project, 1980, unpub.), are all further examples of transference.

The concept of rites of passage, as in the bramble remedy mentioned above, appears in other whooping cough remedies. Crossing water was a suggested Scottish remedy (Beith 1995: 143). Taking a child with whooping cough to the edge of the sea and waiting while the tide ebbed and took the cough with it was another suggestion (Radford and Radford 1974: 341). Another suggestion was to hold the child upside down in a hole made in the ground, afterward filling in the hole. Bread and butter given by a posthumous child or by a woman whose married and maiden names were the same (Radford and Radford 1974: 67) was regarded as a whooping cough cure.

A pleasant-sounding remedy was to walk the child up and down between the rows of a bean field in flower (Taylor MSS; Hatfield MS). Drinking milk from a cup made of the wood of variegated holly was recommended. The water from boiled hay was administered in Essex (E.M., Barking, Essex, 1985, pers. com.). Onion and garlic were used, as well as other vegetables sliced and soaked with sugar to form a cough syrup. Other members of the onion family were also used in whooping cough remedies, such as chives *(Allium schoenoprasum)* (Vickery 1995: 66) and crow garlic *(Allium vineale)* (Bloom 1920: 246). Other plant medicines include blackcurrant *(Ribes nigra)* shoots boiled with licorice and sugar, figs soaked in gin, mulberry *(Morus* sp.) and castor oil, marigold flowers *(Calendula officinalis)*, and "mouse's ear" (probably *Pilosella officinarum)*. Even the gall that grows on rose bushes, and is called a "Robin's pincushion," has been used in an infusion for whooping cough (Taylor MSS). Mistletoe was considered in East Anglia "a sure cure" (Rider Haggard, ed. 1974: 16). Elecampane *(Inula helenium)* was used as the basis of a whooping cough medicine in Sussex (Allen

1995: 66). In the Scottish Highlands, apple, rowan, and brown sugar were given for whooping cough (Beith 1995: 203). A gypsy remedy used wild thyme (Vesey-Fitzgerald 1944: 28).

Almost all these British remedies for whooping cough, and many others as well, are represented in North American folk medicine. In the UCLA folk medicine archive are numerous records of the use of live fish, toads, frogs, spiders, etc. Again, a number of the remedies involve transference; not only does the remedy using donkey hair appear, but riding on a donkey, ass, horse, or bear is suggested. Exhaled breath from various animals, including a guinea pig, has been used. Mare's milk is again recommended, also a tea made from white ants. The remedy involving passing through a natural arch of vegetation in North American folklore is applied to the native "raspberry briar" (probably *Rubus idaeus)* rather than the British blackberry, which though introduced in North America is not native there (Brown 1952–1964, 6: 352). Inhaling smoke, tar, and fumes are all suggested. There are a large number of records of placing a child in a mill hopper and grinding the corn underneath (Brown 1952–1964, 6: 67). Preparations of urine and dung from various animals are also numerous. There are a number of examples of the idea that bread should be received by the sufferer from a woman whose maiden name was the same as her husband's one, and a posthumous child was thought to have the power to cure whooping cough—two ideas familiar in British folk medicine as well.

Other remedies familiar from Britain include an egg dissolved in vinegar and sweetened with honey; onion, garlic, and mouse-ear, and elecampane were all used too. In addition, various plants native to North America but not Britain were used, such as bloodroot, skunk cabbage root *(Symplocarpus foetidus)*, chestnut leaves *(Castanea* sp.), pennyroyal (probably the

American pennyroyal, *Hedeoma pulegioides*), and prickly pear (*Opuntia* sp.). Roots of marshmallow, or flowers of red clover (*Trifolium pratense*) also appear in American folk remedies, though not in British ones. Water in which oat straw has been boiled, sweetened with brown sugar, was another recommendation. Rubbing the soles of the child's feet with hog's lard, or the chest with eucalyptus oil or rum or brandy, sweet oil and onion, was also tried (Meyer 1985: 266–268).

In Native American practice, many of the plants mentioned above have been used in the treatment of coughs generally. The use of skunk cabbage root has been recorded among the Delaware specifically for whooping cough (Tantaquidgeon 1972: 37); the Mohegan are known to have used an infusion of chestnut leaves (*Castanea dentata*) for treating whooping cough (Tantaquidgeon 1928: 265). An infusion of red clover (*Trifolium pratense*) has been used by the Quebec Algonquin to treat whooping cough (Black 1980: 88), suggesting that this remedy reached general North American folk medicine from this source, rather than from Europe.

*See also* **Amulet, Apple, Beans, Bloodroot, Bread, Coughs, Earth, Excreta, Garlic, Holly, Mallow, Mistletoe, Mouse, Onion, Rowan, Snail, Spider, Thyme, Toads and frogs, Transference, Urine.**

### References

Allen, Andrew. *A Dictionary of Sussex Folk Medicine.* Newbury: Countryside Books, 1995.

Beith, Mary. *Healing Threads: Traditional Medicines of the Highlands and Islands.* Edinburgh: Polygon, 1995.

Black, Meredith Jean. *Algonquin Ethnobotany: An Interpretation of Aboriginal Adaptation in South Western Quebec.* Mercury Series 65. Ottawa: National Museums of Canada, 1980.

Black, William George. *Folk-Medicine: A Chapter in the History of Culture.* London: Folklore Society, 1883.

Bloom, J. H. "Modern Folklore of Warwickshire: Cures." *Notes and Queries* 12(7) (1920): 245–246.

Brown, Frank C. *Collection of North Carolina Folklore.* 7 vols. Durham, NC: Duke University Press, 1952–1964.

Leather, E. M. *The Folk-lore of Herefordshire.* London and Hereford: Jakeman and Carver, 1912.

Meyer, Clarence. *American Folk Medicine.* Glenwood, IL: Meyerbooks, 1985.

Mundford Primary School project, 1980, Norfolk, unpublished.

Porter, Enid. *The Folklore of East Anglia.* London: Batsford, 1974.

Prince, Dennis. *Grandmother's Cures: An A–Z of Herbal Remedies.* London: Fontana, 1991.

Radford, E., and M. A. Radford. *Encyclopaedia of Superstitions.* Edited and revised by Christina Hole. London: Book Club Associates, 1974.

Rider Haggard, Lilias (ed.). *I Walked by Night.* Woodbridge: Boydell Press, 1974.

Simpson, Jacqueline. *The Folklore of the Welsh Border.* London: Batsford, 1976.

Tantaquidgeon, Gladys. *Folk Medicine of the Delaware and Related Algonkian Indians. Pennsylvania Historical Commission Anthropological Papers,* no. 3 (1972).

Tantaquidgeon, Gladys. "Mohegan Medicinal Practices, Weather-Lore and Superstitions." *Smithsonian Institution-Bureau of American Ethnology Annual Report* 43 (1928): 264–270.

Taylor MSS. Manuscript notes of Mark R. Taylor in Norfolk Record Office, Norwich. MS4322.

Tongue, Ruth L. *Somerset Folklore.* Edited by Katharine Briggs. County Folklore 8. London: Folklore Society, 1965.

Vesey-Fitzgerald, B. "Gypsy Medicine." *Journal of the Gypsy Lore Society* 23 (1944): 21–33.

Vickery, Roy. *A Dictionary of Plant Lore.* Oxford: Oxford University Press, 1995.

# Willow (*Salix* spp.)

In British folk medicine willow has primarily been used in the treatment of fevers, headache, and rheumatism. Although a member of the clergy, Rev. Edward Stone, is credited with the "discovery" during the eighteenth century of the painkilling properties of willow, he actually learned it from contemporary folk medicine and was responsible only for drawing it to the attention of the medical fraternity. This act in time led to the isolation of salicylic acid and eventually to the development of aspirin. Willow bark tea was drunk in the East Anglian fens for fever (Porter 1974: 52). As recently as the twentieth century, willow bark was still chewed in the Lincolnshire fens to relieve headache, especially due to hangover (Hatfield 1994: 40). There were other minor uses of willow in British and Irish folk medicine, including wart treatment and various skin conditions (Allen and Hatfield, in press). Toothache and earache have both been treated using willow (Vickery 1995: 401). In Cumbria, it has been used for staunching bleeding (Freethy 1985: 133). In Ireland willow has been used to form a hoop through which a child with a hernia was passed; as the sides of the split willow rod grew together, so the child would mend (Hunt 1938: 197). The flowers of weeping willow have been used in Ireland for treating burns (Allen and Hatfield, in press).

In North American folk medicine, similar uses of willow have been recorded. Willow bark tea has been used for fevers (Brown 1952–1964, 6: 191), ashes of burned willow mixed with vinegar have been used to treat warts (Meyer 1985: 263), and a willow stick has been rubbed on a wart seven times and then planted (Brown 1952–1964, 6: 331). Willow ashes have also been used to treat nausea (Smith 1929: 72). Willow bark tea has been drunk for diarrhea (Wilson 1968: 326). An infusion of willow root has been used to treat toothache (Puckett 1981: 462); more magically, a splinter of willow used to prick the gum of an aching tooth was placed over the door (Hyatt 1970, 1: 513). Just as in Britain, willow has been split and a patient with a hernia passed through it (UCLA Folklore Archive 18_5464). For other uses of willows in North American folk medicine, see the UCLA Folklore Archives.

There are very many species of native willows in North America, and many of them have been used medicinally by the Native Americans for treating fevers and rheumatism (Moerman 1998: 798, 774–775). They have also been used for a wide range of other ailments, including dysentery, bleeding cuts and sores, stomach ailments, scrofula, and venereal disease, and as a hair tonic. (For these and other examples of Native American usage, see Moerman 1998: 500–508.) The strength and flexibility of willow wood has been exploited by Native Americans for splinting fractures (Bourke 1892: 471).

*See also* **Bleeding, Burns, Diarrhea, Dysentery, Earache, Fevers, Fractures, Headache, Nausea, Rheumatism, Toothache, Warts.**

## References

Allen, David E., and Gabrielle Hatfield. *Medicinal Plants in Folk Tradition.* Portland, OR: Timber Press, in press.

Brown, Frank C. *Collection of North Carolina Folklore.* 7 vols. Durham, NC: Duke University Press, 1952–1964.

Bourke, John G. *Medicine Men of the Apache.* Ninth Annual Report of the Bureau of Ethnology. 1887–1888. Washington, DC: 1892, 443–603.

Freethy, Ron. *From Agar to Zenry.* Marlborough: Crowood Press, 1985.

Hatfield, Gabrielle. *Country Remedies: Traditional East Anglian Plant Remedies in the Twentieth Century.* Woodbridge: Boydell Press, 1994.

Hunt, William. "County Donegal, Ireland, Parish of Killymard." *Folk-Lore* 49 (1938): 193–197.

Hyatt, Harry Middleton. *Hoodoo, Conjuration, Witchcraft, Rootwork.* 5 vols. New York: Memoirs of the Alma Egan Hyatt Foundation, 1970.

Meyer, Clarence. *American Folk Medicine.* Glenwood, IL: Meyerbooks, 1985.

Moerman, Daniel E. *Native American Ethnobotany.* Portland, OR: Timber Press, 1998.

Porter, Enid. *The Folklore of East Anglia.* London: Batsford, 1974.

Puckett, Newbell Niles. *Popular Beliefs and Superstitions: A Compendium of American Folklore from the Ohio Collection of Newbell Niles Puckett.* Edited by Wayland D. Hand, Anna Casetta, and Sondra B. Thiederman. 3 vols. Boston: G. K. Hall, 1981.

Smith, Walter R. "Animals and Plants in Oklahoma Folk Cures." *Folk-Say: A Regional Miscellany.* Edited by B. A. Botkin. Norman: Oklahoma Folklore Society, 1929.

Vickery, Roy. *A Dictionary of Plant Lore.* Oxford: Oxford University Press, 1995.

Wilson, Gordon. "Local Plants in Folk Remedies in the Mammoth Cave Region." *Southern Folklore Quarterly* 32 (1968): 320–327.

# Witch

The subject of witchcraft, like sorcery, strictly belongs with religion and folklore, but since in the modern mind witches are strongly associated with herbal medicine, it is necessary to consider the subject as it relates to folk medicine. In societies where almost everyone needed, and had some knowledge of, home remedies, anyone possessing especially great knowledge was regarded with awe, reverence, fear, or a mixture of these emotions. Reginald Scot wrote in 1584, "It is indifferent to say in the English tongue, 'she is a witch' or 'she is a wise woman' " (Scot, Discoverie, V, ix: quoted in Thomas 1973: 518). There is no doubt that many of the women branded as witches in the past were really wise women, with perhaps psychological insight as well as herbal knowledge. Although some distinguished between "white" witches who did good and "black" witches who caused harm (Thomas 1973: 316), all types of witch became labeled by theologians in Europe as in league with the devil and therefore deserving of death.

"Witch," therefore, was not a title that anyone would want to earn. Of those actually brought to trial, many had physical deformities; even though mention of this was not made at the trials, it is surely indicative of the fear bred in people by anything unusual or inexplicable (Thomas 1973: 677). It was easier to blame some sudden illness in man or beast on witchcraft than to agree it was inexplicable. A midwife present at the birth of a grossly deformed baby risked accusation of witchcraft, as did the mother herself (Donnison 1988: 17). Once the perception that a woman was a witch had developed, she was a useful scapegoat for any misfortune. To "prove" the charge of witchcraft, confessions were elicited from the accused, who sometimes admitted to flying. Ointments were rubbed onto the skin of the accused, including deadly nightshade *(Atropa belladonna),* one of the effects of which is to create the illusion of flying (R. Vickery, *Flora Facts and Fables,* no. 25, 8). At the beginning of the seventeenth century, persecution of witches was at its height. A few accused women were doubtless entrepreneurs, trading on their abilities and on the fears of those afflicted with illness. Some were supported by their communities due to the fear they inspired. In seventeenth-century Yorkshire, "a woman notoriously famed for a witch, had so powerful a hand over the wealthiest neighbours about her, that none of them refused to do anything she required; yea unbesought they provided her with fire and meat from their own tables" (Thomas 1973: 675; Fairfax 1882: 34). But for every unscrupulous character like this, there were many hundreds of ordinary women who were valued by their communities for their superior knowledge of healing. Shakespeare probably did many of these a disfavor by his portrayal of the witches' brew in Macbeth, an image that has lingered to the present long after we have forgotten the

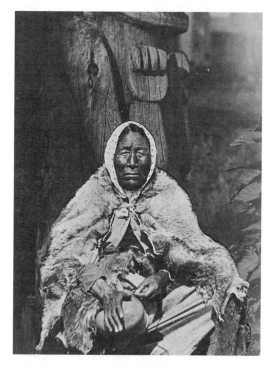

The herb doctor within a Native American tribe, whose knowledge of plant medicine has set him or her aside, is perhaps the nearest equivalent to the British "white witch." (Library of Congress)

extraordinary materia medica in use in official European medicine. The *English Physician* of 1693 lists an amazing variety of animal products, exceeding any fictitious witch's brew. Interestingly, it also reports the opinion of several authors that mercury, worn around the neck as an amulet, protected against "Inchantments and Witchcraft" (Salmon 1693: 8).

Some of the Calvinist settlers in North America brought with them their crusade against witches, and there are several examples of midwives being prosecuted for witchcraft because they used herbs to ease pain. The famous incidents in Salem, Massachusetts, where a minister's children appeared to be possessed and local women were accused of witchcraft, illustrates how witchcraft was a convenient scapegoat for any unexplained and therefore fearful inci-

dent. Epilepsy and mental illnesses were inexplicable and frequently attributed to witchcraft.

At least in England, the image of the village witch survived into the twentieth century. Tongue gives examples of black, white, and "ambivalent" witches in Somerset (Tongue 1965: 63–70). Taylor cites examples of twentieth-century witches in Norfolk (Taylor 1929: 125–133). In rural Norfolk in the 1920s there was a locally famous woman who visited children every springtime. She wore a black Trilby hat and had a bucket containing a syrupy concoction in which little green apples were floating. Every child was dosed with this. Its taste was very bad, but the children were given no choice (Hatfield, pers. com., 1988). In another village, two sisters living in a cottage at the edge of the village were famous for their herbal brews. Children were sent to collect these by their mothers, but they were scared to go alone, as they regarded the women as witches (D. T., Rockland St. Mary, Norfolk, pers. com., 1988). How far this witch image is a product of fairy tales and how far it is a genuine descent from old beliefs is, of course, hard to ascertain, but these examples do illustrate the link even in the contemporary mind between witchcraft and herbal remedies. One lady, recently trained as a medical herbalist, remarked that the children in her village regard her as a witch (S. R., Poringland, Norfolk, pers. com., 2001).

An East Anglian "cure" for witchcraft recorded in the twentieth century involved the fungus that grows on a wych elm *(Ulmus glabra)*; adder's tongue fern leaves *(Ophioglossum vulgatum)*, known locally as "devil's tongue"; "castor" from a horse's leg; and blood from the person who had been bewitched. All this was placed in a stone jug and boiled on a fire made from the wood of the thorn tree. When the whole concoction was burned away, the power of the witch was destroyed (Rider Haggard 1974: 14). Various plants were used to protect against witchcraft, especially the rowan or mountain ash *(Sorbus aucuparia)*. It is still today often planted near houses. Elder *(Sambucus nigra)* was likewise thought to protect from witches; the idea that it is unlucky to cut down an elder still lingers in rural Britain. At some level the memory of this protection still survives even in a world without witches. A number of plants were associated with witchcraft, such as foxglove, known in some areas as "witches' thimbles," and bryony (Thiselton Dyer 1889: 58, 64).

There is no strict equivalent of the witch in Native American healing. Indeed, the distinction between black and white witches implies a separation between the spiritual and the physical or rational. Whereas supernatural powers are feared in European circles, in Native American healing the spiritual and the rational are not separated: both are essential parts of healing. The herb doctor within a tribe, whose knowledge of plant medicine has set him apart, is perhaps the nearest equivalent to the British "white witch." Among the Crow, the term *akbaria* is used to describe such an herbal healer. Shamans who use their powers to cause harm to people are called *agotkon* by the Iroquois (Lyon 1996: 10). They are perhaps closer to the European concept of the black witch.

*See also* **Amulet, Bryony, Epilepsy, Evil eye, Foxglove, Midwife.**

### References

Donnison, Jean. *Midwives and Medical Men.* London: Historical Publications, 1988.

Fairfax, E. *Daemonologia.* Edited by W. Grainge. Harrogate, 1882.

Lyon, William S. *Native American Healing.* Santa Barbara: ABC-CLIO, 1996.

Rider Haggard, Lilias (ed.). *I Walked by Night.* Ipswich: Boydell Press, 1974.

Salmon, William, M.D. *The Compleat English Physician.* London: 1693.

Taylor, Mark R. "Norfolk Folklore." *Folk-Lore* 40 (1929): 113–133.

Thiselton Dyer, T. F. *The Folk-Lore of Plants.* London: 1889. Facsimile Felinfach: Llanerech, 1994.

Thomas, K. *Religion and the Decline of Magic.* Harmondsworth: Penguin: 1973.

Tongue, Ruth L. *Somerset Folklore.* Edited by Katharine Briggs. County Folklore 8. London: Folklore Society, 1965.

Vickery, Roy. "Witches' Flying Ointment." *Flora, Facts and Fables* 25 (2000): 8.

———. *A Dictionary of Plant Lore.* Oxford: Oxford University Press, 1995.

# Worms

As a common affliction of children, at least in the past, this was an ailment frequently treated in domestic folk medicine. One of the commonest treatments was garlic and other members of the onion family. This was either eaten or used as a suppository. In Ireland, wild garlic *(Allium ursinum)* was used as a vermicide (Allen and Hatfield, in press); elsewhere, and in more recent times, cultivated garlic *(Allium sativum)* is used. Other plants used to treat worms include box *(Buxus sempervirens)* (Jobson 1959: 144). Box was still in veterinary use for worming in Dorset in the 1930s (Vickery 1995: 43). In Cumbria, bistort *(Persicaria bistorta)* was used (Vickery 1995: 34), and gathering the plant at full moon was recommended. Bog myrtle *(Myrica gale)*, a plant common in the west of Britain, was used as a worm killer in both Scotland (McNeill 1910: 167) and Wales (Evans 1800: 149). As its common name of "wormwood" implies, various species of *Artemisia* were used to treat worms, especially in Wales and Ireland. Native species of *Artemisia*, such as mugwort and *A. maritimum*, were used, as were introduced species such as *A. absinthium* from southern Europe (Allen and Hatfield, in press). The root of the male fern *(Dryopteris filix-mas)*, was used for worming (Beith 1995: 216), a remedy used by official medicine in the nineteenth century (Allen and Hatfield, in press). A number of gently laxative plants were used in Sussex to purge children of worms, including the juice of carrot *(Daucus carota)*, birch *(Betula* sp.), and fir *(Abies* sp.).

More drastic, and sometimes dangerous, purges included hellebore *(Helleborus* spp.), caper spurge *(Euphorbia lathyris)*, spurge laurel *(Daphne laureola)*, black bryony *(Tamus communis)*, and white bryony *(Bryonia dioica)*. "Wormwort," *Senecio fluviatilis,* also from southern Europe, was introduced by the Romans and became a naturalized source of worming remedies (Allen 1995: 182). In Orkney, fumitory *(Fumaria* sp.) was used for worming humans and animals (Spence 1914: 101), and in Ireland the flowers of gorse *(Ulex europaeus)* were boiled in milk and used for worming children (Vickery 1995: 158). An infusion of hop flowers *(Humulus lupulus)* was a gypsy remedy for worms (Vesey-Fitzgerald 1944: 225). In Gloucestershire, horseradish root *(Armoracia rusticana)* was used (Vickery 1995: 197). Tansy *(Tanacetum vulgare)* was used throughout Britain as a worming agent (see, for example, Taylor MSS, Norfolk).

In North American folk medicine, a similarly wide range of plants were used in the treatment of worms. Some of these are recognizable in British folk medicine too, such as garlic, tansy, wormwood, and birch. (Meyer 1985: 268–271). The root of male-fern *(Dryopteris filix-mas)* is used by the Cherokee for the treatment of tapeworm (Hamel and Chiltoskey 1975: 34), just as in Britain. Other remedies use plants native to North America but not to Britain. Into this category come sassafras, blue flag *(Iris* spp.), witch hazel *(Hamamelis virginiana),* huckleberries, *(Vaccinium* spp.), Canada thistles *(Cirsium arvense),* and pumpkin seeds *(Cucurbita* spp.) (Meyer 1985: 268–271). Some of these remedies are evidently derived from Native American practice; *Cirsium arvense,* for example, has been used as a vermicide by the Abnaki (Rousseau 1947: 155), and the seeds of *Cucurbita pepo* by the Cherokee (Hamel and Chiltoskey

1975: 51). *Sassafras albidum* has been used by both the Cherokee (Hamel and Chiltoskey 1975: 54) and the Iroquois (Herrick 1977: 334). Lavender cotton *(Santolina chamaecyparissus),* on the other hand, is a native of the Mediterranean, and this remedy is presumably imported from there. Jerusalem oak seed was used for worms (Brown 1952–1964, 6: 354). This plant *(Chenopodium ambrosioides),* also known as "wormseed" or "Mexican tea," was used both in folk medicine and herbalism (Crellin and Philpott 1990: 270). Among the Native Americans, it was used by the Houma (Speck 1941: 63), the Koasati (Taylor 1940: 22), the Natchez (Taylor 1940: 22), and the Rappahannock (Speck, Hassrick, and Carpenter 1942: 30). The liquid from boiled mint *(Mentha* sp.) is a remedy of Spanish origin collected in the Pacific Southwest (UCLA Folklore Archives 19_5572). Both the bark and the sap of *Populus tremuloides* were used in treating worms (Meyer 1985: 269)—another remedy also used by the Native Americans and probably learned from them. It has been recorded in use by the Abnaki (Rousseau 1947: 165). Peach, though a native of China, has been used in both folk medicine (Meyer 1985: 270) and Native American practice, among the Cherokee and Delaware (Hamel and Chiltoskey 1975: 47; Tantaquidgeon 1972: 31). Carolina pink *(Spigelia marilandica)* was used in folk practice, and knowledge of its antihelminthic properties was passed on from the Cherokee to a "number of the faculty" (Meyer 1985: 269). It was used by the Creek (Swanton 1928: 669) as well as the Cherokee (Hamel and Chiltoskey 1975: 40). A large number of other plants used by the Native Americans do not seem to have been adopted into general North American folk medicine, such as the infusion of flowers and leaves of boneset used by the Meskwaki (Smith 1928: 214), and the bark of the European spindle *(Euonymus europaeus)* used by the Iroquois (Herrick 1977: 374).

Apart from plant remedies for worms, a number of household substances were recommended, such as salt and water or flowers of sulphur (Meyer 1985: 268), the vapor from hot milk (UCLA Folklore Archives 16_5572), and sugar and coal oil (UCLA Folklore Archives 16_5573).

Worms seem to have attracted a number of superstitions and social taboos, both among the Native Americans and in general North American folk practice. For example, children have been warned that they will get worms if they chew their fingernails and eat them (UCLA Folklore Archives 14_5572); if they pick their noses (Cannon 1984: 138); if they fail to eat all their toast crusts (UCLA Folklore Archives 9_5573); or if they eat too much sugar (numerous records, e.g., UCLA Folklore Archives 5_6063). Among the Native American Jicarilla, it is suggested that eating "forbidden things" will cause worms to grow fast inside one. Even "marrying a Pueblo when young" can cause worms to grow (Opler 1947: 128).

*See also* **Boneset, Bryony, Garlic, Moon, Mugwort, Onion, Peach, Sassafras.**

## References

Allen, Andrew. *A Dictionary of Sussex Folk Medicine.* Newbury: Countryside Books, 1995.

Allen, David E., and Gabrielle Hatfield. *Medicinal Plants in Folk Tradition.* Portland, OR: Timber Press, in press.

Beith, Mary. *Healing Threads: Traditional Medicines of the Highlands and Islands.* Edinburgh: Polygon, 1995.

Brown, Frank C. *Collection of North Carolina Folklore.* 7 vols. Durham, NC: Duke University Press, 1952–1964.

Cannon, Anthon S. *Popular Beliefs and Superstitions from Utah.* Edited by Wayland D. Hand and Jeannine E. Talley. Salt Lake City: University of Utah Press, 1984.

Crellin, John K., and Jane Philpott. *A Reference Guide to Medicinal Plants.* Durham, NC: Duke University Press, 1990.

Evans, J. *A Tour through Part of North Wales in the Year 1798, and at Other Times.* London: 1800.

Hamel, Paul B., and Mary U. Chiltoskey. *Cherokee Plants and Their Uses: A 400 Year History.* Sylva, NC: Herald, 1975.

Herrick, James William. *Iroquois Medical Botany.* Ph.D. thesis, State University of New York, Albany, 1977.

Jobson, Allan. *An Hour-Glass on the Run.* London: Michael Joseph, 1959.

McNeill, Murdoch. *Colonsay: One of the Hebrides.* Edinburgh: David Douglas, 1910.

Meyer, Clarence. *American Folk Medicine.* Glenwood, IL: Meyerbooks, 1985.

Opler, Morris Edward. "Mythology and Folk Belief in the Maintenance of Jicarilla Apache Tribal Endogamy." *Journal of American Folklore* 60 (1947): 126–129.

Rousseau, Jacques. "Ethnobotanique Abénakise." *Archives de Folklore* 11 (1947): 145–182.

Smith, Huron H. "Ethnobotany of the Meskwaki Indians." *Bulletin of the Public Museum of the City of Milwaukee* 4 (1928): 175–326.

Speck, Frank G. "A List of Plant Curatives Obtained from the Houma Indians of Louisiana." *Primitive Man* 14 (1941): 49–75.

Speck, Frank G., R. B. Hassrick, and E. S. Carpenter. "Rappahanock Herbals, Folk-Lore and Science of Cures." *Proceedings of the Delaware County Institute of Science* 10 (1942): 30.

Spence, Magnus. *Flora Orcadensis.* Kirkwall: D. Spence, 1914.

Swanton, John R. "Religious Beliefs and Medical Practices of the Creek Indians." *Smithsonian Institution-Bureau of American Ethnology Annual Report* 42 (1928): 473–672.

Tantaquidgeon, Gladys. *Folk Medicine of the Delaware and Related Algonkian Indians. Pennsylvania Historical Commission Anthropological Papers,* no. 3 (1972).

Taylor, Linda Averill. *Plants Used as Curatives by Certain Southeastern Tribes.* Cambridge, MA: Botanical Museum of Harvard University, 1940.

Taylor MSS. Manuscript notes of Mark R. Taylor, in the Norfolk Record Office, Norwich. MS4322.

Vesey-Fitzgerald, B. "Gypsy Medicine." *Journal of the Gypsy Lore Society* 23 (1944): 21–33.

Vickery, Roy. *A Dictionary of Plant Lore.* Oxford: Oxford University Press, 1995.

# Wounds

Home treatment of wounds right up to the twentieth century in Britain and in North America has been a mixture of basic common sense and, at least apparently, bizarre remedies. Washing the wound in cold water and bandaging tightly seems good advice in any time and place. Applying a live frog, a cow pat, or moldy bread, at least at first sight, seems much more dubious. Official medicine also includes many strange-sounding wound treatments. The list of substances used to treat wounds in Salmon's *English Physician* (Salmon 1693) includes copper, mercury, bee, snail, worm, man (!), camel, cow. Some of these ingredients (including dried mummy!) were included in a seventeenth-century salve made famous by Sir Kenelm Digby. It was designed to treat wounds by sympathetic magic and was applied not to the wound but to the weapon that had caused it. Arising from this idea, folk medicine contains many examples of wound healing wherein the instrument causing the wound is either cleaned or buried, and some of these practices have continued until recent times in both Britain (Newman 1945: 291) and North America (Puckett 1981: 429).

In Sussex folk medicine, from the sixteenth through to the nineteenth centuries, strapping a live frog to a wound was considered to help healing. Frogs under stress release maganins, which might have promoted healing (Allen 1995: 76). To encourage licking of a wound by the patient or by a pet dog sounds unhygienic, but there is evidence that it might indeed be helpful in some cases (Root-Bernstein and Root-Bernstein 2000: 110). Cobwebs were found to be effective at stopping bleeding and encouraging healing, and they have been used within living memory in Britain (Prince 1991: 118) and in North America (UCLA Folklore Archive 1_5589), both in

human and in veterinary practice. Current studies of the structure of cobwebs show that they encourage blood clotting and help seal wounds. The more dubious sounding use of cowpats to treat wounds is a practice that again persisted in country veterinary use as well as for human patients, well into the twentieth century, in Britain (Hatfield 1994: 11) and in North America (UCLA Folklore Archive 4_5437). Other animal products used in wound healing include snakeskin, used in particular for septic wounds (Prince 1991: 101).

Numerous plants have been used for wound healing in British folk medicine. In many cases, the country names indicate their use. "Self-heal" and "all-heal" are names used for *Prunella vulgaris,* a native British plant used in wound healing in both folk medicine and orthodox medicine until the modern period. Woundwort (*Stachys* spp.) is similarly a self-explanatory name, while yarrow, used in healing since the ancients, has among its English country names "carpenter's weed" and "staunchweed." The name "yarrow" is thought to be derived from the Anglo-Saxon *gearwe,* meaning healer (Stockwell 1989: 28). St. John's wort is another plant used for healing throughout Britain. In folk medicine it was often used on its own (Tongue 1965: 35); in orthodox medicine it was one of many ingredients in wound salves, such as the famous eighteenth-century Admiral Wade's balsam. Comfrey has been widely used in wound healing in Britain, as have mallow and elder. Of the plants used to treat wounds in British folk medicine, the petals of Madonna lily (and of other lilies to a lesser extent), steeped in brandy, is one of the more surprising—because, unlike most plants used in traditional remedies, it is not a native. In recent times, castor oil (from *Ricinus communis*) has been used to clean and heal wounds in both humans and animals (M.H., Attleborough, Norfolk, 1990, pers. com.) (Prince 1991: 114). Pine resin has been used in recent times for treating infected wounds (Hatfield MS). Spores from puffballs were dusted onto wounds to arrest bleeding, and the whole fungus was also made into a poultice for dressing wounds. Puffballs were, at least in East Anglia, commonly kept in barbers' shops as well as farm buildings for use in treating cuts in humans and animals.

Fungi have been exploited by folk medicine in another approach to the treatment of wounds. A number of moldy substances, at least some of which probably contained antibiotics, were used in folk medical treatment of wounds. Rotten apples, moldy cheese wrappings, and even purpose-grown mold from copper pennies coated with lard (*Daily Express,* November 19, 1943) are among twentieth-century pre-antibiotic uses of molds. The use of moss, particularly of the bog moss (*Sphagnum* sp.) as a wound dressing in both official and unofficial medicine was recognized on both sides of the Atlantic.

In North American folk medicine, as in Britain, animal products were used in wound treatment. Aside from the cowpats mentioned above, these include mashed roaches (Saxon 1945: 536), fat meat and turpentine (Puckett 1981: 427), beef gall (Brown 1952–1964, 6: 355), and spit (Brown 1952–1964, 6: 355). Soot and the smoke from burning wool are among other miscellaneous wound remedies used in North American folk practice (Brown 1952–1964, 6: 355, 356).

Among plant remedies used as wound healers in North American folk medicine, some are recognizably the same as those used in Britain. During the American Civil War, yarrow gained the name of "soldier's woundwort," from the use of the crushed plant as first aid for wounds in battle (Coffey 1993: 237). Comfrey was used as in Britain for wound healing (Brown 1952–

1964, 6: 355). Elder bark and dandelion leaves were mixed to form a wound ointment (Clark 1970: 34). Other plant remedies used include green tobacco leaves for bullet wounds (Clark 1970: 19) or poultices of American elm bark (*Ulmus americana*) (Vogel 1970: 303). Jimson leaves were cooked in lard to form a wound salve (McAtee 1955: 214). Leaves of geranium were used (Puckett 1981: 505). Chapparal (*Larrea tridentata*), a native of the Southwest, was used in wound treatment there (Micheletti 1998: 81). As in Britain, puffball spores were used (Wilson 1968: 322). Molds were also used. From Missouri there is a record of wet tree mold wrapped over a wound with cheesecloth (UCLA Folklore Archive 24_5574). For a nail wound, moldy bread and sweet milk was recommended (Parler 1962: 754).

Among the numerous plants used for wound healing by Native Americans, heal-all (*Collinsonia canadensis)* has, its name suggests, been used for treating wounds as well as other ailments. Agave (*Agave* spp.) was used by the Mexican Indians (Kay 1996: 88), as was the succulent cactus *Pachycereus pecten-aboriginum* (Kay 1996: 131). More than a hundred different genera of plants were used by the Native Americans to check bleeding, and in excess of a hundred were used as disinfectants (Moerman 1998: 772, 789). Different species of pine were very widely used. The gum from *Pinus edulis* was used to heal cuts in a similar way to that reported in East Anglia, above (Weber and Seaman 1985: 205).

Among nonplant remedies used by the Native Americans are slices of beaver kidney (Van Wart 1948: 576) and maggots (Fisher 1945: 73–73). The latter were purpose-bred and used to clean up infected wounds, just as they were in warfare in the twentieth century in Europe, and as they are once again in the twenty-first century in North American and European hospitals (Root-

Bernstein and Root-Bernstein 2000: 21–30).

*See also* **Bleeding, Comfrey, Cuts, Dandelion, Elder, Mallow, Molds, Pine, Poultice, Puffball, St. John's wort, Sphagnum moss, Spider, Spit, Sympathetic magic, Thornapple, Tobacco, Yarrow.**

## References

Allen, Andrew. *A Dictionary of Sussex Folk Medicine.* Newbury: Countryside Books, 1995.

Brown, Frank C. *Collection of North Carolina Folklore.* 7 vols., Durham, NC: Duke University Press, 1952–1964.

Clark, Joseph D. "North Carolina Popular Beliefs and Superstitions." *North Carolina Folklore* 18 (1970): 1–66.

Coffey, Timothy. *The History and Folklore of North American Wildflowers.* New York: Facts On File, 1993.

Fisher, Anne B. *The Salinas, Upside-Down River.* Rivers of America. New York: Farrar and Rinehart, 1945.

Hatfield, Gabrielle. *Country Remedies: Traditional East Anglian Plant Remedies in the Twentieth Century.* Woodbridge: Boydell Press, 1994.

Kay, Margarita Artschwager. *Healing with Plants in the American and Mexican West.* Tucson: University of Arizona Press, 1996.

McAtee, W. L. "Home Medication in Grant County, Indiana, in the Nineties." *Midwest Folklore* 5 (1955): 213–216.

Micheletti, Enza (ed.). *North American Folk Healing: An A–Z Guide to Traditional Remedies.* New York and Montreal: Reader's Digest Association, 1998.

Moerman, Daniel E. *Native American Ethnobotany.* Portland, OR: Timber Press, 1998.

Newman, L. F. "Some Notes on the Folklore of Cambridgeshire and the Eastern Counties." *Folk-Lore* 56 (1945): 287–293.

Parler, Mary Celestia, and University Student Contributors. *Folk Beliefs from Arkansas.* 15 vols. Fayetteville: University of Arkansas, 1962.

Prince, Dennis. *Grandmother's Cures: An A–Z of Herbal Remedies.* London: Fontana, 1991.

Puckett, Newbell Niles. *Popular Beliefs and Superstitions: A Compendium of American Folklore from the Ohio Collection of Newbell Niles Puckett.* Edited by Wayland D. Hand, Anna Casetta, and Sondra B. Thiederman. 3 vols. Boston: G. K. Hall, 1981.

Root-Bernstein, Robert, and Michèle Root-Bernstein. *Honey, Mud, Maggots and Other Medical Marvels: The Science behind Folk Remedies and Old Wives' Tales.* London: Pan Books, 2000.

Salmon, William, M.D. *The Compleat English Physician.* London: 1693.

Saxon, Lyle. *Gumbo Ya-Ya.* Boston: Houghton Mifflin, 1945.

Stockwell, Christine. *Nature's Pharmacy. A History of Plants and Healing.* London: Arrow Books, 1989.

Tongue, Ruth L. *Somerset Folklore.* Edited by Katharine Briggs. County Folklore 8. London: Folklore Society, 1965.

Van Wart, Arthur F. "The Indians of the Maritime Provinces, Their Diseases and Native Cures." *Canadian Medical Association Journal* 59(6) (1948): 573–577.

Vogel, Virgil J. *American Indian Medicine.* Norman: University of Oklahoma Press, 1970.

Weber, Steven A., and P. David Seaman. *Havasupai Habitat: A. F. Whiting's Ethnography of a Traditional Indian Culture.* Tucson: University of Arizona Press, 1985.

Wilson, Gordon. "Local Plants in Folk Remedies in the Mammoth Cave Region." *Southern Folklore Quarterly* 32 (1968): 320–327.

# Wrinkles

Elderflower water and an ointment made from cowslip leaves were among the folk remedies for the treatment and prevention of wrinkles. A mixture of violets *(Viola odorata)* and goat's milk was highly valued in the Scottish Highlands as a lotion to produce a smooth complexion (Beith 1995: 249–250). A facepack could be made from oatmeal, lemon juice, and cream. Cucumber slices placed on the eyelids were soothing and thought to prevent wrinkles (Souter 1995: 147). The juice of the greater celandine *(Chelidonium majus)* was used to remove wrinkles (Vickery

MSS). In Westmoreland an infusion of butterwort *(Pinguicula vulgaris)* was drunk to procure a smoother skin (Freethy 1985: 128). Wild strawberry leaves *(Fragaria vesca)* were rubbed on the face in seventeenth-century Cornwall to procure a smooth complexion (Deane and Shaw 1975). In Ireland, comfrey juice was thought to be good for the complexion (Logan 1972: 77). In both Scotland and England, May dew was thought to prevent wrinkles (Napier 1879: 170).

In North American folk medicine, washing with cold water was thought to prevent wrinkles (UCLA Folklore Archives 3_5964). Alternatives were to wash with alcohol (UCLA Folklore Archives 7_5964) or urine (UCLA Folklore Archives 4_5964), or a mixture of vinegar and water (UCLA Folklore Archives 8_5964). Face packs to remove wrinkles include cow manure (Parler 1962, 3: 550), a paste of oatmeal and eggs (UCLA Folklore Archives 17_5576), honey and garlic (UCLA Folklore Archives 12_5964), or goose grease (UCLA Folklore Archives 16_5964). Plant remedies for wrinkles include a wash of sassafras tea (Musick 1964: 38), the juice of green pine cones (Beck 1957: 45) or of lily bulbs (Koch 1980: 110), or eating prunes (Hyatt 1965: 161).

There were various folk beliefs concerning wrinkles. They could be caused by counting stars (Espinosa 1910: 414), by letting the moon shine on the face (Brown 1952–1964, 6: 102), or by sleeping with the head raised (Hyatt 1965: 161). The numbers and positions of wrinkles on the face and hands were suggested to indicate how many children the owner would have, or how many spouses, as well as indicating the character of the owner (see, for example, Brown 1952–1964, 6: 26; Hyatt 1965: 167).

*See also* **Comfrey, Cowslip, Dew, Elder, Excreta, Moon, Pine, Sassafras, Urine, Vinegar, Water.**

## References

Beck, Horace P. *The Folklore of Maine.* Philadelphia and New York: J. B. Lippincott, 1957.
Beith, Mary. *Healing Threads: Traditional Medicines of the Highlands and Islands.* Edinburgh: Polygon, 1995.
Brown, Frank C. *Collection of North Carolina Folklore.* 7 vols. Durham, NC: Duke University Press, 1952–1964.
Deane, Tony, and Tony Shaw. *The Folklore of Cornwall.* London: Batsford, 1975.
Espinosa, Aurelio M. "New Mexican Spanish Folk-Lore." *Journal of American Folklore* 23 (1910): 395–418.
Freethy, Ron. *From Agar to Zenry.* Marlborough: Crowood Press, 1985.
Hyatt, Harry Middleton. *Folklore from Adams County Illinois.* 2nd rev. ed. New York: Memoirs of the Alma Egan Hyatt Foundation, 1965.
Koch, William E. *Folklore from Kansas: Beliefs and Customs.* Lawrence, KS: Regent Press, 1980.
Logan, Patrick. *Making the Cure: A Look at Irish Folk Medicine.* Dublin: Talbot Press, 1972.
Musick, Ruth M. (ed.) "Superstitions." *West Virginia Folklore* 14 (1964): 38–52.
Napier, James. *Folk Lore or Superstitious Beliefs in the West of Scotland within this Century.* Paisley: 1879.
Parler, Mary Celestia, and University Student Contributors. *Folk Beliefs from Arkansas.* 15 vols. Fayetteville: University of Arkansas, 1962.
Souter, Keith. *Cure Craft: Traditional Folk Remedies and Treatment from Antiquity to the Present Day.* Saffron Walden: C. W. Daniel, 1995.
Vickery MSS. Roy Vickery. Manuscript notes in his personal possession.

# Y

## Yarrow (*Achillea millefolium*)

As its country name of "soldiers' wound-wort" implies, this plant has been highly valued over the centuries as a wound-healing herb. In addition, an infusion of the plant has been drunk for respiratory complaints, including coughs, colds, and asthma, as well as for rheumatism. The leaves have been pushed up the nose to provoke a nosebleed and thereby relieve headache. Paradoxically, they have also been used to treat nosebleeds (Bardswell 1911: 132). Other uses include chewing the leaves for toothache, a remedy particularly used in Ireland (Allen and Hatfield, in press). The leaves, worn in a shoe, protected the wearer against cramp (Tongue 1965: 38). High blood pressure has been treated with yarrow (Ibbott 1994: 64). Yarrow has been taken as a general tonic in, for example, Shetland (Tait 1947). In some parts of Britain, such as the Isle of Man, the plant was regarded as a panacea (Fargher n.d.). The plant has magical associations too. It was used as a divinatory herb to test whether a boy loved a girl (Page 1983: 41). In Norfolk a sprig of yarrow was traditionally tied to a baby's cradle to ensure its future happiness (Porter 1974: 18).

In North American folk medicine, yarrow has been used in many of the same ways as in Britain. During the Civil War, wounds

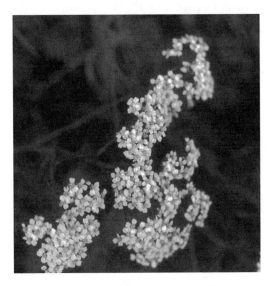

Yarrow is a healing herb valued in both Old and New Worlds particularly for its blood-staunching properties. (Sarah Boait)

were staunched with yarrow (Micheletti 1998: 354). Yarrow tea has been used for treating colds (Lathrop 1961: 13), fever (Levine 1941: 488), indigestion (Browne 1958: 74), and dysentery (Brendle 1935: 171), as well as for preventing nosebleeds (Meyer 1985: 189) or the bleeding of piles (Meyer 1985: 195). As in Britain, it was also used for toothache (Meyer 1985: 47), headache (UCLA Folklore Archives 11_6289), and cramps (Musick 1964: 46). It was regarded as a tonic for the liver (Hendricks 1959: 112) and as good to clear infection from the body (UCLA Folklore

Archives 14_6816). It has been credited with giving long life to anyone who eats it at least once a week (UCLA Folklore Archives 6_6772).

The uses of yarrow by the Native Americans are numerous and varied. They include staunching the bleeding of wounds, piles, nosebleeds, and heavy periods; treating respiratory disorders, fevers, rheumatism, toothache, and headache; and for heart complaints (Moerman 1998: 42–45). At least one tribe regarded the plant as a panacea (Turner et al. 1990: 66). Like the English East Anglians, the Potawatomi credited the plant with the power to repel evil spirits (Smith 1933: 47).

*See also* **Asthma, Colds, Coughs, Cramp, Dysentery, Fevers, Headache, Heart trouble, Indigestion, Menstrual problems, Nosebleed, Piles, Rheumatism, Tonic, Toothache, Wounds.**

## References

Allen, David E., and Gabrielle Hatfield. *Medicinal Plants in Folk Tradition.* Portland, OR: Timber Press, in press.

Bardswell, Frances Anne. *The Herb-garden.* London: A. & C. Black, 1911.

Brendle, Thomas R., and Claude W. Unger. "Folk Medicine of the Pennsylvania Germans: The Non-Occult Cures." *Proceedings of the Pennsylvania German Society* 45 (1935).

Browne, Ray B. *Popular Beliefs and Practices from Alabama.* Folklore Studies 9. Berkeley and Los Angeles: University of California Publications, 1958.

Fargher, D. C. *The Manx Have a Word for It.* Vol. 5, *Manx Gaelic Names of Flora.* Port Erin: privately published (mimeo).

Hendricks, George D., et al. "Utah State University Folklore Collection." *Western Folklore* 18 (1959): 107–120.

Ibbott, Selena. *Folklore, Legends and Spells* (of Gloucestershire). Bath: Ashgrove Press, 1994.

Lathrop, Amy. "Pioneer Remedies from Western Kansas." *Western Folklore* 20 (1961): 1–22.

Levine, Harold D. "Folk Medicine in New Hampshire." *New England Journal of Medicine* 224 (1941): 487–492.

Meyer, Clarence. *American Folk Medicine.* Glenwood, IL: Meyerbooks, 1985.

Micheletti, Enza (ed.). *North American Folk Healing: An A–Z Guide to Traditional Remedies.* New York and Montreal: Reader's Digest Association, 1998.

Moerman, Daniel E. *Native American Ethnobotany.* Portland, OR: Timber Press, 1998.

Musick, Ruth M. (ed.). "Superstitions." *West Virginia Folklore* 14 (1964): 38–52.

Page, Robin. *The Country Way of Love.* Harmondsworth: Penguin Books, 1983.

Porter, Enid. *The Folklore of East Anglia.* London: Batsford, 1974.

Smith, Huron H. "Ethnobotany of the Forest Potawatomi Indians." *Bulletin of the Public Museum of the City of Milwaukee* 7 (1933): 1–230.

Tait, Robert W. "Some Shetland Plant Names." *Shetland Folk Book* 1 (1947): 73–88.

Tongue, Ruth L. *Somerset Folklore.* Edited by Katharine Briggs. County Folklore 8. London: Folklore Society, 1965.

Turner, Nancy J., Laurence C. Thompson, M. Terry Thompson, and Annie Z. York. *Thompson Ethnobotany: Knowledge and Usage of Plants by the Thompson Indians of British Columbia.* Victoria: Royal British Columbia Museum, 1990.

# Yew (*Taxus baccata*)

This tree is notoriously poisonous and has been used only in a limited way in British folk medicine. The fact that as recently as the nineteenth century infusions of its leaves were used to sponge corpses and prevent putrefaction (Rootsey 1832–33) may explain the custom of planting yews in churchyards. A preparation of the twigs has been used in Lincolnshire for kidney complaints (Taylor MSS). The plant has also been used as an abortifacient, but such usage has sometimes proved fatal (Taylor 1848: 790). In Ireland, yew has been used for treating ringworm (Allen and Hatfield, in press). The only part of the plant that is not toxic is the pulp of the fruit. The "berries" were used in treating scrofula, nosebleeds, and heart palpitations in the seventeenth century (Wright 1912: 233).

The English yew has scarcely been used in general North American folk medicine. Both this species and the Pacific yew *(Taxus brevifolia)* and Canada yew *(Taxus canadensis)* have been used by Native Americans to treat a wide range of ailments, particularly respiratory complaints and rheumatism (Moerman 1998: 551–553). The Iroquois used English yew as an abortifacient (Herrick 1977: 264). Pacific yew was used by the Hanaksiala for kidney complaints and by the Tsimshian for treating cancer (Compton 1993: 187). Yew has recently sprung to fame for providing a "new" official treatment for ovarian cancer (Chevallier 1996: 273).

## References

Allen, David E., and Gabrielle Hatfield. *Medicinal Plants in Folk Tradition.* Portland, OR: Timber Press, in press.

Chevallier, Andrew. *The Encyclopedia of Medicinal Plants.* London: Dorling Kindersley, 1996.

Compton, Brian Douglas. *Upper North Wakashan and Southern Tsimshian Ethnobotany: The Knowledge and Usage of Plants.* Ph.D. thesis, University of British Columbia, Vancouver, 1993.

Herrick, James William. *Iroquois Medical Botany.* Ph.D. thesis, State University of New York, Albany, 1977.

Moerman, Daniel E. *Native American Ethnobotany.* Portland, OR: Timber Press, 1998.

Rootsey, Samuel. "Observations upon Some of the Medical Plants Mentioned by Shakespeare." *Transactions of the Medico-Botanical Society of London for 1832–33* (1834): 83–96.

Taylor, Alfred S. *On Poisons, in Relation to Medical Jurisprudence and Medicine.* London: John Churchill, 1848.

Taylor MSS. Manuscript notes of Mark R. Taylor, in Norfolk Record Office, Norwich.

Wright, A. R. "Seventeenth Century Cures and Charms." *Folk-Lore* 23 (1912): 230–236, 490–497.

# Index

# About the Author

Gabrielle Hatfield, Ph.D., is a botanist and folklorist and has served on the committee of the Folklore Society. Her work on East Anglian plant remedies won the Michaelis-Jena Ratcliffe Prize for folklore in 1993. For the past twenty years, she has researched plant medicines in Scotland and England during the eighteenth, nineteenth, and twentieth centuries, work which led to her appointment as an Honorary Research Associate at the Royal Botanic Gardens in Kew. Her publications include *Country Remedies: Traditional East Anglian Plant Remedies in the Twentieth Century and Memory, Wisdom, and Healing: The History of Domestic Plant Medicine.* She is married with four grown-up children, and lives on a farm in Norfolk, England.